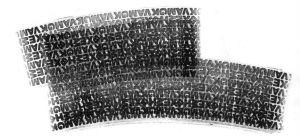

STUTTERING
THEN AND NOW

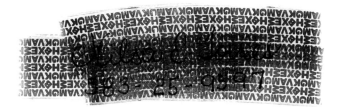

STUTTERING THEN AND NOW

George H. Shames
University of Pittsburgh

Herbert Rubin
University of Pittsburgh

Charles E. Merrill Publishing Company
A Bell & Howell Company
Columbus   Toronto   London   Sydney

Published by Charles E. Merrill Publishing Co.
A Bell & Howell Company
Columbus, Ohio 43216

This book was set in Garamond.
Cover Design Coordination: Cathy Watterson
Text Designer: Mary Henkener
Production Coordination: Linda Hillis Bayma

Library of Congress Catalog Card Number: 85-61552
International Standard Book Number: 0-675-20125-X
Printed in the United States of America
1 2 3 4 5 6 7 8 9 — 91 90 89 88 87 86

Photo credit: Carl Rogers, p. 294, by Nozizwe S.

There are many of our colleagues who have made significant contributions in the area of stuttering but who could not be included in this book. We are aware of and grateful for their scholarship, although they could not participate directly in this volume. We would like to acknowledge each of them by name, but there are just too many. Their work has had impact upon, and in fact is represented in, the contributions of the authors of this book.

Preface

George H. Shames and Herbert Rubin

As we planned this book, our goal was to write a text for the practitioner of stuttering therapy. In reviewing the significant literature we decided that the authors' words are better than ours in characterizing their thinking at a given time. Rather than attempt an exhaustive survey of the literature, we set out to identify the field's most significant and representative figures and to present their most important and exemplary contributions. In doing so we also decided to ask them to evaluate and to update their material from their current perspectives. In a sense they were asked to indicate whether they would say the same thing today, and, if not, why not.

What we want to share with you in this volume is the excitement that we have experienced, first as students and now as participants, in the field of stuttering therapy. This excitement stems from at least two sources: the persistence and complexity of the problem, and the brilliance and persuasiveness of the people who work on it. Some of these pioneers are still active; their careers span as many as seven decades of thought and practice. Although reference to stuttering goes back to the Old Testament and to Greek mythology, practical solutions to the problem are a twentieth-century phenomenon. We thus have the opportunity to tap the minds of these original twentieth-century thinkers. In doing so we seek to recapture for you the excitement that these contributors have generated, looking back and looking ahead. Their powerful thinking has stimulated successive generations of thinkers, who in turn have made significant contributions. Some are included in this volume. As editors who have been influenced by these early contributors, and who are keenly interested and active in this field, we have decided to include some of our own work, without presuming to have had similar impact.

In the chronology of thought, the names Travis, Johnson, Van Riper, and Rogers are the earliest represented here. We decided to include their work because of its significance even if they were unavailable or unable to participate in the current updating. Rogers and Van Riper have graciously designated others to review their original contributions. We are very grateful to Bloodstein, Luper, and

Seeman, who have made significant contributions of their own, for reacting from a current perspective to the pioneering work of their colleagues. These three persons were invited to contribute because of their prior associations and expertise with the work of their predecessors. We also are grateful to Vivian Sheehan for updating the work of Joseph Sheehan.

Recognizing the inherent diversity of the points of view represented here, the disparities in time among them, and the new information now available to us, we have assumed the responsibility of uniting and interrelating the content of the various chapters in this book. As we do so we will attempt to identify common principles and to pose questions to guide the reader through the issues in the theory and management of stuttering. We suspect these principles may be common to many therapies outside the field of stuttering. However, within the field of therapy for stuttering it is important to preserve the unique contribution of each of our authors.

Part of the apparent difference among these authors is the particular perspective each one takes and the way in which he or she discusses a problem. But as we examine the various contributions we are not surprised to find continuities of thought, recurring concepts, and significant areas of agreement that only naturally follow the mutual consultation and sharing of ideas that characterize a community of scholars. One of our purposes is to alert the reader to these commonalities.

One risk of presenting a text with this format is disposing the readers to choose on the basis of convenience or tactical simplicity only one of the different perspectives provided here. Another risk is that in the spirit of eclecticism the reader may try to synthesize a number of incompatible approaches. One good way to avoid these pitfalls is to recognize the underlying principles that enable the reader to compare tactics and rationales for consistency. Strategies and tactics undergo change readily. Underlying principles change more slowly and therefore may not be apparent to practitioners who inadvertently select strategies that contradict the principles by which they have been operating. A third potential hazard lies in changing strategies so readily as to create discontinuities in therapy. Such abruptness jeopardizes the commitment and the credibility of the clinician and also reaffirms the disposition of the client to continually look for a better solution to his problem. A good way to avoid this particular pitfall is to explore and to refine tactics that are compatible with the therapeutic principles one believes in.

We have not been alone in observing that successful therapy results at least in part from a belief in and commitment to the validity of the therapy. This commitment and enthusiasm of the therapist is readily communicated to the client.

If indeed one of the purposes of this book is to help the reader to make a choice, we hope it is made on the basis of careful examination and comparison of the principles and rationales of the therapies represented here.

Indirectly, but of no less importance, a major purpose of this book is to improve the effectiveness of therapy. To do so, we examine each of the approaches presented here from the point of view of the stutterer. To what extent does each author address the questions and the problems that our clients are likely to raise? We hope that each of you by reading, being stimulated by, and reacting to this book becomes a more effective and comfortable clinician. Although between these covers we have gathered a great deal of wisdom, there is also a wisdom and a human experience within each of you that we expect will be stimulated, adding to and enriching the valuable contributions we have presented here. As wise as the words of the contributors may be, only you can translate them into clinical interactions.

Another function of this book is to help resolve for some of you whether in fact you want to work with stutterers. While this population needs help, we must recognize that not every speech pathologist or psychologist is disposed to provide it. If we can help you to make that choice we will also have served.

We have organized the book in three parts: *The Beginnings, Causation and Dynamics,* and *Clinical Management.* In *The Beginnings* we have invited Jack Matthews to provide an overview and reaction to the history of the theory and management of stuttering. Although he has provided therapy for stutterers he brings to this book no particular theoretical or clinical bias. He characterizes himself as an interested witness to the transience and permanence of the recent history of stuttering.

The second part comprises the broad spectrum of ideas about the cause and nature of stuttering. Stuttering appears to be a many-faceted problem, as chapters on physiology, semantics, emotion, and learning would indicate. We necessarily have been selective in inviting contributors who have made unique offerings of historical significance and whose ideas are still enjoying professional attention.

Each author was consulted on the choice of his earlier writing included herein and agreed to provide a current update. Three exceptions are Wingate, Matthews, and Gregory who have each been invited to provide an original manuscript. We recognize that we cannot include all of our colleagues who have made significant contributions to the field of stuttering. The impact of their work is shown in the many references in the following chapters.

The third part of this book is on clinical management. Again, we attempted to provide a comprehensive and representational selection of the current major therapies, selected on the basis of how they have come to be best known. They include counseling, systematic desensitization, modification of stuttering, operant-based therapy, cognitive therapy, and environmental modification. In addition, we have tried to address maintenance and relapse, which can be common to all of these therapies. Except for Gregory, whose chapter deals with environmental modification and counseling, all of these contributors provide updates of previously published material selected in the same manner as the material in Part Two.

Finally, we have provided editorial introductions to each chapter and have tried to integrate these diverse contributions with an editorial introduction to the major sections as well as a general conclusion.

ACKNOWLEDGMENTS

This book is unusual in that it is organized around previously published material. We are, therefore, deeply indebted to the publishers of those articles and chapters that our authors wrote years ago. Their permission to reprint was essential to the production of this volume, but the gracious way in which that consent was provided made our task as editors that much more enjoyable. The cooperating publishers included: The American Speech-Language-Hearing Association, Prentice-Hall, Inc., The Speech Foundation of America, Journal Press, Journal of the Experimental Analysis of Behavior, Houghton-Mifflin Company, Stanford University Press, Elsevier Science Publishing Company, Inc., Charles E. Merrill Publishing Company, and The Monterey Institute for Speech and Hearing. The specific material for which permission was granted is denoted at the beginning of each chapter in which it appears.

We also wish to thank the following reviewers of the manuscript for their constructive comments and suggestions, which significantly influenced the final format and content of this volume: Richard Culatta, University of Kentucky; Stanley Goldberg, San Francisco State University; Elizabeth Webster, Memphis State University; and Gordon Blood, Pennsylvania State University.

Editorial Note: In some instances in this text, the pronoun "he" is used to denote both male and female stutterers. While the majority of stutterers are male, we have chosen this usage only to avoid cumbersome language, and we intend no sexual bias.

Contents

PART ONE   THE BEGINNINGS

---

1   Historical Prologue   *Jack Matthews,* **5**

PART TWO   CAUSATION AND DYNAMICS

---

2   Overview of Part Two: Theory, Research, and Clinical Management—A System of Interactions   *George H. Shames and Herbert Rubin,* **23**

Etiology and Maintenance, 24   Is Stuttering the Disorder or Is It Symptomatic of an Underlying Disorder?, 30   Normal Disfluency, 33   Stuttering as Learned Behavior, 40

3   Physiological and Genetic Factors   *Marcel Wingate,* **49**

Physiological to Psychological, 53   Modern Times, 61   A Brief Personal Perspective, 63

4   Stuttering: Discoordination of Phonation with Articulation and Respiration   *William H. Perkins, Joanna Rudas, Linda Johnson, and Jody Bell,* **73**

Selection of Phonation as the Independent Variable, 74   The Problem, 76   Method, 77   Results, 78   Discussion, 79

POSTSCRIPT   Discoordination of Phonation with Articulation and Respiration   *William H. Perkins,* **82**

Implications for Understanding Stuttering, 82   Effective-Planning-Time Hypothesis, 86   Implications for Therapy, 87

5 **The Unspeakable Feelings of People with Special Reference to Stuttering** *Lee Edward Travis*, **93**

General Statements, 93   The Core Phenomenon of Stuttering, 94   Stuttering as Learned Behavior, 95   The People of This Study, 98   The Old Conditions of Learning, 99   A Sketch of Some Older Training Situations, 100   New Conditions of Interpersonal Relationships, 104   The Unspeakable Feelings, 106   Concluding Thoughts, 115

POSTSCRIPT   Emotional Factors *Lee Edward Travis*, **117**

6 **A Study of the Onset and Development of Stuttering** *Wendell Johnson et al.,* **125**

Introduction, 125   Procedure, 126   Results, 126   Conclusion, 129

POSTSCRIPT   Semantics and Beliefs *Oliver Bloodstein,* **130**

Origin of the Theory, 130   Influence on Later Theories, 132   Influence on Research, 133   Influence on Therapy, 136

7 **Two-Factor Behavior Theory and Therapy** *Gene J. Brutten,* **143**

Behavior Theory, 143   Behavior Therapy, 146   Classical Conditioning: Modification Procedures, 146   Instrumental Conditioning: Modification Procedures, 149   Summing Up and Looking Ahead, 153

POSTSCRIPT   The Two-Factor Theory *Gene J. Brutten,* **155**

Two-Factor Behavior Theory, 157   Two-Factor Behavior Therapy, 168   Epilogue, 178

8 **Theory and Treatment of Stuttering as an Approach-Avoidance Conflict** *Joseph G. Sheehan,* **187**

The Problem, 187   The Conflict Hypothesis, 188   The Fear-Reduction Hypothesis, 192   Treatment, 195   Summary, 198

POSTSCRIPT   Approach-Avoidance and Anxiety Reduction *Vivian M. Sheehan,* **201**

The Research Odyssey, 201   Analysis of Therapy Techniques, 205   Other Clinical Contributions from the Theory, 207   Recent Developments, 208   Conclusion, 209

9 **Operant Stuttering: The Control of Stuttering Behavior Through Response-Contingent Consequences** *Bruce Flanagan, Israel Goldiamond, and Nathan Azrin,* **213**

POSTSCRIPT   Operant Stuttering Update *Bruce Flanagan,* **217**

Zeitgeist, 217   1958 Revisited, 219   Replications, 221   Related Research, 222   Punishment, 224

10   **A Discussion of Nonfluency and Stuttering as Operant Behavior**   *George H. Shames and Carl E. Sherrick, Jr.,* **237**

The System of Operant Analysis, 237   Nonfluency, 238   States of Deprivation and Aversive Stimuli, 239   Stuttering, 241   Implications for Research on Therapy, 245   Summary, 246

POSTSCRIPT   **An Operant Perspective**   *George H. Shames,* **248**

PART THREE   **CLINICAL MANAGEMENT**

---

11   **Overview to Part Three: The Roles of the Client and the Clinician During Therapy**   *George H. Shames and Herbert Rubin,* **261**

Client's Expectations, 261   Changes in Attitudes and Behavior, 263 Conclusion, 270

12   **Environmental Manipulation and Family Counseling**   *Hugo Gregory,* **273**

Points of View, 273   Evaluation Procedures, 277   Environmental Changes, 280   Conclusion, 286   Case Illustration—Jerry, 287   Case Illustration—Jenny, 288

13   **The Attitude and Orientation of the Counselor**   *Carl Rogers,* **295**

A General Consideration, 295   The Philosophical Orientation of the Counselor, 295   The Therapist's Hypothesis, 296   The Specific Implementation of the Counselor's Attitude, 297   Some Formulations of the Counselor's Role, 298   Research Evidence of a Trend, 300   The Difficulty of Perceiving Through the Client's Eyes, 301   The Rationale of the Counselor's Role, 302   The Counselor's Role as Implementation of an Hypothesis, 302 The Client's Experience of the Counselor, 303   A Theory of the Therapist's Role, 304   The Difficulty of Understanding the Perceptions of Another, 306 Some Deep Issues, 307   The Basic Struggle of the Counselor, 308   Unsolved Issues, 308   An Objective Definition of the Therapeutic Relationship, 309

POSTSCRIPT   **Client-Centered Therapy**   *Julius Seeman,* **316**

Some Theoretical Variants of Client-Centered Therapy, 317   The Person-Centered Approach, 319   A Case Analysis, 320   An Illustration of the Therapeutic Process, 323   A Look at the Process, 330   Conclusion, 334

14   **Systematic Desensitization Based on Relaxation**
Joseph Wolpe, **337**

The Conduct of Desensitization Sessions, 339

Behavior Therapy of Stuttering: Deconditioning the Emotional Factor   *Joseph Wolpe,* **343**

Methods of Deconditioning Neurotic Emotional Habits, 344   Behavior Therapy in Stuttering, 345

POSTSCRIPT   Systematic Desensitization   *Joseph Wolpe,* **350**

Revised Schemas for the Mechanisms of Stuttering, 350   The Predominance of the Emotional Factor and the Need for Individual Diagnosis, 352   A Survey of Recent Techniques, 353   Regulated Breathing Methods, 355   Therapeutic Mechanisms of the New Methods, 357

15   **Modification of Behavior, Part One**   *Charles Van Riper,* **363**

Exploring the Problem, 363

Modification of Behavior, Part Two   *Charles Van Riper,* **367**

Calming and Toughening the Stutterer, 367

Modification of Behavior, Part Three   *Charles Van Riper,* **373**

Modifying the Stuttering, 373

POSTSCRIPT   Modifying Stuttering Behavior
Harold L. Luper, **380**

Comments on Modification of Behavior, 382   A Brief Peek at the Crystal Ball, 388

16   **Evolution of a Target-Based Behavioral Therapy for Stuttering**
Ronald L. Webster, **397**

Introduction, 397   Program I, 398   Program II, 398   Variations on Program II, 399   Program III, 400   Program IV, 401   Program V, 401   Program VI, 403   Conclusion, 405

POSTSCRIPT   Stuttering Therapy from a Technological Point of View   *Ronald L. Webster,* **407**

Technology and Stuttering Therapy, 407   General Properties of Technology, 408   Technology and Basic Scientific Principles, 412   Conditions Necessary for Technology Development, 412   Limitations in a Technological Approach to Stuttering Therapy, 413

17   **Operant Procedures Applied to Stuttering Therapy for Children**   *Bruce P. Ryan,* **417**

Case 1, 418   Case 2, 420   Case 3, 422   Case 4, 425   Case 5, 426   Discussion, 427

POSTSCRIPT   Operant Therapy for Children
Bruce P. Ryan, **431**

Introduction, 431   Overt Themes, 432   Covert Themes, 440   Conclusions
and Summary, 442

18   **Stutter-Free Speech: A Goal for Therapy**   *George H. Shames and
Cheri L. Florance,* **447**

The Clinical Relationship, 449   The Phases of Therapy, 449

POSTSCRIPT   A Current View of Stutter-Free Speech
George H. Shames, **454**

Changes in the Format of Therapy, 459   Summary of Changes in Tactics in the
Stutter-Free Speech Program, 459

19   **A Point of View About Fluency**   *Herbert Rubin and
Richard Culatta,* **467**

The Program, 468   Resumes of Therapy, 471   Conclusion, 472
Summary, 472

POSTSCRIPT   Cognitive Therapy   *Herbert Rubin,* **474**

Pragmatics of Stuttering, 476   Psychological Factors, 479   Expectancy, 479
Maintenance, 481   Etiology, 482   Therapy for Children, 483
Conclusion, 484

20   **Maintenance of Fluency: A Review**   *Einer Boberg,
Pauline Howie, and Lee Woods,* **489**

Introduction, 489   Long Term Outcome of Behavioral Treatment Programs for
Stuttering, 490   Discussion, 494   Speculations on Fluency Relapse, 497
Summary, 499

POSTSCRIPT   Relapse and Outcome   *Einer Boberg,* **501**

Increased Interest in Maintenance?, 501   Methodological Issues, 503
Experimental Investigations in Maintenance, 506   New Speculations, 508
Prospects for the Future, 509

21   **Concluding Remarks**   *George H. Shames and Herbert Rubin,* **517**

Introduction, 517   Unresolved Issues, 522

Name Index, 531

Subject Index, 534

PART ONE

THE BEGINNINGS

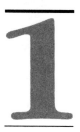

Historical Prologue

Jack Matthews

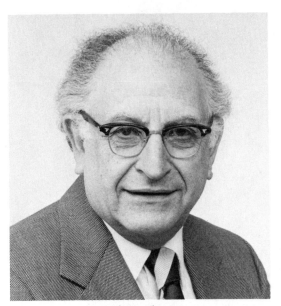

Jack Matthews

The task of preparing a historical introduction to this volume necessarily had to fall to a senior colleague in Speech Pathology who could recall from personal experience and interpret the evolution, major controversies, and differences in perspective over approximately half a century of stuttering theory and therapy. We sought a contributor who could provide an objective history of this field and who was himself not biased or invested in any particular perspective on stuttering. In Jack Matthews we found someone who not only satisfied these criteria, but whose background included research and scholarly activities in social psychology, research design and statistics, general semantics, personality theory and clinical psychology, group dynamics, psychological test construction and measurement, and the quantification of qualitative phenomena. This list is not a representation of casual interest on the part of Professor Matthews; each of these specialties reflects a deep and long-standing involvement on the part of a scholar who has taught, consulted, performed, and supervised research in all of them. As such, he brings the scientific method with its rigorous and critical scrutiny to the field of stuttering.

Matthews has applied his skills to the assessment of clinical effectiveness in stuttering therapy as well as in the fields of cleft palate, articulation disorders, and mental retardation. One of the things his many students recall is the constant questioning, always in a warm but persistent manner: "How do you know that what you say is true?" "What are the data to support your conclusions?"

His leadership role in our profession, exemplified in his past presidency of the American Cleft Palate Association and the American Speech and Hearing Association, provides a sense of history that this introductory chapter requires. It is interesting that Matthews warns us at the outset what we were forced to conclude at the end, contrary to our hopes, that the best we can do is to synthesize contrasting beliefs and practices. We cannot resolve them. And that, indeed, is what the scientific method is about.

Historical Prologue

Jack Matthews

This chapter is a historical prologue for a series of papers in which a number of authorities tell how their ideas about stuttering have changed over the last quarter of a century. What are their views about stuttering in 1985? How do these views compare with views they held 25 years ago? The editors have given me the latitude to go back in history even beyond this 25-year time frame. Where shall we begin and how shall we go about the task?

I propose that we make no attempt to start at the beginning because I don't know the beginning. Instead, let's simply agree that the problem of stuttering has been a part of the human condition for thousands of years. A number of references suggest that Moses stuttered. And why did Demosthenes place pebbles in his mouth as he spoke above the roar of the waves on a Greek beach several thousand years ago? An often-given explanation is that Demosthenese was trying to overcome stuttering. One Greek writer suggested several thousand years ago that the "cure" for stuttering was to "emigrate to the south." Was he suggesting that stuttering was caused by some sort of environmental pressures and that the "cure" was to get away from those pressures? Down through the centuries stuttering has been described as an affliction of humankind. A number of famous men have been identified as stutterers. Stuttering did not seem to have interfered with the accomplishments of some of these individuals.

I choose not to dwell on this early history but instead to start at the time I first began to study speech and its disorders—1934 at Heidelberg College in a small city in Ohio. I propose to recall my early encounters with the literature on stuttering. I'll try to remember some of my associations with individuals who sought relief from what they called stuttering or stammering. I will try to identify changes in the literature in the past 50 years. Frequently it is hard to know if the changes are more in me than in the literature. I'll try to give you enough information about Jack Matthews so you can decide.

I began my college career in chemistry. As a science major I spent a lot of out-of-laboratory time as a debator, an actor, and a participant in oratory and extempore speaking contests. I'm fairly certain that I received a lot of reinforcement from my father, who had been a soapbox orator and theater buff in London.

Dad gave me an interest in and a love of speech and theater. I was also interested in science and when I received a college scholarship in chemistry I decided to become either a chemist or a chemical engineer. Gradually my interests turned more and more to speech and theater, but it was not until my sophomore year that I changed from a chemistry major to a joint speech and political science major.

In retrospect I can't help but wonder whether Dad's avid interest in politics and his having served as campaign manager for political candidates in Canada might have influenced my attraction to political science and persuasion and my choosing a dual major in speech and social science. As I write about my perspective and opinions in the mid-1930s I also speculate about the possible relationship between my father's love of politics and my own involvement in school and community politics as well as politics in professional associations. I'm sharing these speculations in the hope that both of us will realize that our beliefs about stuttering are based on more than research findings and "objective" data. As would-be scientists we want to believe that our present analysis of the causes and treatments of stuttering is based on a logical pitting of one set of facts against competing ones. In spite of the many statements by philosophers of science we still operate much of the time as if we were 100% objective in the process of examining literature to determine issues like the causes and cures of many of humankind's problems. Oliver Bloodstein in his chapter on Diagnosogenic Theory gives us insight into how the strength of Wendell Johnson's personality influenced the approach to stuttering taken by many of his students. In turn we can see how Wendell Johnson was influenced by Korzybski as well as a new zeitgeist that had developed by the 1930s. It was a zeitgeist that gave less weight to heredity and more to social environment as a shaper of human behavior. I commend you to Bloodstein's chapter for a good presentation of the importance of factors other than research findings.

Part of the reason for my delay in declaring a speech major grew out of the attitude of the dean of my college towards leaving "science" and going into a field that might provide fun but little intellectual academic challenge. In looking back on the years 1934–1935 from the vantage point of 1985 I cannot be certain whether my lifelong interest in science may in part have grown out of my trying to demonstrate that I could indeed "do" science.

My first encounter with what today we know as speech pathology was in a course in which I was exposed to the notes my professor took when he was a graduate student at the University of Michigan, where he had studied with John Muyskens, Walter Pillsbury, and Clarence Meader. Pillsbury and Meader had written one of the early (1928) texts on the psychology of language. This psychological interpretation of the laws and phenomena of language had not impressed my professor nearly as much as Muyskens's physiological explanation of speech and language. To my professor, the endocrine system was far more important in understanding communication and its disorders than any Freudian or Watsonian concepts of psychology. I learned from my professor in my first course dealing with speech disorders that if I was to really understand problems like stuttering I would have to spend a year studying gross anatomy. I was literally dragged to Ann Arbor to view the kind of anatomy training I *must* have. It was with Dr. Strong, who insisted not only on his speech students learning anatomical dissection but also on their learning along with medical and dental students. On this trip to Ann Arbor I was permitted to see the laboratory of Professor Muyskens and to see the equipment Muyskens had designed to obtain kymograph records (created on a rotating drum on which a moving pen records the waveform of muscular contractions) of speakers who stuttered, who had accents, or who were normal. Is it any wonder that in 1934 stuttering was for me a disorder that resulted from a defective anatomical-physiological-neurological system? Muyskens had not identified a germ or a virus as the "cause" but I was sufficiently "educated" or "brainwashed" by my professor to be pretty well convinced that by further study of anatomy and physiology with due concern for endrocrinology I might find the cause and cure of stuttering.

My undergraduate college was small and did not have a speech clinic. In fact, the speech department had only one person on the faculty and he was responsible for teaching public speaking, coaching debate, and directing theater productions along with carrying out some clinical activities with students and members of the community who had speech problems. I was allowed to serve as an assistant to my professor in all of these activities, including the search for the cause and cure of stuttering. Because of his heavy load my professor was not always able to see those with speech problems as soon as they came for help. I would sometimes see them to try to arrange a schedule. In the course of making these arrangements I would gather case history information. I can recall how elated but puzzled I was on a number of occasions when I learned that following a conference with me the individual's speech problem disappeared. I was equally puzzled by the number of people who left their sessions with my professor relatively free of stuttering but who months later were stuttering worse than ever.

As more and more people in the small college town learned of my interest in speech and its disorders, I heard more stories from individuals who reported that at one time they stuttered. They would tell me about their early experiences with stuttering but would recount these experiences in speech that was as normal as my own. Again, I was puzzled by the fact that these "cures" took place many times with no help from a speech specialist.

I observed my professor working with stutterers and was struck by the fact that many could speak without stuttering if they whispered. If they read from a manuscript in unison with several others they did not stutter. Often they were able to assume a role in a dramatic reading and do so without stuttering. I puzzled over the relationship between choral reading and the elimination of the physiological problems which I "knew" caused stuttering. How did reading in unison bring about the physiological changes needed to effect a cure?

From time to time I would meet someone who reported that he was a cured stutterer. I would try to find the secret of their cure. These "cured" stutterers almost always reported, "I overcame my stuttering when I developed a sense of confidence." They also reported that on their way towards their cure they had experienced some relapses and went back to a pattern of stuttering. When I probed for the reason of the relapse I was frequently told, "I had a temporary loss of confidence. Once I regained and was able to maintain my confidence my stuttering was cured." As I write these recollections of 1934 I am struck by Perkins's postscript in this book in which he observes: "I have not known many cured stutterers, but those whom I have queried invariably assign their 'cure' to a sense of confidence, and their past relapses enroute to their cure to temporary loss of that confidence."

I must admit that because of this possible link between stuttering and confidence there were a few times when I almost questioned the established doctrine on the cause of stuttering and what had to be done to cure it. But I could not question very much because to do so would be to question my mentor, someone who "knew" the cause and cure of stuttering and could cite many successes attributed to his cure. Despite the fact that I came out of a science background I did not at that time ask for data to support my mentor's claims. Many of the contributors to this volume also had faith in the "cures" of their mentors. How many readers of this volume also have faith in the cures of their mentors? But it's time to jump back again to the mid-1930s, to my small college in Ohio.

Our college library was small, and there was little if anything to read about stuttering or other disorders of speech. Why bother reading when my professor's notes taken from his classes with John Muyskens were available and were repeated in each course in speech I took as an undergraduate? It was not until my senior year that I discovered that on some college and university campuses the endrocine system was not considered to be the key to understanding stuttering.

In 1935 I attended a national meeting of teachers of speech, some of whom were interested in stuttering as well as other topics relating to speech. I heard people like Robert West suggest a number of neurophysiological correlates of stuttering. I heard Lee Travis report on studies of heart rate and breathing in stutterers. Bryng Bryngelson described therapy techniques that involved changing the stutterer's handedness to its original "natural" state. I was greatly impressed by the contributions of Wendell Johnson and Charles Van Riper but was again puzzled that as these men spoke they stuttered.

At the first national meeting I attended in 1935 there were a few former stutterers who were anxious to tell about the cure that had helped them. There were some who reported they had been "cured" a number of times, but after each cure they relapsed into stuttering, sometimes worse than ever. And there were a few who reported that they used to stutter, but they overcame the problem without any therapy. They were suggesting in 1935 what Perkins in his postscript in this volume observes, i.e., they assigned their "cure" to a sense of confidence.

At this national conference of teachers of speech I discovered that there were a number of so-called experts who believed they had found the cause and cure of stuttering and held their views with the intensity of a recent convert to religious cult. They were true believers. All the clinicians I spoke to reported successes for a variety of different clinical approaches. I spoke to no clinicians who could report long-term follow-up results on a series of patients. I met many people who impressed me as being warm and caring, but I did not ask if their concern for their clients might have something to do with the success of their therapy. This thought was somewhat foreign to the kind of training I had received in the chemistry and physics laboratories while I was still "doing" science. So my search continued for the cause and cure of stuttering. Because of the point of view of my undergraduate professor I expected that cause to lie in the realm of the physiological. John Muyskens's concern with the role of the endocrine system was still alive in my thinking even though by my senior year I began to realize there might be other causes. Graduate school would give me the answer—so I thought.

Because of financial need and my own interests, I began my master's degree as freshman debate coach and business manager of the university theater. One half day a week I spent in the speech clinic. This was 1938, and we were quite impressed by the research on cerebral dominance. Although Orton and Travis had written on this topic as early as 1929, it was not until almost 10 years later that I was exposed to their theory. I was impressed. Here was a really scientific explanation of what caused stuttering. Armed with knowledge of cause I should then be able to devise cures. If dominance was at the core of the problem then my diagnostic procedures would have to include reliable and valid methods for measuring dominance. I became expert at building laterality boards to determine the "natural" handedness of clients I saw in the clinic. I became familiar with measures of handedness, "footedness," and "eyedness." Laterality tests became so important in my clinical techniques that I routinely administered a battery of laterality tests to all my clients, including those with foreign accents and lateral lisps. I discouraged my clients from activities that might stress ambidextrous functioning as opposed to unilateral activity geared to strengthening the natural handedness. This meant that many of my clients had to unlearn their right-handed behaviors, because my laterality tests had established that they really were left-handed. With a number of children I was able to reverse the efforts of parents and teachers to shift a child from writing with the left hand to writing with the right hand. With many of these children I was rewarded with reports from parents that following their initial meeting with me they eased the pressures they had been exerting on the "natural" left-handed children and the stuttering had disappeared. Success! I had found the cause and was able to bring about the cure. At the time I never raised the question about what was bringing about the cure. My reading of Orton and Travis and the interviews Bryngelson was kind enough to give me suggested that my success should be credited to restoration of natural laterality. As a 21-year-old convert to the notion that physiology was the key to understanding stuttering I spent little time wondering if there was any relationship between the cures my young stutterers were experiencing and the lessening of parental pressures in many areas besides changing handedness. I had not yet been introduced to parent counseling. Nor did I raise with myself the question of whether some of the speech arts activities (dramatic skits, choral reading, etc.), which I introduced to my young stutterers as a fun break from the monotony of exercises to strengthen the "natural" laterality, might be building confidence. In 1938 I would not consider confidence as a possible variable because it was not a physiological correlate.

So in 1938 I could report that many of the children I treated no longer stuttered. Some continued to stutter and were still being treated as stutterers in the university speech clinic when I completed my master's degree and moved to another campus to begin work on my Ph.D.

In late 1938 I discovered Alfred Korzybski and General Semantics. His *Science and Sanity* had been published in 1933 but was slow to attract much attention in the speech community. I was so intrigued by Korzybski's work that I wrote my master's thesis in the area of general semantics. My thesis attempted to trace some of the origins of the major tenets in Korzybski's formulation of general semantics. Some I was able to trace back to several of Plato's dialogues. I became aware for the first time that a good many "new" ideas of today had been thought about years earlier, in some cases centuries ago. Since then I have come to realize that many of my most astute insights were "stolen" from me by individuals who died before I was born. In part because of my having explored some of the origins of the general semantics movement I began to look at the earlier writings dealing with stuttering and with stammering, a term more frequently employed in an earlier era. I discovered that many have claimed to have found the cause and cure of stuttering. These cures were reported, accepted as fact by many, and later rejected. It was not until many years later that I came to realize what Bloodstein and other contributors to this volume have pointed out, "Theories of stuttering are seldom abandoned because they have been disproved. Most often we just get tired of them." (p. 138).

From Korzybski I learned to recognize that my perception of the world differed from that of others who had had different experiences and might have developed different value systems. It was not until my exposure to Korzybski that I came to realize that stuttering does not mean the same thing to all speech clinicians. For the first time the thought occurred to me that what I wanted my clients to achieve in my "cure" might not be the same goal that other clinicians had for their clients. Boberg's chapter, "Relapse and Outcome," provides a good current statement of these important concepts.

From Korzybski I learned that language—how you label something—can influence how you feel about that thing. I came to realize that when clients talked about their stuttering it was in a context of negative feelings about the speech act and about themselves as speakers. I had tended until this point to focus on the objective speech behavior—what caused it and how to correct it. Until this point, in my thinking I had tended to minimize the possible contribution of clinicians who were interested in helping stutterers feel better about their stuttering and learn to stutter in an easier manner.

Because of Korzybski I also came to question my earlier tendency to separate mind and body and to assume that the cause and cure of stuttering was in the realm of the body as opposed to the mind. It was at this time that I began to seriously question how much I would be helped in my search for the cause and cure of stuttering by delving further into Muyskens's concerns about the endocrine system and Strong's pronouncements from the anatomy laboratory. I was ready to turn my back on cerebral dominance and genetic, biochemical, and physiological theories. A new day was dawning. I was about to discover psychology!

I was attracted to psychology because of some thinking that had been stimulated by reading Korzybski. I got another kind of push from the dean of the graduate school who told me he would not approve a Ph.D. program in speech unless I took at least one third of my work in a field with more "substance." My mentor, G. Oscar Russell, had recently (1936) published the report of an x-ray analysis of tongue and articulatory organ position in the production of vowels. This was an extension of earlier x-ray studies of physiological processes in speech production. He urged me to take my cognate work in either physiology or anatomy but reluctantly he allowed me to elect work in physiological psychology. In time I was given his blessing for courses in statistics and tests and measurements. At a joint meeting of the American Psychological Association, the American Association for Applied Psychology, and the forerunner of the American Speech-Language-Hearing Association, Russell introduced me to Wendell Johnson by saying, "I want you to meet this young fellow. He has some crazy ideas that might appeal to you."

Russell was right. The ideas and the man did appeal to me. Johnson had not only become aware of Korzybski's work but had attended workshops and seminars at Korzybski's institute in Chicago. He helped me to meet Korzybski and to attend the Institute for General Semantics.

Johnson incorporated some key concepts of general semantics into his approach to stuttering. This approach was to become the basis of the semantogenic theory of stuttering, which became the foundation for what became the Iowa approach to therapy. I was influenced by Johnson's ideas and by him as a person. Like many in our field I owe him a great debt for his early encouragement as I was establishing myself in speech pathology. (*See* Bloodstein's chapter "Semantics and Beliefs.") The fact that Johnson held appointments in both speech and psychology certainly was a factor in pushing my own graduate studies in the direction of psychology. This in turn was responsible for my joining the Psychological Research Unit of the U.S. Air Force during World War II.

If there were such an entity as an objective historian we might call on that person to help us decide whether the late 1930s gave rise to an increase in interest in the emotional adjustment and personality traits of stutterers or whether I was more receptive to such approaches at that time. In trying to assess trends in stuttering theory and therapy, it's difficult to separate what is happening "out there" from the many factors that influence what you perceive is taking place out there. My perception is that at the time I returned from the U.S. Air Force Psychological Research Unit to graduate school many people in speech pathology were not getting the answers they had hoped for from the once highly regarded cerebral dominance, biochemical, and physiological theories. Many were turning to psychology for answers and guidance.

In my own case I expected more than I should have from psychology. I was still looking for a cause but now it was in the realm of personality differences rather than differences in physiological measures. Clinically I could see improvement in my clients after they had experienced a series of psychotherapy sessions with me. Wasn't that to be expected? After all, I was on my way to becoming a card-carrying clinical psychologist capable of helping people cope with their personality problems. Regardless of the nature of the psychological pain my clients were experiencing, they needed help from someone who could deal with feelings rather than speech blocks, with self-image rather than vocal cord spasms. All that physical-anatomical-physiological approach was old hat and resulted in some temporary help but no long-term permanent cure. Clearly psychology was the key. With such perceptions about the state of the art in stuttering therapy is it any wonder that when I came to the University of Pittsburgh to establish a graduate program in speech pathology I set it up as a unit within the psychology department? For a number of years this program derived its degree-granting authority from an interdisciplinary committee representing psychology, speech, medicine, dentistry, and education. Administratively it was housed in psychology.

During this period we compared stutterers with nonstutterers on a variety of psychological rather than physiological measures. We found less and less evidence to support our original notions of the psychological differences we were sure were present and causing stuttering. I was reluctant to accept such negative findings and blamed the results on poor research design, insensitive measures, etc., rather than questioning the assumption that psychological problems caused stuttering. An earlier fixation on physiological causes had been replaced by the belief that the answer would come from psychology.

During the early years of the speech pathology training program at Pitt, I had my first encounter with "Dr. J," a practitioner who some would call a fraud and a quack but who also had supporters among some physicians and parents of children whom he had "cured" of stuttering. "Dr. J's" techniques included a vibrating device applied externally to the throat, warm baths, warm beverages, yeast, reassurance, dramatic readings, and selected use of prayer. Because he was licensed as a lay minister no one questioned his competence in the use of prayer. Because he was head of the speech clinic in one of the largest children's hospitals in the eastern United States few questioned his competence in the area of speech until several pediatricians became concerned that some children who were being treated for stuttering with baker's yeast complained of stomach discomfort from the large amounts of gas generated by the yeast. I began to see a number of children whose stuttering had initially improved, but later had worsened, after "Dr. J" had exercised his therapy techniques. Some members of the hospital staff were concerned that "Dr. J," who did not have a M.D. degree, was coming very close to practicing medicine. Some hospital staff had serious questions about many of "Dr. J's" practices. On the other side of the coin were strong statements of support from the highly respected head of the hospital's pediatric service who could recount numerous children who had been cured by "Dr J." This is not the place to discuss the steps taken to find out about "Dr. J's" training. It may be of interest to reveal that I found that "Dr. J" had no degree at all, that the European universities he claimed to have attended were nonexistent and that his formal education ended with high school. "Dr. J" was removed from his post at the hospital and changed his activities from "curing" stuttering to "curing" cerebral palsy and mental retardation.

My encounter with "Dr. J" puzzled me but also caused me to question some of my own behavior. I was puzzled how someone with "Dr. J's" lack of the usual credentials could reach such a responsible position and be able to make strong claims about the success of his therapy. I could not be sure that he was deliberately deceiving parents when he reported that he had been able to help many children who stuttered—that indeed he could identify large numbers who experienced a "cure" for stuttering after he worked with them. True, some of his patients relapsed, but this was also true of some of my patients. In fact, at this stage in my career I had already participated in several professional programs in which a number of experts in stuttering told of "my worst clinical failure."

My concern over the case of "Dr. J" led me to investigate a famous (some might refer to it as infamous) "stammering school" located in a large midwestern city. They advertised extensively and promised to cure stuttering. Among the various therapy techniques they employed was teaching their clients to speak in time with a metronome. The metronome was replaced by moving the arm to describe a figure **8** in the air and uttering a word each time the hand reached the center of the figure **8**. Gradually the finger was substituted for the hand. It was possible to demonstrate dramatic reduction in stuttering; in fact, some "permanent" cures for stuttering could be claimed and substantiated by this school. We all know, however, that most of these "cures" were followed by relapse. The uncomfortable aspect of my pondering the record of this "stammering school" and of "Dr. J" was that I could produce little data to demonstrate that my record was much better than theirs. I had come to realize that a number of people were going to overcome stuttering without any outside help. I also had to face up to the fact that a sizable number of my clients initially improved but subsequently relapsed into stuttering that was worse than when I first saw them.

The would-be scientist in me said we must find the cause of stuttering and not be detracted from our mission to cure by wasting time treating symptoms. At this time respected speech pathologists like Johnson and Van Riper were reporting therapy approaches that spent much time dealing with symptoms. The Iowa approach was gaining more and more support. It was easy for me to question this approach by telling myself and my students that what we were seeing was the result of the intervention of warm, caring clinicians. I could even dip into the literature of psychology and say, "We are seeing another example of the Hawthorne effect." But while I was discounting the Iowa approach I had the uncomfortable feeling that any successes I might point to in my therapy might also be credited to the Hawthorne effect.

Early in the 1950s I began to see fewer clients and to take on more supervisory and administrative duties. I became director of the University of Pittsburgh's Division of Psychological Services and head of the graduate training program in clinical psychology. In this capacity I came in contact with a number of psychiatrists. At this time, the psychiatric community lived and practiced in two camps. One was neuropsychiatry, in which the knee-jerk hammer was more important than the couch. I was still disappointed with my earlier exposure to the physiological approaches to stuttering and my exposure to Muyskens and the endocrine system. As a Fellow of the Clinical Division of the American Psychological Association I felt more comfortable with the other camp of psychiatry—the one that carried on the work of Freud diluted as little as possible by the inroads of GAP (Group for the Advancement of Psychiatry) or the ideas of Harry Stack Sullivan.

I was thrown into contact with these psychoanalytically oriented psychiatrists in several ways. They served as consultants in our clinical psychology training program. They taught courses in psychodynamics both in our psychology department and in our school of social work. From time to time I would also work jointly with a colleague from psychiatry who wished to discuss a patient who stuttered and showed considerable "resistance." I became impressed over several years with the large number of patients who were in analysis and whose stuttering behavior underwent little change. In almost every instance I was told that the real problem was in the patients "resistance." During this period I also saw a number of clients who had either completed analysis or had terminated analysis after several years. When these patients approached me it was usually with a statement such as, "I finished four years of analysis" or "I've spent over ten thousand dollars on analysis." They might continue, "I know I hate my father but is there anything you can do to help me stop stuttering? I have some insights into my feelings and my relationships with my family but I'm still stuttering." These people were asking for help with their symptoms. I was seeking the cause of their problem. Analytical psychiatry was going after the neurosis. The analysts too were concerned with cause rather than symptom. Meantime, in Iowa City, in Minneapolis, and in Kalamazoo concerned and creative speech pathologists were not only paying attention to symptoms but were telling their clients, "You are a stutterer and will always be a stutterer. Now let's see if there are some easier ways to stutter and let's see if you can develop a better attitude towards yourself." Much as I admired Johnson, Van Riper, and Bryngelson as people and as clinicians I could not accept what was later to be known as "Iowa therapy."

But eventually I moved in the direction of accepting and using much of "Iowa therapy." Why? One factor was my increasing conviction that neurosis was not the cause of the problem with most stutterers. My experience with patients with a variety of psychological problems other than stuttering made me question more and more the efficacy of analytical therapy. Within clinical psychology, approaches other than the traditional analytical were being employed. Carl Rogers's client-centered therapy was gaining support not only within clinical psychology but also in the other helping professions.

I was pushed by another force to reexamine my unwillingness to focus on symptoms. Within our school of social work were several faculty who were exploring psychological approaches other than analysis. Throughout most American schools of social work psychology courses were presented from a psychoanalytical point of view. The one exception was at Penn, where another point of view was emerging. The people in this camp came to be known as functionalists. My colleagues at Pitt began to interact with their colleagues at Penn and in the course of several years the few Pitt functionalists had joined the dissenters from psychoanalysis at Penn. This is not the place to list in detail the philosophical differences which separated the functionalists from the Freudian-oriented practitioners. The two groups differed on the question that had been bothering me in stuttering therapy: How much attention should we devote to symptoms and their treatment as opposed to cause and its removal?

I was attracted to the functionalists as people. I was having little success in finding the cause of stuttering. I saw some exciting results growing out of the use of Rogerian techniques by a wide variety of professional workers. I was also impressed by several studies that compared various psychotherapy interventions and found no evidence to show that any one was any better, or worse, than any other. The key variable seemed to be the relationship established between client and therapist. If the relationship was good the outcomes seemed equally good regardless of the therapy employed. Then too there were studies suggesting that just being put on a waiting list or allowing a year to pass produced results that were comparable to what came out of a variety of different therapy interventions.

From my medical friends who had one or two degrees in psychology I got reports that a large number of their patients would get better even if no medication was prescribed. These physician friends were not bothered by treating symptoms. They sought causes but often could not find a cause. Their patients hurt but seemed to get some relief from the attention the physician gave to symptoms and relief of symptoms. I was told that often the treatment of symptoms provided a period of relief and reassurance which did not interfere with the body itself "curing" the disease. I knew from my clinical experience and that of my colleagues that some former stutterers reported that they used to stutter and that they have never had any speech therapy. Would I be hurting such an individual—one who was going to get better on his own—if I tried to give him some relief from the symptoms that brought him to my office?

It was at this point in my growth as a speech pathologist that I added to my concern about finding the cause of stuttering some concern with dealing with symptoms. It was also at this point that I became frustrated in not being able to know: (a) Who will get better with no therapy? (b) Of those whose speech improves who will be doing well 2 years from now? (c) Are the results of an Iowa approach any better than any one of the therapy interventions used by speech pathologists who start out with different notions about the cause of stuttering? My inability to answer these questions led me to believe that the literature on stuttering lacks sufficient concern for evaluating therapies. This belief has led me to spend more time in recent years pondering problems of program evaluation and therapy evaluation rather than examining the arguments in support of a given theory of stuttering or a particular therapeutic approach. There were several experiences that led me to become more concerned with evaluation than I had been earlier in my career. Some were in areas related to speech pathology, some in other fields.

Let's examine some "cures" which later came to be questioned and in some cases discarded. In 1954 Kurtzke and Berlin first reported on the beneficial effects of isoniazid on patients with multiple sclerosis. Shortly after their publication, isoniazid was on its way to becoming the miracle drug it had proved to be in the treatment of tuberculosis. As a consultant to the Veteran's Administration in speech pathology and in clinical psychology I became acutely aware of the pressure of veterans' organizations to improve not only the speech of the multiple sclerosis patients we were working with but also their coordination, feelings of well being, etc. We were criticized because we were not keeping up with "new developments" in the field and were failing to use the effective treatment being used in New York hospitals. As a result of such pressures a group of neurologists, psychologists, and speech pathologists carried out an evaluation of isoniazid on 186 patients from 11 hospitals. Burgi, Everson, and I (Matthews, 1960) were able to report within 5 years of the original claims of the Kurtzke and Berlin study that isoniazid did not result in improvement in the speech of multiple sclerosis patients. The complete report on this evaluation study of the effects of isoniazid showed similar negative results for all of the variables examined. The "miracle" drug had lost its magic when subjected to careful study but not until many false hopes were raised.

In a similar tradition glutamic acid was claimed as a cure for mental retardation. A careful evaluation study of its effects was carried out in Western Psychiatric Hospital and at Polk State School. Again the miracle did not hold up.

Prefrontal lobotomy was hailed as a new breakthrough for neuropsychiatry and was widely employed before it was carefully evaluated. Today there are many professionals who are concerned about the harm done by the use of this procedure, which in time was found to be of no value. Not only were false hopes raised but in some instances real and potential damage was done to patients.

In the area of cerebral palsy we have lived through the "cures" of icing, carbon dioxide, and brushing. In cleft palate we went through the era of bone grafting. In each instance the cure was announced or inferred from a report in a respectable journal or presented at a professional meeting. The new approach was picked up and used for several years before evaluation studies determined that the cure was not a cure. In some cases we were seeing a placebo or Hawthorne effect. In other instances there were flaws in the original research that was presented. With the exception of the fabricated data Schmidt published on increasing the IQ of mentally retarded children in the Chicago public schools I know of no deliberate fabrication of evidence to support a particular therapy intervention.

Because of my increasing awareness of the absence of long-term follow-up studies of various approaches to stuttering I found myself able to resist becoming a true believer of either the learning theory or the operant conditioning approaches to stuttering. I have tremendous respect for Wischner's attempts to combine the insights of Hull and Spence in learning theory with Johnson's work in stuttering. Wischner's search for a scientific explanation of the stuttering process and the clinical uses of punishment is to be commended. Had Wischner's work appeared 20 years earlier I might well have jumped on the bandwagon and embraced Wischner's approach as the answer. To Wischner's credit I must observe that from the time we first discussed stuttering in the Psychological Research Unit of the air force in 1942 until he left the University of Pittsburgh 30 years later I never heard him claim he had *the* answer or *the* approach to stuttering.

cation of operant conditioning. Again, if Skinner had published 20 years earlier I might have seized upon operant conditioning as the answer. (*See* Ryan's chapter "Operant Therapy for Children".) My failure to say, "This is it!" to these ideas says more about me than about their formulation. Also, my unwillingness to embrace cognitive approaches as the final word on stuttering speaks to my growing skepticism of finding *the* answer rather than questioning the creativeness and the validity of these approaches.

I recognize some of my biases but I'm sure that some are more obvious to the reader than to me. I realize that in general my world is a happier place for me if I know the cause of the phenomena I observe. But you may not derive as much satisfaction as I do from knowing causes. As a former debater and debate coach, I may be unduly concerned with definitions. Perhaps that's why I am bothered by the fact that although stuttering means different things to different people there is a tendency from study to study and clinician to clinician to assume that stuttering is stuttering is stuttering. Perhaps we need a dozen new terms to describe a variety of speech behaviors that differ with age of speaker, type of stress in the speaking situation, visual components, etc. By the early 1950s I had become convinced that we were making claims for therapy outcomes that were not being substantiated. I worked with several of my graduate students to develop instruments that could be used to measure outcomes (Schaef & Matthews, 1954; Matthews, 1955; Matthews, 1959).

As one with an early concern for both the necessity and the worth of evaluation I may be too critical of our failure to recognize that the goals of therapy often differ widely. Some therapies strive for fewer blocks. Others seek less stress or struggle in blocks. Some are concerned with helping the stutterer feel better about himself and his speech. No one of these is the "right" goal but any attempt at evaluating therapy must begin with a clear-cut notion of the goal of therapy.

I suggest a great deal more attention to long-term evaluation of therapy. Such evaluation requires agreement on items to include in the definition of stuttering as well as agreement on the parameters to measure after therapy. Although we have reports of satisfactory reliability of ratings within a single clinic we lack reports on rating reliability from clinic to clinic. I hope more evaluation is carried out by people who do not have a vested interest in the outcome of the therapy.

I am impressed by the methodological sophistication displayed by the work of Andrews on meta-analysis. He and his group are to be congratulated for their efforts to bring together the variety of studies that have tried to evaluate the effectiveness of stuttering therapy. No matter how sophisticated Andrews's analytical techniques are, there is no escaping the fact that he brings together studies that do not agree on the definition of stuttering or the goals of therapy. He integrates well-designed studies with ones with serious weaknesses in methodology. In reading Andrews (1980, 1983)—which I strongly recommend—bear in mind the popular folk-formula: g in $= g$ out (garbage in $=$ garbage out).

Andrews sounds a more optimistic note than I believe is justified when he concludes, "For 10 years there has been good evidence that a planned and disciplined approach to therapy is effective." (Andrews, 1983). I admire Andrews's statistical analysis but am unwilling to accept the overall inference that the battle against stuttering is almost won. I am more inclined to accept Boberg's caution from his chapter "Relapse and Outcome": "We may wish to postpone our victory celebrations for yet awhile."

In looking back on 50 years' exposure to the field of stuttering I chose to share my shifting views during my entire career to date. Some of these shifts came about as styles or fads came and went in the field. Some of what I reported as "real" changes may simply have been my perception of what was happening. Perhaps in some cases this stemmed from what I wanted to see or what I needed to see to justify my own existence.

I must be on guard against my own skepticism. If indeed a new explanation of the cause and cure of stuttering does appear I must be open to recognizing its validity and not simply assuming that it is another premature, unsubstantiated claim. I hope we can all remain receptive to evidence that evaluates the effectiveness of our therapy. In my judgment we are rediscovering the wheel in many of our approaches. Our claims often go beyond what we can deliver. Nevertheless, the search for answers must go on. In the chapters which follow you will have a chance to observe our most recent searches to understand and treat stuttering.

REFERENCES

Andrews, Gavin, Guitar, Barry, & Howie, Pauline. (1980). Meta-Analysis of the effects of stuttering treatment. *Journal of Speech and Hearing Disorders, 45,* 287–307.

Andrews, Gavin, Craig, Ashley, Feyer, Anne-Marie, Haddinott, Susan, Howie, Pauline, & Neilson, Megan. Stuttering: A review of research findings and theories circa 1982. *Journal of Speech and Hearing Disorders, 48,* 226–246.

Bloodstein, Oliver. (1975). *A handbook on stuttering* (rev. ed.). Chicago: National Easter Seal Society for Crippled Children and Adults.

Korzybski, A. (1933). Science and sanity: An introduction to non-Aristotelian systems and general semantics. New York: International Non-aristotelian Library Publishing Co.

Kurtzke, J. F., & Berlin, L. (1954). The effect of isoniazid on patients with multiple sclerosis. *American Review of Tuberculosis, 70,* 577–592.

Matthews, Jack, & Bendig, A. W. (1955). The index of agreement: A possible criterion for measuring the outcome of group discussion. *Speech Monographs, 22,* 39–42.

Matthews, Jack, & Burgi, Ernest J. (1959). A suggested instrument for evaluating speech therapy with cerebral palsied adults. *Journal of Clinical Psychology, 15,* 143–146.

Matthews, Jack, Everson, Richard, & Burgi, Ernest J. (1960). The effects of isoniazid on the speech of patients with multiple sclerosis. *Journal of Speech and Hearing Disorders, 25,* 38–42.

Perkins, William (Ed.). (1980). Strategies in Stuttering Therapy. *Seminars in Speech, Language and Hearing, 1,* 277–409.

Schaef, Robert, & Matthews, Jack. (1954). A first step in the evaluation of stuttering therapy. *Journal of Speech and Hearing Disorders, 19,* 467–473.

Shames, G. H., & Egolf, D. B. (1976). *Operant conditioning and the management of stuttering.* Englewood Cliffs, NJ: Prentice-Hall.

Shames, G. H., & Florance, C. L. (1980). *Stutter-free speech: A goal for therapy.* Columbus, OH: Charles E. Merrill.

Travis, L. E. (1957). The unspeakable feelings of people with special reference to stuttering. In L. E. Travis (Ed.), *Handbook of Speech Pathology.* New York: Appleton-Century-Crofts.

Van Riper, C. (1971). *The Nature of Stuttering.* Englewood Cliffs, NJ: Prentice-Hall.

Williams, D. E. (1971). Stuttering therapy for children. In L. E. Travis (Ed.), *Handbook of Speech Pathology and Audiology.* Englewood Cliffs, NJ: Prentice-Hall.

PART TWO

CAUSATION AND DYNAMICS

2

Overview of Part Two
Theory, Research, and Clinical Management—
A System of Interactions

George H. Shames and Herbert Rubin

Overview of Part Two
Theory, Research, and Clinical Management—
A System of Interactions

George H. Shames and Herbert Rubin

From biblical times to the present stuttering has defied explanation. What it is and where it comes from are the issues addressed in this section. Theories of stuttering have arisen from people's desire to understand complex and inconsistent behaviors, rather than to stimulate further inquiry. Historically, the need to relieve the painful and embarrassing condition of stuttering was more important than comprehending its origin. The people were more important than the problem. Even current theories of the origin of stuttering are assessed in terms of their ultimate relationship to alleviation, although there was a time when a great deal of thinking and research focused on etiology. Much of this work was done at the State University of Iowa in the 1940s. The focus at that time ranged through genetics, neurophysiology, behavioral psychology, and general semantics as bases for understanding the origins of stuttering. Wendell Johnson, one of the leaders at Iowa, and father of the semantogenic theory of stuttering, is reputed to have used the metaphor of a cow stuck in some barbed wire. In such a situation, would you sit down with the animal and take a developmental history? Would you interview the cow to determine how she got into this predicament and how she feels about it? Or would you pull out your wirecutters and relieve the beast from her misery? What Johnson was questioning was the role of theory and its relevance to therapy. He was participating in the final stages of the classic nature versus nurture controversy that had engrossed many of the great thinkers of the preceding century. By the mid-1950s this controversy had been largely abandoned in favor of a compromise. Recently, however, advances in genetics, in particular genetic engineering, have focused some researchers on the prepotence of inheritance as a factor in human behavior. The chapters that follow in this section, written over a 40-year time span, reflect these changes in perspective.

What is a theory, and why do we devote so much of this volume to theories of stuttering? A theory provides a statement of relationships among events. It simultaneously attempts to explain data and to generate researchable hypotheses, which in turn provide additional data. A theory is a framework for asking cohesive questions in a systematic way. In this sense a theory determines what you look for and see, and therefore determines the form of your data. However, it is still possible to observe events and react to them without a theoretical orientation. For thousands of years stuttering has been observed, recorded, and treated without theoretical direction. No attempt to explain data and generate hypotheses was involved in placing pebbles in the mouths of stutterers or in surgically removing sections of their tongues. These treatments reflected simple associations, but no framework for asking cohesive questions in a systematic way. Stuttering attacks the senses. Ancient practitioners and lay listeners alike could see and hear stuttering with little theoretical constraint because they wanted to do something about it. Why suddenly, in the middle of the twentieth century are we so concerned with the theory of stuttering? As with medicine and psychology, the technology of research has profoundly affected our thinking about ancient problems. Although Mendel and Pasteur provide isolated historical examples of carefully controlled research, they were precursors of the widespread application of the scientific method to theory validation. Another possible explanation for the recent emphasis on stuttering theory is the history of relative ineffectiveness of therapy for this eminently practical problem. If more stutterers had been "cured" by a few, if not a single treatment strategy, would so many theories have been developed? In other words, at least some of our current theories of stuttering seem to have arisen from the need to explain the poor and inconsistent results of therapy, and to generate better strategies of clinical management. This relationship between the number of theories and the effectiveness of therapy may reflect our expectation that a theory about stuttering should provide statements about its therapy in addition to explanations of its origin and dynamics. One final point we should note at this time is the significant number of theorists, researchers, and practitioners who themselves stutter. Apart from the unavoidable issue of bias, since none of us can be completely objective about ourselves or our behaviors, it is possible that professionals, as stutterers, are more highly motivated to explain, study, and alleviate the problem of stutterers. They may feel a special responsibility. Although they may share the label and the problem, their theories range from genetic and physiological differences through emotional causes to such environmental influences as developmental, semantic, and learning factors.

ETIOLOGY AND MAINTENANCE

It may be important to distinguish between the origins of stuttering and those factors that maintain stuttering after its original appearance. The origins are usually impossible to observe and difficult to reconstruct, and reports often reflect the bias and the interpretation of the informant. In addition, an emphasis on etiology during clinical management may function to divert the clinician and the stutterer from dealing with the issues at hand. Questions like "If I only knew why I stutter" may be a form of clinical resistance and only serve to delay therapeutic progress. A prolonged attempt at finding what caused the problem may be futile and frustrating, an exercise in creative imagination. Beyond this, it can actually have the deleterious effect of supporting a belief system that is antitherapeutic, as might be the case in the "inevitability" of stuttering as an interpretation of a genetic theory of origin. On the other hand, although the process by which stuttering is maintained may be very similar to its origins, it is usually directly observable and therefore subject to verification. If we agree that theories are verifiable by the results of research, then we should try to sort out research that has addressed the origin of stuttering from research on the dynamics of stuttering (which has been related to etiology only by deduction) from research on maintenance factors (which may have etiological significance for moments of stuttering). The sorting out of these issues is especially important in the chapters in this section. The reader must recognize whether a particular theory of stuttering deals with origins, maintenance, dynamics, or a combination. Failure to do so in the assessment of any reported research makes interpretation of the results difficult and vulnerable to error. On the other hand, separating out these three aspects enables us to interpret research and its implications for prevention and the development of therapeutic tactics as well as strategies for environmental change.

Why, since our stated interest is the alleviation of stuttering, do we concern ourselves with etiology at all? In fact, behaviorists, who are necessarily data-oriented, do not concern themselves with etiology. And the "data" that etiological thinkers work with are introspective reports based on memories of events long past. An alternative etiological approach is to observe the dynamics of stuttering that differentiate stutterers from normal speakers and to reason from these differences about the probable origins of the disorder. Neither of these kinds of data comes out of "experimental" studies which, by definition, require controlled manipulation of independent variables. Given these difficulties, there is yet value in exploring the etiology of stuttering. One manifestation of this value is the numerous clinical strategies such theories have generated.

Prevention

Perhaps, however, the most important reason to investigate etiology is that if we identified the origins of the problem we would have a basis for preventing it. To help understand the impact of the issue of prevention, let us look at just one of the theories discussed in this chapter, Johnson's diagnosogenic argument. If he was correct in stating that the majority of young children become developmentally disfluent during their preschool years, the significance of so many youngsters having in their behavioral repertoires speech patterns that can easily be shaped into stuttering is overwhelming. His theory offers both an explanation of how the problem develops and how it can be prevented. Probably the most effective and widespread preventative strategy used in this country has been Johnson's "Open Letter to the Mother of a Stuttering Child" (1949). This publication became the basis for most of the content and much of the style of parental counseling for the last 40 years. Johnson's strategy was truly preventative in that his counseling and his research on the diagnosogenic theory focused on the "normal" behavior of developmental disfluency, rather than waiting for the appearance of pathological behavior before beginning intervention. Once the strategy is used to remedy nonnormal behavior, the process is one of alleviation and not prevention.

Johnson's approach represents a field study based on historical case reports. More recently, however, Brookshire and Eveslage (1969) and Halvorson (1971), demonstrated in a laboratory situation what can be construed as an analogue of the etiology of stuttering. Each of these experimenters demonstrated that the typical decremental effects of punishment can be reversed. Typically, in the laboratory, when stuttering is followed by contingent punishment, its frequency is reduced. However, in these experiments, when stuttering was followed by both punishment and positive reinforcement for the next fluent word, stuttering was observed to increase beyond the levels it had been reduced to during punishment alone. In the home when punishment is in the form of admonishments about disfluency followed by praise for slowing down and being fluent, we have the paradigm for establishing stuttering suggested by the laboratory studies. Also, when the punishment is delayed and appears to the child to be random, its subsequent contingent use in the same form can be rendered less effective in reducing the undesirable behavior. Still a third source of information about the etiology of stuttering are clinical studies that have manipulated specific variables such as the quality of parent–child verbal interactions (Egolf, et al. 1972; Kasprisin-Burrelli, et al. 1972). Both of these clinical studies have focused on maintaining factors which could have significance for the etiology of the problem.

Other more recent studies which have continued to emphasize the importance of parent–child interaction in the development and maintenance of disfluency, and consequently of establishing and maintaining fluency (Adams, Johnson, Gregory & Hill), have been reported in Perkins (1980). In each case the parents have been formally involved in observing, describing, and eventually identifying patterns of behavior, both their own and their child's, surrounding instance of fluency and disfluency. What is clear from these clinical and laboratory studies is that not only can patterns of disfluency be reversed in the home, but also that stuttering can actually be prevented by adopting explicit child-rearing practices that contain contingencies for effective communication. We are suggesting that parents must arrive at a balance between their natural instincts and the current culturally determined standards of child rearing, replete with endless lists of *dos* and *don'ts*. If these two motivating forces have not been reconciled by the parents, they may create conflict that can overwhelm and immobilize them.

Parents may be faced with the same perplexing questions that clinicians have been struggling with in applying the research data to clinical management. From the research literature and clinical case studies, we can pose four independent variables that reflect different approaches to the prevention of stuttering: (a) Don't punish normal disfluency. (b) Don't reinforce fluency that immediately follows an instance of disfluency. (c) Ignore instances of disfluency. Don't react to the manner of the child's speech. And, more positively, (d) React to the content, in particular the feelings communicated by the child. Compatible with any of these four independent strategies is a fifth consideration that emphasizes establishing an unhurried, noncompetitive, patient, listening atmosphere in the home that gives the child a chance to talk. However, the application of these data to research in the prevention of stuttering is made especially difficult because definitive research in this area should be longitudinal, and because the multiplicity of interactive variables in the home environment have not been, and perhaps cannot be, studied in the laboratory. Isolating a single specific variable in the laboratory, and experimentally studying its effects on either fluency or disfluency is quite different from observing the effects of that same variable within a complex natural environment.

Another important issue to resolve in the study of prevention is whether the large group of disfluent preschool children encompasses one population or two, a developmentally disfluent but normal population, and a higher risk population of genetically or environmentally predisposed youngsters. In the chapters that follow, Johnson, Flanagan, and Shames, reflecting semantic and operant aspects of etiology, represent proponents of a one-population theory of stuttering. Only implicit in the work of Perkins, Travis and Wingate is a two-population theory, although it has been made explicit by Adams (1980) and by L. Johnson (1980). If there are two populations, one normal and one abnormal, then our professional attention should be directed primarily, if not exclusively, toward the high-risk group, since the normal children are likely to outgrow their disfluency without intervention. Criteria offered by clinicians like Adams and L. Johnson to differentiate these two populations of disfluent children include both qualitative speech behaviors such as the presence of prolongation and the schwa vowel during repetitions, and quantitative speech behaviors such as the number of repetitions per disfluency and the overall percentage of disfluency. The research strategies to resolve the one- versus two-population issue would logically include tentatively identifying two groups of children and observing them over time, without intervention, to see if they develop as predicted. Although this approach would verify the differentiating criteria, the ethical questions raised by a nonintervention strategy preclude its application. Another research strategy involves intervention to verify the effectiveness of prevention tactics, whereby two or more high-risk groups would undergo different management programs. Still a third research strategy would be a direct investigation of genetic differences. If successful, such a study would provide the ultimate criterion for identifying a high-risk population. Since we obviously are far from having available such criteria, most clinicians choose a conservative approach to prevention by counseling the parents who are concerned about their children's disfluency, and occasionally by treating these children directly.

Clinical Management

The impact of stuttering theory has been far greater in the realm of treating the problem than identifying its origins or its prevention. Theories of etiology and maintenance focus our attention on events that are considered to be important and how they relate to one another. Each substantive theory directs us to look for, evaluate, and manage specific components of the stuttering problem as identified by these theories. These components could be as complicated as interactions between parents and children, and as circumscribed as repetitions or pause time in speaking. For example, Bloodstein's anticipatory struggle theory focuses on anticipation, and therefore the emergent therapy deals with the client's anticipation of a stuttering block; Sheehan's theory of approach-avoidance conflict focuses on the stutterer's vacillations between silence and speaking, while Johnson's semantogenic theory addresses parents' evaluation of their children's "normal" disfluencies. While perhaps the most valuable contribution of theories of stuttering has been identifying the components of the problem to address in therapy, another less apparent contribution has been the prospects for outcomes and the clinical strategies that have been derived for achieving the goals of therapy. These prospects on outcomes seem to be part of therapeutic climates that lead to such diverse and alternative convictions as reversiblity, where on the one hand stuttering can be completely eliminated or "cured", but on the other hand, stuttering can only be reduced in severity and the client must adapt to his identify as a stutterer, albeit in a more controlled and less severe state. Clinicians should be aware of the atmospheric baggage they hold as practitioners of a particular therapy, whereby they consciously or unconsciously persuade the client to adopt their convictions, both by modeling these convictions and by their rhetorical behavior in therapy. How the clinician and the client talk about what they are doing in therapy may be as important in effecting changes in attitude as the client's reactions to his increased fluency.

The relationship between a particular theory and the relevant therapeutic management may be one of three kinds. First, it may be stronger between the theory and the pertinent events of the problem than what the practitioner actually does in therapy. This appears to be the case with both approach-avoidance conflict theory and with two factor theory. Second, the relationship between the theory and what is done in therapy may be more predictable and consistent, as appears to be the case with semantogenic theory, cognitive theory and psychoanalytic theory. Finally, we have the behavioral theories that suggest strategies of management with very little relationship to theories of origin or identifying critical behaviors. Behavioral theories borrow from the observations of substantive theories of stuttering the events they are going to address, and freely apply their strategies across the broad range of those substantive theories. Many of these strategies have come out of experimental studies in the laboratory and have the goal of reducing the frequency of stuttering. They have employed such tactics as punishment of disfluency, reinforcing fluency, and reinforcing responses that compete with disfluency, including increasing the duration of fluent utterances, as well as reinforcing thematic content that is incompatible with stuttering. We have to be careful to avoid the indiscriminate application of laboratory procedures to the clinical situation for at least three reasons: (a) The kinds of controls and isolation of variables available in the laboratory may not be appropriate or possible in the clinic. (b) Laboratory demonstrations typically do not address generalization and transfer of behaviors outside of the laboratory. (c) Caution must be exercised in using punishment procedures in the clinic because their effects are likely to be both temporary and induce negative emotional side effects.

From the client's point of view, laboratory research studies are of little or no interest. The value of etiological theory to stutterers lies in the explanation it provides of why they began to stutter in the first place, an explanation that is acceptable both to the client and to society at large. Perhaps the most important aspect of this explanation is the label itself, which includes tacit assumptions about its origin (e.g. genetic, physiological, emotional). With identifying an individual as a stutterer comes membership in a social minority that carries certain attributes and privileges. One is the concept of handicap, of an affliction beyond

the individual's control, which makes the behavior in question more s
ceptable than voluntary behaviors, such as spitting. Such an analysis place _
tering in the same category as a physical tic, which enjoys similar social
toleration. There are mores and a system of behaving, a social protocol, already
established for living with the stuttering problem. Not only the stutterer, but each
of us has a traditional role to play in the social ritual, which differs somewhat for
children and adults.

Parental explanations of stuttering, which often include traumatic events of
an emotional or physical nature, thinking faster than he can speak, pressures of
stress or excitement, imitation of another child, nervousness, inherited tendencies, etc. imply simultaneously a neutral or innocent role for the parents and an
excuse for the child. All three come to view the incipient stutterer as a victim,
helpless in the face of external and internal events, which they see as beyond their
control. The social ritual allows only the parent (or grandparents) to interrupt a
disfluent child with solicitious suggestion, albeit without conviction, to stop and
start over again, take a deep breath, slow down, and think before you talk, etc.
How does the child reconcile the contradictory messages that on the one hand
he can't help it, but on the other are specific things to do to "try"? And what does
he understand of the nature of his speech problem and what he can do about it?
Talking about stuttering is a social taboo. Even in households with disfluent children, overt commentary is the exception rather than the rule. Taboo subjects
tend to surround themselves and the members of the problem with a sense of
shame and guilt which, together with a sense of victimization and helplessness,
can continue through adolescence into adulthood.

For adult stutterers the social ritual proscribes any comment about disfluent speech, with the possible exception of the stutterer himself, in the form of
a joke or an excuse. Neither family nor friends risk the embarrassment of commentary, as if they were confronting the emperor without his clothes, conspira-
tors in denial. The social denial by both stutterer and listeners, combined with
the aversiveness of stuttering itself, can lead to a perceptual distortion by the stutterer, where he does not recognize that he just blocked. The observation that
many stutterers avoid eye contact during a block supports the notion of perceptual defense whereby a stutterer arranges not to confront his listener, and his listener's possible reactions, to the aversive experience. The "possible" reactions of
the listener are largely projected and fantasized by the stutterer. In fact, most listeners, especially adults, play out their roles of polite, noninterruptive
collaboration.

It is clear that theories of origin have an influence on the client and family,
as well as on the clinician. For the client and family, theories can provide much-
needed explanations for understanding the nature of the problem. For the clinician, they can provide a conceptual system that links origin, dynamics, and therapeutic strategy.

Research

One of the most widely acknowledged purposes of theory is its heuristic value,
its ability to generate researchable hypotheses. Research methodology can en-

compass observational field studies, clinical studies, and highly controlled laboratory experimental studies. In addition, research in stuttering has addressed its origins, dynamics and maintenance, prevention, and strategies and tactics of therapy, as well as the reliability and validity of measurement. Stuttering has also been studied indirectly with respect to correlates such as personality, demographic factors, and physiological, social, and cultural variables. Each of these issues has come in for its share in research, although recently less has been directed toward the study of origins and more toward therapy and its outcome. Each theory provides the researcher with a system for asking questions. These can be substantive, as in the effect of parent evaluation upon disfluency, or procedural, as in the comparison of the effects of different schedules of reinforcement. Some theories are more heuristic, either because they are more attractive or more provocative than others. Although we think of theory as the stimulant of clinical or laboratory study, on occasion clinical or field observation stimulates the generation of theory. This appears to be the case in relating stuttering to clinical observations of hostility, indirectly expressed. As a matter of fact, the influence of clinical observation has been much more powerful than research findings in developing therapeutic programs. One major exception to this rule is research in identifying and measuring behavioral variables and applying principles of conditioning, especially operant conditioning. The study of such variables as positive reinforcement, punishment, and self-control procedures and their schedules of application has been directly translated into clinical strategies. The only qualification, to which we have referred earlier, is the reluctance to use laboratory punishment procedures in the clinic because of their undesirable consequences.

Aside from research in behavioral management strategies, much of the investigation in the laboratory into the nature of the stuttering block appears to have little relevance for what goes on in therapy. One reason for this lack of transfer is the complexity of behavioral analysis and the objective framework of the scientist, which are difficult for the stutterer to appreciate. Most clients and many clinicians prefer instead to deal in the subjectivity and synthesis of the stuttering experience. Another reason is that research into the stuttering block focuses on behavior that can be eliminated with the snap of a finger or on establishing a competing response. Conversely, clinicians seem to ignore information coming out of the laboratory that could relate to how they view the problem of therapy. The ideal, of course, is a system whereby there is mutual stimulation among the observations of the clinicians, systematic clinical research, highly controlled laboratory research, and theory of management, as differentiated from theory of origin.

IS STUTTERING THE DISORDER OR IS IT SYMPTOMATIC OF AN UNDERLYING DISORDER?

Some of the theories introduced in this chapter suggest that stuttering is indicative of a more basic pathology, much in the way that a fever is a sign of infection. The issue of symptom versus behavior is not limited to the area of stuttering; it has long been a topic of controversy in the fields of psychiatry and psychology.

Whether we view certain human problems within the context of a medical or a behavioral model is not merely a semantic distinction, and it is not a superficial distinction. These models are frameworks that reflect ways of thinking about the problem and what you do about it. The medical model suggests an underlying disease, the only overt evidence of which may be its symptoms. The behavioral model on the other hand argues that overt, ostensible behaviors can be independently manipulated and do not necessarily represent underlying conditions. Therefore, having successfully altered the frequency of observable behaviors, we have resolved the problem in the behavioral model, whereas in the medical model unless the underlying condition is alleviated the problem remains. Freud's concept of defense mechanisms suggests that some behaviors may function to protect the individual from confronting threatening material that is buried in the unconscious. It is possible to view these defenses as symptoms of that repressed material. Eliminating these symptoms can lead to three possible consequences. The first is a successful confrontation with the underlying condition, eliminating the need for a defense. In the event the individual is not ready to confront the repressed material, either the second consequence, psychologic trauma, ensues, or the third consequence occurs, a new defense or symptom is selected. The first consequence illustrates the successful elimination of a symptom. The second consequence is deemed unlikely by many psychotherapists who argue that if an individual is not ready to confront an issue, you can't make him or her do so. The third consequence leads us to the consideration of relapse. Although relapse is a term used by psychotherapists and behaviorists alike, while the psychotherapist views neurosis as involving unconscious defense mechanisms, the behaviorist views neurosis as being maintained by specific neurotic behaviors.

Blanchard and Hersen (1976) characterize two types of neurosis. One type is maintained by behavior designed to reduce anxiety and therefore to lessen distress. This type of neurosis has been most frequently addressed by behaviorists. Relapse is not expected following successful treatment of this type of neurosis since the patient is freed from his neurotic symptom and now has a broader, more direct, less neurotic repertoire of behaviors for reducing his distress. The second type of neurosis is maintained by secondary gain, i.e. "through external social reinforcers that the patient receives contingent upon evidencing his/her symptoms. These secondary gain processes predominate in hysterical neuroses and conversion reactions" (Shames, 1981). With this type of neurosis "simple symptom removal should lead to relapse as the patient tries to seek ways to sustain this secondary gain from society" (ibid). It has been this type of neurosis in which psychotherapists have seen relapse, largely in the form of symptom substitution. With respect to stuttering, however, relapse most often takes the form of the return of the original behaviors rather than the appearance of new behaviors. Another confounding issue is that stuttering has been interpreted as involving both anxiety reduction and secondary gain, which raises the questions of the appropriateness of the bipartite neurotic model, the homogeneity of stutterers, and the absence of a sound theoretical model of stuttering. We are indeed caught up in a controversy of symptoms versus behavior, for which we have no theory and no research, especially in the area of relapse. Even in the anxiety reduction model of stuttering most speech pathologists have considered only anxiety related to the anticipation of stuttering (Wischner, 1950; Sheehan, et al., 1962; Bloodstein, 1958). One notable exception to this pattern is Travis's chapters. He emphasizes basic underlying anxiety as a major component in the problem of stuttering, although he does not address either reducing that anxiety or the anxiety related to anticipating stuttering. Instead, Travis discusses stuttering as the result of a conflict between the desire to express strong unacceptable feelings and the fear of the consequences of their expression. Although the models provided by psychotherapy and behavioral psychology appear to be both relevant and useful, they do not seem to account for the issue of symptom versus behavior in the area of stuttering. We have much to do yet in the formulation of theory, the study of relapse, and in the distinction and relationship between the two types of anxiety.

When clients attempt to explain their stuttering they often find it more acceptable to characterize it as a habit than as a neurotic symptom. The connotative loading of the term "habit" includes emotional neutrality, triviality, and automaticity of the behavior, a safe and innocent way of describing the stutterer's role. One distinction between types of habit that the layperson often blurs is their adaptiveness. No one denies the adaptiveness of such habits as the sequence of putting on clothes or brushing teeth. Neither is there much question about the maladaptiveness of nailbiting or overeating. However, it is very difficult to identify a neurotic habit that is exclusively maladaptive, i.e. with no positive consequence for the individual. Let us reexamine the "habit" of stuttering. The act of stuttering does not save time or energy, and therefore cannot be classed in the category of purely adaptive habits. Stutterers are quite willing to acknowledge the maladaptive aspects of their problem. In fact, that is all they tend to see. It holds them back at school, limits their employment opportunities, restricts their social interactions, and imposes apprehension, embarrassment, and other negative feelings. We, as speech pathologists, on the other hand, recognize in addition the less obvious secondary gains that tend to maintain the stuttering behavior; the relief from speaking responsibility, the manipulation of a social situation, the sympathetic, protective reactions of the listener, and perhaps the opportunity to express hostility in a safe and indirect manner. However, when the speech pathologist confronts the stutterer with the suggestion of benefits accruing from the problem, there is often strong active resistance and occasionally even emotional breakdown. These reactions range from denial to anger to tears, indicating that the idea of secondary gain is both significant and threatening to them. What is it that is so unacceptable? Although there may be many explanations, the one that seems most plausible is related to the universal feeling of helplessness that stutterers report. Any suggestion that attacks that concept threatens to deprive stutterers of their innocence, their sense of being handicapped, and instead, places them in the role of having some responsibility for their behaviors. As such they become manipulators, and hardly worthy of the sympathy, nurturing, and love that a truly handicapped individual inspires. If, in fact, stutterers are accountable for their disfluency, then would they not also experience guilt?

Whether a habit is seen as adaptive or maladaptive may vary with the perspective of the individual, stutterer or nonstutterer. The same behavior can be viewed as adaptive by one person and maladaptive by another. For example, word substitution is seen as adaptive by the stutterer because he avoids stuttering, and maladaptive by the speech pathologist because the stutterer fails to deal with the problem directly. On the other hand, when a stutterer struggles overtly in the act of speaking he recognizes the inefficiency of the effort being put forth, as well as the embarrassment experienced, but society may see as adaptive the stutterer's persistence in the valiant struggle to communicate against an apparently significant handicap. Unwittingly, society may be maintaining a problem by becoming a part of the adaptive network.

The concept of stuttering as an adaptive or maladaptive habit is not treated in the chapters that follow, and is not part of any major current theory of the maintenance of stuttering. In the 1930s and 1940s both Dunlap (1932), emphasizing negative practice, and Hull (1943) formulating a measure of habit strength, identified intervening variables to relate to the overt behavior. Although many stutterers continue to view their problem as a habit, those current theories of stuttering that deal with the internal state of the stutterer (psychodynamic, genetic, and cognitive) do not. Behavior theory, which probably accounts for most of the clinical service provided today, does not deal with the internal states of the stutterer and does not account for stuttering as a habit. Interestingly, if it did, it would necessarily invoke Hull's concepts of deprivation and drive reduction, of habit incentive and habit strength. Just as the intervening variables critical to the concept appear to have lost favor, so the concept of an underlying disorder of which stuttering is a symptom seems to be yielding to a view of stuttering as primarily an independently manipulable behavior.

NORMAL DISFLUENCY

One issue that all theory of human disorders must address is whether the behavior in question differs from normal behavior in kind and in degree. With regard to stuttering, this issue becomes especially significant because there are two relevant behaviors that appear in the repertoires of both stutterers and of nonstutterers: developmental disfluency, and those pauses, interjections and fragmentations that are associated with the processes of composing and editing our utterances. (Shames & Sherrick, 1963; Goldman-Eisler, 1968) Another issue all theories of stuttering should account for is the spontaneous fluency of young children before the appearance of developmental disfluency, and the spontaneous fluency of all stutterers at some time or other as a part of their daily experience. In other words, a comprehensive theory of stuttering must account for both the disfluency of normal speakers and the fluency of stutterers.

Developmental Disfluency

Developmental disfluency refers to a phase of normal speech and language development characterized primarily by numerous regular and effortless repetitions of initial syllables and words of which the child seems to be unaware. These disfluencies never appear with the onset of speech. Rather we have observed, and parents report, that children acquire their first words and even their first short phrases fluently. When significant disfluency is first described, it is almost universally in the context of longer phrases and sentences. Whether developmental disfluency is a universal phenomenon is open to question. Certainly it is a frequent phenomenon according to parental reports. But few studies have involved detailed observations of large numbers of children during the significant age range of two to four years (Colburn & Mysak, 1982; Yairi, 1983). On one hand there are recognized developmental milestones associated with this age that suggest a relationship with the appearance of disfluency; on the other there is a host of individual explanations pertinent to events in a particular household. A universal explanation might relate developmental disfluency to the child's attempts to master new and increasingly complex linguistic skills, in particular grammar and syntax (Colburn & Mysak, 1982). Another universal explanation might be a relationship between psychosexual development and speech wherein disfluency is interpreted as an oral fixation or retentive behavior (Glauber, 1958). The background against which we are examining those disfluent behaviors we have labeled developmental is, of course, one of essentially fluent speech. Young children have been consistently fluent before the onset of noted disfluencies, and they continue to be fluent much of the time, often predictably and consistently (singing, speaking in unison, in monologue and talking to infants or animals) even after the diagnosis of stuttering.

Determining the dimensions of fluency is much more difficult than doing the same for disfluency. Disfluency has been described with well-defined benchmarks such as part- and whole-word repetitions, pauses, interjections, and prolongations (Johnson, Darley, & Spriestersbach, 1963). These are the behaviors; disfluency is always a judgment made about behaviors. Fluency, on the other hand, seems to be a judgment made in the absence of these behaviors and, therefore, suffers from a lack of definition about the size of the fluent unit. Where disfluency is a specified event, fluency is a nonspecified chain of events that may include phonemes, words, phrases, and prosodic contours. Another way of looking at the problem of the dimensions of fluency is from the perspective of figure and ground. Disfluency is a figure viewed against the background of fluency; fluency seems to be just the background, and therefore a qualitative concept, always more than the sum of its parts. Thus we are convinced that we cannot talk about fluency as a response in the same manner that we talk about disfluency as a response.

How does stuttering theory deal with this issue of determining the dimensions of fluency and disfluency? Generally, stuttering theory has ignored explanations of fluency. Instead it has attempted to explain the onset and maintenance of disfluency, with the clinical consequence of reducing and modifying stuttering rather than strengthening fluency. Stutterers report that their efforts are directed toward trying not to stutter, rather than trying to be fluent. Van Riper supports this philosophy in his caution to clients that they not seek fluency, because to do so will result in further anxiety and tension, which result in failure (1954). From another point of view Van Riper's caution is justified in that fluency is not a well-defined behavior and that the stutterer would otherwise end up seeking an elusive, qualitative judgment from both the listener and self. Because of his history of tracking stuttering, the stutterer may be poorly disposed to make a judgment about his own fluency. Johnson et al. (1963) did categorize specific forms of disfluency, but they also emphasized the global perception of a listener that something is wrong with the speaker. Quite independently of the disfluency or fluency of the child, according to Johnson, the listener's perception reflects his or her semantic evaluational system which results in the label "stutterer." His theory stated that some parents disregard the pervasive background of fluency, and choose instead to focus upon the more circumscribed event of disfluency. Darley (1955) described these parents as perfectionistic and demanding, and who may have been sensitized by a family history of stuttering.

For Johnson, developmental disfluency was a universal that could lead into stuttering, given a conducive environment. However, he did not identify any intermediate stages. What Johnson called developmental disfluency, Froeschels (1921) described as incipient stuttering and Bluemel (1932) identified as primary stuttering. It is likely that all three were referring to the same behavior. The proliferation of terminology resulted in confusion among speech pathologists, as illustrated by Glasner and Vermilyea (1953). This confusion extended beyond the labels ascribed to disfluent behaviors to the criteria on which the labels were based and to the selection of clinical strategies. Van Riper (1954) attempted to resolve the overly simplistic dichotomy of primary and secondary stuttering by introducing the concept of transitional stuttering to describe the changes in behavior, feelings, and level of awareness that the child undergoes as he becomes a confirmed stutterer. The more closely people looked, the more behavioral detail they described, resulting in Bloodstein's (1960) outline of four developmental phases of stuttering. In 1971 Van Riper identified four alternate tracks on which stuttering developed differently for different individuals. In one way the increased descriptive detail was beneficial in that both differences and commonalities among stutterers could be identified. On the other hand, the focus on stuttering, in particular on its early identification, seems to have eroded the role of developmental disfluency and its environmental context as postulated by Johnson (1942). Our professional emphasis during the last decade seems to be one of treatment rather than prevention. In the process of detailing disfluent behavior with increasing elaboration we have failed to describe and to account for fluency.

Johnson's message when he used the term "developmental disfluency" was that there is nothing wrong with your child. Wischner (1950) stated that stuttering is the stutterer's attempt to avoid the parental reactions that follow spontaneous disfluency of concern, disapproval, and admonition. In other words, he saw stuttering as an active attempt to avoid developmental disfluency and its social consequences. Bloodstein (1958) elaborated on both Johnson's and Wischner's views of the child's reactions to his developmental disfluency. Bloodstein's concept of "anticipatory struggle" further describes how developmental disfluency can be perceived negatively by the child and can lead to attempts to avoid or force through the anticipated disfluency. That forcing constitutes both the struggle and the stuttering. For all of those theorists who invoke the concept of developmental disfluency as a factor in the onset of stuttering, the developmental aspect suggests a normal and universal behavior.

On the other hand, when we think about the speech of a preschool child as incipient stuttering or primary stuttering, and talk to the parents about it in the same way, we are communicating a very different message. That message is that a problem exists, and that there is the prospect of its becoming worse. Additionally, there is a message for the clinician and the theorist that raises again the question of whether we are dealing with a single population of normally disfluent children or two populations, one of which is highly predisposed to become stutterers.

Conditioning theory has not focused on the origins of stuttering for the most part. Brutten and Shoemaker (1967) constitute an exception to this observation by virtue of their identification of the breakdown of fluency in young children as a consequence of autonomic reactions to environmental stress. This breakdown is viewed as the initial stage of stuttering. Their theory did not account for nor recognize the concept of developmental fluency as a precursor to stuttering. Shames and Sherrick (1963), who did focus on the origins of disfluency as well as stuttering, applied the principles of operant conditioning to the theory of Johnson based on his view of the role of developmental disfluency and the environment in the onset of stuttering. Like Brutten and Shoemaker, they discussed the dynamics of conditioning but depended on the observations of their predecessors with regard to the specific units of behavior that were being considered. In the clinic, however, the operant-based practitioners have focused on fluency as a goal, if not as behavior. They have attempted to increase fluency by reinforcing progressively longer utterances and intervals of time during which a speaker is fluent (Rickard & Mundy, 1965; Shaw & Shrum, 1972).

Applying an exclusively quantitative criterion such as number of words or total speaking time subordinates a significant qualitative criterion such as phrase or sentence integrity, which has more linguistic validity. Brown (1945) and Bloodstein (1974) did take into account linguistic criteria in both developmental disfluency and stuttering, although their loci tended to focus on single words or parts of words rather than on the longer linguistic units of phrases or sentences. There may be important information about both fluency and disfluency that is integral to these longer linguistic units and obscured by a simple count of smaller units such as words or time intervals. For example, if for a particular speaker all disfluencies occur on the first word of a phrase or sentence, any quantification of events after the first word and before the period at the end of the sentence would not be an accurate representation of the individual's fluency. In the attempt to seek the most reliable datum we must beware of the implications for the validity of the variables being studied. The selection of these variables is always arbitrary to some point. We should recognize that the ancestry of operant conditioning can be found in the experimental laboratory with its associated priorities on tight control, precise measurement, and variables that can be managed in those circumstances. Ease of measurement and operational procedures should not blind us to the significance of variables that are not as easily measured and managed but which may be as valid or more so. Such issues as overt versus covert events, qualification and quantification, the operation of discriminative and situational stimuli, and the experimental and clinical control of multiple versus isolated variables point up the differences between field observation and laboratory studies. Both are important, and both contribute to our discipline, but they yield different information. It is up to us to determine how that information can be applied in both research and clinical management.

Normal Disfluency

The main difference between normal disfluency and developmental disfluency, which we also see as a normal phenomenon, seems to be the relative reaction of listeners. Developmental disfluency attracts attention to itself while normal disfluency does not. More specifically, it appears that the feature of developmental disfluency that makes it outstanding is the number of repetitions per word, often 6 or more. An additional factor that makes developmental disfluency more noticeable is the greater number of words on which disfluencies occur. Where developmental disfluency usually occurs within a circumscribed time (a matter of weeks to a few months at the most, sometime during the preschool years) normal disfluency continues throughout life. Observations of disfluency in both children and adults have yielded a range of 1% to 3%, which most researchers agree on as normal. The figure is probably higher for children for whom Johnson (1959) calculated a percentage of disfluency of slightly over seven. He further categorized forms of disfluency, eight types in all, which have been useful in illustrating the great variety of disfluencies among and within speakers.

One possible explanation of the differences in fluency from speaker to speaker is that some of us are more skillful verbally than others. Specifically, those speakers with greater mastery of the language can be expected to be the most fluent. Since complete mastery of one's language is never fully attained, however, some degree of disfluency is likely to be found in all normal speakers. For these reasons we can expect more disfluency among children, who are neophytes in learning the system. However, as we become more mature and sophisticated linguistically, disfluencies may become more subtle, taking the form, for example, of interjections like "well" and "you know" rather than the more elemental word repetitions of childhood. Another explanation of the presence of disfluency at all stages of language development is the need for redundancy in linguistic processing. Repeating elements of language, or introducing noncommunicative elements or paraphrasing elements already spoken serve to reduce the amount of linguistic information processed per unit of time, thereby easing the task of speaker and listener alike. The form that some of these disfluencies take, especially interjections, and the rate at which we speak, which also affects the task of linguistic processing, are largely culturally determined. Expressions like "I mean," "like," "you know what I mean," and "man" are all ways of slowing the rate of linguistic processing in a subtle manner, of which both speaker and listener are usually unaware. Some of these terms may be slang, and all of them are faddish and ephemeral, and often come and go as a subcultural phenomenon. In addition to linguistic processing there is an editorial function of disfluency. Unlike written language, our speech tends to be fragmented, characterized largely by repetitions, incomplete sentences, and revisions. The fragmenting seems to be part of a composing process that requires ongoing review, a feedback operation that involves repeating the initial part of an utterance before completing it. If, in the process of review, the speaker decides to revise or change the sentence already begun, we are left with an incomplete fragment and a substitute sentence. This operation can happen more than once within a single sentence for some speakers, sometimes punctuated with interjections of the kind just discussed. The process of linguistic encoding is facilitated by rate reduction and review, and from the point of view of the listener, the process of linguistic decoding may be similarly facilitated.

Every stutterer knows that he or she is one. How do we as listeners distinguish between a stutterer and disfluent normal speaker? We do not have direct access to the self-image, the anxiety or the expectations that a stutterer experiences. All we can react to is the overt form and frequency of a speaker's disfluency. The more subtle forms of normal disfluency, like sentence fragments, interjections, or word and phrase repetitions, are not likely to attract a listener's attention unless their frequency is unusually high. However, if the form of disfluency is unusual, like sound repetitions or prolongations, or if their intensity or duration attract attention, we are likely to identify the speaker as a stutterer. Johnson's eight categories of disfluency (1963) include interjections, sound and syllable repetitions, word repetitions, phrase repetitions, revisions, incomplete phrases, broken words, and prolonged sounds. Of these, Johnson found that four categories distinguished normal children from stutterers statistically. The critical forms of disfluency were sound or syllable, word and phrase repetitions, and prolongations. The overall proportions of disfluency were significantly different between the two groups, almost 18% for the stutterers and just over 7% for the normal children. Therefore, it is not possible to determine whether the qualitative difference in form or the quantitative difference in frequency is the more striking feature of stutterers' disfluency. The interesting and useful question we would like to be able to answer is, "Can we predict stuttering later in life from the disfluency of children?" Also, keeping in mind Johnson's diagnosogenic argument, to which aspect of children's disfluency do parents react: form, frequency, or both? With respect to form, we have already seen that fragmenting words by either repetition or prolongation of sounds or syllables is most indicative of stuttering and most striking to parents. With respect to frequency, children are clearly more disfluent than adults and stutterers more disfluent than normal speakers. While Johnson's nonstuttering children were disfluent a little more than 7% of the time, the convention we usually apply to normal adult disfluency is a limit of 3%. Since all of us are disfluent some of the time, the more obvious criterion of 0% disfluency for normal speech is unreasonable. Researchers and clinicians, who find it difficult to determine whether a specific instance of disfluency involves stuttering, find it convenient to use a range of 1–3% disfluency as an acceptable goal of therapy in part because this frequency lies within the realm of expected normal disfluency. A simple quantitative criterion like percentage of disfluency has the added advantage of avoiding qualitative judgments which seem to be more difficult to make.

The Two-Population Theory of Stuttering

Earlier in this chapter we briefly discussed, under the heading of Prevention, the question of whether disfluent children can be divided into two populations, one of which develops into stutterers and the other of which is likely to outgrow their disfluency without intervention. The significance of this question goes beyond the issue of prevention. It has implications for theories about the origin of stuttering, for clinical management decisions, for the concept of predisposition, and for how you would go about distinguishing between the two populations, if indeed there are two.

The issue of two populations is a theory in its own right, although it is predicated on the earlier concept of developmental disfluency. What Johnson saw as a developmental universal, something manifest by all children, although to different degrees, recent researchers (e.g., Adams, 1980) argue that the differences among disfluent preschool children are differences in kind, not merely in degree. In other words, some of these youngsters are incipient stutterers who, without intervention, will not outgrow their disfluency. This theory is not the only one that involves the notion of two populations, however. Any genetic or physical theory of the origin of stuttering implies two populations: stutterers and nonstutterers. Most of the research in the 1930s and 1940s was designed to differentiate stutterers from nonstutterers on the basis of physiological, psychological, and anatomical factors. What is different about the two-population theory is that it focuses on disfluent children during a particular period in their development. Johnson said that children who become stutterers are just like other children in all respects. What is different for them is the way their parents react to their disfluency. Two-population theorists, however, imply that Johnson failed to distinguish differences among these youngsters. Johnson clearly believed that there was only one population of disfluent children. On the other hand, those of us who employ concepts such as incipient stuttering or primary stuttering as an interpretation of childhood disfluency are invoking a two-population theory. The research in which we engage to differentiate these two populations on the basis of attributes of their disfluency should eventually validate or invalidate the theory. As with any other theory, however, validation or invalidation will depend upon how it accounts for the variability of clinical success that ranges from failure to total reversibility in confirmed older stutterers.

From the point of view of the practitioner, whether you have resolved the question of one population or two, selecting a management strategy often commits you to a resolution. This commitment may be a conscious one, as when counseling the parents of a disfluent youngster, or unconscious, for example, in selecting children to work with. With limited clinical resources it sometimes becomes necessary to provide therapy for those with more urgent needs, postponing or withholding treatment from those who may outgrow their problem without intervention. Having decided to offer therapy for a disfluent child, the next issue is whether to work directly with the child, to counsel the parents, or both. Exclusive parent counseling has been the strategy of choice for the youngest disfluent children, and it has been our most successful strategy out of all therapy provided for disfluency. Granting responsibility for managing their children to the parents we counsel emphasizes the importance of environment rather than questioning the normality of the child. The overwhelming success of this strategy provides clinical data to support the one-population theory of stuttering. Conversely, deciding to work directly with the disfluent child can mean either of two things: the child may be older and well on the way to becoming a stutterer by the time he is evaluated professionally, or something in the form or frequency of the child's disfluency suggests that this is not merely a developmentally disfluent child, but an incipient stutterer. Even if the parents are counseled simultaneously, the theoretical implication is that the child comes from a separate population that predisposes stuttering. Predisposition to stutter, rather than environmental factors, becomes the central issue of management.

Johnson worked hard to prevent the child's awareness of having a speech problem and specifically to prevent the child from labeling it. Johnson, and others following him, felt that the principal ingredient in the success of exclusive parent counseling for early disfluency was preventing awareness on the part of the child. However, other compatible explanations for the success of early indirect intervention include the resilience and flexibility of children in their formative preschool years. Even those theorists who disagree with Johnson's focus on awareness, and who instead counsel parents to confront their children about their speech assume the basic normalcy of the child and therefore subscribe to a single population theory of stuttering.

Unfortunately, one of the facts of life in therapy for confirmed stutterers is the high frequency of relapse. While there may be many reasons for relapse, Boberg (1979) relates it to a heavy genetic loading. Clinicians who subscribe to the likelihood of relapse prepare their clients for it, teach them to expect it, and teach them how to manage it when relapse occurs. Emphasis on relapse, or on the inevitability of stuttering, clearly supports a two-population theory.

Even if the two-population theory of stuttering proves to be valid, the presence of a genetic or environmental endowment does not ensure that a child will become a stutterer. We must still resort to the concept of predisposition, which means that some environmental input is necessary for the problem to materialize. The catch, of course, is that if environmental input is the critical etiological determinant of stuttering, then predisposition may function merely as a theoretical explanation for factors that have not been clearly demonstrated. Other arguments for the significance of environmental input include the observation that stuttering appears long after birth and after the child has begun to speak. Whether or not a child is predisposed to stutter, the behavior itself seems to be acquired.

STUTTERING AS LEARNED BEHAVIOR

Learning theory as applied to the problem of stuttering will be discussed from three different points of view in the chapters that follow. Brutten's two-factor theory of stuttering addresses its origins, Sheehan's approach-avoidance conflict theory addresses the question of the moment of stuttering, Shames's operant conditioning perspective addresses the process of how normal disfluencies are shaped into stuttering behavior.

Learning theory carries with it a specific system for observing, manipulating, and describing behavior. While the general assumptions about learning theory include dealing only with manifest events, some of the theory employs mediating constructs that are not directly observable. These constructs are necessarily inferred, the primary example of which in the field of stuttering is anxiety. The chapters by Brutten and Sheehan rely heavily on that construct, although in very different ways. Where Sheehan views reducing anxiety as strengthening stuttering behavior, Brutten sees the increase of anxiety associated with the act of speaking as strengthening stuttering behavior. In both cases the authors are invoking an inferred construct to explain overt behavior. The operant perspective, represented by Shames, addresses more the overt aspects of stuttering.

When we think about the acquisition of any behavior we should try to understand its origin, its development, its stabilization, and its strengthening. With respect to the origin of stuttering, we can only speculate about how stuttering was acquired by any one child. For ethical reasons, we cannot verify experimentally the conditioning process of acquiring stuttering. We may not subsequently be able to undo the damage wrought. Therefore, although the history of conditioning comes from the learning laboratory, it cannot be expected to contribute experimental data to support its theoretical speculations about origin. Experimental verification requires introducing and withdrawing specific events to determine their effect on the behavior in question. However, when we study normal adult subjects, beyond the age where stuttering is likely to develop, we can address the issues of shaping, stabilization, and strengthening in a laboratory context. A great deal of useful information has come from such studies. Adult stutterers and nonstutterers alike have been subjects in these temporary research projects with no long-term negative impact. Stuttering, like any other form of behavior, can be observed to change over time. These changes include, overtly, the form and frequency of disfluency and associated behaviors, and, covertly, the feelings and attitudes related to stuttering. The adult who stutters is not like the child who stutters. The differences between them are the result of shaping processes. Shaping starts with a response evident in the repertoire of an individual, and proceeds with the modification of that response by differential reinforcement. The term *differential* is used because in the process of shaping we are concerned with changing a response from some primitive form to a more desirable one. We differentiate some aspects of the response from others by selective reinforcement and extinction. Comparing the primitive form of the response to the target or desired response we can then plan to shape one from the other by successive approximation to the target. While it may be tempting to explain developmental phenomena such as the acquisition of fluency or of walking as the result of shaping procedures, it is difficult in these examples to isolate the role of maturation. Therefore we reserve the term *shaping* for those procedures in which we can demonstrate unequivocally the effects of specific reinforcement and extinction operations. The acquisition of stuttering, however, is not a developmental phenomenon, nor is the clinical acquisition of fluency, both of which have been described as shaping operations. Having said this, we should point out that the clinical acquisition of fluency has been based on a solid experimental foundation. The acquisition of stuttering, on the other hand, has not been submitted to a formal experimental analysis, and therefore only by conjecture can it be described as a shaping procedure. The lack of experimental data about the shaping of stuttering in childhood fortunately has not been an obstacle to clinicians who modify the home environments through parent counseling. Without really knowing the details of the shaping process, clinicians have guided parents in identifying those practices that either exacerbate or ameliorate disfluency. The next step clinically is to help the parents to discontinue some practices, e.g., telling the child to "take a deep breath and start over," and to substitute competing responses such as responding to the content instead of the manner of the child's comment.

Stabilization refers not so much to a process as to a point where the frequency of a particular behavior has reached a relatively stable level. Strengthening, on the other hand, refers to increasing the frequency of occurrence of a particular behavior. Both stabilization (establishment) and strengthening rely upon the same four experimental procedures that serve as the basis for all learning theory: positive reinforcement, negative reinforcement, punishment, and extinction. When these experimental operations were first applied to the study of stuttering in the laboratory (Flanagan et al., 1958), many people were surprised at their success and their simplicity. It was demonstrated that the frequency of stuttering could be manipulated by providing consequences contingent upon its overt appearance, and independently of any attention to anxiety or other covert processes. To the additional surprise of many of us, some of these consequences were aversive, indicating that punishment is effective in reducing stuttering in the laboratory (Siegel, 1970). Both punishment and anxiety are basic to a number of theories of the origin of stuttering that are discussed in this section. If punishment is also effective in reducing stuttering outside of the laboratory, we have serious questions to ask those theorists who see punishment as a cornerstone in acquiring and maintaining stuttering. Similarly, if stuttering can be manipulated outside of the laboratory without reference to anxiety, then we must also ask serious questions about the critical role of not only anxiety, but also of other feelings and attitudes. Heretofore, these covert variables have been presumed to be controlled by the autonomic nervous system, best understood in the context of classical conditioning and not subject to cognitive, voluntary, or instrumental control. It was in this context that Brutten and Shoemaker stated that the aspect of stuttering based on classical conditioning is reduced by weakening the association among the variables of unconditioned stimulus, conditioned stimulus, and the conditioned response. Brutten and Shoemaker's theory and the resultant therapy incorporate both anxiety and punishment but stop short of the experimental operations that have been demonstrated to be effective in strengthening or reducing stuttering. Recent research in biofeedback has blurred the boundary between classical and operant (instrumental) conditioning by demonstrating operant control over autonomic responses such as heart rate and blood pressure (Blanchard & Epstein, 1978). Therefore, the role of classical conditioning in the acquisition of stuttering, independent of instrumental considerations, must be questioned. Additionally, when biofeedback tactics are applied to kinesthesis during the act of stuttering, muscle sensation is enhanced, resulting in manifest control over speaking (Guitar, 1975). Although the constructs coming out of classical conditioning help guide clinicians in identifying relevant covert variables such as anxiety, we continue to rely on operant procedures to manipulate these variables. Whatever the theory of stuttering may be relative to its origins or dynamics, when it is submitted to experimental verification it is studied by means of the four conditioning operations of positive reinforcement, negative reinforcement, punishment, and extinction.

The manipulation of stuttering in the laboratory is far different from manipulating that behavior outside of the laboratory. Transfer and maintenance are critical clinical issues as well as being theoretical and research goals. Clinicians have been aware for some time that it is one thing to alter a stutterer's fluency in the controlled environment of the clinic but quite another to transfer, generalize, and maintain that fluency under other, more natural controls and circumstances. As a result they have developed tactics for facilitating transfer of control, many of which are based upon principles of conditioning (Van Riper, 1954; Ryan & Van Kirk, 1974; Shames & Florance, 1980). However, such has not been the case for laboratory experimentation in which specific tactics are tested and variables studied that appear pertinent to processes of transfer and maintenance. The theory of the problem of stuttering does not lie merely in its origins or dynamics; a comprehensive theory must account for its elimination, either spontaneously or through therapeutic intervention.

Ideally, theory, research, and clinical management interact in ways that provide mutual stimulation and information. Clinical observation can provide inductive data for developing theory which, in turn, generates hypotheses that can be tested, which then provide further data for clinical management. As you read the following chapters on the theory of stuttering it will be useful to keep this ideal interaction in mind, as well as the many issues we have raised concerning etiology and maintenance, developmental disfluency, normal disfluency, stuttering as a symptom of something else, or stuttering as learned behavior. We should note that in the chapters that follow the authors are updating their thinking about theories of stuttering that were originally formulated from a few years to decades earlier. Those formulations were based on information that was available at that time as well as the thinking and experience of the theorist. The update reflects an attempt to recast and to reevaluate that theory in the context of current information and current thinking. The chapters cover the spectrum of theory but have not been written in relation to one another. Therefore it is a challenge to the reader to interrelate and to integrate this material in the different time perspectives involved.

In the coming chapters there is a broad range of theoretical perspectives, including stuttering as an inherited predisposition, as a manifestation of underlying emotional disturbance, and as a conditioned response. While it is tempting to seek a single explanation of the problem of stuttering, there may be more than one explanation, and there may be more than one kind of stuttering. We must take into account the observation that some approaches seem to be more effective with some stutterers than others and vice versa. This is not a bad state of affairs if we could match each stutterer with an ideal management program, but unfortunately we must also take into account the number of stutterers who seem not to benefit, beyond temporary relief, from any management program. The preponderance of relapse in such cases suggests either that there is an invariant underlying disorder, possibly genetic, or that the secondary gains of stuttering are so powerful that they overshadow the short term gains of fluency. Another factor to bear in mind is spontaneous recovery, which may be an indication of the opposite dynamic whereby the gains of fluency progressively overshadow the conditions that had been reinforcing stuttering. It is quite possible that we will never be able to determine whether stuttering has a single or multiple causes. In many ways this situation parallels that of other human disorders such as asthma, tics, schizophrenia, and depression, where many theories co-exist, and more theories continue to be spawned by the failure of any one theory to explain everything and by the differential success of various therapies (i.e., psychopharmacological, behavioral, psychoanalytic, counseling, and experiential/encounter groups). In terms of delivery of service it may not be important that we do not arrive at a single explanation for the problem of stuttering. However, if indeed there are different kinds of stuttering problems, which lend themselves to different theoretical explanations, we may be facing the greatest challenge of all, that of differential diagnosis of individuals. This approach leads to the selection of a theoretical explanation which, in turn, binds us to a particular therapy for a particular stutterer. The implication of this is that no one theory will explain everything. No one therapy will be a panacea for all stutterers. It may be judicious at this point, instead of seeking out one theoretical chapter that is most compatible with your own thinking, to remain open to the possibility that several of these points of view may be valid, albeit for different individuals or groups of stutterers.

REFERENCES

Adams, M. (1980). The young stutterer: Diagnosis, treatment and assessment of progress. In W. Perkins (Ed.), *Strategies in stuttering therapy.* New York: Thieme-Stratton, Inc.

Blanchard, E., & Epstein, L. (1978). *A biofeedback primer.* Reading, MA: Addison-Wesley.

Blanchard, E., & Hersen, M. (1976). Behavioral treatment of hysterical neurosis: Symptom, substitution and symptom return reconsidered. *Psychiatry, 39,* 118–129.

Bloodstein, O. (1958). Stuttering as an anticipatory struggle reaction. In J. Eisenson (Ed.), *Stuttering: A symposium* (pp. 3–69). New York: Harper.

Bloodstein, O. (1960). The development of stuttering: II Developmental Phases. *Journal of Speech and Hearing Disorders, 25,* 366–376.

Bloodstein, O. (1974). The rules of early stuttering. *Journal of Speech and Hearing Disorders, 39,* 379–394.

Bluemel, C. (1932). Primary and secondary stammering. *Quarterly Journal of Speech, 18,* 187–200.

Boberg, E., Howie, P., & Woods, L. (1979). Maintenance of fluency: A review. *Journal of Fluency Disorders, 4,* 93–116.

Brookshire, R., & Eveslage, R. (1969). Verbal punishment of disfluency following augmentation of disfluency by random delivery of aversive stimuli. *Journal of Speech and Hearing Research, 12,* 383–388.

Brown, S. (1945). The loci of stuttering in the speech sequence. *Journal of Speech and Hearing Disorders, 10,* 181–192.

Brutten, E., & Shoemaker, D. (1967). *The modification of stuttering.* Englewood Cliffs, NJ: Prentice-Hall.

Colburn, N., & Mysak, E. (1982). Developmental disfluency and emerging grammar. *Journal of Speech and Hearing Research, 25,* 414–427.

Darley, F. (1955). The relationship of parental attitudes and adjustments to the development of stuttering. In W. Johnson and R. Leutenegger (Eds.), *Stuttering in children and adults.* Minneapolis: University of Minnesota Press.

Dunlap, K. (1932). *Habits: Their making and unmaking.* New York: Liveright.

Egolf, D., Shames, G., Johnson, P., & Kasprisin-Burrelli, A. (1972). The use of parent-child interaction patterns in therapy for young stutterers. *Journal of Speech and Hearing Disorders, 51,* 222–232.

Flanagan, B., Goldiamond, I., & Azrin, N. (1958). Operant stuttering: The control of stuttering behavior through response-contingent consequences. *Journal of Experimental Analysis of Behavior, 1,* 173–177.

Froeschels, E. (1921). Beitrage Zur Symptomotologie des Stottereres. *Monatsschr. Ohrenheilk, 55,* 1109–1112.

Glasner, P., & Vermilyea, F. (1953). An investigation of the definition and use of the diagnosis "primary stutterer." *Journal of Speech and Hearing Disorders, 18,* 161–167.

Glauber, P. (1958). The psychoanalysis of stuttering. In J. Eisenson (Ed.), *Stuttering: A symposium,* pp. 71–119. New York: Harper.

Gregory, H., & Hill, D. (1980). Stuttering therapy for children. In W. Perkins (Ed.), *Strategies in stuttering therapy.* New York: Thieme-Stratton, Inc.

Goldman-Eisler, F. (1968). *Psycholinguistics: Experiments in spontaneous speech.* New York: Academic Press.

Guitar, B. (1975). Reduction of stuttering frequency using analog electromyographic feedback. *Journal of Speech and Hearing Research, 18,* 672–675.

Halvorson, J. (1971). The effects on stuttering frequency of pairing punishment (response cost) with reinforcement. *Journal of Speech and Hearing Research, 14,* 356–364.

Hull, C. (1943). *Principles of behavior, an introduction to behavior theory.* New York: Appleton-Century-Crofts.

Johnson, L. (1980). Facilitating parental involvement in therapy of the disfluent child. In W. Perkins (Ed.), *Strategies in stuttering therapy.* New York: Thieme-Stratton, Inc.

Johnson, W. (1949). "An Open Letter to the Mother of a Stuttering Child," YOU AND YOUR CHILD, April 1941. Reprinted in *Journal of Speech and Hearing Disorders, 14,* 3–8.

Johnson, W. (1942). A study of the onset and development of stuttering. *Journal of Speech Development, 7,* 251–257.

Johnson, W. (1961). Measurements of oral reading and speaking rate and disfluency of adult male and female stutterers and nonstutterers. *Journal of Speech and Hearing Disorders, Monog Supplement, 7,* 1–20.

Johnson, W., Darley, F., & Spriestersbach, D. C. (1963). *Diagnostic methods in speech pathology.* New York: Harper and Row.

Johnson, W., et al. (1959). *The onset of stuttering.* Minneapolis: University of Minnesota Press.

Kasprisin-Burrelli, A., Egolf, D., & Shames, G. H. (1972). A comparison of parental verbal behavior with stuttering and nonstuttering children. *Journal of Communication Disorders, 5,* 335–346.

Rickard, H., & Mundy, M. (1965). Direct manipulation of stuttering behavior: An experimental-clinical approach. In L. Ullman and L. Krasner (Eds.), *Case studies in behavior modification.* New York: Holt, Rinehart and Winston.

Ryan, B., & Van Kirk, B. (1974). The establishment, transfer and maintenance of fluent speech in 50 stutterers using delayed auditory feedback and operant procedures. *Journal of Speech and Hearing Disorders, 39,* 3–10.

Shames, G. H. (1981). Relapse in stuttering. In E. Boberg (Ed.), *Maintenance of fluency.* New York: Elsevier, North Holland, Inc.

Shames, G. H., & Florance, C. (1980). *Stutter-free speech: A goal for therapy.* Columbus, OH: Charles E. Merrill.

Shames, G. H., & Sherrick, C. E. (1963) A discussion of nonfluency and stuttering as operant behavior. *Journal of Speech and Hearing Disorders, 28,* 3–18.

Shaw, C., & Shrum, W. (1972). The effects of response-contingent reward on the connected speech of children who stutter. *Journal of Speech and Hearing Disorders, 37,* 75–88.

Sheehan, J., Cortese, P., & Hadley, R. (1962). Guilt, shame and tension in graphic projections of stuttering. *Journal of Speech and Hearing Disorders, 27,* 129–139.

Siegel, G. (1970). Punishment, stuttering and disfluency. *Journal of Speech and Hearing Research, 13,* 677–714.

Van Riper, C. (1954). *Speech correction—principles and methods.* New York: Prentice-Hall.

Van Riper, C. (1971). *The nature of stuttering.* Englewood Cliffs, NJ: Prentice-Hall.

Wischner, G. (1950). Stuttering behavior and learning: A preliminary theoretical formulation. *Journal of Speech and Hearing Disorders, 15,* 324–335.

Wischner, G. (1952). An experimental approach to expectancy and anxiety in stuttering behavior. *Journal of Speech and Hearing Disorders, 17,* 139–154.

Yairi, E. (1983). The onset of stuttering in two and three year old children. *Journal of Speech and Hearing Disorders, 48,* 171–177.

3

Physiological and Genetic Factors

Marcel Wingate

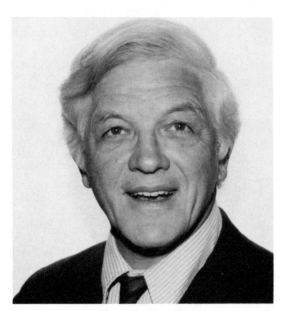

Marcel Wingate

Mike Wingate has become the conscience of our scholarly thinking about stuttering. He has over the years raised significant questions about the most basic beliefs and assumptions in this field. He has forced many of us to re-examine such initially unquestioned tenets as the learning basis of stuttering, Johnson's Diagnosogenic Theory, and even the basic definition of the disorder. His persistence in raising these questions has drawn battle lines between members of our profession, often as the result of his presenting data that does not support a popular point of view.

Wingate has offered an explanation of stuttering as a problem involving the stutterer's difficulty in performing phonetic transitions, in particular the voiced–voiceless alternation. He has also offered a definition of stuttering that has become widely accepted in the field. He states that the core features of stuttering which have universal applicability are: "(a) Disruption of the fluency of verbal expression, which is (b) characterized by involuntary, audible or silent, repetitions or prolongations in the utterance of short speech elements, namely: sounds, syllables, and words of one syllable. These disruptions (c) usually occur frequently or are marked in character and (d) are not readily controllable." (*Journal of Speech and Hearing Disorders,* 1964, p. 488).

In this chapter he presents a strong case for physiological dynamics and genetic etiology as the basis of stuttering. This particular perspective has become increasingly popular in recent years, in large part as the result of Wingate's scholarly activity. He has carved out a special role as an interpreter of the theoretical state of the art and, in addition to his courageous questioning of longstanding beliefs and his taking on the heavyweights in our field, he has managed to identify the significance of research data from diverse points of view. He is as at home with a learning curve or with a genealogical analysis as he is with a sound spectrograph. His ability to interrelate data coming from these differing theoretical perspectives provides us with an overview that we would like to see as the fruition of a history of scholarly activity.

Physiological and Genetic Factors

Marcel Wingate

This book is intended as a kind of near-term retrospective on stuttering, focusing on how the positions of various authors have changed over approximately the past 20 years. A focus of this kind is timely since there are increasing signs of a considerable shift in direction of inquiry into stuttering. In recent years, literature particularly in the major journals of the field of stuttering reflect a trend toward considering stuttering to reflect some physiological aberation.

It is important to recognize, however, that the investigation of stuttering as essentially a physiological anomaly is not a new trend. Rather it represents the resurfacing of a direction of inquiry which, for all practical considerations, has been essentially submerged for about 40 years. Throughout the 19th century stuttering was understood by most respected authorities as essentially a physiologically based disorder; this understanding carried over into the 20th century, as reflected in the early experimental research on stuttering: Halle (1900), Ten Cate (1902), Fletcher (1914), Robbins (1919), Anderson (1923), and Travis et al. (1925–1937).

However, this long-term interest in the physiology of stuttering, moving, in the first decades of this century, toward the refinement in understanding that can come only through careful research, was subverted within a few years by the rapid development of an alternative interest—the psychological. This shift in focus of interest can be portrayed graphically by tracing the course of experimentation in stuttering over a span of 20 years in the second quarter of this century. Figure 3-1 represents data compiled by Sortini (1955) who extracted from the relevant literature published between 1932 and 1951 the articles that reported experimental research on stuttering. Sortini separated the articles by content into the following seven categories: laterality, physiology, neurophysiology, genetics, psychology-behavior, personality, and miscellaneous. The curve for physiological studies drawn in Figure 3-1 represents a combined compilation of the first four categories; the curve for psychological studies is based on the fifth and

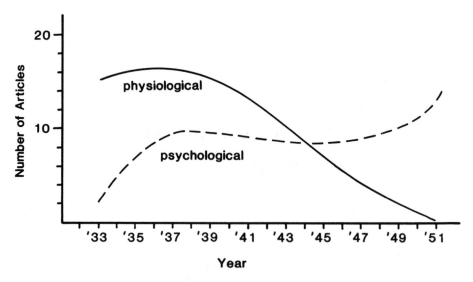

Figure 3-1. Course of interest in psychological versus physiological factors in stuttering between 1932 and 1951 as reflected in relevant publications. Based on data from A. J. Sortini, Twenty years of stuttering research, *Journal of the International Council of Exceptional Children, 21,* 1955, pp. 181–183. Reprinted with permission.

sixth categories combined. Clearly the shift is quite dramatic.[1] The intersection of the two curves indicates that 1944 was the critical year, but one should consider that the data represented do not take into account publication lag which, overall, probably amounted to one to two years. This point is not crucial but of interest relative to the dates identified later in this chapter.

It is important to realize that this clear shift in focus did not result because the physiological study of stuttering did not yield sufficiently compelling or impressive findings. Rather, the change reflected the steadily increasing influence of several circumstances that developed in the first quarter of the century that not only occasioned the preoccupation with a psychological study of stuttering but also bent many of the physiological findings to an interpretation in psychological terms.

The most important of these circumstances were: first, the advent of dynamic psychology, which followed rapidly from the writings of Sigmund Freud that appeared at the turn of the century; second, the birth and vigorous growth of behaviorism, proceeding from John B. Watson's "manifesto" delivered as his presidential address to the American Psychological Association in 1915; third, the development of speech pathology and audiology as a discipline, beginning in the mid-1920s at the University of Iowa; and fourth, the involvement of individuals who were (a) stutterers and who (b) also had training in the "new" psychology.

The psychological hypotheses of Sigmund Freud had a certain intrinsic appeal simply because they were startling and dramatic. Appearing as they did in

---

[1]A literal extrapolation of the two curves would yield a distorted representation of subsequent experimental publications in stuttering. However, although a certain minimal level of physiological investigation persists the bulk of work done in the next three decades was clearly psychological in orientation.

the Victorian era they were shocking and revolutionary, but they also offered revelation and relief. Relief was provided through the resulting cracks in the rigid, repressively moralistic codes of behavior inherent in the mentality and decorum of the Victorian era. Revelation derived from the (actually renewed)[2] affirmation of nonconscious mental activity and its potential influence in our lives, and, as well, in the emphasis on the (long-realized) importance of one's emotions for behavior and well-being. Freud's ideas had another, fundamental, appeal: by giving sex such a prominent role the whole theory focused on a topic in which almost everyone is perennially interested. Subsequent developments in dynamic psychology did not all retain the focus on sex but, in one way or another, invoked the concepts that human behavior and personality reflect dynamic forces within the psychology of the individual.

Freud's ideas were accepted more readily in this country than in Europe. His first direct exposure to the American public came from a series of lectures he was invited to give at Clark University in Massachusetts. For the American audience the whole idea of explaining mental health, personality, and behavior in terms of dynamic psychology had special appeal. In this open culture of no traditional social class levels and in which a dominant feature of creed is that all men are created equal, one could expect to find favor for a point of view that supported the belief that what a person becomes is mainly determined by environment. Moreover, the important role attributed to anxiety in Freud's conjectures also appealed to the American mind. As noted in a whimsical but quite accurate essay that appeared in the 1966 issue of *Time* magazine:

> As the Frenchman worries about his liver and the Englishman complains about his catarrh, the American is concerned with his mental health. No other nation has so high a quotient of mind probers of one kind or another; . . . ("Pop-Psych," 1966).

The intense and long-term appeal of dynamic psychology in the United States is reflected in the persistence with which American psychiatry has followed psychoanalytic doctrine. As late as 1964 a British psychiatrist (Sargent, 1964), writing on the differences in psychiatric treatment in the United States and England, noted that:

> The psychoanalytic dominance in the United States is a state of affairs which prevails in no other country in the world at the present time, except perhaps in Israel, where American psychiatric influences have been increasingly felt in recent years.

The concepts and emphases of dynamic psychology were soon incorporated into explanations of stuttering, contributing substantially to the trend toward explaining stuttering as a purely psychological problem. That there was not then, nor has there been since, any substantial evidence to support a psychodynamic conception of stuttering remained entirely beside the point.

The work and ideas of John B. Watson had an even greater influence on efforts to explain stuttering as a psychological problem. Although Watson's actual academic career in psychology was quite brief it is widely recognized that no

---

[2]Contrary to too-frequently stated claims, Freud did not "discover" the unconscious. Other writers, long before him, were aware of and discussed nonconscious mental activity.

American has had a greater influence, or a more lasting one, on American psychology—and on related disciplines. Again, the behaviorism movement[3] proffered concepts having a basic appeal to the American mind. The tenets of behaviorism, centering on stimulus and response as the basic unit of psychology, placed almost exclusive emphasis on the role of environmental factors as determinants of behavior. Behaviorism conveyed the heady promise of eventual ability to predict and control behavior; additionally, its S-R formulations carried the attractive implication of scientific objectivity and precision.

It is of particular significance that Watson's interests focused on the learning of emotional reactions in humans. He hypothesized that psychiatric disorders, such as phobias, hysterical symptoms, and tics, as well as more normal "defense mechanisms," could be explained in terms of conditioning (Watson, 1916a, b). He proposed that "the method of conditioned reflexes" could explain how "the three basic emotions" of fear, rage, and love are modified in the course of development and become associated with many events and objects (Watson & Morgan, 1917). His report (Watson & Rayner, 1920) on the fear conditioning of the infant Albert became widely known and extensively cited. Summaries and discussions of the study appeared in a wide variety of popular literature and textbooks in abnormal, developmental, and general psychology,[4] where it was presented as illustrating the relationship between fear and learning.

Unfortunately, the little Albert story is a classic example of the kind of distorting circumstantial influences that are under discussion here. Recently Harris (1979) has presented evidence that the little Albert story is more legend and folklore than the scientific demonstration it is assumed to have been. Harris carefully reviewed Watson's writings and subsequent references to, and use of, the Albert study, from which he presents convincing documentation that the little Albert story is a myth that generations of psychologists have told and retold to each other over the past 60 years. Harris notes,

> Unfortunately, most accounts of Watson and Rayner's research with Albert [including Watson's own accounts] feature as much fabrication and distortion as they do fact. From information about Albert himself to the basic experimental methods and results, no detail of the original study has escaped misrepresentation in the telling and retelling of this bit of social science folklore.

Moreover, the study had a number of serious methodological flaws. Although these flaws were duly noted by a few critical reviewers of the period, the standard treatment was to accept the story as told and to pass it on, often with attractive embellishments. And, "as behaviorism's influence grew, even relative skeptics seem to have been willing to devote more attention to the Albert study." Harris commented that,

> There has undoubtedly been some distortion due to the simple retelling of the Watson and Rayner study, but *a more dynamic influence on textbook accounts*

---

[3]Behaviorism is primarily a conception of what psychology should be; what constitutes the proper subject matter of psychology. It rejected all forms of mentalism and introspection in favor of observable events that could be dealt with in S-R terms.

[4]It also figured prominently in more esoteric sources, where it has served as the model, or font, of certain (even contradictory) theoretical efforts to explain human behavior. For example: Wolpe, 1958, 1973; Eysenck, 1960; Seligman, 1970.

seems to have been the authors' opinions of behaviorism as a valid theoretical viewpoint [italics added].

The same influence also came to bear heavily on the explanation of stuttering.

PHYSIOLOGICAL TO PSYCHOLOGICAL

The psychological influence on the interpretation of stuttering found expression as early as 1914 in a publication titled "An experimental study of stuttering" (Fletcher, 1914). Fletcher, a psychologist who also stuttered, reported a study in which the "main problems" were: "1. to describe stuttering in terms of its physiological manifestations; 2. to enumerate and describe the associated mental conditions; and 3. to ascertain, if possible, the part played by these mental states in its causation." To this end he studied the breathing, vocalization, articulation, and accessory movements of stutterers, certain other "psychological" functions such as volumetric, heart rate, and galvanic changes, and several measures of objective and subjective emotions. His analyses of the latter measures, in particular, were related in his discussion to information from other sources in the psychological literature that dealt with attitudes, imagery, and attention.

Fletcher's findings clearly revealed many physiological irregularities in his stutterer subjects, which he duly reported. However, consistent with the aim stated as the first sentence of the article, he interpreted his findings as reflecting psychological processes centering particularly in the emotions of "fear, anxiety, or dread, or shame or embarrassment." In consideration of the historical relevance of this publication as the first example of a powerfully developing trend, Fletcher's conclusions are reproduced here.

1. The motor manifestations of stuttering are found to consist of asynergies in the functioning of the three musculatures of speech—breathing, vocalization, and articulation.
2. Accompanying these asynergies there are also to be found tonic and clonic conditions of other muscles which are not involved in normal speech. These accessory movements tend to become stereotyped in each individual.
3. Stutterers are found to differ widely in type of asynergy, and particularly in accessory movements. It is, therefore, impossible to assert that any form of breathing, of articulation, or of vocalization constitutes the essence of stuttering.
4. Besides the motor manifestations of stuttering there are other accompanying conditions which consist in disturbances of pulse-rate, and of blood distribution, and in psycho-galvanic variations; these changes appear before, during, and after the speaking interval. The intensity of these manifestations is found to vary approximately with the severity of the stuttering.
5. The essential condition of the rise of stuttering seems to be a complex state of mind, which should be classified generically as feeling, in the wider sense of that term (138; 227). It is to be noted, however, that the quality rather than the intensity of these feeling states governs the rise of the defect. Certain forms of excitement, such as that incident to speaking in public, for example, caused stuttering to disappear entirely in over fifty per cent of our cases.
6. In general the feelings that tend toward inhibition or depression, such as fear, anxiety, or dread, or shame or embarrassment, are the ones that are most

likely to be the precursors of stuttering. Probably all these attendant mental states operate in a vicious circle in that they act as both cause and effect. The writer is of the opinion that in general the permanent condition of nervousness that is thought to be characteristic of stutterers should be regarded as effect rather than cause.

7. The states of feeling that have to do with the production of stuttering vary in degree from strong emotions to mere attitudes or moods. These latter are often so slight in degree that it is difficult for the subject to report their presence, and yet by the logical "method of difference" it seems necessary to consider their presence as a causal factor.

8. In addition to states of feeling, stuttering seems to be affected by the quality of mental imagery, by attention, and by association. All movements that, like those of speech, are incapable of clear and detailed imaginal representation in consciousness are, in the same way as speech, liable to functional disorders that are analogous to stuttering. When the stutterer's attention can be distracted from his speech his stuttering generally ceases. The affective and emotional experiences associated with the pronunciation of sounds, rather than the nature of the sounds themselves, determine the rise of stuttering.

9. Stuttering, therefore, seems to be essentially a mental phenomenon in the sense that it is due to and dependent on certain variations in mental state. Hence the study of stuttering becomes a specifically psychological problem; and it seems evident that a detailed analysis of all the various aspects of the phenomena of stuttering will furnish important contributions to general psychology.

It is certain that Fletcher had an influence on the course of thinking in the period marking the origins of the discipline of speech pathology.[5] He was a visiting professor of psychology at Iowa for the academic year 1923–24 and the summer session of 1924. During that time he directed the university's first graduate theses, addressed to stuttering;[6] according to Moeller (1975), p. 20) "it was with these two theses that the Iowa research program in stuttering began in earnest, to continue without interruption to the present." Moeller also reported that Travis said Fletcher probably inspired him "to pick up stuttering as a really important research problem." However, Travis's early work with stuttering led him to appreciate it, and to continue to investigate it, as an anomaly that is basically physiological.

The psychological influence was not yet being applied widely to the explanation of stuttering. Anderson (1923), reporting experimental work from the psychological laboratory of the University of Wisconsin, described his findings straightforwardly as differences, without attendant interpretation as psychologically based phenomena,[7] thus:

---

[5]The disciplines of speech pathology and audiology can be said to have originated at Iowa, during this period, and launched substantially from a base of research effort in stuttering. See Moeller, 1975.

[6]The master's theses of M. M. Font, "A comparison of free-associations of stutterers with those of normal speakers," and M. B. Hebenstreit, "Effect on motor control of negative instruction in the case of stutterers." Abstracts of these theses appear in Johnson and Leutenneger, 1955.

[7]It is pertinent to note that Anderson thanked Joseph Jastrow and Clark L. Hull for their "encouraging interest and valuable suggestions during the progress of this work." The reader should recognize Clark Hull as the author (in the 1930s and later) of a very influential general theory of behavior that elaborated the basic stimulus-response concepts of Watson's behaviorism. In the early 1920s, however, Hull's interests were in aptitude testing and hypnosis. It is also relevant to note that Hull's student and closest associate, Kenneth Spence, was professor of psychology at the University of Iowa from 1938 to 1965. One final note: Anderson did not stutter.

In sum, the results of several tests give evidence that stutterers differ from certain other people not merely in speech reactions but in other types of reactions which have no apparent connection with speech. Thus, there is objective evidence that stuttering and allied disorders are something more than defects of speech.

Travis (not a stutterer) is acknowledged as the first person specifically trained in the discipline of speech pathology and audiology.[8] In his years at Iowa he was always involved in experimental work in the laboratory, even developing some of his own equipment. His earliest publications (Travis, 1922, 1924a, 1924b) reported research on, essentially, variability of human auditory threshold as a function of psychological state in normal and psychologically disturbed individuals. In his first study of stuttering (Travis, 1925) he expected that the emotionally arousing conditions he employed would produce greater variability in voice features of stutterers than in the normal subjects; instead, he found evidence of muscular fixation in the stutterers. This study, and the next one (Travis, 1926) were a prelude to his *Studies in Stuttering* series, a sequence of five studies published from 1927 through 1929. The subtitles of this series clearly reflect their content: I. Disintegration of the breathing movements during stuttering; II. Photographic studies of the voice in stuttering; III. A study of certain reflexes during stuttering; IV. Studies of action currents in stutterers; and V. A study of simultaneous antitropic movements of the hands of stutterers. His interest in lateral dominance in stuttering, which followed from his association and work with Orton, was signalled in Orton's introduction in the *Studies in Stuttering* series:

> In the course of a study of certain cases of strephosymbolia in 1925, I noted that among my first series of fifteen cases there were three patients who stuttered or who had formerly done so and four others whose speech had a peculiar laboring hesitancy like that of one who has been broken of stuttering. There are a number of instances recorded in the literature of the onset of stuttering when a normally left-handed child is coerced into using the right hand for writing and of recovery when the use of the left hand is permitted.

Travis's interest in the role of lateral dominance in stuttering is undoubtedly the focus for which his years at Iowa are best remembered. However, over the eight years following *Studies in Stuttering* Travis's work led to over a dozen more publications on stuttering, ranging from the assessment of body type (Travis & Malamud, 1933) to the study of electrical potentials of the brain (Travis & Knott, 1937; Travis & Malamud, 1937). Most of this work had a physiological orientation and, overall, yielded encouraging results.

In 1938 Travis left Iowa, and this period of outstanding and significant contribution to the understanding of stuttering came to an end. The psychological eclipse had already started at Iowa and in a very few years Travis hastened the shadowing of his own bright work through the publication in 1940 of "The need for stuttering" (Travis, 1940). In this, and a subsequent statement (Travis, 1957), he implicitly repudiated his earlier achievement. The change represented a capitulation to the psychological influence that was still gaining momentum from

---

[8]Johnson (Johnson & Leutenegger, 1955, p. 7) wrote, "It is probably essentially true that he (Travis) was the first individual in the world to be trained by clearly conscious design at the doctoral level for the definite and specific objective of working experimentally and clinically with speech and hearing disorders."

its beginnings earlier in the century. He would explain later, to Moeller (1975, p. 75):

> I maintained my interest in cerebral dominance until I came to USC. At USC I had a big clinic and almost no laboratory so I did much more clinical work than at Iowa. And I had to get results. So I began to shift from this neurological thinking and approach to [a] psychological [one]. I picked out the modified psychoanalytic treatment as probably the best concept to work with[9] and teach with. We began to look at stuttering more as a psychological than a physiological thing.

So, Travis's shift in orientation was not occasioned by a lack of evidence from physiological investigation, or by contradictory findings from psychological studies; the change was essentially happenstance, a circumstantial event. It is of considerable interest that, in the same interview (Moeller, 1975, p. 75) Travis also said,

> We still find that the relationships between the two hemispheres of stutterers differ from the same relationships of nonstutterers. We have always found some evidence of disturbed cerebral dominance in stutterers. But I still don't know what to do about them.

Travis's contribution to the study of stuttering should not be remembered simply, or even predominantly, in regard to lateral dominance. His research included some of the earliest significant experimental investigation of malfunction in the speech production processes of stutterers, a topic to which research effort is finally returning.

As noted earlier in this chapter, the psychological eclipse of the physiological orientation to stuttering had already begun at Iowa shortly before Travis's departure. The development of this influence was due almost entirely to the writings of Wendell Johnson.

Johnson originally went to Iowa for help with his stuttering and to finish college. He stayed on to earn the advanced degrees (by 1931) and to eventually become a member of the speech pathology faculty. His early work in stuttering either yielded evidence that supported a physiological explanation of stuttering or presented no notable contradictions to it (for example: Johnson, 1932, 1933, 1934, 1935). In fact, as late as 1936, reporting a study of the relationship of psychological factors to stuttering severity (Steer & Johnson, 1936), the authors wrote,

> It is obvious to any student of the subject that stuttering is a matter of organic function and that it is specifically a matter of the function of muscles, nerves, and the brain. There is nothing in the results of this study which implies any contradiction of that statement. . . . [and] it is necessary to distinguish between the stability of the stutterer's speech mechanism which is due entirely to fundamental constitutional factors, and the instability of the stutterer's speech mechanism which is due to superimposed and transitory emotional and psychological factors.

However, sometime in the mid-1930s, Johnson became indelibly affected by the notions of general semantics. Also, he and Knott (also a stutterer) had begun to

---

[9]Not, in my view, a wholly satisfactory explanation. Several psycholanalysts, including Freud himself, have acknowledged that stuttering is not amenable to psychoanalysis.

use, as formulative data, their introspections of their own stuttering (see Moeller, 1975, p. 75ff).[10] Then, in 1937, they authored the first article in a series head-titled *Studies in the Psychology of Stuttering.* The series, directed by Johnson, consisted of 19 articles published between 1937 and 1944. The first article (Johnson & Knott, 1937) identified the phenomena of stuttering adaptation and the so-called "consistency effect," phenomena which were to be the object of a long line of subsequent research pursuing a psychological interpretation of stuttering. Johnson and Knott interpreted the data of the first study in stimulus-response terms, an interpretation that was not only repeated, but elaborated and extended, in many publications that appeared over the next 40 years.

It is imperative to recognize that the interpretation offered by Johnson and Knott was just that; in fact, it was bald conjecture. There was nothing in the data nor in the experimental procedure[11] that clearly suggested principles of learning. In addition, there were serious flaws in the collection and analysis of the data, flaws that also were repeated in the subsequent research (Wingate, in press). But, evidently no complaints were registered, no skepticism expressed, and the movement to explain stuttering as a psychological problem gained momentum.

Two publications, both literature reviews, which appeared in 1944, were probably the capstone of the movement that subverted and submerged physiological study of stuttering. The first article (Hill, 1944a) was addressed to biochemical investigation; the second (Hill, 1944b) dealt with physiological findings. Both reviews were quite thorough and thoughtful, and the author correctly pointed out certain limitations in some of the work bearing on biochemical and physiological study of stuttering. However, the thrust of his analysis was essentially analogic. Of the 49 references in the article on biochemical findings (Hill, 1944a) only 20 dealt directly with stuttering; and of the 126 references in the article on physiological investigation (Hill, 1944b) only 50 were addressed to stuttering. Hill extracted from those reports that did not deal with stuttering the indication that certain bodily processes are associated with physical exertion or emotional arousal. He then argued that the anomalous physiological findings in studies of stutterers could be understood as resulting from psychological influences. Thus:

> In all instances where differences between stutterers and normal speakers purportedly were obtained, the differences were compared with and shown to approximate closely changes in so-called normal persons during muscular activity and affective behavior. (Hill, 1944a)

Hill thus repeated, in reference to a much broader range of data, the kind of analysis and interpretation made by Fletcher 30 years before him. Hill, like Fletcher and Johnson, was a stutterer trained in psychology. Evidently, like Johnson at least, personal attitudes played a role in his orientation:

> The phenomena of stuttering can well be explained if principles of normal behavior are adhered to without attempting to make the stutterer a unique animal in the universe. (Hill, 1944a).

[10]The method of introspection was soundly repudiated by behaviorism, the concepts of which Johnson employed beginning at least with the 1937 article initiating the *Studies in the Psychology of Stuttering* series.
[11]The method employed in this study was borrowed from earlier work by Van Riper and Hull (1955) who, although obtaining similar results, had accounted for them quite differently.

HEREDITY COMPROMISED TOO

It has been known for some time that stuttering runs in families and that the incidence of familial occurrence is substantial. Makuen (1914) considered heredity to be "the most important factor in the etiology of stuttering"; he noted that approximately 40% of the 1000 cases he had studied had other stutterers in the family. Bryant (1917) reported that in his clinical experience with 20,000 cases of stuttering over half had relatives who stuttered.

The data from such clinically based reports were augmented in the 1930s by a number of studies addressed directly[12] to inquiry into the familial incidence of stuttering (Nelson, 1939a, 1939b; Wepman, 1935, 1939; West, Nelson, & Berry, 1939). These studies identified the incidence of stuttering among relatives of stutterers as compared to the family incidence of stuttering in comparable numbers of normal speakers. The findings from these studies indicated that, on the average, stuttering occurred about six times as often among relatives of stutterers than in the families of normal speakers. Overall, the evidence seemed to clearly indicate genetic transmission even though the pattern of such transmission was not clear and, in fact, did not appear to conform to Mendelian "laws" of inheritance.

Then, in 1940, a publication by Gray (1940) offered the explanation that the recurrence of stuttering along family lines is due to a kind of "social heredity."[13] The Gray study (done at the University of Iowa and directed by Wendell Johnson) focused on the pedigree of a stuttering family which, in terms of geographical locale of residence, could be described as containing two "branches"—the Iowa branch and the Kansas branch. The two branches also differed in incidence of stuttering, the Iowa branch having considerably more stutterers than the Kansas branch (Figure 3-2). As stated by Gray:

> The study was designed to answer questions regarding the distribution of stuttering within the family, the definite similarities or differences among the stutterers, former stutterers, and nonstutterers, and the nature of the evaluations or assumptions expressed by members of the family regarding stuttering.

However, the data base was quite uneven, since "A limited amount of information [was] obtained concerning the Kansas branch." Nonetheless we can accept that the identification of stutterers in the two branches of the family was accurate. The data regarding stuttering incidence were the essential base for the study and its conclusions, which were:

> It seems reasonable to doubt[14] that a sheer hereditarian [genetic] hypothesis would account readily for the difference in incidence of stuttering between the Iowa and Kansas branches of the family, . . .
>
> [and]
>
> The stuttering in this family might be regarded as semantogenic. . . . Briefly, this family might with some reason be regarded as "stuttering conscious," quick to diagnose as stuttering the hesitant, repetitious first speech attempts of children

---

[12]Additional supportive data was contributed by studies whose genetic interest in stuttering focused on other matters; for example, Bryngelson (1935), Bryngelson and Clark (1933), West (1937).

[13]The term "heredity" is used in similar fashion in other contexts, for example the "hereditary titles" of aristocracy.

[14]The reasonableness of this doubt was not made clear, and it was certainly not obvious to objective assessment.

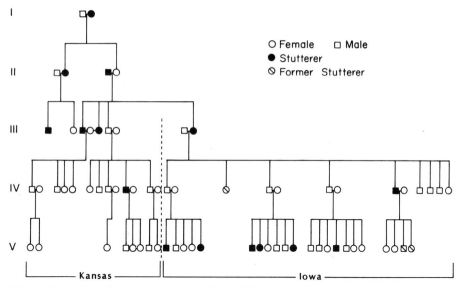

Figure 3-2. A pedigree of stuttering; the "X" family. From M. Gray, The X family: A clinical and laboratory study of a "stuttering" family. *Journal of Speech Disorders, 5,* 1940, 343–348. © 1940, the American Speech-Language-Hearing Association, Rockville, Maryland. Reprinted with permission.

learning to talk, and prone to develop in the child the familial anxieties and generally negative evaluations regarding hesitant or repetitive speech.

Data in support of the latter conclusion were neither adequate nor defensible. To the contrary, Gray mentioned later in the article that:

There were certain members of the family whose beginning speech was regarded as "non-fluent," and some of these were diagnosed as stutterers, while some were not.

In other ways too the material presented in the article fails to support, or actually contradicts, the interpretation proposed by Gray. First of all, it is by no means unique to find expression of a genetic characteristic over several generations of one "branch" (or more) of a family but not in another "branch" of the same family. Figure 3-3 shows a pedigree of Huntington's chorea, an inherited disorder of the nervous system marked by degeneration of the basal ganglia and cerebral cortex. Manifestations of the disorder are not evident until the affected individual is between 30 and 40 years old. A single dominant autosomal gene is responsible for this hereditary disorder. Note that individuals in generations II, III, and IV in the lines following from the unaffected siblings 3, 6, and 7 in generation II do not evidence the disorder. Also, generations III, IV, and V following from sibling 8 in generation II also do not evidence the disorder. Similar patterns of genetic transmission are to be found for many other conditions.[15] The pedigree presented by the "X" family is entirely consistent with a pattern of genetic transmission.

Moreover, there are even more specific contradictions to the social heredity interpretation. The anxiety-about-disfluency conjecture cannot credibly explain the recurrence of stuttering in the "X" family pedigree. First, how can an influence that is presumably so pervasive, yet simultaneously so vague, as a set of

[15]For example: precocious male maturity; Leber's disease (optic atrophy); white forelock.

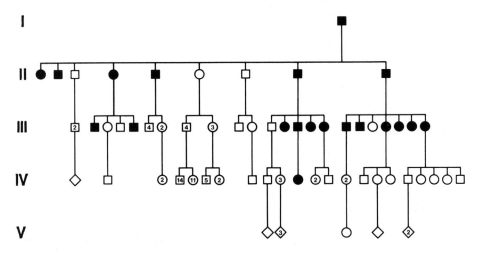

Figure 3-3. A pedigree of Huntington's chorea. From Fuller and Thompson (1960, p. 96). Squares indicate males; circles, females; diamonds, the sex was unknown to the recorder. Numbers in the symbols record the number of siblings not listed separately. Solid symbols indicate affected individuals. Spouses (unaffected) are not recorded. Reprinted by permission of John L. Fuller.

attitudes and anxieties about speech be so specific in their effect? Note that in the fourth generation of the Iowa branch only three of nine children (2, 4, and 5)[16] stuttered. The first and third children (both boys) did not stutter, nor did children 6 through 9 (three of the four being boys). If stuttering were induced in siblings 2, 4, and 5 through "generally negative evaluations" of the "hesitant, repetitious speech attempts of children learning to talk" then how did siblings 1, 3, 6, 7, 8, and 9 escape this influence? In particular, if such influence is expressed through parents' anxieties, why did it not affect a first child, whose developmental achievements are typically scrutinized more carefully than those of later children? Also, even if one were to claim that negative parental attitudes were somehow dormant or suppressed for the first child, one should expect that sibling 2, or at least siblings 4 and 5, should have sent the negative evaluations into vigorous action. Why, then, shouldn't siblings 6, 7, 8, and 9 also stutter? Similar questions can be asked about other sibling relationships among generations II through V, in both branches of the family; in no instance can the social heredity conjecture provide an explanation.

Another fact that cannot be explained by the social heredity conjecture is that the occurrence of stuttering skips generations. For example, the first and third children in generation IV of the Iowa branch did not stutter, but their mother and some of their children did. The skipping is also evidenced in one line of the Kansas branch where its appearance alternates over generations II through V. How can negative evaluations and anxieties have an effect in one generation, not be evident in the next generation, yet reappear in the third or subsequent generation? The assumptions, qualifications, and rationalizations needed to make the facts of familial incidence fit the social heredity conjecture would create a preposterous fabrication that would be rationally indefensible.

[16]We will consider child 2 as stuttering (even though she is identified by Gray as a recovered stutterer) since she stuttered as a child.

The occurrence of trait in only certain individuals in any particular generation and its appearance or absence in successive generations are entirely consistent with the facts of genetic transmission. The fundamental principle of genetics is that genes segregate during the biological processes leading to the creation of a new individual. Because of segregation any particular gene may or may not be passed on to progeny. Clearly, then, a child who does not receive a particular gene cannot transmit it to succeeding generations. The facts of stuttering occurrence in the "X" family are clearly accountable in terms of genetic transmission. In contrast, the social heredity explanation is not consistent with, and cannot accommodate, the facts of stuttering recurrence. Anyone knowledgeable in the field of genetics could be expected to dismiss the Gray paper on grounds that an absurd conclusion had been reached through total ignorance of, or indifference to, the basic facts of genetics, which were well known long before the time of the Gray article.

Once again, like the interpretation offered by Johnson and Knott for the phenomena of stuttering adaptation and stuttering recurrence, the psychological interpretation of familial incidence of stuttering evidently elicited no objection or expression of skepticism. In fact, certain writers (see Bloodstein, 1981, pp. 96–98; Taylor, 1976, p. 345) still accept the interpretation as credible. Evidently others also continue to believe that the social heredity account, articulated by Gray, has substance; for example, Kidd (1984a) remarked recently that "over the last twelve years I have continued to be confronted by this absurd paper" from persons who apparently considered it to have merit.

Comparable to psychologists' recounting of the legend of Little Albert, stuttering has had its own folklore that has been told and retold from one generation to another.

MODERN TIMES

The reappearance of interest in physiological factors in stuttering has been evident only in the past few years. In fact, except for isolated instances, as recently as 1970 there was ample reason to point out the persisting preoccupation with a psychological orientation to stuttering and to note that this orientation had encouraged redundant investigations that contributed little to understanding the disorder (Wingate, 1970b). Moreover, if one reviews the appropriate literature sources over the past decade one will still find a heavy overloading of the so-called "operant" focus on stuttering. Actually, the operant work reflects primarily a simple methodological matter; as far as contributing to understanding the nature of stuttering, this line of literature hardly does more than repeat, in barely altered vocabulary, the explanatory notions expressed repeatedly since the behaviorism movement developed its devoted following over 40 years ago.

In recent years, however, an interest in nonbehavioristic study of stuttering has gradually increased. Remarkably, and somehow quite appropriately, one significant dimension of this renewed interest in physiological investigation of stuttering has been the attention addressed to the matter of laterality (for example: Curry & Gregory, 1969; Andrews et al. 1972; Lussenhop et al. 1973; Zimmerman & Knott, 1974; Sussman & MacNeilage, 1975; Rosenfield & Goodglass, 1980).

Concepts of laterality and methods of investigating it have become more refined than they were earlier, and these refinements (though still crude relative to the complexity in organization of the central nervous system) have underlaid a more sophisticated study of laterality. Some findings of this recent research have been equivocal; however, the bulk of the work has yielded evidence that clearly indicates that stuttering involves some kind of anomalous function in the central nervous system.

Research of a related nature, designed to explore central nervous system functions not specifically pertinent to the matter of laterality, has yielded additional evidence of central nervous system anomalies in stuttering (for example: Sayles, 1971; Stromsta, 1972; Cooper & Allen, 1977; Hall & Jerger, 1978; Toscher & Rupp, 1978; Moore & Haynes, 1980; Decker et al. 1982).

After the publication of two articles that proposed an integral account of how the well-known ameliorative conditions affect stuttering (Wingate, 1969, 1970a), much investigation has been addressed to laryngeal function and voicing in stuttering (for example: Adams & Reis, 1971, 1974; Freeman & Ushijima, 1978; Cross et al. 1979; Reich et al. 1981; Watson & Alfonso, 1982; Cross & Luper, 1983). Again, the bulk of this research has yielded evidence of anomalous laryngeal and voicing function in stuttering. Other related areas of study (for example: Shapiro, 1980; Zimmerman, 1980) have revealed anomalies in other dimensions of speech-related function.

In sum, recent research in the several areas of investigation reviewed above concur in providing a substantial body of evidence that stuttering represents, in a variety of ways, the product of aberrations in physiological function.

Revival of significant attention to the heredity of stuttering has developed only recently, although one analysis of hereditary factors in stuttering (Garside & Kay, 1964) appeared in 1964 as a chapter in a monograph reporting the findings of several studies of stuttering (Andrews & Harris, 1964). The genetic analysis presented by Garside and Kay was, expectedly, more sophisticated and comprehensive than those of the earlier era of the 1930s. Again, the basic findings corroborated the previous evidence of an increased incidence of stuttering in the families of stutterers. The data were discussed as compatible with either of two modes of genetic transmission: polygenic inheritance, or inheritance by a common dominant gene with a multifactorial background. In both cases sufficient allowance was made for the possible secondary involvement of environmental factors (although full psychological and environmental explanations of stuttering transmission were considered "unsatisfactory for want of evidence.")

The contribution made by Garside and Kay to the investigation of genetic dimensions of stuttering evidently aroused little interest, possibly because it was immersed in a context having a clear behavioral orientation. The authors of the monograph revealed a preference to view stuttering as learned behavior, invoking such traditional learning theory notions as conditioned stimuli, anxiety, reinforcement, anticipation, and avoidance. In a representative summary statement (Andrews & Harris, 1964) the authors wrote:

> We have seen that from an aetiological point of view stuttering can be regarded as the product of certain adverse environmental factors acting upon a genetic matrix. From the pathogenetic point of view there is reason to believe that these causal

factors operate by distorting the pattern of learning speech. In the five studies reported in this monograph there is certain indirect evidence that stuttering is probably a complex learned habit. (p. 163)

Recent years have seen the most active expression yet of interest in the heredity of stuttering, represented almost exclusively in the work of Kenneth Kidd, a human geneticist whose research in other areas of behavior genetics led to an interest in the heredity of stuttering (Kidd, 1977, 1980, 1983, 1984b; Kidd et al. 1978; Kidd et al. 1980; Kidd et al. 1981; Gladstein et al. 1981; Seider et al. 1982, 1983; Cox & Kidd, 1983). As in the heredity studies of 40 years ago, Kidd's findings also confirm the clinical evidence that stuttering "runs in families." More important, however, is the fact that the methods of modern human genetics are being applied knowledgeably to the analysis of such findings. Kidd's analyses show that two different genetic models, the multifactorial-polygenic model or the single major locus model, provide a good fit to the data of stuttering occurrence. The fact that two alternative models can accommodate the data does not qualify or compromise the basic evidence of the genetic factor in stuttering. Although, at the present time, Kidd's analyses include the possibility that some environmental influences may contribute to the occurrence of stuttering, those who cling to a psychological interpretation of stuttering can find little comfort in this possibility. "Environmental" includes intrauterine conditions, natal circumstances, diseases, drugs, metabolic processes, accidents, et cetera; psychosocial contributions are likely to be minimal. Both of the models discussed by Kidd indicate that the genetic component in stuttering is much more important than a nongenetic component.

A BRIEF PERSONAL RETROSPECTIVE

My formal involvement with stuttering began in 1956 with a study that was originally intended to test whether the instrumental escape or the instrumental avoidance learning paradigm offered the better model of stuttering. The findings indicated that neither model conformed well to the realities of stuttering phenomena. This experience constituted my first, and quite impressive, confrontation with the fact that extant explanations of stuttering did not coincide very well with the realities they were presumed to explain. The experience was to lead to further realization of the very considerable lack of concordance between what was known about stuttering as compared to popular efforts to account for it (see Wingate, 1962a, 1962b, 1962c; 1966b, 1966c). Moreover, various "definitions" of stuttering could be seen to be little more than statements of presumed etiology that ignored, took for granted, or implicitly repudiated the speech features of stuttering—the very features that have always been the basic realities of stuttering (Wingate, 1964; 1965; 1976, Ch. 4). It seemed to me that inadequate attention was directed to stuttering as a speech event, and that the most defensible direction to move in the study of stuttering was to investigate it as a defect in oral language expression, which it most clearly seems to be (see Wingate, 1976, Ch. 9, for a specific analysis of the nature of this evident defect). These considerations, in relation to the findings from certain studies of language factors in stuttering (reviewed in Wingate, 1979a, 1979b) led to the hypothesis that stuttering reflects anomalies in functions underlying oral language expression, particularly the prosodic dimensions. Evidence supporting this hypothesis emerged in results obtained in a series of relevant studies (Wingate, 1966a; 1967a; 1967b; 1979a; 1981; 1984b). Other research has indicated the existence of anomalies in related areas of expressive language (Perozzi, 1970; Wingate, 1971; 1982; 1984a).

Although we can hope to eventually understand the nature of the stuttering act, the incoordinations which are its overt manifestations, it has seemed to me that such understanding will require the prior appreciation of more abstract (central) dimensions of the disorder based in the psychophysiology of this manifestly aberrant function. Our knowledge of such dimensions will be largely inferential and conceptual, but a coherent and internally consistent conceptualization should lend itself to verifiable demonstration in externally observable events.

REFERENCES

Adams, M., & Reis, R. (1971). The influence of the onset of phonation on the frequency of stuttering. *Journal of Speech and Hearing Research, 14,* 639–344.

Adams, M., & Reis R. (1974). Influence of the onset of phonation on the frequency of stuttering: A replication and reevaluation. *Journal of Speech and Hearing Research, 17,* 752–754.

Anderson, L. O. (1923). Stuttering and allied disorders: An experimental investigation of underlying factors. *Comparative Psychology Monographs, 1,* 1–78.

Andrews, G., & Harris, M. (1964). *The syndrome of stuttering.* London: Heinemann.

Andrews, G., Quinn, P. T., & Sorby, W. A. (1972). Stuttering: An investigation into cerebral dominance for speech. *Journal of Neurology, Neurosurgery and Psychiatry, 35,* 414–418.

Bloodstein, O. (1981). *A handbook on stuttering.* Chicago: The National Easter Seal Society.

Bryant, A. F. (1917). Influence of heredity in stammering. *Journal of Heredity, 8,* 46–47.

Bryngelson, B., & Clark, T. B. (1933). Left-handedness and stuttering. *Journal of Heredity, 24,* 387–390.

Bryngelson, B. (1935). Sidedness as an etiological factor in stuttering. *Journal of Genetic Psychology, 47,* 204–217.

Conture, E., McCall, J., & Brewer, D. (1977). Laryngeal behavior during stuttering. *Journal of Speech and Hearing Research, 20,* 661–668.

Cooper, M. H., & Allen, G. D. (1977). Timing control accuracy in normal speakers and stutterers. *Journal of Speech and Hearing Research, 20,* 818–830.

Cox, N. J., & Kidd, K. K. (1983). Can recovery from stuttering be considered a genetically milder subtype of stuttering? *Behavior Genetics, 13,* 129–139.

Cross, D. E., Shadden, B. B., & Luper, H. L. (1979). Effects of stimulus ear presentation on the voice reaction time of adult stutterers and nonstutterers. *Journal of Fluency Disorders, 4,* 45–58.

Cross, D. E., & Luper, H. L. (1983). Relation between finger reaction time and voice reaction time in stuttering and nonstuttering children and adults. *Journal of Speech and Hearing Research, 26,* 356–361.

Curry, F. K. W., & Gregory, H. H. (1969). The performance of stutterers on dichotic listening tasks thought to reflect cerebral dominance. *Journal of Speech and Hearing Research, 12,* 73–82.

Decker, T. N., Healey, E. C., & Howe, S. W. (1982). Brainstem auditory electrical response characteristics of stutterers and nonstutterers: A preliminary report. *Journal of Fluency Disorders, 7,* 385–401.

Eysenck, H. J. (1960). Learning theory and behavior therapy. In H. J. Eysenck (Ed.), *Behavior therapy and the neuroses: Readings in modern methods of treatment derived from learning theory.* Oxford, England: Pergamon Press.

Fletcher, J. M. (1914). An experimental study of stuttering. *American Journal of Psychology, 25,* 201–255.

Freeman, F., & Ushijima, T. (1975). The stuttering larynx: An EMG, fiberoptic study of laryngeal activity accompanying the moment of stuttering. *Haskins Laboratories Status Report on Speech Research,* SR-41. New Haven: Haskins Laboratories.

Freeman, F. J., & Ushijima, T. (1978). Laryngeal muscle activity during stuttering. *Journal of Speech and Hearing Research, 21,* 538–562.

Fuller, J. L., & Thompson, W. R. (1960). *Behavior genetics.* New York: Wiley.

Garside, R. F., & Kay, D. W. K. (1964). The genetics of stuttering. Chapter 7 in Andrews, G., & Harris, M. *The syndrome of stuttering.* London: Heinemann.

Gladstein, K. L., Seider, R. A., & Kidd, K. K. (1981). Analysis of the sibship patterns of stutterers. *Journal of Speech and Hearing Research, 24,* 460–462.

Goodstein, L. D. (1958). Functional speech disorders and personality: A survey of the research. *Journal of Speech and Hearing Research, 1,* 358–377.

Gray, M. (1940). The "X" family: A clinical and laboratory study of a "stuttering" family. *Journal of Speech Disorders, 5,* 343–348.

Hall, J. W., & Jerger, J. (1978). Central auditory function in stutterers. *Journal of Speech and Hearing Research, 21,* 324–337.

Halle, M. Ueber storungen der athmung bei stottern. (1900). *Monatschrift fur Spracheilkunde, 10,* 225–236.

Harris, B. (1979). Whatever happened to Little Albert? *American Psychologist, 34,* 151–160.

Hill, H. (1944). Stuttering: I. A critical review and evaluation of biochemical investigations. *Journal of Speech Disorders, 9,* 245–261. (a)

Hill, H. (1944). Stuttering: II. A review and integration of physiological data. *Journal of Speech Disorders, 9,* 289–343. (b)

Howie, P. M. (1981). Concordance for stuttering in monozygotic and dizygotic twin pairs. *Journal of Speech and Hearing Research, 24,* 317–321.

Johnson, W. (1932). The influence of stuttering on the personality. *University of Iowa Studies in Child Welfare, 5* (Whole No. 5).

Johnson, W. (1933). An interpretation of stuttering. *Quarterly Journal of Speech, 19,* 70–75.

Johnson, W., & Duke, L. (1935). Changes in handedness associated with onset or disappearance of stuttering: Sixteen cases. *Journal of Experimental Education, 4,* 112–132.

Johnson, W., Knott, J. R. (1937). Studies in the psychology of stuttering: I. The distribution of moments of stuttering in successive readings of the same material. *Journal of Speech Disorders, 2,* 17–19.

Johnson, W., & Leutenegger, R. R. (Eds.). (1955). *Stuttering in children and adults.* Minneapolis: University of Minnesota Press.

Kidd, K. K. (1977). A genetic perspective on stuttering. *Journal of Fluency Disorders, 2,* 259–269.

Kidd, K. K. (1980). Genetic models of stuttering. *Journal of Fluency Disorders, 5,* 187–202.

Kidd, K. K. (1983). Recent progress in the genetics of stuttering. In Ludlow, C. and Cooper, J. (Eds.), *Genetic Aspects of Speech and Language Disorders.* New York: Academic Press, 1983.

Kidd, K. K. (1984). Personal correspondence, (a)

Kidd, K. K. (1984). Stuttering as a genetic disorder. In Curlee, R., & Perkins, W. (Eds.), *Nature and Treatment of Stuttering: New Directions.* San Diego: College-Hill. (b)

Kidd, K. K., Heimbuch, R. C., & Records, M. A. (1981). Vertical transmission of susceptibility to stuttering with sex-modified expression. *Proceedings of the National Academy of Science, 78,* 606–610.

Kidd, K. K., Kidd, J. R., & Records, M. A. (1978). The possible causes of the sex ratio in stuttering and its implications. *Journal of Fluency Disorders, 3,* 13–23.

Kidd, K. K., Oehlert, G., Heimbuch, R. C., Records, M. A., & Webster, R. L. (1980). Familial stuttering patterns are not related to one measure of severity. *Journal of Speech and Hearing Research, 23,* 539–545.

Lussenhop, A. J., Boggs, J. S., LaBorwitt, L. J., & Walle, E. L. (1973). Cerebral dominance in stutterers determined by Wada testing. *Neurology, 23,* 1190–1192.

Makuen, G. H. (1914). A study of 1,000 cases of stammering, with special reference to the etiology and treatment of the affliction. *Therapeutic Gazette, 38,* 385–390.

Moeller, D. (1975). *Speech pathology and audiology: Iowa origins of a discipline.* Iowa City: University of Iowa Press.

Moore, W. H., Jr., & Haynes, W. O. (1980). Alpha hemispheric asymmetry and stuttering: Some support for a segmentation dysfunction hypothesis. *Journal of Speech and Hearing Research, 23,* 229–247.

Nelson, S. E. (1939). Personal contact as a factor in the transfer of stuttering. *Human Biology, 11,* 393–401. (a)

Nelson, S. E. (1939). The role of heredity in stuttering. *Journal of Pediatrics, 14,* 642–654. (b)

Orton, S. T. (1927). Studies in stuttering. *Archives of Neurology and Psychiatry, 18,* 671–672.

Orton, S. T. & Travis, L. E. (1929). Studies in stuttering: IV. Studies of action currents in stutterers. *Archives of Neurology and Psychiatry, 21,* 61–68.

Perozzi, Joseph A. (1970). Phonetic skill (sound mindedness) of stuttering children. *Journal of Communication Disorders, 3,* 207–210.

Pop-Psych, or, "Doc, I'm fed up with these boring figures." (Oct. 7, 1966). *Time,* pp. 38–39.

Reich, A., Till, J., & Goldsmith, H. (1981). Laryngeal and manual reaction times of stuttering and nonstuttering adults. *Journal of Speech and Hearing Research, 24,* 192–196.

Robbins, S. D. (1919). A plethysmographic study of shock and stammering. *American Journal of Physiology, 48,* 285–323.

Rosenfield, D. B., & Goodglass, H. (1980). Dichotic testing of cerebral dominancy in stutterers. *Brain and Language, 11,* 170–180.

Sargent, W. (1964, July). Psychiatric treatment here and in England. *The Atlantic Monthly*, pp. 88–95.

Sayles, D. G. (1971). Cortical excitability, perseveration, and stuttering. *Journal of Speech and Hearing Research, 14,* 462–475.

Seider, R. A., Gladstein, K. L., & Kidd, K. K. (1983). Recovery and persistence of stuttering among relatives of stutterers. *Journal of Speech and Hearing Disorders, 48,* 402–409.

Seligman, M. E. P. (1970). On the generality of the laws of learning. *Psychological Review, 77,* 406–418.

Shapiro, A. J. (1980). An electromyographic analysis of the fluent and dysfluent utterances of several types of stutterers. *Journal of Fluency Disorders, 5,* 203–231.

Sheehan, J. G. (1958). Projective studies of stuttering. *Journal of Speech and Hearing Disorders, 23,* 18–25.

Sheehan, J. G. (1970). Personality approaches. In Sheehan, J. G. (Ed.), *Stuttering: Research and therapy.* New York: Harper and Row.

Sortini, A. J. (1955). Twenty years of stuttering research. *Journal of the International Council for Exceptional Children, 21,* 181–183.

Starkweather, C. W., Hirschman, P., & Tannenbaum, R. S. (1976). Latency of vocalization onset: Stutterers vs. nonstutterers. *Journal of Speech and Hearing Research, 19,* 481–492.

Steer, M. D., & Johnson, W. (1936). An objective study of the relationship between psychological factors and the severity of stuttering. *Journal of Abnormal and Social Psychology, 31,* 36–46.

Stromsta, C. (1972). Interaural phase disparity of stutterers and nonstutterers. *Journal of Speech and Hearing Research, 15,* 771–780.

Sussman, H. M., & MacNeilage, P. F. (1975). Hemispheric specialization for speech production and perception in stutterers. *Neuropsychologia, 13,* 19–26.

Taylor, I. (1976). *Introduction to Psycholinguistics.* New York: Holt, Rinehart, and Winston.

Ten Cate, M. J. (1902). Ueber der untersuchung der athmung bei sprachfehlern. *Monatschrift fur Spracheilkunde, 12,* 247–259, 321–341.

Toscher, M. M., & Rupp, R. R. (1978). A study of the central auditory processes in stutterers using the Synthetic Sentence Identification (SSI) test battery. *Journal of Speech and Hearing Research, 21,* 779–792.

Travis, L. E. (1922). Studies in dissociation: Changes in the auditory threshold induced by crystal gazing. *Journal of Experimental Psychology, 5,* 338–346.

Travis, L. E. (1924). Suggestibility and negativism as measured by auditory threshold during reverie. *Journal of Abnormal and Social Psyhology, 18,* 350–368. (a)

Travis, L. E. (1924). A test for distinguishing between schizophrenoses and psychoneuroses. *Journal of Abnormal and Social Psychology, 19,* 283–298. (b)

Travis, L. E. (1925). Muscular fixation of the stutterer's voice under emotion. *Science, 62,* 207–208.

Travis, L. E. (1926). A phono-photographic study of the stutterer's voice and speech. *Psychological Monographs, 36,* 109–140.

Travis, L. E. (1927). Studies in stuttering: I. Disintegration of the breathing movements during stuttering. *Archives of Neurology and Psychiatry, 18,* 673–690.

Travis, L. E. (1927). Studies in stuttering: II. Photographic studies of the voice in stuttering. *Archives of Neurology and Psychiatry, 18,* 998–1014.

Travis, L. E. (1940). The need for stuttering. *Journal of Speech Disorders, 5,* 193–202.

Travis, L. E. (1957). The unspeakable feelings of people with special reference to stuttering. In Travis, L. E. (Ed.), *Handbook of speech pathology,* New York: Appleton-Century Crofts.

Travis, L. E., & Fagan, L. B. (1928). Studies in stuttering: III. A study of certain reflexes during stuttering. *Archives of Neurology and Psychiatry, 19,* 1006–1013.

Travis, L. E., & Herren, R. Y. (1929). Studies in stuttering: V. A study of simultaneous antitropic movements of the hands of stutterers. *Archives of Neurology and Psychiatry, 22,* 487–494.

Travis, L. E., & Knott, J. R. (1937). Bilaterally recorded brain potential from normal speakers and stutterers. *Journal of Speech Disorders, 2,* 239–241.

Travis, L. E., & Malamud, W. (1933). The relationship between physical habitus and stuttering. *Psychological Bulletin, 30,* 726, Abstract.

Travis, L. E. & Malamud, W. (1937). Brain potentials from normal subjects, stutterers, and schizophrenic patients. *American Journal of Psychiatry, 93,* 929–936.

Van Riper, C. (1971). *The nature of stuttering.* Englewood Cliffs: Prentice-Hall.

Van Riper, C., & Hull, C. J. (1955). The quantitative measurement of the effect of certain situations on stuttering. In W. Johnson (Ed.), *Stuttering in Children and Adults.* Minneapolis: University of Minnesota Press.

Watson, B. C., & Alfonso, P. J. (1982). A comparison of LRT and VOT values between stutterers and nonstutterers. *Journal of Fluency Disorders, 7,* 219–241.

Watson, J. B. (1916). Behavior and the concept of mental disease. *Journal of Philosophy, 13,* 589–597.

Watson, J. B. (1916). The place of the conditioned reflex in psychology. *Psychological Review, 23,* 89–116.

Watson, J. B., & Morgan, J. J. B. (1917). Emotional reactions and psychological experimentation. *American Journal of Psychology, 28,* 163–174.

Watson, J. B., & Rayner, R. (1920). Conditioned emotional reactions. *Journal of Experimental Psychology, 3,* 1–14.

Wepman, J. M. (1935). Is stuttering inherited? *Proceedings of the American Speech Correction Association, 5,* 39–52.

Wepman, J. M. (1939). Familial incidence in stammering. *Journal of Speech Disorders, 4,* 199–204.

West, R., Nelson, S., & Berry, M. F. (1939). The heredity of stuttering. *Quarterly Journal of Speech, 25,* 23–30.

Wingate, M. E. (1962). Evaluation and stuttering: I. Speech characteristics of young children. *Journal of Speech and Hearing Disorders, 27,* 106–115. (a)

Wingate, M. E. (1962). Evaluation and stuttering: II. Environmental stress and critical appraisal of speech. *Journal of Speech and Hearing Disorders, 27,* 244–257. (b)

Wingate, M. E. (1962). Evaluation and stuttering: III. Identification of stuttering and the use of a label. *Journal of Speech and Hearing Disorders, 27,* 368–377. (c)

Wingate, M. E. (1964). A standard definition of stuttering. *Journal of Speech and Hearing Disorders, 29,* 484–489.

Wingate, M. E. (1965). A reply to "A definition in search of data and a theory." *Journal of Speech and Hearing Disorders, 30,* 200–202.

Wingate, M. E. (1966). Prosody in stuttering adaptation. *Journal of Speech and Hearing Research, 9,* 550–556. (a)

Wingate, M. E. (1966). Stuttering adaptation and learning: I. The relevance of adaptation studies to stuttering as "learned behavior." *Journal of Speech and Hearing Disorders, 31,* 148–156. (b)

Wingate, M. E. (1966). Stuttering adaptation and learning: II. The adequacy of learning principles in the interpretation of stuttering. *Journal of Speech and Hearing Disorders, 31,* 211–218. (c)

Wingate, M. E. (1967). Slurvian skill of stutterers. *Journal of Speech and Hearing Research, 10,* 844–848. (a)

Wingate, M. E. (1967). Stuttering and word length. *Journal of Speech and Hearing Research, 10,* 146–152. (b)

Wingate, M. E. (1969). Sound and pattern in "artificial" fluency. *Journal of Speech and Hearing Research, 12,* 677–686.

Wingate, M. E. (1970). Effect on stuttering of changes in audition. *Journal of Speech and Hearing Research, 13,* 861–873. (a)

Wingate, M. E. (1970). Stuttering, 1970: Where do we stand? *Journal of Speech and Hearing Research, 13,* 5–8. (b)

Wingate, M. E. (1971). Phonetic ability in stuttering. *Journal of Speech and Hearing Research, 14,* 189–194.

Wingate, M. E. (1976). *Stuttering: Theory and treatment.* New York: Irvington-Wiley.

Wingate, M. E. (1979). The first three words. *Journal of Speech and Hearing Research, 22,* 604–612. (a)

Wingate, M. E. (1979). The loci of stuttering: Grammar of prosody? *Journal of Communication Disorders, 12,* 283–290. (b)

Wingate, M. E. (1981). Sound and pattern in artificial fluency: Spectrographic evidence. *Journal of Fluency Disorders, 6,* 95–118.

Wingate, M. E. (1982). Early position and stuttering occurrence. *Journal of Fluency Disorders, 7,* 243–258.

Wingate, M. E. (1984). Language factors in stuttering. Unpublished research. (a)

Wingate, M. E. (1984). Stutter events and linguistic stress. *Journal of Fluency Disorders, 9,* 295–300. (b)

Wingate, M. E. (in press). Adaptation, consistency, and beyond. I: Limitations and contradictions. *Journal of Fluency Disorders.*

Wolpe, J. (1973). *The practice of behavior therapy* (2nd ed.). New York: Pergamon Press.

Wolpe, J. (1958). *Psychotherapy by reciprocal inhibition.* Stanford, California: Stanford University Press.

Zimmerman, G. (1980). Articulatory behaviors associated with stuttering. *Journal of Speech and Hearing Research, 23,* 108–121.

Zimmerman, G. N., & Knott, J. R. (1974). Slow potentials of the brain related to speech processing in normal speakers and stutterers. *Electroencephalography and Clinical Neurophysiology, 36,* 47–51.

Stuttering: Discoordination of Phonation with Articulation and Respiration

William H. Perkins, Joanna Rudas, Linda Johnson, and Jody Bell

Postscript
Physiological Dynamics—Discoordination of Phonation

William H. Perkins

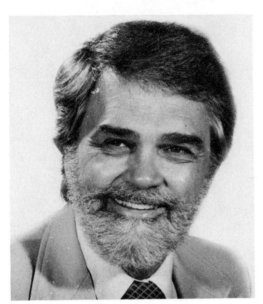

William H. Perkins

There was no question that Bill Perkins should be one of the authors of this book. Our problem was which of his many contributions to select. Perkins was initially trained in the traditional thinking about stuttering. He later was influenced by psychoanalytic interpretations of the problem, and then went on to study and support an operant perspective. Most recently he has come to view stuttering as a voicing disorder and has focused his attention on its physiological aspects. He has emphasized the integra-

tion of respiration, voicing, and articulation in both the etiology and the management of stuttering. Perkins has reduced stuttering anxiety to uncertainty about voice onset, and consequently focuses therapy on tactics that promote greater confidence in the stutterer's ability to initiate voicing.

We asked Perkins to select what he thought was a significant theoretical statement from among his previous writings. He chose the article reprinted herein, which we were delighted to accept because it appears to be a forerunner of much research in the succeeding ten years that has dealt with laryngeal dynamics. Like so many in this book, Perkins is a leader in the field of Speech Pathology. He has been the editor of the *Journal of Speech and Hearing Disorders* and helped raise the standards and quality of that publication. He recently was awarded the Honors of the American Speech-Language-Hearing Association. Perkins has always been generous with his time and his energies as teacher, consultant, and clinician. He is an active researcher and is both editor and author of numerous books and publications. In particular, his book *Human perspectives in speech and language disorders* (1978) brought a down-to-earth, personalized view of communication disorders, presenting technical information in case-study format. It is this personal emphasis that comes through in his chapter that follows, presenting the psychological aspects of physiological events. Like others in this volume, Perkins does not see the stutterer as becoming a normal speaker. Treatment, therefore, becomes a compensatory strategy.

4

Stuttering: Discoordination of Phonation with Articulation and Respiration

William Perkins, Joanna Rudas, Linda Johnson and Jody Bell

University of Southern California, Los Angeles

Complexity of phonatory and respiratory adjustments was systematically simplified in 30 adult stutterers under three speaking conditions: voiced, whispered, and articulated without phonation. Stuttering was reduced considerably when whispering and was practically eliminated when articulating silently. The possibility that stuttering consistently results from complexity of phonatory coordinations with articulation and respiration was strongly supported. Increased speaking rates under conditions that decreased stuttering seemed to be evidence that efficient rhythmical flow of speech is facilitated by simplification of phonatory and respiratory adjustments.

Rational analysis, clinical investigation, and systematic research are lending support to an old suspicion: many of the abnormal disfluencies judged as stuttering involve problems of smooth coordination of phonation[1] with articulation and respiration (Travis, 1931). After reviewing the vast literature of stuttering, Van Riper (1971) concluded that the core of the disorder is a disruption of timing of the motor sequences of sound, syllable, and word production. He suggested that the marked reduction of stuttering during whispering and its elimination during pantomimed speech could be attributed to the high degree of conscious articulation at slower speech rates that permit synchronization. He also proposed the alternative that this puzzling reduction of stuttering "could be accounted for on the basis of a simplified synergy (the absence of voice and/or airflow)..."

Adams (1974) has offered a physiologic and aerodynamic analysis of stuttering and fluency. He proposed that fluency is dependent on smooth coordination of activities of the respiratory, phonatory, and articulatory systems. He suggested "that the muscles and forces that promote control, and coordinate subglottic pressure, glottal resistance, and supraglottal pressure are the major determinants of both fluency and stuttering." Discoordination of these elements would be manifested as difficulty in achieving transglottic pressures that would promote the precisely timed glottal airflow and vocalization required to facilitate smoothly articulated speech. Thus, discoordination of elements of speech does not cause stuttering, it is stuttering.

Because evidence of disrupted motor timing can be found during stuttering at all levels of the speaking system, the possibility exists that each level could serve as a focus of difficulty that triggers discoordinations with other levels of the system (Adams, 1974). In other words, respiratory mistimings could disrupt phonatory and articulatory processes, and conversely oral articulatory or phonatory mistimings could impair the smooth management of subglottic, transglottic, and supraglottic pressures required for fluent speech.

---

[1]Phonation is used in a generic sense in this report to identify any laryngeal adjustments made to coordinate the breath stream with utterance of syllables. Hence, it will refer to whispered as well as voiced speech. For convenience, we will use the term articulation to identify supraglottal processes, even though phonation also includes an articulatory function. Respiration will refer to subglottic processes. Thus, phonation will be used to differentiate laryngeal from subglottic and supraglottic activities.

Note: From *The Journal of Speech and Hearing Research, 19,* 1976, pp. 509–522. Reprinted with permission.

SELECTION OF PHONATION AS THE INDEPENDENT VARIABLE

Simplification of the phonatory process was selected as the independent variable in this experiment for several reasons. A practical consideration was that the complexity of phonatory valving required for generating a breathstream that can be modulated for speech can be systematically altered. Intelligible speech can be produced not only with a normally voiced and voiceless breathstream, but also with a whispered breathstream or, for viewers who can lip-read, with oral articulatory movements produced without breathstream management for speech. Neither vocal tract articulatory processes nor subglottic respiratory processes permit equally as systematic alterations as those that can be made in the phonatory system. Admittedly, respiration for maintaining alveolar pressure can be achieved with a variety of muscular activities (Hixon, 1973). Similarly, variation is permissable in articulatory adjustments provided they remain within limits of producing intelligible speech. Such respiratory and articulatory alterations, however, do not appear to be easily varied systematically.

An extension of this argument is that the phonatory process appears to be the only one that permits progressive simplification of motor coordinations, either in rate or number of adjustments to be coordinated. Speech normally flows at roughly 14 ± 2 phonemes per second, about twice the speed at which individual articulators can be controlled (Lenneberg, 1967; Stetson, 1951; Miller, 1951; Hudgins and Stetson, 1937). Hence, the necessity of coarticulatory overlapping of vocal tract movements to achieve such rates. No alteration in articulation would conceivably simplify the complexity of these coordinations. The rate at which they would have to be made and the number of distinctive features that would have to be controlled would presumably remain constant regardless of articulatory adjustment. The same reasoning would seem to apply to respiration. The necessity of maintaining sufficient alveolar pressure to produce a typical average of five to seven syllables per second along with various prosodic stresses within a phrase would also appear to be relatively constant irrespective of respiratory adjustment (Lenneberg, 1967; Daniloff, 1973).

Complexity of phonatory coordinations, on the other hand, is progressively simplified by changing from normal voicing to whispering to articulating si-

lently, as shown in Figure 4-1. Normal speech requires that the vocal folds be abducted and adducted for voiceless and voiced sounds, respectively. Voiced and voiceless sounds are often produced alternately, as in the nonsense phrase, *put it off a ketchup*. Thus, glottal openings and closings can occur at the same rate as articulatory movements. Moreover, prosodically appropriate pitch and loudness adjustments must be made for each voiced sound. These adjustments require precise adduction and vocal fold adjustments of effective mass, elasticity, and viscosity.

With whispering, both number and rate of adjustments are simplified. For a loud whisper, the tips of the arytenoids are firmly approximated while the posterior borders are separated, thereby creating a glottal chink. The vocal folds are adducted tightly enough to prevent vibration; any adjustment in which cord resistance exceeds subglottal pressure is sufficient (Pressman, 1942; Perkins, 1971b). Softer whispers can involve sufficient adduction of the cords to generate turbulence from airflow through the glottis, but not sufficient for the cords to be set into vibration (Broad, 1973). Spectral pitch and loudness are probably determined by respiratory adjustments of subglottal pressure or by adjustments of the glottal chink, or both. They can occur, potentially, as rapidly as from syllable to syllable. Because only a voiceless breathstream is generated through the glottis, no adductory/abductory movements are needed between phrase initiation and termination.

With silent articulatory movements (lipped speech), further phonatory simplification along with respiratory simplification is achieved. The breathstream is managed independently of speech needs. Whether the vocal folds are abducted or adducted, or are tense or lax is immaterial; prosodic and voiced/voiceless requirements are eliminated. Phonation and respiration need not be coordinated with articulation.

Rational analysis provides another reason for studying effects of simplifying phonation. Logically, laryngeal valving would seem to be the most complex process to coordinate for fluent speech. That voiced/voiceless phonatory coordinations are more complex than subglottic respiratory and supraglottic articulatory adjustments seems reasonable. Whereas normal high-speed supraglottal articulation can be achieved by overlapping movements of a variety of vocal tract structures at slower speeds, phonatory abductory/adductory movements must be capable of occurring at high-speed articulatory rates. No alter-

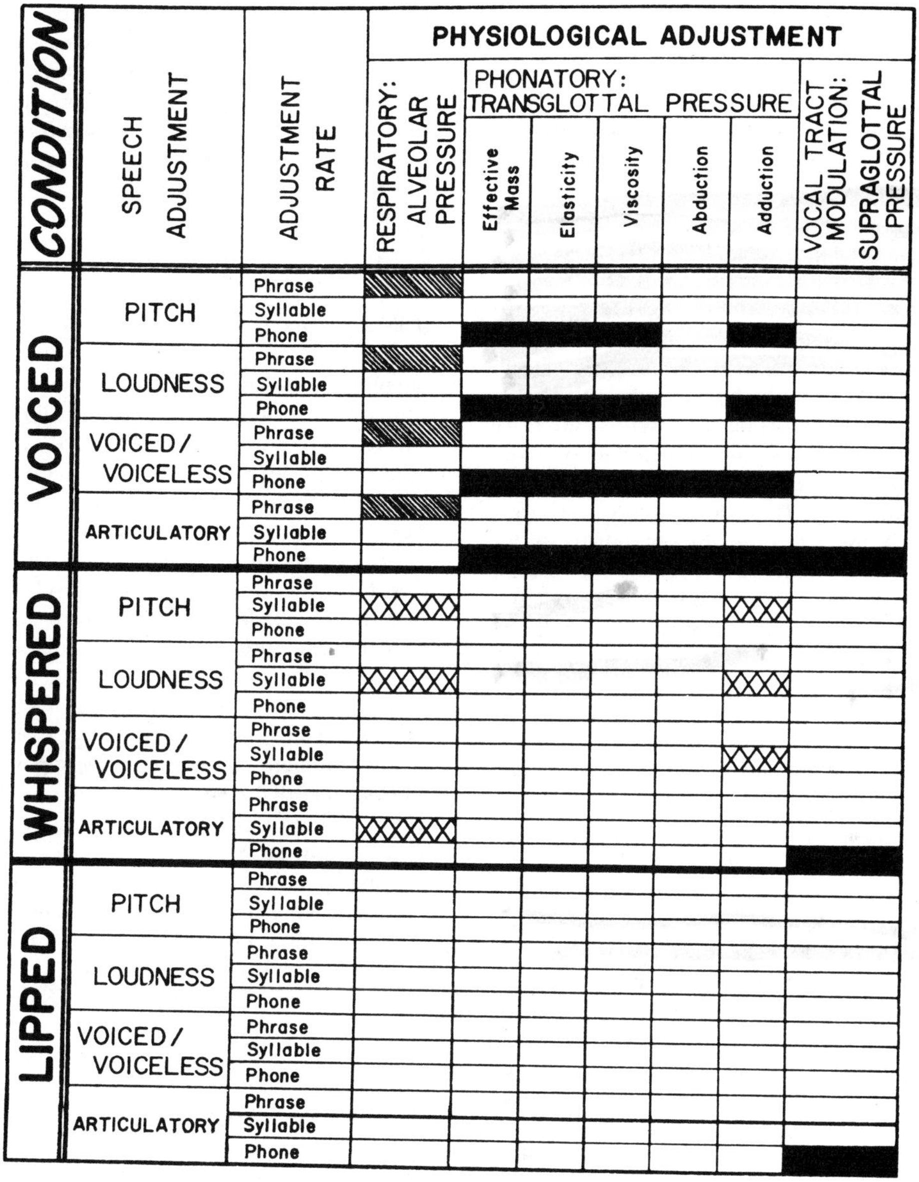

CONDITION	SPEECH ADJUSTMENT	ADJUSTMENT RATE	PHYSIOLOGICAL ADJUSTMENT						
			RESPIRATORY: ALVEOLAR PRESSURE	PHONATORY: TRANSGLOTTAL PRESSURE					VOCAL TRACT MODULATION: SUPRAGLOTTAL PRESSURE
				Effective Mass	Elasticity	Viscosity	Abduction	Adduction	
VOICED	PITCH	Phrase	▨						
		Syllable							
		Phone		█	█	█		█	
	LOUDNESS	Phrase	▨						
		Syllable							
		Phone		█	█	█		█	
	VOICED/ VOICELESS	Phrase	▨						
		Syllable							
		Phone		█	█	█	█	█	
	ARTICULATORY	Phrase	▨						
		Syllable							
		Phone		█	█	█	█	█	
WHISPERED	PITCH	Phrase							
		Syllable	✖					✖	
		Phone							
	LOUDNESS	Phrase							
		Syllable	✖					✖	
		Phone							
	VOICED/ VOICELESS	Phrase							
		Syllable						✖	
		Phone							
	ARTICULATORY	Phrase							
		Syllable	✖						
		Phone							█
LIPPED	PITCH	Phrase							
		Syllable							
		Phone							
	LOUDNESS	Phrase							
		Syllable							
		Phone							
	VOICED/ VOICELESS	Phrase							
		Syllable							
		Phone							
	ARTICULATORY	Phrase							
		Syllable							
		Phone							█

Figure 4-1.   Number and rate of physiological adjustments involved in speaking aloud (voiced), whispering, and articulating silently (lipped). The slowest adjustments are from phrase to phrase ▨▨▨ , the most rapid are from phone to phone ████ (about 14 ± 2 per second) and in between are syllable to syllable adjustments ✖✖✖ (about 6 ± 2 per second).

native laryngeal mechanism exists for opening and closing the glottis, so movements of these structures cannot be overlapped at slower speeds to achieve high speeds; presumably, they must be capable of moving at about twice the speed of articulatory structures. Moreover, the small size of laryngeal structures suggests that they must be controlled with greater precision than supraglottal structures.

Too, the dynamic interrelations among muscular and aerodynamic forces for managing glottal vibratory characteristics would seem to be much more intricate than the pharyngeal, labial, lingual, and velar constrictions, occlusions, and cavity shapings used to modulate the breathstream. For these adjustments, the essential requirement is to position the structures in the vocal tract. By contrast, vocal fold vibrations are dependent on effective vocal fold mass, elasticity, and viscosity adjustments that must be coordinated with subglottal and supraglottal pressures to maintain the precise transglottal pressure that will produce the desired pitch and loudness of each syllable (Adams, 1974; Moore, 1968; Perkins, 1971a).

As for a comparison of phonatory with respiratory complexity, the contrast would seem to be even greater. Both in precision and rate of control, the difference seems sharp. Thoracic structures are large. Their speech task is to maintain a breathstream for the duration of each phrase. Presumably, the fastest adjustments that might have to be made are for loudness from syllable to syllable, a rate less than half that of phonetic articulation. Timing of respiratory muscle contraction is apparently a relatively slow process that has to do primarily with maintaining steady alveolar pressure against a background of declining relaxation pressure (Draper, Ladefoged, and Whitteridge, 1959; Hixon, 1973; Netsell, 1973). Thus, respiratory processes seem to be less complex to coordinate than supraglottal articulatory processes and certainly than phonatory processes.

Finally, a growing body of evidence points to laryngeal functions as being crucial in stuttering. Wingate (1969) concluded from his review of the literature that stuttering is reduced by "artificial" fluency because "the stutterer is induced, in one way or another, to do something with his voice that he does not ordinarily do." Adams and Reis (1971, 1974) demonstrated that difficulty initiating phonation is "an important predictor of stuttering—certainly more powerful than such variables as word length and grammatical class." Brenner, Perkins, and Soderberg (1972) found that neither silent rehearsal with articulatory movements nor whispered rehearsal reduced stuttering in normal speech as much as aloud rehearsal. They suspected that the differences were due to complexity of the phonatory processes rehearsed in each condition. Most recently, Adams and Hayden (1976) showed that stutterers are slower than normal speakers in a nonspeech task of initiating and terminating phonation. They thereby supported their alternate explanation that the direction of causation of stuttering disfluencies is from phonation to articulation, not vice versa. Direct evidence of phonatory involvement has been provided by Freeman and Ushijima's (1975) demonstration that abductor/adductor reciprocity is disrupted during moments of stuttering.

THE PROBLEM

This experiment was undertaken to determine the effects on stuttering and speech rate of systematically simplifying the complexity of phonatory and respiratory coordinations for speech. The foregoing analysis led us to suspect that complexity of phonatory adjustments can trigger discoordinations of the activities seen in the prolongations, repetitions, and hesitations of stuttering. Although these motor discoordinations occur at a physiological level, they can best be observed at a behavioral level (Perkins and Curlee, 1969; Perkins, 1971a). Prolongations and hesitations are identified by listener judgments of inappropriate durations of phonetic elements. Physiological correlates of these judgments have not yet been determined, so no criteria yet exist for recognizing phonetic discoordinations physiologically. The purpose of this study was not to reveal biological details of motor discoordinations in the speech system directly, but rather it was to determine by observing speech behavior if the discoordinations of stuttering were affected by alternations in phonation and respiration. Efficient research strategy dictated determining first if the general outline of our suspicions was defensible before pursuing this lead in detail.

We reasoned that if laryngeal adjustments were progressively simplified without systematically varying articulatory targets,[2] we should be able to determine whether or not complexity of the phonatory process is related to stuttering. If it is not, then stuttering should not be affected from one treatment

[2]We assumed that the speaking system functions as a dynamically integrated unit in which a change in glottal resistance alters the balance of subglottic, supraglottic, and transglottic pressures. Thus, respiratory and articulatory adjustments could presumably accompany experimental manipulations of phonation. Speech disfluency would, therefore, reflect physiological discoordinations in the whole speaking system, not just in the isolated phonatory portion of the system that would be systematically varied. The fact that articulatory targets were held constant would not imply that the same vocal tract adjustments would necessarily be made to produce target sounds from one experimental condition to another.

condition to another. If it is, then frequency of stuttering should be reduced during whispering and eliminated during silent articulation without phonation.

An explanation for reduction of stuttering with reduced phonatory complexity could be inferred from speech rate. If Van Riper's (1971) suggested explanation is accurate that whispering and silent articulation require greater concentration, then speech rate should be retarded, as he suspects, and coordinations would thereby be facilitated. If his alternate explanation is accurate that simplification of phonatory complexity facilitates synergic coordination of the speaking system, then speech rate should at least be maintained if not increased.

METHOD

Subjects

Twenty-five male and five female subjects who stuttered when whispering were used to determine the effects on frequency of stuttering during reading under three speaking conditions: voiced, whispered, and articulated without phonation. The subjects consisted of stutterers awaiting initiation of treatment at the University of Southern California Center for the Study of Communicative Disorders at the time of the study. They ranged in age form 14 to 67 and represented a wide range of educational, ethnic, and socioeconomic backgrounds. In general, they appeared to constitute a representative sample of stutterers found in a large metropolitan area.

We had determined from a pilot study of 15 subjects that in four of them whispering consistently reduced stuttering to zero. Without exception for these subjects, stuttering remained at zero when articulating without phonation. Because the effects of reducing "off-on" phonatory adjustments as is accomplished in whispering could be inferred from the effects of all-voiced passages used by Adams and Reis (1971, 1974), the crux of this experiment was to ascertain the effects of further simplification of phonatory and respiratory complexity by articulating without phonation. Obviously, a determination of the effects of this condition in comparison with the condition of whispering could not be made in subjects who did not stutter when whispering. Accordingly, stuttering during whispering was a subject selection requirement for this investigation. Other requirements were that subjects be free of neuro- or laryn-

geal pathology, that they meet criteria for speaking under the three treatment conditions, and that they not attempt to use syllable prolongation procedures.

Procedures

Each subject read three 130–131 syllable excerpts from the "Rainbow Passage," a different one under each treatment condition. Conditions were systematically rotated across passages as the data were gathered originally. We selected the first 30 subjects who qualified for the experiment. This rotational arrangement was thereby somewhat imbalanced; seven were accepted from the voiced-lipped-whispered (V-L-W) order, 11 from L-W-V, and 12 from W-V-L. The fact that a Friedman two-way analysis of variance of percent syllables stuttered revealed no significant order effect ($p < 0.05$) in a pilot study of these procedures suggests that the experimental results were not seriously confounded.

Three judges made independent measures from frontal head and chest video recordings (without sound) for 10 subjects each. The resulting 90 passages were analyzed to obtain measures of stuttering and rate. Stuttering was defined as any syllable disfluency—prolongation, repetition, hesitation, or interjection. The measure of stuttering used was percent syllables disfluent, and the measure of rate was syllables per minute.

Reliability among judges was determined in advance of the experiment by having them measure 30 passages in common, 10 voiced, 10 whispered, and 10 articulated without phonation. Because the counts were made using video without sound, the judges were never certain of which condition was being viewed. To test ability to lip-read a wide range of types of speech and stuttering, each passage was from a different subject. The intraclass correlations among these judges were 0.99 for both syllables per minute and percent syllables disfluent.

The reason for using video measures only was to obtain comparable measures of the voiced and whispered conditions with the silent condition of articulation without phonation. To ascertain whether or not stuttering and rate could be judged validly by visual stimuli alone, another set of measures, video with sound, was used to determine the relationship of visual with audiovisual measures. Comparing these two sets of measures, Pearson product-moment coefficients for both percent syllables disfluent and syllables per minute were higher than 0.98 for both whispered and voiced conditions. These correlations were high enough to give us confidence that visual cues were sufficient to approximate the audiovisual information normally used to judge stuttering.

The rate measure of syllables per minute can be deceptive as a description of articulatory rate. A typical method of measurement is to record time at the beginning and end of speaking and count the number of syllables spoken. The problem with this method is that the resulting measure can be so strongly affected by duration of stuttering and pauses between phrases that variations in articulatory rate can be obscured. Because syllable prolongation is a powerful means of reducing stuttering (Curlee and Perkins, 1969), a slight prolongation could reduce the severity or frequency of prolongations and hesitations enough to increase the rate measure considerably. The result, paradoxically, would be that an increase in syllables per minute would have been accomplished by a retarded articulatory rate.

To meet this objection, a measure of syllables per minute was computed from the elapsed speaking time for the total number of syllables in the passage. Speaking time was measured by manually activating an electric timer with a telegraph key that was depressed for the duration of each syllable. An instance of stuttering was counted as comparable to one fluent syllable regardless of the number of syllable repetitions or duration of moments of stuttering. The key was not depressed during pauses between phrases. The measured speaking rate thereby reflects the speed at which the stutterer was attempting to speak irrespective of time consumed by pauses and stuttering.

RESULTS

Inspection of subject performance in Table 4-1 shows unambiguously that syllable disfluencies were progressively reduced as the complexity of phonatory and respiratory coordination was simplified. One-tailed t tests of the predicted differences between correlated means show that stuttering was reduced significantly ($p < 0.001$) from 24.6% syllables disfluent in the voiced condition to 10.3% in the whispered condition. In the silently articulated condition, stuttering was further reduced significantly ($p < 0.001$) to 0.8% syllables disfluent in comparison with the whispered condition. All subjects stuttered less without phonation than when whispering, and the

three exceptions (CM, RH, and TM) to a reduction of stuttering from voice to whisper were slight.

The possibility that reduced stuttering might be attributed to a slower speaking rate was rejected. A randomized block design showed that significant ($p < 0.01$) differences did exist; speaking rate increased progressively with simplification of phonation. Dunn's multiple comparisons showed a significantly faster ($p < 0.01$) syllable rate during whispering (209.6 syllables per minute) in comparison with voiced speech (176.6 syllables per minute), and a rate (237.2 syllables per minute) while articulating without phonation that was significantly ($p < 0.01$) faster than the whispered rate.

Table 4-1. Percent syllables disfluent of subjects under three treatment conditions arranged in order of voiced condition severity.

Subject	Voiced	Whispered	Lipped
DH	5.4	1.6	0.0
AI	6.9	3.1	1.6
LZ	7.5	6.0	4.7
RH	8.2	9.0	0.0
LF	10.5	2.3	1.6
TM	12.9	13.2	0.7
BW	13.2	5.4	2.3
AS	13.9	3.7	0.0
CM	14.2	11.8	0.0
CM	15.6	16.9	3.1
TR	16.0	6.9	0.0
JM	18.1	1.5	0.0
JH	20.0	10.0	0.0
RB	20.2	12.3	1.5
FM	21.9	10.9	0.0
RP	22.1	4.6	1.5
LD	23.5	12.5	0.0
SS	24.2	15.8	0.0
RD	24.4	3.0	0.7
DP	25.6	3.8	0.0
MK	29.4	7.6	0.0
FH	29.7	19.8	2.8
JS	29.8	4.7	3.1
RP	29.9	7.5	0.0
MW	37.4	9.7	0.8
LL	38.9	25.4	0.0
LB	39.7	16.3	0.0
KS	42.9	1.6	0.0
CB	61.2	55.4	0.8
RH	70.5	7.6	0.0

DISCUSSION

The most striking feature of these results is that they are practically invariant. Twenty-seven of 30 subjects showed a reduction of stuttering from the voiced to whispered condition (the three exceptions differed by 1.3% syllables disfluent or less). All 30 without exception showed further reduction from whispering to silent articulation. Of these, 17 reduced syllable disfluency to zero; for the remainder, the highest frequency was 4.7 percent syllables disfluent. Even this measure was probably high because we used a strict criterion of syllable disfluency. As a result, many of these disfluencies would probably be judged as normal rather than stuttered.

Clearly, some condition existed during this experiment powerful enough to exert almost complete control of stuttering. Such other variables as influence abnormal disfluency must somehow exert their effects through that condition. Whatever the ultimate explanation, it must account for these results.

The explanation that seems to fit the evidence best is that stuttering is a function of complexity of phonatory coordinations with articulatory and respiratory processes. The fact that phonatory complexity was progressively simplified, as the independent variable, was demonstrably accomplished. All subjects met criteria for speaking under voiced, whispered, and silently articulated conditions which, of necessity, required the physiological simplifications of laryngeal adjustments discussed earlier. Because this was the only variable that was deliberately altered systematically, and because reductions of stuttering consistently followed these simplifications, the cause-and-effect relation seems likely.

Additional evidence that supports a discoordination hypothesis is revealed by a split-half analysis of the data in Table 4-1. Subjects were rank ordered according to percent syllables disfluent under the voiced condition. The mean for the least severe half was 13.6% syllables disfluent under the voiced condition, 7.6% during whispering, and 1.0% during silent articulation. The mean for the most severe half, on the other hand, was 35.3% during voicing, 12.7% during whispering, and 0.5% during silent articulation. The point to note is that silent articulation reduced syllable disfluency somewhat more effectively for the most severe than for the least severe. This inverse relation between voiced and lipped conditions is also seen in the slightly negative, but not significant, Spearman rho correlation (− 0.10). Such results

suggest that discoordination is more likely to be at the core of severe than mild stuttering. To the extent that factors other than discoordination contribute to stuttering, they may play a proportionately larger role, and accordingly may be more apparent when complexity of speech coordinations is minimized, in mild than severe stutterers.

Effects of these simplifications in phonatory complexity cannot be easily explained as the result of increased conscious effort and deliberate articulation. If this had happened, the articulatory rate would have been retarded. Instead, it accelerated progressively from voiced to whispered and from whispered to silently articulated conditions. Subjects were given no instructions regarding rate, so they apparently spoke faster spontaneously as complexity of their phonatory adjustments was simplified. This fits with the explanation that the problem is one of coordinating phonation with articulation and respiration.

Whether complexity of articulatory or respiratory adjustments could also trigger discoordinations of the speaking system cannot be conclusively affirmed or denied by this study. The fact that oral articulatory and respiratory discoordinations disappeared when phonatory complexity was simplified sufficiently only demonstrates the possible causal role of phonation. It does not eliminate the alternative that articulatory and respiratory processes could serve the same role.

Adams and Hayden's (1976) work, which is supported by our results, does bear on this issue, however. They tested alternative explanations of stuttering being caused, as one possibility, "by excessive speech mechanism constriction and tension" that interferes with quick initiation of phonation, and as the other possibility, by delays in voicing that prompt "oral articulatory" repetitions and prolongations. They tested the alternatives by measuring "the time it took stutterers to initiate voicing while not stuttering." They were significantly slower than nonstutterers in initiating and terminating voicing. Adams and Hayden reasoned that this result should not occur if oral articulatory processes caused stuttering, because the experimental tests of voicing were conducted when subjects did not stutter. Their finding does not conclusively rule out the possibility that complexity of supraglottal articulatory processes could trigger stuttering, but they weigh heavily against it.

Because we had to rely on subject compliance

with our instructions, the possibility that intervening variables produced the results obtained cannot be categorically excluded. One possibility, the distraction effect, seems unlikely, though, because silent articulation invariably reduced stuttering more than whispering, yet both are atypical methods of speaking. To make the case for distraction, one would have to argue that silent articulation was more distracting than whispering for all subjects, or that it was more deliberate and slower than whispering or voicing. The first argument seems implausible, and the second is contradicted by the evidence; speaking rate accelerated under this condition.

A somewhat more plausible alternative is that communicative responsibility was reduced. Other explanations may also be possible, but to be competitive they must account for highly consistent results. Unlike research trends that permit varying operation of innumerable conditions, invariant effects point strongly to consistently related causes. Admittedly, a variety of psychological variables, such as communicative responsibility, may have operated in our subjects' compliance with instructions. The possibility, however, that each subject had practically the same uncontrolled psychological reaction to each experimental condition, and that this reaction determined the frequency of stuttering hardly seems credible. Equally unlikely is the argument that a variety of reactions produced consistent effects on stuttering in all subjects. Still, further work is needed to determine definitively the relevance of such alternative explanations.

We favor viewing complexity of phonatory coordination with articulatory and respiratory processes as the determinant of our results because systematic alterations in this variable yielded remarkably consistent effects on stuttering. If this explanation is to be pursued, two major directions are pertinent. One is to determine why stutterers have more difficulty coordinating phonation with articulation and respiration than do nonstutterers. Have they simply never learned the coordinations of normal speech, are they merely at the low end of the normal distribution of endowments of skill in coordinating the speaking processes, or are they below normal limits for this skill? If poorly endowed, is this characteristic transmitted genetically? What are the neurological correlates? Does the problem resemble dysarthria or apraxia; is cerebral dominance involved; is Schwartz's (1974) analysis of the laryngeal reflex that he suspects is at the core of stuttering supported by evidence; is the auditory system involved, and if so,

how? These only suggest the wealth of leads that are open.

The other major direction is to determine how other variables that affect stuttering are related to phonatory coordinations. Some of these relations seem reasonably apparent. The work of Adams and his colleagues (1971, 1974, 1976) on voicing initiation is supported by our results and fits readily within the general framework of phonatory discoordination with subglottal and supraglottal processes. Similarly, the possibility that adaptation is a rehearsal effect also fits within this framework. It was from the research of Brenner et al. (1972) that the lead for the current investigation was obtained. They suggested that the reason stuttering was significantly less with aloud than with whispered or silently articulated rehearsal was that speaking aloud permitted practice in coordinating phonatory with articulatory movements.

Somewhat more speculative is the possibility that delayed auditory feedback reduces stuttering by enforcing a slow enough articulatory rate to permit fluent coordination of speaking system movements. Although Adams et al. (1973) and Ingham, Martin, and Kuhl (1974) have studied the effectiveness of slow speaking rate in the reduction of stuttering, the method of testing rate in both studies differed critically from the clinical procedure used to establish fluency. Adams and his associates had stutterers speak one word per second, whereas Ingham and his colleagues set a slow target rate that stutterers matched. No instructions were reported in either investigation as to how these slow rates were to be achieved. Our clinical experience with over 200 stutterers with whom rate control procedures have been used is that most must be instructed in the desired technique of prolonging syllables as the method of slowing rate. With this technique, fluency as well as reduction of the disruptive effect of delayed auditory feedback (DAF) is virtually assured. Conversely, no other rate control technique we have observed has insured fluency. This impression is buttressed by some experimental evidence that stutterers who slow their rate of speech by pausing between syllables articulated at a normally rapid rate continue to stutter (Brenner, 1969). Each pause seems to provide a potential opportunity for discoordinated initiation of the breathstream at the beginning of each syllable. When articulatory rate within the syllable remains rapid, regardless of time between syllables, coordination of speaking system movements, in theory, would not be facilitated as much as they would be by prolonging duration of the syllables. A DAF retarded rate, then, may reduce stuttering to the extent that it facilitates phonatory synergy with articulatory and respiratory processes.

Our results are also congruent with Bloodstein's (1974) hypothesis that stuttering reflects tension and fragmentation in "executing the motor plan of some element of speech." We are proposing that phonatory coordinations especially are among these elements, and that the linguistic factors that Bloodstein has described are related to stuttering by virtue of motor planning difficulties in coordinating phonation with articulation and respiration.

Some of the most profitable leads may well come from Wingate's (1966, 1967, 1969) work on voice and prosody. He has demonstrated that prosody is functionally related to stuttering and has proposed that its effects, along with those of singing, "shadowing," and choral speaking can be attributed to something the stutterer does differently with his voice. All of these activities are noted for their powerful capacity for reducing stuttering. Details of how they are linked to voice remain to be investigated. That they somehow simplify the complex motor planning required for coordinating phonation with articulation and respiration is tempting to consider.

REFERENCES

Adams, M., A physiologic and aerodynamic interpretation of fluent and stuttered speech. *J. fluency Dil.,* **1,** 35–47 (1974).

Adams, M., and Hayden, P. The ability of stutterers and non-stutterers to initiate and terminate phonation during nonspeech activity. *J. Speech Hearing Res.,* **19,** 290–296 (1976).

Adams, M., Lewis, J., and Besozzi, T., The effects of reduced reading rate on stuttering frequency. *J. Speech Hearing Res.,* **16,** 671–675 (1973).

Adams, M., and Reis, R., The influence of the onset of phonation on the frequency of stuttering. *J. Speech Hearing Res.,* **14,** 639–644 (1971).

Adams, M., and Reis, R., The influence of the onset of phonation on the frequency of stuttering: A replication and reevaluation. *J. Speech Hearing Res.,* **17,** 752–754 (1974).

Bloodstein, O., The rules of early stuttering. *J. Speech Hearing Dis.,* **39,** 379–394 (1974).

Brenner, N., Effects of types of rehearsal on frequency of stuttering. Doctoral dissertation, Univ. of Southern California (1969).

Brenner, N., Perkins, W., and Soderberg, G., The effect of rehearsal on frequency of stuttering. *J. Speech Hearing Res.,* **15,** 483–486 (1972).

Broad, D., Phonation. In F. Minifie, T. Hixon, and F. Williams (Eds.), *Normal Aspects of Speech, Hearing, and Language.* Englewood Cliffs, N.J.: Prentice-Hall (1973).

Curlee, R., and Perkins, W., Conversational rate control therapy for stuttering. *J. Speech Hearing Dis.,* **34,** 245–250 (1969).

Daniloff, R., Normal articulation processes. In F. Minifie, T. Hixon, and F. Williams (Eds.), *Normal Aspects of Speech, Hearing, and Language.* Englewood Cliffs, N.J.: Prentice-Hall (1973).

Draper, M., Ladefoged, P., and Whitteridge, D., Respiratory muscles in speech. *J. Speech Hearing Res.,* **2,** 16–27 (1959).

Freeman, F., Ushijima, T., Laryngeal activity accompanying the moment of stuttering: A preliminary report of EMG investigations. *J. fluency Dis.,* **1,** 36–45 (1975).

Hixon, T., Respiratory function in speech. In F. Minifie, T. Hixon, and F. Williams (Eds.), *Normal Aspects of Speech, Hearing, and Language.* Englewood Cliffs, N.J.: Prentice-Hall (1973).

Hudgins, C., and Stetson, R., Relative speech of articulatory movements. *Archives Neeanderlaise de Phonetique Experimentale,* **13,** 85–94 (1937).

Ingham, R., Martin, R., and Kuhl, P., Modification and control of rate of speaking by stutterers. *J. Speech Hearing Res.,* **17,** 489–496 (1974).

Lenneberg, E., *Biological Foundations of Language.* New York: John Wiley and Sons (1967).

Miller, G., Speech and language. In S. Stevens (Ed.), *Handbook of Experimental Psychology.* New York: John Wiley and Sons (1951).

Moore, P., Otolaryngology and speech pathology. *Laryngoscope,* **78,** 1500–1509 (1968).

Netsell, R., Speech physiology. In F. Minifie, T. Hixon, and F. Williams (Eds.), *Normal Aspects of Speech, Hearing, and Language.* Englewood Cliffs, N.J.: Prentice-Hall (1973).

Perkins, W., *Speech Pathology: An Applied Behavioral Science.* St. Louis: Mosby (1971a).

Perkins, W., Vocal function: Assessment and therapy. In L. Travis (Ed.), *Handbook of Speech Pathology and Audiology.* New York: Appleton-Century-Crofts (1971b).

Perkins, W., and Curlee, R., Causality in speech pathology. *J. Speech Hearing Dis.,* **34,** 231–238 (1969).

Pressman, J., Physiology of the vocal cords in phonation and respiration. *Arch. Otolaryng.,* **35,** 355–398 (1942).

Schwartz, M., The core of the stuttering block. *J. Speech Hearing Dis.,* **39,** 169–177 (1974).

Stetson, R., *Motor Phonetics.* Amsterdam: North-Holland (1951).

Travis, L., *Speech Pathology.* New York: Appleton (1931).

Van Riper, C., *The Nature of Stuttering.* Englewood Cliffs, N.J.: Prentice-Hall (1971).

Wingate M., Prosody in stuttering adaptation. *J. Speech Hearing Res.,* **9,** 550–556 (1966).

Wingate, M., Slurvian skills of stutterers. *J. Speech Hearing Res.,* **10,** 844–848 (1967).

Wingate, M., Sound and pattern in "artificial" fluency. *J. Speech Hearing Res.,* **12,** 677–686 (1969).

Discoordination of Phonation with Articulation and Respiration

William H. Perkins

The prospect that phonatory coordinations are pivotal to speech timing and its major disorder, stuttering, is far from new. The discoordination hypothesis, to which this is the postscript, was developed out of a preliminary exploration of one possible reason why phonation seems to be basic to articulation and respiration in stuttering. That research was not intended to be a definitive test of the central role of phonation in the coordination of speech. Instead, that role was posited. Accordingly, the underlying assumption of that research has not been tested directly, nor rigorously.

This caveat is probably of greater importance to the clinical implications of this postscript than to the understanding of the nature of stuttering. That understanding will be gradually revealed as scientific inquiry unravels the problem, caveat or no caveat. But clinical applications tend to take the hypotheses on which they are based as given facts. Instead of assuming validity of the rationale, a much safer and more profitable alternative is to use clinical application as a test of the underlying hypothesis. With this preamble, I'll now discuss the implications of the discoordination hypothesis for understanding the nature of stuttering, and then with its implications for treatment.

IMPLICATIONS FOR UNDERSTANDING STUTTERING

Laryngeal Role in Stuttering

Investigations of the role of the larynx in stuttering reflect remarkable ambivalence. On one hand, it is the larynx, not the vocal tract nor chest wall, that has attracted most of the attention in the research of the last dozen years at least. This attraction announces in no uncertain terms the conviction of investigators that somehow the larynx plays a key role in stuttering, presumably more fundamental than articulation or respiration. On the other hand, hardly a report of this re-

Parts of this postscript are reprinted by permission of the publisher from Implications of Scientific Research for Treatment of Stuttering—A Lecture by William H. Perkins, *Journal of Fluency Disorders*, 6:2, pp. 156–157, 158–162. Copyright 1981 by Elsevier Science Publishing Co., Inc.

search can be found that does not hasten to hedge that role by pointing out that phonation is not an independent element of speech, isolated from respiration and articulation. Proper acknowledgment is given to the possibility that these latter two elements may be just as important as phonation; after all, speech would not occur at all if phonation were not coordinated with them. Still, the persistent interest in the larynx attests to the suspicion that it is somehow involved in the cause of stuttering. Let us review the gist of the evidence that supports this argument.

What we now have is a reasonably good description of how laryngeal functioning of stutterers compares with that of nonstutterers during stuttered and fluent speech, mainly in adults, but also in children. The discoordinations of stuttering, described physiologically in a relatively small number of subjects, involve mistiming and excessive contraction of laryngeal and supraglottal muscles, particularly the disruption of reciprocity of abductors and adductors. Also, laryngeal behavior tends to vary with the type of stuttering. From this evidence, whether supraglottal discoordinations precede or follow laryngeal discoordinations is not determined.

Closely related to this physiological work, and a major topic of research, are descriptive studies of voice onset time (VOT), voice termination time (VTT), and voice reaction time (VRT). Generally, but far from invariantly, children and adults who stutter are slower than nonstutterers in VOT and VTT during fluent speech, apparently because of slower movement during articulatory transitions. By contrast with these descriptions of VOT and VTT, which involve readings ranging from nonsense syllables to the *Rainbow Passage,* VRT measures reflect how rapidly voice can be initiated and terminated. This ability is clearly improved with practice, but with the practice effect removed stutterers are still slightly slower than nonstutterers on oral and manual, as well as on vocal, responses with auditory stimuli, but not with visual.

Experimentation with stuttering has demonstrated that it is invariably reduced when phone rate is slowed, but only inconsistently reduced when syllable or word rate is slowed. Similarly, use of an all-voiced breath stream, which removes abductory-adductory coordination, reduces stuttering, but with numerous exceptions. Whispering, which removes control of the vibratory adjustments as well as abductory-adductory control, reduces stuttering with only a few exceptions. Lipping, which removes coordination of respiratory and laryngeal management of the breath stream with vocal tract articulatory movements, reduces it with no exceptions. By contrast, reducing the number of vocal tract movements to be coordinated does not affect stuttering, but imposing a metronomic rhythm on speech invariably does. Normal rhythms of speech probably have equally robust effects, but this is based on clinical impression, not experimental research. Finally, the adaptation effect, which is far from invariant, is specific to the motor gesture practiced, so whispered, and especially lipped, rehearsal do not improve fluency much during normally voiced speech.

Discussion of singing, choral speaking, shadowing, masking, and DAF (delayed auditory feedback) have been omitted because laryngeal involvement in re-

Postscript   4

ductions of stuttering they produce is a matter of inferential conjecture, not experimental demonstration.

What does all of this mean? Investigations of laryngeal performance during fluent and stuttered speech, and of stutterers and nonstutterers, have provided valuable information about various things that happen in the larynx during stuttering. We now have confirmation of our assumption that the observable discoordinations of stuttering are indeed manifested in laryngeal dissynchronies. This evidence constitutes a part of the physiological definition of stuttering; it characterizes the laryngeal component of stuttering. It cannot, therefore, cause the thing of which it is an integral part.

The VOT and VRT studies, on the other hand, suggest causation. It seems logical to suspect that if stutterers cannot initiate voice fast enough to keep up with their vocal tract movements, discoordination could result. But this interpretation carries with it several problems. First, the evidence suggests that stutterers are not faster with vocal tract responses than they are with laryngeal responses. Second, dysarthrics exhibit even slower coordination abilities, but this disability affects their speech differently from stuttering. Third, the slow response times are not invariably associated with stuttering, which would seem to exclude this condition as necessary for abnormal disfluency. Finally, if we grant the possibility that slow VOT and VRT could reveal a causal factor of stuttering, that possibility must await experimental confirmation before any clinical potential should be contemplated. Admittedly, manipulating VOT and VRT experimentally may be impossible, but comparisons of stutterers and nonstutterers and of stuttering and fluency do not permit us to infer that differences observed descriptively are the cause of stuttering.

Considering the state of existing evidence, we have virtually no basis for excluding alternative explanations of any hypothesis proposed. The method I adopted was to use the evidence as signposts, varying in clarity and size, by which to select stronger, in preference to weaker, leads. The most incontrovertible lead, cast in broadest form, is that stuttering is a discoordination of muscular and/or aerodynamic coordinations among the phonatory, articulatory, and possibly respiratory systems. That these coordinations are facilitated by slowing phone rate with prolongation of syllables is also firmly established. Equally certain is the reduction of stuttering by changing laryngeal action from voiced-voiceless to whispered to lipped.

An attractive possibility is that coordination of tracheal, transvocalis, and vocal tract airstream management is a primary determinant of fluency. When the airstream is changed from voiced-voiceless to whispered, stuttering diminished almost 60% on the average, but with a few exceptions. When no airstream is used, leaving only vocal tract movements to coordinate, stuttering virtually disappears without exception.

That as an aerodynamic coordination problem, respiration, phonation, and articulation are inseparable systems is an idea championed by many. Changes in place, extent, rate, and speed of vocal tract constrictions affect, in all probability, transvocalis air pressure and flow. The question regarding fluency, then, is the extent to which airstream management movements of one system (respiration, phonation, or articulation) affect the coordination of airstream management movements of the other systems.

Experimental evidence indicates that when laryngeal management of trans-vocalis aerodynamics must be coordinated with vocal tract airstream management movements, stuttering tends to occur. With no airstream to manage in lipped speech, even those who stutter most severely have no difficulty with fluent articulatory movements, generally at faster rates. By making no systematic change in vocal tract articulation and by changing laryngeal management from lipping to whispering, stuttering increases over 90%; by changing from whispering to voiced-voiceless speech, it increases almost 60%.

Although vocal tract occlusions will impede and terminate vocal fold vibrations by raising vocal tract pressure to the level of tracheal pressure, no evidence from articulatory experimentation indicates that changing the rate of vocal tract adjustments will disrupt timing of transglottal aerodynamic management. Admittedly, the possibility is not excluded. Still, if a significant effect were possible, some evidence of it would presumably appear as the number of vocal tract constrictions, with attendant aerodynamic changes, is changed experimentally by as much as 18%. Presumably, such vocal tract changes do alter transglottal aerodynamics, but apparently not in a manner that discoordinates laryngeal timing.

This is the evidence that most clearly implicates the larynx in some causal way to stuttering. It indicates that difficulty of coordination of vocal tract, trans-vocalis, and possibly tracheal aerodynamics is a function of the type of air stream generated at the larynx. Other less invariant evidence supports this hypothesis. For example, when an all voiced airstream is used in comparison with a voiced-voiceless airstream, stuttering is reduced, on the average and with many exceptions, about 25%. This compares with more than twice that much reduction when whispering is used in place of voiced-voiceless phonation.

Two alternatives are apparent that separately or together could account for why a voiced-voiceless airstream is more difficult to coordinate than a whispered airstream. One is the possibility that the more frequent voice onsets complicate the coordination. The other is that fortis-lentis fluctuations in driving pressure, which are about twice as great for voiceless as for voiced plosives and sibilants, are greater and pose more complex coordination problems with a voiced-voiceless airstream than with one that is whispered or continuously voiced.

Why a voiced, in comparison with a voiceless, airstream is more than twice as difficult to coordinate also requires consideration. An obvious possibility found in voiced, but not voiceless, speech is the management of loudness and pitch with vibrating vocal folds. The fact that tracheal aerodynamic changes are consistently associated with loudness changes, and to a much less extent with pitch, supports this speculation. Typically, loudness and pitch vary from syllable to syllable to meet stress requirements of pronunciation and expressive requirements of effective communication. Thus, with a continuously voiced airstream, tracheal aerodynamic variations necessary to produce desired loudnesses and

Postscript   4

pitches would be expected to occur from syllable to syllable, thereby complicating coordination of transglottal aerodynamics with vocal tract aerodynamics for management of articulation. Whether such aerodynamic variation complexities are, in fact, functionally related to stuttering remains to be determined.

Running through the laryngeal literature is the tacit, and sometimes explicit, implication that the disfluencies of stuttering are spelled d-y-s, not d-i-s. If stuttering is an organic problem genetically transmitted, then, conceivably, it should be subject to medical treatment, provided we could ever track down the components of the speaking system that are dysfunctional. The possibility that this component is the larynx has had several of us baying in pursuit. I lost enthusiasm for this chase a few years ago, however, when I found reports on a couple of stutterers who were laryngectomized and still stuttered.

May, I say, parenthetically, that we badly need hypotheses about stuttering that can be disproven, preferably with an N of 1. We're a bunch of scientific string savers. Old theories of stuttering never die; they don't even fade away. We cart them around for generations as excess baggage, presumably on the assumption that they will eventually be proven correct. But science does not proceed by proof; it proceeds by disproof. Our blackest mark as scientists is that we have failed to formulate hypotheses, let alone theories, that could be disproven with empirical evidence. We get high marks for effort and high marks for technical ingenuity, but the fact that we are still tromping around on much the same ground that has been stomped on for half a century is embarrassing. In addition, we tend to build our explanations of stuttering backwards. We have a proclivity for formulating neurophysiological models from which we speculate about their application to behavior that has not even been demonstrated to be causally related to stuttering. I am astounded that we are so thoroughly impressed with speculative physiological formulations that lead to nothing but *maybes* and *perhaps.*

In any event, if there is organic dysfunction, as there may well be at least in some stutterers, the dysfunction almost certainly involves some neural component that controls the larynx, but it is not in the larynx itself. Because we see physiological evidence of laryngeal discoordination, we seem tempted to conclude that this is evidence of organicity. In point of fact, we have no evidence of pathology. What we have is evidence of mistiming of neural control of the speech mechanism, particularly as it affects the airstream. Such evidence does not rule out organic causes, but they can just as easily be accounted for as faulty learning or noise in the neural circuitry induced by psychic stress.

EFFECTIVE-PLANNING-TIME HYPOTHESIS

Three independent analyses of the scientific evidence have led to what is essentially the same conclusion about the central problem of stuttering. Gavin Andrews and his colleagues, after analyzing virtually all of the corroborated facts of stuttering, concluded that inadequate central processing capacity is the subsoil of stuttering (1983). They hypothesize that because of diminished capacity, stutterers are limited in their ability to deal with the relationship between motor speech output and its associated feedback. In a commentary on this *tour de force,* Ray Kent reviewed these facts from a neuropsychologic perspective (1983). He concluded that conditions that induce fluency "lead to a reduction of uncertainty in the temporal pattern of speech motor control." Both of these conclusions are remarkably similar to the one my associates and I reached that we called the effective-planning-time hypothesis (Perkins, Bell, Johnson, & Stocks, 1979). We proposed that stuttering diminishes as the amount of effective planning time for phonetic-voice-onset coordinations increases.

What these conclusions have in common provide the foundation for the clinical implications that will be discussed next. If, indeed, coordination of phonetic voice onset is a basic problem for stutterers, then any condition that compensates for inability to coordinate these onsets at normally rapid speech rates should facilitate fluency. An obvious method of compensation would be to slow the speed with which transitions are made from sound to sound. Another method would be to reduce the number of physiological coordinations required. By such reduction, effective planning time for the remaining coordinations would be increased proportionately. This was the method investigated that led to the discoordination hypothesis.

Still another method of increasing effective planning time is to increase predictability of voice onset, thereby reducing the need for the planning time required if onsets were unpredictable. At least three techniques seemingly may accomplish this purpose. One is rhythm: the stronger the pattern, the more predictable the onsets. Another is frequency of voice onsets to be managed: as the number of onsets decreases, effective planning time increases for remaining onsets. The work of Adams and his colleagues (1973) shows that reducing frequency of onset does tend to reduce stuttering, but not as powerfully as the preceding compensatory techniques. Similarly, location of voice onset in a phrase could affect predictability. Those onsets between sounds within a phrase could be predicted by virtue of linguistic structure, whereas onset of the first sound in a phrase is relatively more indeterminate and should require more effective planning time. The early work of Johnson and Brown (1935), in which they found that 90% of stuttering occurred on the initial sound of a word, supports but does not confirm this possibility. Presumably, competition for phonetic planning time would be greater in phrases with complex grammar than in those with minimal linguistic structure. Evidence of this possibility is in the finding that stuttering is reduced when phrases are of one-word length (Adams et al., 1973), and that it tends to occur on accented syllables of polysyllabic words (Brown, 1938). Thus, the ground work is laid for applying this concept to therapy of stuttering.

IMPLICATIONS FOR THERAPY

If the foregoing formulation is granted, but the caution holds that this formulation has not been adequately tested, then any clinical procedure that effectively generates more time for the planning of temporal programs of speech should facilitate fluency. This theory accounts for why so many different types of therapy are

Postscript 4

effective. If confidence is linked to a sense of certainty, which seems reasonable, then anxiety and apprehension are linked to uncertainty. Conceivably, the fundamental cause of stuttering could be erosion of confidence to express oneself openly and fluently. More heretically, the "cure" of stuttering, then, would be development of confidence in oneself and in the ability to express ideas directly and fluently. Translated into neuropsychologic terms, this is equivalent to saying that stuttering develops as uncertainty in the planning and timing of spoken messages increases. Conversely, stuttering recedes as certainty of expression increases effective planning time for speech processing. Unfortunately, the evidence for this speculation is only clinical impression. I have not known many cured stutterers, but those whom I have queried invariably assign their "cure" to a sense of confidence, and their past relapses enroute to their cure to temporary loss of that confidence. None have claimed a cure from use of fluency-inducing techniques, even though use of those techniques may give them confidence that they can sound like normal speakers.

Ironically, much more is known from research about effects of fluency-inducing conditions than about effects of confidence. Prolongation of syllables is a direct method of increasing motor speech planning time; it is universally effective in establishing a fluent drone. Shortening phrase length reduces linguistic processing time, as does simplifying grammatic structure. Whispering reduces the number of phonatory coordinations to be dealt with, and rhythm provides a predictably pattern for their processing. Presumably, choral reading, shadowing, and signing reduce stuttering for these same reasons. Predictable as these conditions are as means of establishing fluency, my impression is that they work as compensatory techniques. I doubt that they are basic to the onset of stuttering, or to recovery from it. They may, however, facilitate both.

Implicit throughout this discussion is the assumption that some constitutional condition underlies stuttering. Whether it involves defective neural circuitry or mistimed neural processing in a normal mechanism is not known.

What difference does this make clinically? Mainly, it affects our expectations of how much recovery from stuttering can be anticipated and how we approach the problem of onset of stuttering. If stutterers are constitutionally limited in the facility with which they can achieve fluency, then presumably they would have to rely more heavily than normal speakers on compensatory skills, such as rate control, rhythm, and breath flow to speak fluently or stutter fluently, whichever approach you prefer. By the same token, young children beginning to speak in connected phrases would be at greater risk of having the fluent flow of speech fragmented in ways that invite the judgment of stuttering than would children whose constitutional facility for fluency is greater.

REFERENCES

Adams, M., Lewis, J., & Besozzi, T. (1973). The effect of reducing rate on stuttering frequency. *Journal of Speech and Hearing Research, 16,* 671–675.

Andrews, G., Craig, A., Feyer, A., Hoddintot, S., Howie, P., & Neilson, M. (1983). Stuttering: A review of research findings and theories, circa 1982. *Journal of Speech and Hearing Disorders, 48,* 226–246.

Brown, S. (1938). Stuttering with relation to word accent and word position. *Journal of Abnormal and Social Psychology, 33,* 112–120.

Johnson, W., & Brown, S. (1935). Stuttering in relation to various speech sounds. *Quarterly Journal of Speech, 21,* 481–496.

Kent, R. (1983). Facts about stuttering: Neurophysiological perspectives. *Journal of Speech and Hearing Disorders, 48,* 249–255.

Perkins, W. (1978). *Human perspectives in speech and language disorders.* St. Louis: C.U. Mosby.

Perkins, W. (1981). Implications of scientific research for treatment of stuttering—a lecture. *Journal of Fluency Disorders, 6:2,* 155–162.

Perkins, W., Bell, J., Johnson, L., & Stocks, J. (1979). Phone rate and the effective planning time hypothesis of stuttering, *Journal of Speech and Hearing Disorders, 22,* 747–755.

5

The Unspeakable Feelings of People with Special Reference to Stuttering

Postscript
Emotional Factors

Lee Edward Travis

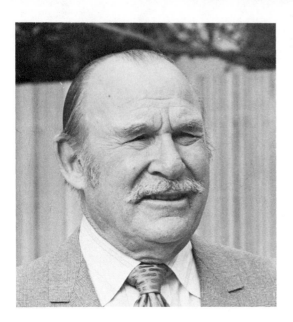

Lee Edward Travis

Lee Edward Travis has been affectionately and respectfully referred to as "the father of the profession." It is alleged that some 50 years ago he participated in a conference in an office at the State University of Iowa, surrounded by wise academicians, and became part of a conceptualization that has now come to be known as "Speech Pathology." His was a founding that went far beyond the topic of stuttering. Yet his primary focus of theorizing, research, teaching, and clinical activity has been on the problem of stuttering. It was with Travis that so many of the authorities on stuttering studied. The list is long and illustrious and includes such people as Van Riper, Johnson, and Bryngelson, to name only a few who shared Travis as their mentor.

Travis's own thinking about stuttering has ranged through cerebral dominance and genetics to learning and psychoanalysis. He combines the rigors and critical attitudes of science with a sensitivity to the meter and feelings of psychoanalytic therapy. He hears the music as well as the words of people in trouble, and combines art and science in his varied encounters with people who stutter. As Dr. Travis reviews his history for us, we easily see a willingness to change, and a responsiveness both to his own curiosity and to new information.

Travis's training and emphasis in the psychoanalytic aspects of stuttering provided a revolutionary change, not only in his own thinking, but in stuttering theory in America. The powerful impact of his chapter reprinted from the *Handbook of speech pathology,* which he also edited, can be attributed to his eloquence and to his leadership in the field, in addition to its startling content. Not only was Travis a past president of the American Speech and Hearing Association, but he was also a recognized scholar in neurophysiological research. His switch in conviction in 1957 represented a dramatic and courageous personal as well as professional change. And now, almost 30 years later, Travis again demonstrates that courage in his openness to acknowledge his doubts about the significance of the psychoanalytic view of the origin of stuttering. In this process he has, in fact, come full circle to re-embrace the neurophysiological basis for stuttering. He sees the need to differentiate the cause of stuttering from its effects on the speaker, and this has led him to see therapy as a compensatory experience that at best manages those effects. There is no cure.

5

The Unspeakable Feelings of People with Special Reference to Stuttering

Lee Edward Travis

Stuttering is the consequence of the young child speaking with his mother and father. In his words he sought their appraisal of him. In his utterances he asked to be known and to be understood. In their reply they told of his unacceptability in his current verbalized form. He would need to change, either in his deep parts or in the verbal expression of them. As he continued to talk, not knowing quite what to do about himself, he began to hesitate and to stumble a little and to repeat. Now his mother and father were no longer so critical and rejecting of him and his telling, but were actually supportively concerned. He must need their love and they would give it to him. He must need their attention and they would give that also. He did need these things, their love and their attention, but not for the reason his parents gave them, not because he stuttered.

GENERAL STATEMENTS

May I propose that stuttering is based upon an interchange between the speaker and the listener, an interaction between what is in the speaker's mouth to say and what is in his listener's ear to hear. The main troubles of the stutterer are derived from the complimentarity and mutual exclusiveness of orders of opposite sign given simultaneously by an authority. By every seemingly normal and natural appearance the parents want their child to talk early and to talk

well. It may be really that they are too ambitious for him in these areas. Yet by a frown and a glance and even by a verbal message he is asked if not ordered not to talk now, or that way, or about that subject matter. As the parents and the child define a relationship between them they work out together what type of communicative behavior is to take place in the relationship.

In the beginning of speech in the child, was not speech meant to be pure impulse perfect in every motion like the walk of the cat? The child did not know that he talked, let alone how he talked. One day his mother called his attention to his speech, however, and he knew for the first time that he talked, and never again would he not know that he knew. From then on he was responsible, and possibly terribly responsible, too responsible for his speech revelations. He was initiated young into the monitored ways of life and his confidence and simplicity were checked. Something had gone wrong, something possibly undefined, but something in some way was his fault; he had done it. He was to blame. He was responsible. From now on he must make speech happen. No longer or ever again will it just happen of itself. He must through pain of thinking and choice decide the course of his declarations. Always now he will move with some anxiety, because he can never know what is right and when something will go deeply and strangely wrong.

Stuttering may be considered as an advertisement

Note: From L. E. Travis "The Unspeakable Feelings of People with Special Reference to Stuttering" in HANDBOOK OF SPEECH PATHOLOGY AND AUDIOLOGY, L. E. Travis, Ed., © 1971, pp. 1009–1033. Reprinted by permission of Prentice-Hall, Inc., Englewood Cliffs, N.J.

of some form and degree of placing the speaker under taboo (Frank, 1961). In stuttering, the speaker is experiencing an interdiction laid upon his performance in saying words to another. In his speech blocks he is signaling his ostracism imposed upon him by his company of listeners. Stuttering is a special case of the universal conflict between closeness and distance, involvement and autonomy, intimacy and autism. His experiments in closeness have been too painful to stand and he has suffered a reaction of self-banishment. He has settled for a minimum relatedness which does not include free talking about his thoughts and feelings. Rightly or wrongly he has interpreted the responses of another as adversive.

In a significant way parents place the child in a paradoxical position in teaching him to talk. Conflicting levels of message occur when the verbal statements of parents qualify their tone of voice, body movement, or contextual situation incongruently (Haley, 1963). Stuttering is the reciprocal to the parents' verbal requests. They ask the verbal symptom of their child, thereby participating in its appearance and its maintenance. Their verbal demands contain qualifications of themselves. Saying this another way, the parents teach the child how (by his stuttering) to circumscribe their management of his behavior, particularly of his verbal behavior. Stuttering is thus responsive behavior occurring in an interpersonal context. It will not stop on command because it is a style of maneuvering other people, although the results may be stressful to everybody.

Like all other developmental deviations, stuttering tends to be self-perpetuating. The interpersonal pattern between child and parent that flowered the stuttering originally trained the stutterer to prefer his stuttering relationship with other people as well. His experiences with all people continually confirm his stuttering reactions to them, for his stuttering is not dependent only upon an intrapsychic deviation, but also upon current interpersonal experience. Between people who speak and those who listen, stuttering tells of excuses and explanations in the preservation of the speaker's self-esteem. The symptom is the advantage enjoyed by the stutterer in gaining control of what is to happen in a relationship with someone else. The obvious trouble in speaking may represent considerable distress to the stutterer subjectively, but much distress is preferred to living in an unpredictable world of social relationships over which he may otherwise have little or no control.

In the control of a relationship stuttering is symptomatic because neither the stutterer nor the listener necessarily senses this to be true. On the contrary, the stutterer circumscribes the behavior of the listener while denying that he is doing so. The stutterer denies responsibility in the control of the listener, but nonetheless controls him, blaming his control on something else, the stuttering, over which he insists he has no control. Stuttering is assured since parents and others, including speech therapists, dance to the stutterer's tune of stuttering and thereby perpetuate his stuttering behavior. What works now started the stuttering in the first place. The start was when the child speaker was told either implicitly or explicitly by his parents to try to say something that he had been told not to say. And he would never be quite clear what it was that received such paradoxical treatment. What exactly was it that he should and should not say? His guilt was all the more disquieting since the nature of his crime was usually unstated. "You know what I mean," "you know very well what you have done," "you know why I punish you," "we both know your problem," are all common statements to the child facing reprimand. He has an obscure and gnawing sense of being profoundly in the wrong, though for no discernible reason. May he avoid if possible the feeling that his very existence is an affrontery to his parents and even to others. Finally, may he avoid the feeling that just to be alive is both a fault and his own fault.

THE CORE PHENOMENON OF STUTTERING[1]

Neurophysiologically, speech is a modification of expiration. In the organism at rest, normal breathing movements consist of an active inspiration followed by a passive expiration. It is evident, however, that with speech, an inspiration which is always active is followed also by an *active* expiration. The speaker regulates the rate and amount of expiration and properly modifies it to form sounds and sound combinations to suit best the purposes of his speaking. In modifying the outgoing breath stream for goals of vocalization and articulation, the speaker does one es-

[1]This section, The Core Phenomenon of Stuttering, and the next section, Stuttering as Learned Behavior, are based upon the author's article, A Theoretical Formulation of Stuttering, which appeared in *Western Speech,* 23, Summer, 1959.

sential thing—for varying periods of time he partially or completely obstructs this breath stream by the partial or complete approximation of juxtaposed structures in the pathway of the outgoing air column. The primary structures used in this process of modification are the vocal cords, tongue, velum, hard palate, alveolar ridge, teeth, and lips. In one sense, these structures used in relationship to each other present a series of air valves which may completely or partially block the passage of air. The movements of these and other structures in proper temporal and spatial relationship to each other constitute the so-called speech movements—the movements necessary for the production of speech sounds. When the speaker is performing normally, the alteration and control of the outgoing breath stream are appropriate to the intention of communication.

As we have noted, the speaker is constantly blocking the outgoing breath stream in various degrees and for varying lengths of time. The length and completeness of the blocks determine, partially at least, the rate and rhythm of speech. If juxtaposed structures, such as the vocal cords, back of the tongue and velum, middle of the tongue and hard palate, tongue tip and upper front teeth, upper front teeth and lower lip, or the two lips were to continue the approximation beyond certain time limits, speech would be altered in rate and rhythm. Some sounds would be prolonged if the approximation of juxtaposed structures were of the improper length for the production of that sound, and other sounds would be completely absent if the approximation of the juxtaposed structures involved was complete. For example, if a speaker continued the correct approximation of the structures involved in the formation of (s) beyond the desired or standard time limit, a continuous hissing sound would be produced. If, on the other hand, he carried the approximation of these same structures too far, made a complete block and held it, then no sound at all would be forthcoming.

These examples pertain to the prolongation or the complete blocking of a single sound. The repetition of a sound, a syllable, a word, or even of a phrase may occur as an expression of the same fundamental overmodifying process. May it be concluded, then, that the core of the phenomenon known as stuttering may be conceived neurophysiologically as an overmodification of the outgoing breath stream by a series of air valves? This overmodification is, essentially, a prolongation of the proper degree of approximation of juxtaposed structures or a prolongation of the complete approximation of these structures, resulting in varying degrees and kinds of blocking of the forward flow of speech. The stutterer experiences a perseveration or an exaggeration, or both, of the functioning of the speech valves. It is as though he were unable to manage the air stream by means of these valves; they close too tightly, or too long, or repetitively in violation of his purposes. Crudely, the defect may be described as "sticky valves." To the discomforture of the stutterer the valves stick. This is unintentional or involuntary, and it interferes with and interrupts the stutterer's management of the valves. When it is occurring, the stutterer may struggle with it and manifest the well-known secondary symptoms. After this uncontrollable sticking has occurred sufficiently often in interpersonal relationships, the stutterer establishes anticipatory reactions to possible future occurrences. As a consequence of the anticipatory, current, and consequent reactions, a whole constellation of thoughts, feelings, and acts are built around the core phenomenon of "sticky valves." Thoughts of suicide, feelings of inadequacy, and acts of grimacing are family members of this constellation.

The word "stuttering" then can be used to denote the overmodification of the outgoing breath stream by a series of air valves. It would seem that explanations of anticipatory, current, and consequent reactions to the nuclear phenomenon are not too difficult. Although the core phenomenon itself is difficult to explain etiologically, we shall concentrate our main efforts to do just that.

STUTTERING AS LEARNED BEHAVIOR

The basic assumption is made that stuttering is established and maintained by learning. According to current learning theory as I am able to understand it (Hilgard and Bower, 1966), this assumption appears to be logically tenable. Too, in paying deference to learning as a psychoneurological process, one is paying deference to psychology, and to glands, nerves, and muscles; in short, to psychophysical issues. In the simplest possible statement, some cue or set of cues is bound with stuttering in such a way that the appearance of the cue evokes the stuttering. The process binding the cue and the stuttering response is gearlike. The following formula should clarify this:

(1) Cue (listener, real or imaginary) → Activation of unadmitted feelings and thoughts → Fear of the revelation of these inadmissibles → Defense against revelation of these inadmissibles (stuttering) → Reactions to stuttering (secondary stuttering).

On occasion, possibly on many occasions, the stutterer will want to talk, to say or reveal some thoughts or feelings to another person. He will want to tell his mother something, something of his observations or feelings; and in these instances the communication process originates from within; the process has an intrapsychic origin. On other occasions the sight, sound, or presence of his mother or her verbal relationships with him will stimulate him to talk to her. The communication process now has an interpsychic origin. In the first example, the drive or need or anxiousness to speak may arouse the unadmitted feelings and ideas which, in turn, would arouse the fear of them, the fear of their revelation, and the child will honor the fear and defend against the threat of telling by saying nothing. This idea may be expressed in the following formula:

(2) Need or desire to communicate → Activation of unadmitted thoughts and feelings → Fear of revelation of these inadmissibles → Defense against the revelation of these inadmissibles (silence) → Shyness, delayed speech, unsociability (secondary symptoms).

Although clinically we consider this second child to be a delayed-speech case, in a sense he is a stutterer. Under pressure to talk, from both within and without, his symptom may change, superficially, from speechlessness or delayed or unintelligible speech to stuttering as a defense. Whether the first factor in formulae (1) and (2) is intrapsychic or interpsychic, the defense is the same: a defense, silence or stuttering, against the revelation of feared thoughts and feelings.

Although the stimulus to speak may be an inner desire (intrapsychic), it may lead to the cue (another person) that in turn starts the chain reaction leading to stuttering. This idea may be formulated as follows:

(3) Need or desire to communicate → Cue-producing response (noting another person) → Activation of unadmitted thoughts and feelings → Fear of revelation of these inadmissibles → Defense against revelation of these inadmissibles (stuttering).

The real significance of the cue (parent, sibling, friend, teacher, lover, anybody, or any number of people) is its vigilance. It must first of all be alive (stutterers have little, if any, trouble addressing inanimate objects); in addition it needs to be human (stutterers have little or no trouble addressing animals); and finally, and above all, it needs to listen. The listener is the trigger for most stuttering. Possibly the deeper meaning of listening is that it implies understanding, discovery, and detection on the part of the listener of that which may lead to punishment and condemnation of what was understood about the speaker. Notoriously, the stutterer is relatively untroubled when speaking in unison with others where everyone is talking and no one is listening. Conversely he is troubled, relatively very much, before an audience where everybody listens and only he speaks. The audience multiplies the danger that the speaker will be found out. The stutterer may have trouble even when speaking alone, for he is speaking to an imaginary listener, or listeners, or to himself. We must realize that a speaker is also his own listener and at times his most vigilant one, affording an evaluation often more severely critical than that afforded by others. So regardless of whether the vigilance is from within or from without, we hold it to be the provocation of stuttering.

Too, we believe that stuttering itself—the overmodification of the outgoing breath stream—is not, in the ordinary sense, learned by the child or taught by the parents. The stutterer does not "imitate" the stuttering of others. He never hears it, or hears it so infrequently in relation to relatively fluent speech, that to assign any importance to the idea that stuttering is learned by empathizing with other stutterers is absurd. Equally absurd is the thought that parents or siblings give the young speech-learner examples of stuttering to imitate. Even those few stuttering parents whom we know have little or no difficulty in communicating verbally with their children. Stated more technically in terms of learning theory, parents do not make stuttering speech as such worthwhile. It is not rewarded and hence learned in this simple fashion. Instead parents actually punish stuttering; or more accurately, they punish the child for stuttering almost as though it were a naughty act. Yet stuttering occurs in the first place without example, and more puzzling still keeps on occurring, even increasing in frequency and severity without example, and without obvious reinforcement. The answer to this enigma is to be found in the stand that stuttering is not an excitatory ore release response, but an inhibitory one, and that the punishment it incurs is less than the punishment the inhibited response would have received had it not been inhibited. In this sense stuttering is rewarded, relatively, as being the lesser of two pains. The stutterer accepts the punishment for his stuttering in order that he will not receive a greater punishment for speaking the truth. Punishment of stuttering is a reward for not revealing the guilty secrets which one has judged to be dangerously threatening. Punishment of stuttering may make the stuttering worse as a symptom to the listener but really better to the speaker in the sense of developing it as a defense. This is to say that stuttering when punished is a success (reward) in that it keeps the punitive agents off the track of the really dreaded feelings and thoughts seeking expression through speech. The more severe and the more obvious this camouflage (stuttering) becomes, even by being attacked and condemned, the more effective it will be in reducing the fear and anxiety cued by the arousal of the real culprits—hate, lust, exhibitionism, voyeurism, etc. Punishment and even certain kinds of would-be therapy may increase the tendency for the punished act (stuttering) to occur, since in a real sense stuttering is being rewarded thereby, in shifting the vigilance of the listener (self or another) away from the detection of the really dreaded feelings and thoughts of the speaker.

Current theory presumes that drives, feelings, and thoughts seek release through responses. When these responses, including speech, are punished, fear will be learned and will act consequently to motivate its own responses to keep these punished acts from occurring. Now the person has two opposing sets of drive response dynamics. One set is composed of a wish, a feeling, or a thought and an appropriate response for the realization of the wish, feeling, or thought. The other set is composed of the fear of the appropriate response and some response for the realization of the fear. More concretely, the child has a wish, feeling, or thought to express verbally. He speaks his mind and is punished for doing so. The pain scares him, scares him for speaking simply and plainly what he felt and thought. He is now trapped. He is caught in a dilemma. If he wants to say something and cannot for fear of being punished, what is he to do when both the need to speak and the fear of speaking either persist throughout the day or are being activated constantly by his surroundings? If he speaks he is punished and frightened. If he does not

speak he is frustrated. Either condition is, relatively speaking, untenable. There is, however, a way out: a compromise between speaking the truth and keeping silent. He can guard, monitor, and screen carefully his verbal output, to honor somewhat both the need to speak his mind and the fear of speaking it.

The responses motivated by fear have a central core of flight. To reduce the fear which produces an unpleasant tension one seeks to separate himself from the fear-producing stimulus. The separation need not always mean fleeing literally from something. At important times it may mean the inhibition of acts, including thoughts and feelings, that may lead to something. One need not always retire from a frightful situation; one may simply inhibit the thoughts and feelings about it and remain there physically. In a manner of speaking the thoughts and feelings flew away, were chased away, or possibly more revealing still, one flew away from them. Of the many ways to think about the significance of stuttering, in a real sense it is a partial success at telling the truth and simultaneously a partial success at silence. Tragically, in the end one learns to fear his own wants, feelings, and thoughts, and he acts to flee from them or to destroy their expression by various means, including stuttering. The conflictual relationship between responses motivated by such drives as aggression, sex, and messing, and those motivated by fear intensifies the struggle of all drives for expression and leaves the host in possession of soil fertile for the fostering of symptomatic behavior.

Possibly too obviously we have not come to grips with today's most perplexing question about stuttering—its selection by the child as his choice of symptom. Why exactly does anybody, the child in his early days and the adult in his more mature ways, tell everyone of his troubled soul by settling for such a personally and socially handicapping means as stuttering? Why does not this child, along with all children, reveal his misgivings about himself in some other language—in enuresis, asthma, lying, or stealing. He could wet in the dark, wheeze behind a cold, or lie or steal in relative inconspicuousness. But he must always stutter in public, in plain sight and sound of a vigilant listener. In some way and by somebody who mattered dearly he must have been convinced that the cost of stuttering was relatively reasonable. Some extremely significant person told him so clearly by word, by inflection and quality of voice, by lifting an eyebrow, by a pained expression, by seeking a speech teacher, or by some other unmistakable sign that what now was perceived only as nonfluency, but what later would come to be known as stuttering, had a peculiarly misleading value. Three absolutely necessary ingredients had to be present simultaneously to form stuttering: fearfully disavowed thoughts and feelings, nonfluency, and a diagnostician. The expanded concept may be expressed in the following formula:

(4) Need to speak (internally or externally aroused) → Activation of disavowed feelings and thoughts → Fear of these feelings and thoughts → Non-fluency → Internalization of diagnosis of stuttering → Stuttering.

When a child is convinced that his parents are convinced that he is just stuttering, then a certain relief follows in the stuttering. The stuttering is misleading the diagnostician and successfully serving the purpose of obscuring, if not entirely covering, the really dreaded preoccupations with speaking the truth. Really stuttering is a manifestation of a fear to speak the truth to oneself or about oneself to another. It occurs most frequently in those families that place a high premium upon the truth and then punish its verbalization. To the extent that a child can be self-conscious comfortably, he will not stutter.

THE PEOPLE OF THIS STUDY

This chapter reports a picture of some people obtained from the psychotherapeutic situation. The therapist is given a unique opportunity to view and to experience the mental life of another person who is in the throes of a struggle to solve vital intrapsychic and interpersonal problems. The psychotherapeutic relationship affords a naturalistic approach to an increased understanding of the magnificent mental processes of man. Before some of the manifestations of these processes, the therapist stands in awe and in humility. Before others he stands in sheer ignorance. Even at a time when there are those who feel that little is left to learn in therapy, the present writer believes that only an humble beginning to an immensely significant approach to humanity's problems has been made. It seems true that some main highways have been cut through the forest, but it seems equally true that untold riches remain as mysterious as ever away and beyond the beaten paths.

Some people have enough misery to drive them to enter into therapeutic negotiations. In their misery they have sufficiently high motivation to get them to talk long enough and honestly enough to explore the wonderfully intricate details of themselves in relatedness. Imagine the average person who is indistinguishable from the mine-run of people spending three or four hours a week for two to three years talking freely and almost interminably about himself. He just would not do it because he has no need or motivation to do it. Mainly, he is not miserable enough. Then, too, there will have to be someone who has the motivation and the patience to listen for all of these hours and months and years, one who has the training and experience to understand and accept what he hears.

In most instances where human behavior is studied, in the laboratory, at the party, in the parlor, motives are slight and the situation is trivial. In psychotherapy just the opposite is true. Not only are motives strong, but the situation is crucial. For the patient it is either a continued life of sickening anxiety and misery or a new life of peace and happiness. Such urgency brings every resource of the patient and therapist into play in the interpersonal relationship of therapy where the patient will reveal and sense himself more completely than he ever has in the past and more than he ever will again in the presence of another. The patient must tell all and the therapist must cope with the most vexing and vital issues of interpersonal relationships.

The label of "patient" misleads many people. For the purpose of this chapter, the patient is one who is so anxious and miserable that he seeks help. According to other criteria, he may not be as maladjusted as others who do not go into therapy, but the way *he* sees and feels himself makes him a patient. Our patients should not be considered basically different from other people. Rather, they are a group of people who differ from other people in the degree of motivation for psychotherapy.

The clearest common feature of the people we studied was misery. In a way and to a degree they were all miserable. Their misery was enough to drive them to seek help. They expressed their misery in the various complaints of irrational fears and anxieties, stage fright, distaste for life, homosexuality, sexual frigidity, alcoholism, primary hypertension, asthma, ulcer, and stuttering. Some had more of one complaint than another, but all were miserable. In a word, their lives did not agree with them. Psychological burps and belches threatened to expose their emotional indigestion.

Actually 65 people were studied, and their productions and reactions form the basis for the materials of this chapter. These people were observed in the psychotherapeutic situation for a total of approximately 13,000 hours. Some were seen for as little as 10 hours and some for as much as 400 hours. The average number of hours was about 200. Thirty of these people complained mainly of stuttering. Thirty-five complained of the other conditions listed above. Further breakdown of these people seems unnecessary for the main theme of this chapter. All of these people were adults ranging in age from 16 to 50 years. There were 27 females and 38 males.

Our special respect will be paid to those 30 individuals who complained of stuttering. Most of them felt severely handicapped in speech, and not only undertook therapy but persisted in the therapeutic relationship up to 400 hours for some individual cases. Some stutterers for one reason or another, including insufficient motivation, discontinued therapy early. No statistical comparisons will be made between those who came for stuttering and those who came for some other reason, such as homosexuality or sexual frigidity. Some broad comparisons will be noted and evaluated, mainly to stimulate further study rather than to draw any final conclusions.

We are impressed with the obvious: that stutterers are human beings and that as such they have a great deal in common with other people, even in the manner of speaking. Both introspective and objective observations convince us that most people stutter. Only a few people are sufficiently miserable over their speaking relationships, however, that they bring their problem to therapy under the label of stuttering.

THE OLD CONDITIONS OF LEARNING

A symptom is a remark about the culture in which that symptom developed. It is a reflection upon the nurturing influences of the home and community in which the person was reared. According to his lights, the patient was right in adopting a response or a set of responses known as a symptom. He found along the way that to react symptomatically reduced drives and tensions. His symptom was thus rewarded or reinforced, and in this sense learned (Dollard and Miller, 1950, p. 15).

Our people came to us because of what happened to their basic needs and drives as they grew from birth. Originally, *in utero,* their environment was relatively perfectly comfortable and complete. It met relatively perfectly and completely their growing demands. There were no discomforts, deficiencies, or frustrations. And then they were born: physically, mentally, and emotionally helpless. They were extremely weak in every way but one, the need to live. Their desire to eat, to eliminate, to breathe, and to be comfortable was great. Their means of satisfying these living needs were utterly dependent upon those who cared for them. Their very existence was entirely at the mercy of their elders, at the mercy of the physical, emotional, intellectual, economic, and social conditions of the adult giants around them. Only in infancy and childhood were our people's own capacities to control their lives so meager, ineffectual, and pitiful.

It ought not to be surprising, then, that acute emotional conflicts occurred in the earliest days of our people. These people, as children, had no tolerance for delay of the satisfaction of their needs. They could not yet learn to wait, to reason, to hope, to plan. Rather, they were compelled by all-consuming drives, tensions, and discomforts to action—crying, twisting, flaying. They could not think, talk, or reason, or control either themselves or their environment. Between them and their adult teachers was a tremendous gap. They had to be fed, picked up, hauled around, cleaned, and protected. And how were these things done? Here was the critical issue. At this time what may be done for good or for bad may never be undone. What was lacking may never be made up. What pain was given may never again be taken completely away. These possibly tumultuous interpersonal relationships furnished the soil for unverbalized and hence unconscious emotional conflicts. Only when these people learned to talk and to think could the impact of these circumstances be reduced.

Had our people, as helpless children, been handled with the greatest indulgence, they would not have served as subjects of this chapter. Could they have had the greatest support from parents during the earliest weeks, months, and years of their lives, they would not have stuttered. Their savage drives should have been kept at the lowest possible level by the attentiveness of their parents. Every supportively encouraging effort should have been made by the parents to teach the child to talk and to think in order that he might in turn learn to wait, hope, reason, and plan.

But the parents of our people did not keep the strongest drives of their children at a low level of urgency and they did not know how or they did not resolve to impose the burdens of a civilized life in a tolerable and reasonable way. Instead our people, as children, were treated as emotional and intellectual little adults. Adult powers to control their drives and feelings were assumed. Incompatible demands were made and utterly impossible checks and tasks were set. Unlearned and at times unlearnable discriminations were expected. Heavy sanctions were applied for mistakes and failures.

The conditions of the stutterer's early life created his stuttering. They proved hostile and painful to the expression, verbal and otherwise, of his drives, and he feared rejection and punishment if he tried honestly to express himself. He feared criticism of his true thoughts and words. He felt that others expected him to be unbearably good in thought and in word. Too, through his failure to be received for what he was, he had suffered wounds to his self-esteem. He had generalized from specific, unacceptable thoughts and words to the unacceptability of himself as a whole. Not only were his expressions unworthy, but he himself was unworthy as well. His old repressions were continually reinforced by the current contempt of others. No one understood him and he was not capable of understanding himself. In listening to their stuttering child, parents might have felt deservedly miserable in realizing that they were listening to themselves.

Stuttering may be defined as an advertisement of strong, dimly admitted motives of which the stutterer is deeply ashamed. Repression falls on the verbal expression of these motives and may fall on all words and sentences lest they might lead to these motives. When any person stutters, he is blocking something else besides what you and he might think he is trying to say; something else that is pressing for verbal expression but which will be intolerable to you and to him alike should it be uttered.

A SKETCH OF SOME OLDER TRAINING SITUATIONS

With our stutterers, the culture took a position on their various infant and child needs. It took the position, a traditional one, that their drives should be tamed relatively early and firmly. This was accomplished mainly by setting up in the child, fear, shame, and guilt in opposition to drives, urges, and wants. This opposition of forces, such as fear against drive, resulted in dilemmas which produced acute emotional conflicts. Then our people as children inhibited many cue-producing responses which would have mediated thinking, feeling, and talking. In short, they repressed the conflicts. Unfortunately, this learned management of conflicts (repression) did not solve the dilemmas permanently. The emotional paralysis of repression had to be continually maintained in the face of environmental factors which kept threatening to reactivate the conflicts. As these situational stimuli pecked away at these children, rewarding drive one time and fear another, the children were constantly taxed to keep the painful and anxiety-producing conflicts low. One manifestation or advertisement of this taxing effort was stuttering. Before the eyes and ears of their parents, our people showed in stuttering speech the operation of opposing feelings: sexual curiosity and the shame of it, hostility and the fear of it, and desire to mess and the embarrassment over it.

Possibly there are innumerable ways and combinations of ways by which society imposes its will through the acts of the parents. Yet it seems clear that we can group these ways into a certain limited number of clusters. We may be accused of overemphasizing these relatively few situations. Our excuse for seeming to do so is that the situations listed are clinically and experimentally documented (Travis and Baruch, 1941, Ch. 7; Dollard and Miller, 1950, Ch. 10). Certainly our general thesis will not be altered by substituting or adding other situations.

Crying

Crying is the child's first powerful response. It is assumed to be a response to some need or discomfort. The baby's or child's cry is also a powerful stimulus to its elders, producing empathically anxiety in the mothering ones (Sullivan, 1953, Ch. 3). It amounts to a demand or command upon those who are in a position of responsibility to the child. The culture takes the position that a child should not cry, at least not much. The members of the culture vary in their ways of meeting this position, and the way it is met determines important habits and traits in the child.

Crying may be thought of as the first cue-producing response. Its purpose is to attract stimuli that will relieve tension. In general, it should be honored as the one simple thing the child can do to get results and as the first small unit in the child's control of the world. Not to reward or reinforce crying is to teach the child that there is nothing it can do to relieve tensions, discomforts, and pain of the moment. Such training may lay the foundation for apathy and not trying something else, such as speech, when in need or in trouble. Too frequently a child is recognized only when its cry is violent. It may learn from this to respond all out of proportion to its needs and to become excessively demanding. It will fail to learn such discriminations as small needs are met by smaller demands. Possibly most important of all, when a child is left to "cry itself out" or is slapped for crying, it may learn too well that it is unloved and unwanted and that its world, the parents or family, is hostile and spiteful. Further, the fear, anxiety, and hostility existing with the futile crying will become associated with the original need for crying; to the darkness, the isolation of the nursery, the absence of parental stimuli, and other current things, acts, and relationships. So the child may become anxious when hungry (the original drive for crying), afraid of the dark or of quietness, nervous or angry when left alone, and so on. And as it grows, the parents may complain of a shy, or apathetic, or excessively demanding, or retarded and inhibited child, and later on of a socially handicapped adolescent and adult. To cry when in need, when hurt, lonely and devastated, and to fail to get available help will leave long and lasting adverse effects.

Feeding

Hunger is probably the strongest living need. Everything else depends upon the satisfaction of the hunger drive, which is an urgent, incessant, all-consuming, and timeless force producing intense activation. In the early years of life, the hunger drive and the strong responses it excites are completely incompatible with the child's ability to cope with them. He is utterly dependent upon somebody else for the management of his problem. He cannot wait, or talk to himself, or hope, or plan. He can only cry, now.

The culture takes a stand here, too. Mainly it is that the child shall be fed, but fed predetermined amounts of food, on schedule. In addition, the child shall be fed, but only under certain conditions (i.e., being alone, or after being good, or only if he will eat quickly and neatly). For rigid cultural standards governing the satisfaction of the hunger drive, the child has little or no tolerance. He cannot tell time. He cannot distract himself with feelings and thoughts and words about the future. He cannot understand the meaning of delay, or the limited amount of milk, or the conditions of its forthcoming. But he is acquiring much important learning. He may be learning that effort, particularly vocal effort, does not pay. He may learn that he is not wanted or loved. He may learn to fear the dark or being alone. He may learn to "over-react" because he is fed only after his most violent responses. On the other hand, the feeding experience can be the occasion for the child to learn to like others and to be with them; to learn that he is desirable and wanted; to learn that his needs are appreciated; and to learn that his reactions, particularly his vocal ones, are helpful. The seemingly "natural" and innocuous feeding situation is fraught with important and emotional consequences. Too many people, including parents, do not see this. They see little if anything at all to worry them. Yet observant students may see the child becoming apathetic, apprehensive, and shy, and failing to develop appropriate verbal skills. The tragedy is that much of this learning is secret. The child cannot label the experiences which it is having at this time. It cannot talk about them or talk them out. It portrays them in ways that we label as apathy, or speechlessness, or fearfulness, or sociability, or confidence. What was not labeled and not verbalized at these early times cannot well be reported later. In therapy only shadows and echoes of these early and deep feelings appear. Patient and therapist glimpse only their contrails. They emerge mutely interwoven into the fabric of conscious expression.

Toilet and Cleanliness Training

Although possibly not as strong as the hunger drive, the drive to eliminate is nevertheless persistent and commanding and at times takes precedence over every other need. Bowel and bladder tensions may exert a priority right upon the interests and efforts of the organism.

The child begins with an innocent interest in his feces and urine. He may handle and play with fecal material. There is no evidence of an innate revulsion toward the acts or the products of elimination. Quickly, in some instances during the first few months of life, his natural and naive eliminative behavior runs into the cultural patterns lying in wait. These patterns will demand that he deposit his excretory materials only in a prescribed and secret place and that he keep his body clean in doing so.

These patterns will demand, too, that he limit to the bare essentials any verbal reference to these issues so that this subject matter is closed out and excluded from social reference for life.

More often than not, instead of the child being led gently and supportively by example into meeting the cultural goals of elimination and cleanliness, it is doused with hostile, punitive, and loathing parental attitudes when it displays its naiveté or fails to honor cultural demands. The culture sets its task as the building within the personality of the child barriers of loathing and disgust for urine and feces. To construct these inward barriers, the child must put himself in a conflict situation. He must pit one set of feelings against another set. He must desire and loathe the same thing at the same time. A swelling bladder or bowel produces a strong drive that the child wishes to honor. The pain of losing the parents' love and of their punishment if he does honor this drive naturally places the child in a state of great anxiety. To salvage something from this dilemma, the child has to turn on the drive or on the parents or both. This management of a conflict situation is loaded with possible future emotional sickishness. If he turns on the drive with fear, loathing, and disgust, he will repress it in certain ways and to certain degrees. In the future he may become constipated, he may cry when eliminative demands call him, or he may become afraid of the toilet itself. If he turns on the parents, he may become defiant and stubborn, or furtive and sneaking, or attempt struggling with them, or possibly resort to biting and slapping them.

Whatever course or combination of courses the child may select to follow in the face of harsh and hasty toilet and cleanliness training, he will be the loser. On the basis of a pursuing, all-seeing, punishing parent, the child may be making as few responses as possible, certainly not adventuring forth. Being unable to discriminate between parental loathing for his penis and anus and their excreta, and loathing for himself, he adopts feelings of unworthiness, insignificance, and hopeless sinfulness. These feelings and reactions are of particular interest to the speech pathologist. Any child laden with guilt, fear of its guardian, loathing for its excretory organs and their functions, and feelings of wretched awfulness cannot be expected to acquire and risk verbal, adventuresome communication. It has too much that it must not talk about. It will learn to speak less well or not at all because it does not remain close and warm and free in a give-and-take relationship to those very people who could teach it to talk well.

Sex Training

Sex is an ever-recurring conflict element. Hourly feelings, reactions, and words confirm this statement. This is not so because sex is the strongest drive. Certainly under specific circumstances, pain, fear, and hunger outrank it. Even some secondary drives such as ambition and pride can be stronger than sex. It appears that sex is so universally implicated because it is so universally attacked and inhibited. In no other instance is an individual asked to block completely the expression of such a strong drive for such a long period of time; the culture demands for all practical purposes a completely sexless child.

Conscience and custom weigh most heavily upon sex. Too many people do not guess that children have a sex life and that guilt and shame are a crushing burden to lay on a child's mind. But the guilt will not always crush or hold. Although there are taboos which dare not be broken, children and adults learn interesting ways to break them. They lie or cheat; become impotent or inverted; develop anesthesia or paralysis; and speak not at all or block in their attempts at verbal utterance. It is around sex that the culture builds its biggest moral junk pile. Sex, or rather its place, has been cast in the leading role in interpersonal relationships. Society is split into boy and girl, man and woman, male and female, masculinity and femininity. Sex typing become inextricably involved with sex rejection and sex acceptance. Is the baby a boy or a girl; is the child a sissy or a tomboy; is the adult a homosexual or a lesbian? That there is such wondering is telltale.

Cultural management of sex often ends in the greatest misgivings that the individual can have in regard to himself and others. His sexual feelings can come to evoke intense anxiety. They can come to arouse loathing and nausea for his sexual anatomy and physiology. They can lead him into feared relationships with others where defensively he may close up and escape. The individual can come to despise and reject parts of himself and to generalize from the parts to the whole.

The extensions of his feelings may become puzzling if not amazing. Because of masturbation taboos he may dread to be alone. Because of homosexual taboos he may be afraid of men. Because of incest taboos he may be fearful of women. These fears may lead him to be afraid to be. And even if he should try, he will have trouble in talking his way out. His teachers have been niggardly about giving him names for sexual organs, sexual feelings, and sexual acts. What names they may have given him were powerfully emotionally loaded. But, anyway, he was harshly intimidated relative to talking or feeling or thinking about sex at all. It became remote, inscrutable, and maleficent. Some way or other, though, he did learn something. He did acquire some words and thoughts. When they occurred to him, however, especially when the possibility of doing anything about them occurred to him, his conflict was keener both by arousing drives and by cueing off the anxiety attached to them. He was pained when he thought about sexual matters and relieved when he stopped. The result was repression. This was just not good management. The person was victimized. He lost, possibly forever, the opportunity to use higher mental activities in solving conflicts involving sex and authority. In the future he could see the unreasonableness of his sexual inadequacies and his crippled interpersonal relationships based upon those ineptnesses, but he could not do anything about them. No amount of reasoning, or logic, or pleading helped. Some people find that help through the renaming and reestablishment and reevaluation of these bygone feelings and events can come only by succeeding in the weary work of psychotherapy. Some people find in therapy that sex conflicts lurk behind the all-too-innocent appearing speech block. They may also find it possible to accept cheerfully and amiably a degree of authority and threat without the defensive measure of stuttering.

Anger-Fear Situation

We may assume that anger responses are produced by the innumerable and unavoidable frustration situations of child life (Dollard, Doob, Miller, and Sears, 1939). We could certainly recommend a regimen of child care to minimize frustration situations, but our big quarrel here is with the management of anger responses when they do occur. Society takes a firm and consistent stand toward the responses of anger in inhibiting them by fear and pain and allowing them reign only in a few circumstances of play and self-defense. Parents resent and fear the anger and rage of a child; and the culture, since it is dominated by parents, accepts and even rewards the virtuous chastisement of the rebellious youngster. Possibly it would not be so harmful if anger and anger alone could be inhibited or extinguished by fear and pain. But universally anger is associated with toilet and cleanliness training, eating, sleeping, sex, and all the other learning situations in the home. So we come to have such combinations as anal and oral sadism, and sex-

ualized agression. The fear and pain that was meant for the anger and its responses became attached to all feelings, drives, thoughts, and words that were in the child's consciousness at the time. Too, those people and things and relationships that were present became connected to the fear and anxiety responses of the child. Thus fear and anxiety became attached not only to anger, but to all the other emotional responses which the child might have been making at the time, and to all the cues of the situation in which the responses were occurring. After this learning has occurred, the cues produced by any emotion of anger may set off anxiety responses which will outstrip not only the emotional responses of anger themselves but all the associated feelings and emotions. This produces conflict, and repression results to relieve the situation. When anger with its partners in pluralistic marriage is repressed, it is constantly exposed to reactivation, and as it stirs to subject the person to pain and humiliation, the counterforces of fear and guilt arise to hold it down. Among other evidences of this fear is stuttering, the inhibition of speaking for fear of revealing anger and its several associates.

Summary of Some Older Training Situations

We have sketched some training situations where conflicts abound in our culture. In these situations particularly, the child's drives meet frustration, condemnation, and derogation. At first, the conflicts are between the wanting child and society, especially his parents. The conflict is quickly internalized, however; it is between two of the child's incompatible drives or between the two contradictory sets of responses to these drives. Parents and the culture instill fear, anxiety, shame, and the need to please in the child to block his sex, anger, and messing responses. Thus their child comes to own pairs of conflicting motives, drives, and responses. He will have such pairs as sex-anxiety, anger-fear, and messing-shame. Society is on the side of the second member of each pair. It not only induces anxiety, fear, and shame; it acts to perpetuate them. These feelings are not pleasant to the child. They are unpleasant. They are to be avoided. But how? It appears that the child need make only one response to relieve or reduce his fear and anxiety: *stop thinking* (Dollard and Miller, 1950, p. 203). He stops thinking about anger, or sex, or messing. He is aided in this response by the fear and anxiety which seem to have an innate tendency to stop thinking and speaking. With awareness of sex or anger or messing gone, unpleasant fear is likewise gone, and the child is learning or has learned to forget or to repress. His stopping thinking or his forgetting or repressing has been rewarded by the removal of an unpleasant feeling and the installation of a feeling of well-being once gain. Repression is really not "good" learning, however. It is a deficit development. Stopping thinking and feeling are costly. Repression leaves gaps, holes, and deficiencies in the personality structure; importantly in social relationships. As stimuli, especially social ones, arouse feared and dreaded responses, the repressed person exhibits hesitancies, blocks, and awkwardness. The range and richness of his responses will be lessened. Rigid, repetitious, and tried-and-true responses will predominate his repertoire. Repression falls alike on all responses, including speech, that may arouse fear and anxiety. When it is impossible to avoid speaking, consistently for some people, and at times for all people, stuttering blocks will be necessary lest the sentences lead to strong motives of which the speaker is deeply ashamed or terribly frightened. (Reference to Fig. 5–1 may help clarify these concepts.)

NEW CONDITIONS OF INTERPERSONAL RELATIONSHIPS

As we have seen, there is the strongest likelihood that the conditions of the stutterer's early life created his speaking difficulties. The main conditions were the methods of his parents in transmitting the spirit of the culture to him. The parents not only induced in the child the drives of fear, guilt, and shame as checks on the child's primary drives, but they and their help-

Figure 5–1. Crude schematic representation of the internalization (introjection) of the cultural forces of fear and condemnation and their inhibition (repression) of the drives, feelings, and thoughts of the child. The compromise expressions of these opposing systems may result in symptoms including stuttering. Phase I—The needs of the very young infant gain satisfaction from the culture. The very young baby's wants are generally met. Phase II— The beginning of the taming or domestication of the older infant's biological drives, generally by fear and pain. The conflict is between the baby and his environment, between the inside and the outside. Phase III—To cope better with the internal-external conflicts of Phase II, the child (one to three years of age) begins to adopt the negative attitudes and values (internalize, introject) which the culture has expressed relative to his wants and feelings. The conflict is beginning to be internalized, to be between action systems within the child. He is beginning to be split. Phase IV—By three, the child has made the inhibitory forces of fear and condemnation which originally belonged to the culture more completely his own to oppose his drive and feeling system. He is now more split, having parts of himself disavowed by other parts. External cultural inhibitions still help his internal inhibitory forces to control his now repressed wants and feelings and thoughts. Phase V—Through the ever-waxing and waning of both sets of the internal oppositional forces in their relation to environmental factors, compromise or symptomatic expression may occur (including stuttering).

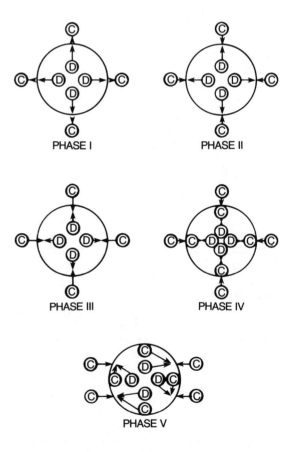

PHASE I

PHASE II

PHASE III

PHASE IV

PHASE V

D – Drives, feelings, even thoughts of child
C – Cultural forces of fear, pain, condemnation
C – Cultural acceptance of infant's wants

ers in society perpetuated these checks. The parents and society aligned themselves behind not only the establishment of fear and its derivatives but the continuation of these inhibiting and anxiety-producing forces. So the patient not only had effective help in acquiring or learning conflicts and repression within himself but strong support in maintaining them. Under these conditions his stuttering, the manifestation of his conflicts, was likewise fostered. In his search for help with his speech, the necessary conditions of unlearning and new learning were usually not found and he continued in his stuttering ways. On the basis of principles and practices borrowed from psychoanalysis and learning theory, our stutterers were subjected to conditions which reversed essentially the old conditions of their rearing. We offered the stuttering individuals conditions which in certain crucial respects were in striking contrast with those of their previous life.

The New Parent

The patient entered into interpersonal relationships with a person of prestige who paid strict, favorable, and sympathetic attention and who held out strong hope of help. This person felt and showed exceptional permissiveness, no condemnation, total tolerance, and complete composure. He made one important demand: the patient must do his best to say everything that came to his mind, to strive for complete self-revelation. For failing to do this at times the patient was not condemned but constantly encouraged to be under high obligation to succeed. This person, the therapist, was a new experience for the patient. He loomed large in contrast with the patient's parents, teachers, relatives, bosses, and other fellow members of society. He never became frightened or punitive or ashamed of anything that the patient said. He never gossiped, or became impatient. He set his patient free from the restraint of logic, and cross-examination; and when the occasion demanded, he fearlessly stepped in and said things which the patient could not say for himself (see Chapter 9 [of *Handbook of Speech Pathology and Audiology*] for a more complete exposition of these points).

The Extinction of Repressing Forces

The patient talked about frightening topics. He talked about shameful and embarrassing feelings and experiences. He expressed anxiety. For these revelations

he was not punished. The feared and shameful motives and feelings were completely accepted. The fear, shame, and guilt were not rewarded by words or expressions from the therapist of condemnation or nonacceptance. Therefore they were extinguished. The extinction generalized to weaken the motivation to repress other related topics that were too frightening and shameful to discuss or even contemplate before. On the other hand, sexual, angry, and messing feelings were rewarded. They came back and out easier and easier to be channeled for future usefulness. The patient was helped to place these helpless past conditions of childhood and contrast them with his present interpersonal relationships. As fears were reduced by reassurance and extinction (unrewarded), at first the most lightly repressed thoughts and feelings began to appear. In generalizing, the patient adventured further to risk greater fears, and since they too went unreinforced, more strongly repressed and inhibited responses occurred.

The Reward of Discovery and Admission

Simultaneously with the unrewarding of fear and consequently its extinction, there is the reinforcement of the discovery and admission of repressed thoughts and feelings. The patient is accepted, even praised, for his painful and anxiety-producing revelations. Whereas before he has received severe disapproval (reward of fear and consequent further repression of primary drives), he now receives calm approval. The rewarding of his repressed materials and the unrewarding of his repressing forces bring him great relief and the feeling of a striking intervention in his life of conflict and anxiety.

Concluding Thoughts

Under these conditions, admittedly sketchily and schematically presented, the unspeakable feelings of the stutterer were discovered. It is hard, if not impossible, to be fair to the great richness, wide variety, beautiful intricacy, and strict lawfulness of the phenomena to be reported. In the author's attempts to present these matters to students and colleagues, he has met with awe, doubt, and even hostility on the part of his listeners. Two colleagues doubted that human beings could possess, let alone express, such thoughts and feelings. Our reaction was that we had not in any way given the materials to the patients; that the productions were their very own. Of course our reaction could have been that even had we suggested the unbelievable thoughts and feelings, they still would have had to come from a human being. Our purpose in reporting findings obtained under the conditions of certain new interpersonal relationships is to spur thought and research in the area of impaired communication between people.

THE UNSPEAKABLE FEELINGS

Through the processes we have delineated, the child comes to a day when he has strong and important feelings that are conflicting and ambivalent. In a general way, these feelings may be grouped into two opposing camps; the primary drives and their derivatives in one camp, and fear and its derivatives in the other. Assigning to fear both an inherent and an acquired function of inhibition of thought, feeling, and action, it is the basic repressing force. Its victims are primary drives of eating, elimination, sex-curiosity, and anger, and their elaborations. Large constellations of behavior become built up around these opposing camps. The child becomes to a degree split. He is racked with wanting and fearing the same thing. Into interpersonal relationships he carries his civil warfare. First one and then the other of his opposing feelings are tugged and pulled. If inhibited wanting is enticed out of hiding, fear and anxiety arise to hold it down. If fear is enhanced, the child becomes all the more paralyzed in thought, feeling, and action. In either instance, fear is the predominately felt drive and all responses, particularly thinking and speaking, are thwarted. Out of this soil stuttering flowers. Thoughts must not be thought; feelings must not be felt; and words must not be spoken.

In what form and complexity do the uncommunicable thoughts and feelings reside within the person? Are they familiar to our senses and understanding? Do they conform to logic and to space and time-binding? Some of the answers to these questions will appear in the materials that follow. More important than the answers may be the puzzles that emerge. Could we hope that to be puzzled might lead not necessarily to the right answers but to the right questions?

In discovering and expressing unspeakable feelings and thoughts, the patient approaches his task gingerly. Anxiety and fear make it impossible for him, even with the therapist's heartiest support, to realize easily and quickly the existence and operation of his most important feared and condemned forces. He has suffered greatly in putting away naughty, childish behavior and he is not about to release it. He has paid dearly for what self-esteem he now possesses, and it will take great patience and effort on the part of both him and his therapist to get him to risk his present painfully gained position. But bit by bit, advancing a little and slipping a little, risking and testing, he learns more and more who he is, what he really wants, and how to discriminate, label, and channel.

The patient's first successes are in sharing conscious misgivings. He is guilty over his socially disrespectful thoughts. He is ashamed of some of his anger and sex feelings. Fear plagues him. These he tells, and they are accepted. He, too, is accepted. He risks more of his known frailties, meannesses, and littlenesses. Over and over these are accepted and he is honored for his honesty of expression. As fear is unrewarded and consequently reduced relative to these more lightly inhibited feelings, more heavily repressed feelings share in the fear reduction and commence to stir. They stir and rise up into the dim light of recognition. It is not enough that they move in the shadows. They carry protective armor against even the recognition that might occur in the dusk. To continue the simile, as fear is reduced, the light of recognition increases and the opaqueness of the armor decreases. The result is a clearer understanding of what the patient really is saying. An example may help to clarify this. Relatively early in therapy an adult male stutterer spoke slowly and painfully as follows.[2]

---

[2] The author is sensitive to the likelihood of the reader's resistance and reactions of anxiety and even disgust to some of the recorded utterances of stutterers in therapy. Could it not be that both the author's sensitivity and the reader's disturbance focus the significance of unspeakable thoughts and feelings in the etiology of stuttering? Might there not be a positive relationship between the unreadability and the unspeakability of certain materials? If the reader has trouble in reading another's words, how much more trouble must the speaker have had in speaking them. It is to be hoped that we, the author in presenting and the reader in accepting communications from areas in interpersonal relationships, will share a deeper understanding of the stutterer's problem.

Then, too, the author has purposely adopted an objective and scientific attitude in reporting accurately samples of the raw data from which its implications and conclusions were drawn. If he makes an inference that people may stutter as a defense against the possibility of saying certain customarily unspeakable things, it becomes important to know what these things are. He could have reported simply that the stutterer has thoughts and feelings of which he is deeply ashamed and the possibility of their verbalization causes him to stutter. Is it not more honest that the author report what he found under certain conditions (therapy) and let the reader have the opportunity to draw his own conclusions?

Now I'm in my old room at home and some long object is here. Over at the opposite wall is a large hump. It is a large woman's body lying there. It has no head, but arms and legs. An extraordinary thing is, it has large breasts. I have an idea it ought to have a head but I won't let that head be there. Now head comes and it has long black hair hanging down and it is my mother. I remember away back in the old days that my mother had this long black hair, three feet long. Everything now looks very far off. Huge objects all around, but very far off. I feel small and one object moves in close. I'm afraid it is going to crush my legs. I didn't have time to mention that when I saw my mother lying there naked I felt guilty and uneasy. That huge object over there I'm afraid is going to crush my legs. What am I afraid of? That huge object? I'm lying there so small. Hands are here somewhere. I feel terribly empty and hungry.

From this production, neither he nor his therapist knew what the long object was. Both of them came to know what it was, however, that began as the large hump. Against the inhibitory forces of the patient it could appear first only as an indistinguished hump. In this form, not too much anxiety was raised over it and consequently the force of the repressed thoughts and feelings pushed further to reveal a woman. For the moment, who she was, was too much. The patient's anxiety could tolerate her nudity and her breasts but not her identify. So she was headless. The struggle between the opposing camps of feelings continued with the repressed thoughts and feelings getting the better of the repressing forces of anxiety. And then the head with its long black hair hanging down appeared. With this much out, the identity of the woman who formerly was headless and originally appeared as just a hump became clear. She was his mother. For the discovery of this fact, he paid a price. Threats assailed him. He became small and afraid, empty and hungry. His inhibiting fears were not wont to resign without a struggle and they left him with a knowledge all right, but a guilty knowledge. He knew something now that he should not have known. He knew that once consciously and more recently unconsciously he had desired his mother in a socially unacceptable and dreaded manner. With the therapist's support and his own good discriminating powers, however, he held his knowledge to use in the future to gain more understanding still.

Repressed feelings rarely emerge singly. They generally come in two's and three's. Sexual and messing preoccupations may appear together, or one or both may accompany anger. And essentially always fear and anxiety are present. Later in his therapy, the same stutterer whose production was used above said:

There is a place here with a lot of gravel. Water running through a river bed. A man comes walking along through this water which comes from a cave. It runs in between two ridges of ground. These two ridges turn into two legs. The rest of the body that was lying there now sits up. Now it stands up and leaves a little pile of feces on the ground. Then a hand throws a basket of feces over the head of this person. I grab his hands and pull on his arms and try to throw him over. We wrestle and I throw him over into this water. He gets up all covered with light and dark spots. I grab his head and throw him in again. He comes out all black this time with a long, black, cat-like tail. I throw him in again and he comes out a bear. I rush out and he tries to bite me. But I throw him in again. This time it's very thick mud and he has a hard time climbing out. I note that his legs have become very slender and pretty and I pull him out and he becomes a woman. She also has a long, thin tail like a cat. I try to clean the mud off her and hold her close to me and stick my penis into her. She shrivels up and disappears. Then I look up and there's a house looking like army barracks. She's in the doorway of this house and she has a long tail, long ears, and web feet with hair all over her. She turns into an ugly animal. Queer thing—there's a tree here and a large window and other things, but always in front of me is this ugly animal. Everywhere I look, she's there. I look down at my legs and they have turned into the hind legs of a horse. I have long ears like a horse. Dog here too like a French poodle, long, thin, and queer. I grab the dog by the throat and shake him and throw him down on the ground. He turns into my brother.

Hostile feelings arose against the man (father?), the woman (mother?), and the dog (which turned into his brother). Actually, he did have a younger brother. Messing and sexual feelings emerged. Fear and anxiety existed throughout this production. To help make the repressed hostile, sexual, and messing feelings palatable, the father and mother were not clearly recognizable. Further, they and his brother were given animal characteristics, because bestial feelings deserve only bestial objects. Even he had to become animallike, with the legs and ears of a horse, in order to tolerate or excuse his primitive feelings.

The young man whose productions we have been citing was the older of two boys. he was two years old when his brother was born and was held out of school until his brother was old enough to enter with him. On the patient's part, the rivalry between the two brothers was keen. We never saw the younger brother. The parents, especially the mother, were strong, exacting, and highly monitoring. Their attitudes toward the sex, eating, and toilet training of their boys were strict and inflexible. Their social goals were high and no effort was spared to attain them. The patient began to stutter early, about a year

after the birth of his brother, and developed a very severe stuttering. He was practically speechless when
he came to us, being able to produce around 50
words an hour during continual efforts to speak in his
early hours of therapy. His primitive feelings were
strongly repressed and fixated at an early developmental level. They remained infantile and childish
because of being repressed so early and harshly, and
they could not be modified and channeled by the
subsequent experiences of later childhood and early
adulthood. Upon coming to us at 25, he was generally
constipated, picky in his eating habits, and had never
had a date.

This short historical background has been given
in order that we might better appreciate the following productions. They were his total verbal output for
fifty minutes of continuous effort to speak. The bulk
of the time was occupied in stuttering blocks which
were characterized by an extremely tight pursing of
the lips. The therapist could write down easily every
word the patient said.

Large object, man's legs, He has loose pair of pants on. I
reach up under his pants and grab his penis. It is large
and soft. I pull on it and pull it off. This man stands up
and reaches out as though asking for his penis back. I
don't want to let him have it. He reaches out and tries
to grab it. I put my hand on his face and push him away.
He opens his mouth and cries. All this happens on the
lawn of our old home. Across the field mother comes
running. She is real large, larger than the house. The
man is my brother. She comes over and I hold out my
hand with the penis in it to show her what I had. He's
over there hollering and waving his arms. Suddenly I
squat down and take a crap and feces come out in a
long ribbon—like toothpaste being squeezed out of a
tube. I look up and overhead is a long, thin lamp post. It
walks in and out among tangled ribbons of feces. It almost trips. It does trip and falls over with a crash. I leap
on it. This ribbon of feces still hangs out of my anus. The
lamp post has arms and I hold them. It also has a
penis and I kick that and break it off. It also has hair and
I reach up and grab a handful and pull it off. A hat
comes off with the hair. On the upper end of the post
are eye glasses like father's. I hit it in the head that is
made of glass. The whole front of the head is broken in.
I run my hands over the lamp post looking for other
protuberances that I can break off. I roll it over and it
has a pair of buttocks and between them an anus. I run
my hand and arm up the anus and spread my fingers
out inside and grab intestines and tear them out
through the anus. I shake my fist in front of father's face
and cram fistfuls of intestines into his face and say "how
do you like that?" I grab him by the throat and order
him to stand there. He tries to fall over but I hit him so
hard that the lamp post is bent. He stand up there bent
over. His head is low enough that I hit him in the head
if he does anything wrong. He cries and wipes intes-

tines out of his eyes. All over the place are trees standing around with their hands on their hips with the
attitude that I should be ashamed of myself. A head
floats in the air. I grab for it. It has long black hair that I
hold in my arms. It's only a head. I stick my penis into
the neck. The lips on the head kiss me. Liquid runs out
between the lips and all over my front. I put my
thumbs into the eyes and pull out the eyeballs and play
with them in my hands. But they are hooked onto the
head with two long white cords. The head isn't angry
at me for playing with the eyes. I replace one eye and
try to pull the other one off completely by breaking the
cord. The head opens its mouths and shows lots of
teeth. It tries to bite my penis off but I believe it can't.
As I look at the head it becomes very ugly. A hole is
through its lower jaw so that by looking into the mouth
I can see the bottom. I grab the ears and throw the
head to the ground and stamp on it. It rolls around on
the ground, all covered with blood and dirt, I try to
clean it off but it's hard to do since the dirt is in the
eyes, hair, and mouth. I want to wash it off but there is
no water. So I urinate on it but this doesn't clean it very
well. Besides, it turns yellow. I look up and there is father, very large and heavy and angry. He has a club. I
look closely at the club and it is my brother. Father
brandishes my brother like a club and I feel he is trying
to hit me. I try to strike my father but he holds my
brother out real close to me so that I can't get at my father. I reach out and pull out two large handfuls of hair
from my brother's head. The places where I pulled the
hair out are bleeding. I try to replace the hair but I get
it on crooked and it grows like that and my brother has
these two uneven places on his head pointing up like
horns. His ears are pointed and his nose is long and he's
like an elf that I thought of as a kid. He has wings. All
this time father has been holding my brother out at me.
Father has a long pencil between his fingers. I grab it
and stab him through the penis and push the pencil on
all the way through until it comes out the other end.
His legs shrivel up and turn into a horse's legs. He turns
into a horse hooked onto a wagon with its wheels all
broken. The horse looks queer too, as though made out
of a fluid, and he's not firm. He keeps changing his
shape.

At first blush, the feelings and acts revealed in such
products are unacceptably raw to our conscious selves. And this is exactly the point. Many people, including stutterers, are numbly and dumbly involved
in such culturally unbearable mental materials that
are repressed and, therefore, consciously undetecta-
ble. Nevertheless, their presence is felt in a gnawing
anxiety that has its peak moments handled by some
symptom, including stuttering. Before therapy our
stutterer did not know that he wanted to bite off his
brother's penis and show it to their mother as if to say,
"Look what I have done. Now you have only one
whole son. Brother is weak and impotent, I am strong
and potent. Only I can deserve your complete respect." Before therapy he did not know that he had

equally strong if not stronger feelings of aggression and destruction against his father. He wanted to destroy him in a most thorough and brutal manner. And as it was with his brother, his father too would snivel and beg for mercy in the face of our stutterer's pent-up rage. After each savage but successful attack upon his competitors, brother and father, his mother would appear. Is it not true that she is the real issue? With the brother she appeared clearly as the mother. Her only distortion was her enormous size, "larger than the house." Her role here was not too important, mainly to see what he had done. With the father, she appeared only as a head floating in the air. Here her role was extremely important. She was made to receive his primitive, sexualized aggression. In proportion to the importance and unacceptability of his casting of his mother, she was distorted, finally ending as an ugly, yellow, dirty head.

Finally, to justify the venting of his spleen in one fell swoop, our patient has the father threaten him with a club that is the brother. Our patient's wrathful retaliation is so right now since both of his competitors are a menace to him. He can justifiably save his life and strikes out to do so. To get at the father he must destroy his weapon, the brother. The outcome is humiliating to his antagonists. The brother becomes an elf with horns, pointed ears, and a long nose; and the father, a formless, spineless horse hooked to a broken-down wagon.

It is our contention that these strong anal and sexual aggressions of antisocial quality grew out of the important training situations of infancy and early childhood. Because of the pain and anxiety meted out by the parents in temporal and spatial relation to the patient's expression of early instinctual drives, he repressed (drive reduction by stopping thinking and feeling) these drives and the interpersonal relationships connected with them and henceforth carried them as unconscious, motivating forces. When these forces taxed the patient's repressing or inhibiting forces (fear and anxiety) to the limit, other defenses were called into action. When these defenses in turn could not hold, a final stand was made through stuttering. Stuttering may be conceptualized then as a final defense or block against the threatening revelation through spoken words of unspeakable thoughts and feelings. It may be visualized as a sieve through which some materials and force can pass, emerging in reduced amount and altered form. Both the repressed feelings and the restraining force (sieve or stuttering) derive some satisfaction. The former does get out, albeit in reduced amount and al-

tered form, and the latter does hold even if it has to give a little. Certainly it held to the extent that few, if any, of the listeners really knew what the stutterer said when he stuttered. If the unspeakable thoughts and feelings of the stutterer are strong and plentiful, his stuttering will be severe, because as a defense it must be equal to or better than the forces defended against.

According to clinical observation stutterers, both children and adults, are well-spoken. That is, they speak words that are highly socially proper and acceptable. As a group they do not speak "mean" thoughts and feelings to others or about others. They are polite and respectful. They are "good" people. What they say in the interpersonal relationships of everyday life is in sharp contrast with what they say in the interpersonal relationships of therapy. This great incompatibility of conscious and unconscious mental content may be a factor in the stutterer's problem.

Mr. Brown, 45, was a brilliant businessman with legal training and experience. To others his stuttering appeared inconsequential. To him it was catastrophic. His professional life was being ruined by his unbearable anxiety in verbal communication which was an absolute essential in his business. All his life he has had an ineluctable need to please and be loved and respected and he has succeeded, at least as far as others are concerned, in realizing this need. Indeed, by all others he is a most admired and respected man. In therapy, impressing upon him the attitude that nothing is to be feared or hated but only understood, he communicated many times the following content and feeling:

I'm chopping wood with an axe. I shudder. Splinters hit me in the eyes and that gave me a shudder. Two of us chop off our toes and this makes me a shudder. We look alike and act in unison. We dig a V-shaped ditch and plant radishes and they grow up very rapidly. We have to plant them very quickly and get away because they grow so fast. I kick this other guy in the rear and this gives me a shudder. I want to split him in half and this gives me a shudder. I do it and each half turns into a whole person. Branches grow out of the ears and I cut them off and I shudder. I see a penis and it is sliced lengthwise. Cut-off, smaller penises are marching towards me and I fight back at them with a stick or sword but they get bigger and bigger, too big to subdue. Some of them urinate like a shower and I run away but a big man catches me and brings me back and I have to sit there. Finally, penises all lie down and I can get up and walk over them. Big man doesn't care, but I mustn't get too far out of his sight. If I go too far a big penis rises up in front of me. He puts a big penis to watch over me. I shudder. I feel hemmed in. I walk away and come to that V-shaped ditch and a person is lying in it. I cross over and climb stairs and big man sees me. I'm still within his reach. I'm washed off and someone urinates on me. All this makes me wince. I hide inside the branches of a tree. I get out and penises are all around me like a fence and I shudder. They start spraying. I can't get away. I slide down into a river and wash off and feel safer. I swim under logs like penises lying on water. I go into a cave and a nude woman is there, and I feel secluded and safe. Animals are roving outside but I feel safe. They look in but it's dark and they can't see me. I have to defecate and I do it right there. This makes me shudder. A messy deal. Snakes come out of rock. I feel antagonistic.

I'm in a train, and instead of going into a tunnel, it goes into a large reptile's mouth. We back up and try again and go into another reptile's mouth. I'm surrounded by reptiles wagging their tails. They get closer and closer and I go up a tree, safe for awhile but someone chops the tree down. I'm still safe like in a womb. Wish I could get away, out into the sun. I'm getting awfully tired. Another reptile is after me. I'm getting worn out. This awfully hard. That's the way it used to be. I shouldn't feel that way now. Snake comes up and I'm too tired. It grabs my hand. I run up a tree but that's a snake too (breathing hard). I want to give up but I can't. Remember running home from school when I had defecated in my pants. Remember a man who approached me with his penis out. Don't remember what we did. Other boys there. Maybe we touched his penis. Maybe with our mouths. Don't remember. See a vision of this. I'm so tired. This is so hard (breathing heavily). One big penis I'm particularly afraid of. Wish I could sleep. I try not to see it. I just wish it would let me alone.

There is a treasure-trove of exquisite design in this production. We should be remindful that it, as well as every other similarly obtained projection, is not a production of intellection. Mr. Brown did not consciously construct this adventure. He did not know what he would say during the therapeutic hour. He had no plans for the hour, other than to be there. Under the obligation to speak absolutely freely, the feelings, ideas, and words given above came to him. They came at about the rate of slow conversational speech. He did not look ahead, or plan ahead, or structure what came. Rather, he simply reported what came into consciousness as it came. His attention was focused upon his stream of consciousness, which seemed to flow involuntarily. Some anxiety existed throughout. Anxiety peaks occurred at those times when he would say, "this gives me a shudder," or "this makes me wince."

This stutterer adds exemplification of the almost monotonous regularity of the existence, in these people, of raw and culturally disowned feelings and ideas in the areas of sex, elimination, and hostility. The presence and influence of these unconscious preoccupations were afflictive and uninviting in interpersonal relationships, particularly in communication. In stirring from their servile state, to which they never willingly submitted, they gum the gears of verbal output. Too full of such terrorizing longings, it is no wonder that Mr. Brown dared not speak fluently. His fear and anxiety were not over the possibility of stuttering speech. They were over the threat of the telling in talking, of giving himself away in his words. He was never afraid of his stuttering per se. Really, he was afraid that his stuttering, as a defense, would not hold. He was afraid of possible loopholes in his stuttering and the consequent probability that his blocking utterances were not capable of fulfilling their purposes of defending against words conveying unspeakable feelings and thoughts.

Conflicts and defenses incident to the attempted achievement of sex-typing were seen frequently in the productions of Faith, a relatively severe stutterer of 20. She reported:

> I see a man walking toward me with a child under each arm—a boy and a girl. I call to him and he drops the children and I see he has a very large sexual apparatus in his pants which frightens me and which he is going to use against me as a weapon. The children are for a "come-on." I use pubic hair as a weapon of defense against him but it is futile. So I cut half my hair off my head to make me have half of a man's haircut and I put hair on my chest and it grows so that I'm part man to defend myself. Then I become half male and half female, with half a penis and half a vagina and these halves make love to each other. The right half of me is man and the left half of me is woman. The man-half bends over onto the woman-half which doesn't do anything, just remains passive. The right hand which is the man's hand starts tickling the sole of the left or woman's foot, and goes on up over the leg, mostly over the back of the legs and on up over buttocks, especially around the anus and then continues the tickling all over the woman-half.

Somewhat later in therapy she found herself swimming into shore with a strong, overhand crawl stroke executed by her long, strong arms (in reality she is small and does not swim). Waves beat against her but she got into shore strong and fresh and with a penis. Her breasts were exposed like a man's chest. As she stood there she lost the penis and a brassiere covered her breasts. But as she continued to stand there on the shore she became more and more interested in the girls and developed a penis again. She went into the toilet and her penis melted away and she sat down and urinated like a woman. These reversals in sex-typing kept occurring: a penis would appear and then disappear; hair on her breasts would come and go; a butch hair-cut and long hair would alternate. She would be first a woman, then a man; or half female and half male. Sometimes her sex role, whether male or female, was in relation to others; while at other times she was complete within herself, her male half relating to her female half. A third variation was for her to have complete male and complete female sexual organs at the same time and to relate to a similar person, each person behaving at the same time both as a male and as a female.

Actually, this girl's father was not a strong masculine figure. But from an early day the mother had instilled within her daughter the feeling that for a woman sex was cruel and painful and that man was a bestial creature preying upon women for his own selfish satisfactions. The patient has had three husbands and has never experienced orgasm. Her latest husband often calls her his little man.

Brimful of ambivalence in a most important interpersonal relationship with both men and women, it may be surprising that her only apparent trouble was stuttering. To have the larger force of her unacceptable preoccupations funnel through oral communication, rather than through some other expressive avenue, might account for the original severity of her stuttering. As her anxiety was reduced as she discovered, accepted, and realigned these conflictual feelings, her speech became remarkably improved and her role as a woman more firmly established.

Repeatedly, our stutterers engaged in anthropomorphism. Time and again they would ascribe human characteristics to things not human. They would express feelings, words, thoughts, and acts of a conflict in the form of objects and object relationships. Unacceptable feelings and desires would be concentrated in objects, their location, and their movement. This process may be clearer if we give some examples.

Glass tube filled with tiny microbes lowered into my throat. A swab saturated with argyrol is inserted down my throat. Steady flow of talk keeps flowing from me like accumulation of junk. A mass of gold trinkets is in my mouth, back of my lower teeth. I am a storage house, a vault. I expectorate a ball-like object that remains rolling in my throat. A dentist's mirror probes my teeth and enters my throat. I'm crying and between sobs, toffee-like substance moves back and forth in my mouth. Orifices and tubes and the words vital and potent. Now I'm pushing something up in my throat, using both hands. It's a window and I can't, it's too heavy. Hot stove pipe and a big boat in my throat. Honeycomb

in my throat. Cells of the honeycomb are really breathing cells. A broom sweeps my throat. Spitting out and vomiting coins, muddy water and junk such as nuts and bolts. I want to explode all the antiquated things— junk, old coins, chewing gum, a lump of coal, horseshoe. It was necessary to stifle everything and choke to death all my life. I've been afraid of expelling anything, as though I took a deep breath and held it all my life. I've inhaled, but I've never exhaled. I've sucked in all my desires and cravings. I'm a volcano erupting and pitching all the junk out.

Many hours later, the patient whose examples we have been citing did not need to use so much anthropopathy as a defense against the realization and expression of her feelings. She could speak more directly as follows:

I'm raring to go places emotionally. I'm not scared like I used to be. You kissed me and put your tongue into my mouth and I had an orgasm. It felt just like a stuttering spasm except the fullness and constriction was in the vagina instead of in my throat. I feel that in order for me to speak I must take my panties off and keep my vagina uncovered. It's crazy to hesitate to say anything now. My breasts have grown up. They're full and I'm happy. They're not flabby like they used to be. Hair around my vagina is no longer unclean. It is sweet and wanted. I have no need for stuttering anymore. I'm grown up. My breasts and vagina feel so good. Once when we started I made a vow I'd never discuss sex or religion with you. I exhale through the vagina pure, clean air. I cough up not coins which are obsolete but circles—little emotional feelings and sexual cravings. They come up from my vagina and out through my mouth. I open up the orifices and tubes of my body and feelings, desires and cravings come out. I'm burning up, I'm on fire, I'm alive. I don't have to stutter anymore. Damn it, I can talk as well as you. All my life I thought my body was well but my speech organs were sick. Now the most normal part is the speech part.

This person, in her early forties, came into therapy with a very severe stutter. She was an uneducated, restricted, and economically and socially limited virgin. As she dwelt in the protective shadow of her aging mother, life was passing her by. A combination of external circumstances, including the death of her mother and the remarriage of her father, and internal forces, drove her to seek help, first in a speech clinic and finally in individual therapy. Considering many factors, her age, the severity and duration of her stuttering, her highly restricted upbringing, her limited physical and educational capabilities, her success in therapy was phenomenal. From a halting beginning she progressed to a fluent conclusion. For example, toward the end she said:

Suddenly I see my father and I hate him. He is responsible for me having no husband, no home, and no children. Now I see my hairline structure [pubic hair] and it doesn't disgust me anymore. I'm riding nude on a bare-back horse and the horse becomes my father and I hate him and I hate you too, terribly, sitting there coldly trying to figure me out in a professional way. I lie here on the defensive. I've been belching him up for years, my hate for him. I don't need to stutter him up anymore. Through lip service I was supposed to love him but I didn't, I was lying. It was sinful to hate your father. It was a commandment to love thy father and thy mother. This lie I stuttered.

Still closer to the end she proclaimed:

I can go up to a prominent person and talk without any feeling of ill-at-ease. I just don't care. He and I are just two human beings. Used to have in internal fight, now it's an external fight. I'm ready to go and no home and no education hit me. Formerly when I had a speech spasm or any other trouble I ran home. Now I don't want to hide, I want to come out, to expand, to make my debut. A debut among people. But certain people push me back and I find no refuge in the corner anymore. If my father should die tomorrow I'd cry for the father I used to know or the father he might have been. I feel that Sally is my little sister instead of me being really her little sister. She's away back down the road, so simple and prejudiced. I approach you, I can walk with you.

And at the end:

All the junk and surplus and debris have left me. I'm free and pure. I think of grit and a mouthful of dung and I'll spit it out, defecate through my mouth. I've been defecating and urinating all the years of my life out through my mouth. I was saying all the nasty things through stuttering. I was saying my father was a son-of-a-bitch and my mother was a deluded fool. You held my hand and taught me to talk and I never knew just when you let go and I talked alone.

Eight years have passed since these last words were spoken. During those years her job, which she has handled very successfully, has demanded the meeting of the public at a teller's window and over the phone. Not once, she reports, has she stuttered. Would it be presumptuous to think of her as a "cured" stutterer?

From unexpected people, the expression and communication of the interaction of opposing feelings (want and fear) frequently reveal the magnificence of the mental processes of man. The feelings themselves may be simple, simple want and simple fear of wanting; but the revelation of the conflict is often strangely penetrating and thought-provoking. Our surprising source of the production to follow was a 17-year-old lad who had stuttered severely

since early childhood. In literature, psychology, philosophy, and the social sciences he was extremely naive. His entire life had been spent in activity to satisfy his interest in hunting, ranching, and livestock. He read practically not at all, worked and played mainly alone, and was unsocial, if not antisocial. He knew nothing of such concepts as symbolism, the unconscious, repression, and the like. Theories, principles, and practices of psychotherapy were foreign to him. He did know, of course, what was expected of him; an absolutely free and complete verbalization of his thoughts and feelings. One hour, after he had learned relatively well how to relate in therapy, he spoke as follows:

I see a large body of water. The surface is calm and very smooth, and green and very clear. Then as I see deeper it gets very dark. There seems to be no bottom to it. It gets blacker and blacker the deeper you go. Something is in there like a huge snake. He is very long and winds around and swims along. There are things like weeds, very dense, but no bottom. This eel, or snake, or whatever it is, is the key to something, the guard to a whole new land. The snake goes through an opening that leads to something like a tunnel, and disappears. As I look on the other side, the tunnel comes out into an uncivilized place, with huge reptiles and prehistoric monsters of all sorts in a tangled and dark forest. There is no sky. There is ground with very dark ponds around. All these creatures seemed worried about something. There have been men here before who tried to conquer the animals, to build up civilization but they have all been destroyed. One man is here now. He wears hunting clothes like we have today. He has a rifle but he is just walking among the animals which are of tremendous height and size, as big as our buildings. The animals are all respectful because the man thinks he is the master of them; and the animals have the same feeling, not because he is cruel but because he has broken them. Something in the animals wants to fight back, but something else in them is like horses that have been ridden and broken and know there is no sense in resisting. That's the way this whole setup seems to be. The animals seem to have a feeling of respect but if the man were ever to weaken, or to show by some means that he was not the master of the situation, they would destroy him immediately. This man seems to feel that he wants something harder to break, something that will offer resistance but will be useful after it is broken. But also, he has the feeling that he is afraid to tackle this other situation until he has acquired more confidence by proving that he is a master of things that can fight back and have sense, not human sense, but animal sense. He knew that these things can hurt him physically but can never command him. In these animals once they are broken, as it is with all animals, there is that loyalty of feeling that their master can do no wrong to them. There is a big problem appearing on the scene. It is the girl he wants. He knows that she can never be completely broken because he is afraid of trying to conquer her like he has conquered the animals. There is always the possibility that he might lose control of the situation, and then he would have somebody who would tell HIM what to do. In other words he is afraid that he will not receive from her the same faith in himself that he received from the animals. The question seems to be does he want this human companionship enough to give up his freedom and the respect of the animals?

With our present understanding of the human mind, we would be presumptuous to attempt a full explanation of this communication. Possibly we will be rash to pretend any comprehension of this young man's meaning here, but with the encouragement from the findings of other workers and from this patient's own clearer subsequent communications, we are encouraged to venture some translations of his language into forms more familiar to our current understanding. May we speak for him then as follows?

On the surface I am very calm and unruffled and easily understood. I am quiet and my wants are simple—to be left alone, not to be bothered, to come and go as I please, no fuss, no trouble, no demands upon me. But really, down deeper, I am not so simple and clear to myself or to others. Feelings stir, rebellious feelings, male feelings, conquering feelings. They are powerful and hard to hold in check and ever pressing for expression. I have to be always on the alert to contain them. They are not very smart as human beings go, but they have animal wisdom and demand my constant vigilance to manage their sexual hunger. Only my superior intelligence gives me an advantage. Were it not for this leverage their size and strength would overpower me. I cannot risk any diminution of my already slight superiority. I cannot tackle any other job. I must keep all my energies mobilized to manage my raw, animallike, male feelings; my maturing feelings of maleness, of being a man. If I gave in to these feelings they would weaken me, even destroy me. yet I do want to grow more. I want to reach out with my maleness. I want to test my powers. But as I think this way I become frightened. My feelings go a little too fast. They want to conquer a girl now. This is something different. With great effort I can manage my own sexual feelings. I can control them as long as they are all mine, just mine. But if I let them flow out to another, to a female, can I rule them in relation to her? Can I hold in check both her and me? What will she do to me? I'm fearful that she, being human, will not submit to my will. She may not be mine, all mine. I can keep my feelings all mine. Had I better live alone with them or risk trying to live with her too? I don't know now.

In exploring his big new land of big feelings, he knew that other men had been there before and that they had failed in their conquests. Were not these men the men of his family, or rather his own feelings of the men of his family? He felt that they had failed to crush his feelings, even had been destroyed themselves. (Actually his father was dead.) One man, himself, remained alive. And with great exertion he was not only living but reigning over his feelings. But when his feelings expanded to include women, fear assailed him. Had he not met with trouble, even failure, in controlling his mother, or his feelings about her? Was this trouble or failure to be repeated? So our patient spoke in a strange tongue about his great perplexities; and as he spoke more often, he spoke more plainly until even he understood his speech and his speech troubles.

Before he came into therapy, Allen, a severe stutterer of 16, had the following recurrent dream:

I feel as though I have awakened suddenly. When I look up a huge gorilla is standing over me and reaching out toward me. Then I get out of bed and start running around the room with it chasing me. Although its gets me pretty well cornered, it never quite gets hold of me. I try to go over to my desk to get a knife to kill the gorilla, but it always blocks me. After it chases me awhile I run out into the hall. Although there are people downstairs I am afraid to call them. I fear they will be very angry with me. But downstairs they hear me running around so they come up. As they come up I go into my room to hide from them.

The dream of nightmarish proportions reveals the dreamer's bare management of some of his powerful and dreaded feelings. During the day, conscious control conceals their being; but at night during sleep, with a weakening of his inhibitory forces, they are able to attain an outlet in disguised form. The gorilla is his fearful evaluation of warm, affectional feeling toward his father. When these feelings strive for expression, his fearful learned appraisal of them casts them in monstrous form, and even affords him strength to make an ineffectual attempt to fight. In simplest language, he wants the warmest, most affectional responses from his father. But these wants, he has learned well, are dreadful and when they gain the relative force in sleep to advertise themselves, they are permitted recognition only in caricatural outline. It is informative that in the dream he feared the people (parents) downstairs more than he did the gorilla in his room. He knew in a subtle, subliminal way what the gorilla was; that it was his own wants which had to be concealed from others at all costs. The others were the punitive mentors of his past who had instilled and maintained his fear and dread of his wanting the sexual love of his father.

During the hours of therapy Allen wold have thoughts and feelings similar to those expressed in the dream. For example:

> Now I'm thinking of a huge octopus. It's in a glass cage. It's an awful looking thing. I wouldn't want to be in there with it, although I might as well be. Why do I think of this? It just popped into my head. That is, I might as well be in there with him. Let me think. There is a resemblance between it and my father. The long arms of parents and the long arms of the octopus.

Allen was a brilliant lad whose stuttering was so severe that he was practically speechless. He sucked his thumb and pulled his hair out when he first entered therapy. His parents were exceptionally fine, able, and strong people who enjoyed upper class socioeconomic status. Allen was in continual and futile conflict with them, his school, and constituted law and authority. These conflictual issues came up time and again in his spontaneous and unminded verbalizations.

> A bee is on a streetlight. He's flying all around it trying to get in. He finally finds a hole in it and gets in and sits on the light and it burns him. He gets mad and stings it only it burns his stinger off and that scares him. He tries to get out only he can't find that hole so he dies in there. There's this man and he wants to join the underground in France. He doesn't know how to get into it but finally finds out where they meet and goes there. They grab him and torture him to find out if he's German. He convinces them he isn't so they let him join. He's supposed to blow a bridge with dynamite. He lights it wrong and it blows up too fast and kills him. There's this elephant and he wishes that he were smaller. I don't know why but he does. Finally, somehow he gets to be a tiny elephant. Only then all the big ones kick him around and he wants to be big again, only he can't. There's this flower and it wants to be wheat. It's changed into wheat and is very happy until a horse comes along and eats it. There's a man and he liked to into the freezing compartment in a store. The store owner finally lets this man go in and look around. When he goes in he closes the door behind himself and it locks automatically and he freezes in there. When they find him, he's frozen so they cut him up and sell him as steak. The person who eats him dies from some poison that was in him. There's a dog and he wishes he were a man, so he's turned into a man. On the first day he's drafted into the army and killed in training. Now there's this person who has his hand caught in a washing machine, in those rollers. He tries to get it out but can't and figures it will be easier if he pushes his arm through. He starts to push but finds his arm is attached to his body and he will have to push his body through. He does this and all gets through but his head which he can't get through. He's stuck there. Now there's a person who's a terrific wire walker. He always wears shoes when he is doing this. The manager tells him not to wear shoes this time because people think he has something on his shoes that holds him on the wire. He starts out without shoes and the wire tickles his feet and he falls. There's this man and he swings a sledgehammer around and around, faster and faster. The hammer is tied to his hands and as he swings it too fast he is pulled off his feet into a swamp where there are crocodiles which kill him.

With a plant, an animal, or a man, it is always the same. They want to do something else or be something else and regularly disaster befalls them in the attainment of their wants. In his family of high standards, so very much of his wanting had been blocked with disapproval, fear, and pain. Now at 16 he carries uneasily the repressed conflict of urges and their omnipresent and obdurate counterfeelings of fear and guilt. In the acceptant atmosphere of therapy, his repressed urges and wants were beckoned into being. It appears that they were essentially explorations into new and forbidden roles and relationships and as they enjoyed even disguised realization, their associated, oppositional feelings appeared also. And in every instance the latter won. But this outcome will not always be so. The now maligned feelings will get stronger under the new conditions of learning and simultaneously the restraining and punitive feelings of shame, fear, and guilt will get weaker. His ambivalence of roles, to be this or be that, is further unmasked in the next day's productions.

> There are two people on horses and they have a rope tied around their necks connecting themselves. They want to go in different directions and kick their horses. The two people look exactly alike. They kick their horses and are pulled off and they try to run in opposite directions, only they can't get apart and can't agree on where to go. I think one is trying to go toward a swamp where there are all kinds of birds, crocodiles, and stuff. The one that doesn't want to go to the swamp has a black mask over his face. But he still looks exactly like the other one. These Siamese twins here. One wants to bathe and the other hates to bathe. He won't let the other one take a bath. There is a book and one of the pages wishes it were a different page. If it were a different page it would mix up the book, but still it wants to be a different page. There's this colt that was just born. Its belly button is still attached to its mother and he wants it separated, but mother doesn't because she wants her colt around her. There are two people and they are handcuffed together and they hate each other. They kill each other because they can't get away from each other. There's this spring and it's being kept together, only it wants to get open and can't. Now there's a person driving a black Ford up in the mountains where there are curves. He didn't like to go around the turns so he goes straight over the mountains and smashes into a tree. He had been in prison before and had promised to go straight. He went straight—that's how he interpreted it. There are two

people standing on a fence, and each wants the other one to get off but neither will, so one starts shaking the real thin fence and then the other one starts to shake the fence and they both fall off. There's a person with three arms and he didn't like one of them, so he puts it into a vise and squeezes it thinking it will fall off this way. He succeeds only in crushing the bone. There's a person riding a bicycle and the front wheel wants to go backwards but can't. When he's in the middle of the road, the front wheel comes off and the bike falls and a truck comes along and runs over the man. There's a person in an airplane and he takes off all right, but once he's up the propellers start going in the wrong direction and he flies backwards. He can't see where he's going so crashes into the Empire State Building. He bails out, but his chute catches on a flagpole and his chute is torn. He's held up there. The trouble is, though, that the ropes were tangled around his own neck and he was strangled by his own weight. There are two people with their belts tied together and they hate each other and start hitting each other and both get bloody noses. They are in the ocean and the sharks smell the blood and come and kill both of them.

Toward the end of therapy when her stuttering had become of no consequence, a young woman who had stuttered so severely, spoke as follows:

A geyser is blowing up in the air. A volcano is erupting molten stuff and it's dangerous. People better watch out. Out comes lava, lavatories, bowls and, toilets. Volcano is like an anus sticking up in the air and out shoots all this stuff. Feces, all the insides, like this is anger. All the insides shoot out, tremble all over. All of one gets mad, not just a part. Volcano keeps shooting and spitting up, and feces roll down the side and bury all the houses. I'll go over and tell my mother that I don't need to stutter any more because I know all those words that I saw written on the sidewalks when I was little and wanted to ask her, but was afraid, afraid to know, afraid I was bad, afraid I was naughty. I felt an urge this afternoon to go over and tell her all that has happened. How stuttering is gone and why it's gone.

Throughout therapy, a chief area of concern for her had been elimination. Like any other child, she must have begun the same naive interest in her feces and urine that she had in other parts and products of her body. Undoubtedly she handled and played with fecal material. Without a shadow of a doubt in her case, the day arrived when her mother found her innocent child smearing feces over her own little sweet body, into her beautiful curls and on her clean crib, with vocal abandon. Sharp, punishing, and fear-producing management followed. The baby experienced strong anxiety in relation to her feces and her interest in them. On pain of losing the mother's love and on the further pain of punishment, this baby girl repressed her messing interests and activities. She also

learned to repress verbal reference to these matters, except for slanting and oblique allusions, with the consequence that what began innocently and openly ended up closed out and excluded from the interpersonal relationships of the future. Although repressed, theses interests did not die. Their life was partly saved by the eternal cues of swelling bladder and bowel, odors, noises, and sights. But words must not be spoken. Naughty words, dirty words they became, and they must not be uttered. These words married other words which in turn became contaminated by connubial connection and they too could not be said. Well, where do we end? It is reasonable to assume that in her case we ended with stuttering.

CONCLUDING THOUGHTS

We have used 16 productions of our 30 stutterers. These few were chosen as typical from literally thousands of originations. Every one of our stutterers used the larger share of his therapy in expressing his conflictual feelings through these forms. We have not yet attempted to compare our 30 stutterers with our other group of 35 patients in regard to these productions. We cannot state now that our stutterers gave more, or longer, or more complete, or more diversified originations than did our other group of people. It is our strong clinical feeling, amounting almost to a certainty, that the type of materials we have been presenting is practically exclusively paradigmatic of our stuttering group. The largest proportion of our other patients did not give any such materials. A few gave scattered projections. Those who gave the most did not approximate those stutterers who gave the least. If our feelings stand the test of further study, we may have here an important differentiating factor. It would appear that until such a difference might be established, we should refrain from any consideration of its possible significance.

With almost monotonous repetition our stutterers advertised their unconscious preoccupation with the salvaging of some remnants of their early physical enjoyment. They revealed endlessly a nostalgia for their culturally disavowed, biologically rooted pleasures of sucking, eating, evacuating, and exploring. So frequently their revelations told of their lonely longing for the most primitive, raw, and earthy sensory and motor enjoyments and delights. When early training began its attack upon these pleasures of the flesh, our stutterers must have had three purportful reactions: anger, which met with triumphant counter-anger and which ended in being repressed by fear; a loss of oneness with themselves; and finally, a crippling of interpersonal relationships, significantly with the parents. Their productions portrayed these early reactions. They, the stutterers, did release in therapy hostility; they showed disabling vacillation about themselves, and they manifested fears about others. We were not there to see for ourselves when the parents made their attacks and the stutterers made their reactions, but under the conditions of therapy, the stutterers provided proof that the attacks and the reactions had occurred.

As seen through the feelings and thoughts of our stutterers, the parents, particularly the mothers, were highly monitoring of their children's behavior. In the stutterers' productions or originations, and in their conscious and recovered memories, the mothers were felt as harsh disciplinarians who held their offspring to excessively high standards of conduct and who used shaming and anxiety-dousing tactics in the socializing of their children. The accuracy of our stutterers' feelings are borne out by the studies of Moncur (1951, 1952) who found that the mothers of stutterers were more dominant than the mothers of nonstutterers. In the therapeutical process with our stutterers there emerged clearly, possibly a still more significant implication. It was that the father was relatively weak and passive. We may express this feeling more poetically and say that the stutterer's mother sang an operatic aria while his father hummed a lullaby. It is possible that this relatively greater strength of the mother operated adversely in the sex-typing of the child. An ambivalence of the sexual role was a constant worry at the unconscious levels of our stutterers.

Note may be made of the clinical outcome of psychotherapy with our stutterers. It must remain at this writing, however, as only a note. Our study can hardly be considered as proving anything—most of all, favorable clinical results. We may say though that those stutterers who recovered and expressed what we have termed unspeakable feelings and thoughts did enjoy increased speech fluency and less anxiety over speech blocks. Eleven adult stutterers (seven men and four women) had at least 150 hours each of psychotherapy with us. Of these, five (four men and one woman) were helped greatly; and six (three men and three women) were "cured." We may put psychotherapy in the worst possible light by stating that just as good results might be forthcoming if a stutterer talked to anybody about anything for at least 150 hours. We do not feel that it deserves this harsh dismissal. From the day-to-day, anxiety-producing recoveries and expressions and the consequent reductions in anxiety and speech blocks, we feel on the contrary that therapy was a dynamic, curative process for those stutterers who had the motivation and courage to drive them on.

REFERENCES

Dollard, J., Doob, L., Miller, N., and Sears, R. 1939. Frustration and aggression. New Haven: Yale.

Dollard, J., and Miller, N. 1950. Personality and psychotherapy. New York: McGraw-Hill.

Frank, J. 1961. Persuasion and healing, Baltimore: Johns Hopkins.

Haley, J. 1963. Strategies of psychotherapy. New York: Grune & Stratton.

Hilgard, E., and Bower, G. 1966. Theories of learning. New York: Appleton-Century-Crofts.

Moncur, J. 1951. Environmental factors differentiating stuttering children from non-stuttering children. *Speech Monogr,* 18, 312–325.

Moncur, J. 1952. Parental domination in stuttering. *J. Speech Hearing Disorders,* 17, 155–165.

Sullivan, H. 1953. The interpersonal theory of psychiatry. New York: Norton.

Travis, L., and Baruch, D. 1941. Personal problems of everyday life. New York: Appleton-Century-Crofts.

Emotional Factors

Lee Edward Travis

Intellectually, I am the consequence of the confluence of three streams of thought: experimental psychology, neuropathology and psychoanalysis. From Carl E. Seashore, dean of the Iowa University Graduate School, I learned how to approach problems in human behavior scientifically. I became glued to the laboratory full of beautiful instruments for the study of sensory and motor functions of humankind. Here I anticipated finding out exactly what stuttering was. Before stuttering, during stuttering, and after stuttering I would note and record the stutterer's sensory thresholds and movements. In relation to the stutterer's speech trouble, I wanted to know what was going on in the brain and in the speech muscles.

I learned a good many things. Among them was that the stutterer may try to talk in inspiration, the intercostal muscles and diaphragm may function in opposite directions during stuttering, the deep tendon reflexes become exaggerated during severe speech blocks, and brain waves differ from normal during stuttering.

From Dr. Samuel T. Orton, a neuropathologist and the director of the Iowa Psychopathic Hospital, I learned how to interpret these various laboratory results. His thought was that all the data indicated a reduction for some reason or other in cortical control of speech during stuttering. I came to think of stuttering as caused by aberrant interhemispheric relationships. Maybe there was a substantial bilateral cortical representation of the speech function. Possibly the brains of stutterers are without a particular asymmetry necessary for dominant control of structures producing speech. In the bilateral representation for speech one cerebral hemisphere could interfere with the speech performance of the other.

If bilateral cortical representation of the speech function is the culprit in stuttering, we may ask if it is a problem in behavior genetics. Is there a gene that causes stuttering? Here we are asking if the stutterer was born without sufficient asymmetry, a condition caused by factors operating before birth. But maybe the lack of sufficient asymmetry is the consequence of cultural or organic interventions in the development of enough cerebral dominance for normal speech.

117

Postscript   5

This whole line of thinking about stuttering and its nature ended for me in 1938 when I left the laboratory of the University of Iowa and all its glittering gadgetry to enter the clinic at the University of Southern California, with its fierce demand for cures. I put a small notice in the newspaper about opening a clinic for stutterers. Dozens of them came, and I was transformed rather abruptly from a laboratory researcher to a kind of guru therapist, from a scientific investigator to a kind and loving healer, from a student of neurophysiology to a student of human conflicts and anguish. At Iowa I had studied the stutterer's body; USC I studied his mind and soul.

The third strain of influence in my education now came into prominence. Instead of the laboratory, it was the couch. At Iowa, alongside Dr. Orton's strong emphasis on the organic nature of all psychological ills, there existed a lively interest among the psychiatrists in Freudian psychoanalysis. I joined the discussion groups on psychoanalysis even to the extent of being analyzed myself. At USC I swung full circle back to psychoanalysis in my thinking about stuttering. Hour after hour was spent with individual stutterers in the one-to-one psychoanalytic relationship. I also spent considerable time with stutterers in psychoanalytically oriented group situations. The essence of this work at USC over a period of several years is presented here.

At the University of Iowa my interest in stuttering was mainly in its nature. Mostly I led my students in the instrumental determination of what was occurring in the brain and the speech muscles of the stutterer during stuttering and compared these results with what went on in these same structures during the normal speech of both the stutterer and the normal speaker. I was not concerned with treatment. The students and I joined in a project of shifting the handedness of a number of stutterers over a period of an academic year with no observable positive results. This type of treatment appears to be consistent with the cerebral dominance theory of stuttering. Why it didn't produce cures remains to be determined.

Had I undertaken the treatment of stuttering from the standpoint of the cerebral dominance theory, I might have put the stutterers in a program of learning to manage their speech equipment properly under strict voluntary control. I would have asked stutterers to take charge of their bodies in speaking rather than let their bodies take charge of them in the form of stuttering. I would have thought that their strong volitional effort might serve to strengthen speech dominance.

I think that stuttering is a truly psychosomatic disorder. The problem is not that one factor or the other, constitutional or environmental, is the culprit, but rather, how much of one or of the other. If there is a great lack of cortical asymmetry in the first place, then re-educational procedures may be relatively ineffective. If the stuttering is built on very small aberrant interhemispheric relationships, then environmental influences could be effective in its treatment. What the stutterer inherits is a greater probability of stuttering under the conditions permitting its development. The stutterer was formed from genes that developed a neural arrangement predisposing him or her toward stuttering. In a sense the stutterer has two problems: the basic underlying abnormal organic condition and personal reactions to the expression (stuttering) of that condition.

In treating the person who stutters we should think of a physiotherapist treating a person with a club foot. The therapist can do nothing about the organic condition itself, leaving that job to the orthopedic surgeon, but can do a great deal for the person who has the abnormality. The patient can learn to accept the condition's limitations and to compensate for the clumsy movements of the affected foot. So it can be with the stutterer, except brain surgery has never been considered seriously in the treatment of stuttering. Rather we choose to work with the troubled speaker to effect a change in the management of the peripheral speech mechanism, and in the stutterer's attitudes about himself as a handicapped person. We try to help the stutterer gain voluntary control of his speech parts, to increase self-confidence, to succeed at interpersonal relationships, and to establish the best knowledge possible of himself as an individual and a member of society. Sometimes the patient comes to speak with no or with less stuttering.

Today when my thoughts turn to the mystery of stuttering and the secrets of its nature and treatment, I am convinced that the avoidance and escape behavior, emotional arousal, speech fears, unspeakable feelings, and expectancies of stutterers are all the belated consequences of a basic, underlying cause of the disorder. The basis of most current theories of stuttering is imbedded in these belated consequences. And so could it be said of some of the therapeutic approaches. They treat the reactions of the stutterer to the handicap of stuttering and not to its real cause. In my most dogmatic moments of thinking about stuttering, I feel there is no elimination of its real cause short of drugs or brain surgery. From my own experience with drug treatment for stuttering, I do not consider it effective. For most, if not for all of us, the results of neurosurgery are currently too dangerously uncertain to warrant its use. I think we need further intensive laboratory and genetic studies of the biology of stuttering before neurosurgery can even be considered seriously. But why can't we make some postmortem studies of the brains of stuttering victims? Might not some neuropathology be found to shed light on the this troublesome problem in speaking?

Our presupposition is that the stutterer differs significantly from the normal speaker only in his neuro-anatomical organization for speaking. He has faulty equipment responsible for oral language. In no way is the stutterer personally responsible for the deep and underlying causes of not speaking like others; nor are parents, or culture. True, parents may unwittingly have supplied through their genes the faulty tools for speech. The obstetrician might have inadvertently hurt the stutterer's brain during delivery. In these cases we may place responsibility, but not on certain other aspects such as environment and culture. I have always thought that if I were a stutterer for the reasons most often listed as the culprits, I would be ashamed of myself and quit immediately. I have expressed such feelings to three of my beloved and famous stuttering students, Wendell Johnson, Charles Van Riper, and John Knott. They have smiled and forgiven my implied evaluation of their explanations of why they stuttered.

The stutterer's reactions to the affliction may make the stuttering appear

Postscript 5

worse. They may make the stutterer seem to be shy, even autistic or antisocial. They may limit choices in employment. They may reflect doubts on what is about to be said, doubts on how personal thoughts will be received, even doubts on how the stutterer will be viewed. These are not the cause of stuttering or the reason for its continuation. They are the stutterer's ways of handling the behavioral manifestations of an unseen damage to, or a lack of proper development of the brain centers for speech. Not only may stuttering be faults in the mechanics of speech, but also faults in the meaningfulness or consciousness which give meaning to what is produced by nerves and muscles. One may ask if the stuttering symptom is mainly a verbal expression (blocking, repeating) with the perceptual or meaningful level in the communicative process playing a minor role in the abnormality. Both earlier and later investigations have found that the motor output of stutterers and normal speakers is different during speech processing. The resultant theory is that the aberrant interhemispheric relationships of the stutterer result in the creation of a mistiming of nerve impulses to the bilateral speech muscles. By itself, this idea neglects any consideration of the possible disturbances in the subjective aspects of oral communication, such as meaning in all its powerful and multidimensional glow. In the middle of a stuttering spasm where is the stutterer as a self-regarding, conscious member of society? Maybe he is off somewhere suffering from a degree of automatism that in turn reduces consciousness of the meaning of the speaker–listener relationships. Normally the two halves of the brain work closely together as a functional unit with one half having leading control. When this unitary function is rendered defective, commonly by trouble in one side, both hemispheres are impaired. Our own current thinking about the nature of stuttering is that the unitary function of the two cerebral hemispheres is deficient. This deficiency is from a birth injury, early brain insult, developmental irregularities before and after birth, and genetic forces. However it may have occurred, it expresses itself in both the motor and mental functions of oral communication. In a stuttering spasm the peripheral speech structures behave contradictorily and as parts rather than as a whole, and the ingredient of consciousness in speaking is either absent or diminished. As a result, stuttering speech becomes unintelligible and senseless, and both the speaker and the listener are left dangling.

In a lifetime of trying to understand stuttering I have trod two strikingly different paths to its hiding place. I have placed the stutterer in the role of an object, of a mechanism, essentially disregarding him as a conscious, living social human being. I was concerned almost completely with the stutterer's brain and muscles as they were revealed in their electrical discharges, which in turn were detected and measured by beautifully sensitive and accurate instruments. My subject was really a passive object of study, hardly personally involved in a relationship with me.

Then I have placed the stutterer in the role of a patient in psychotherapy to explore the wonderfully intricate details of self. I invited stutterers to reveal and sense themselves more completely than they have ever done before or may ever do again in the presence of another.

These two attacks upon the mystery of stuttering gave two different sets of data to be interpreted. One set told of the body; what it did when the individual stuttered. The other set spoke of the mind; what it did with the stuttering. In 1931 *(Speech Pathology)* and later in 1978 *(Journal of Speech and Hearing Disorders),* I wrote that stuttering is due to an aberrant interhemispheric relationship, to a lack of cortical asymmetry, and to a lack of one hemisphere taking a dominant role in the control of the bilaterally innervated speech structures serving spoken language. In 1957 *(Handbook of Speech Pathology)* and later in 1971 *(Handbook of Speech Pathology and Audiology),* I held that stuttering is the speaker's attempt to prevent the verbal expression of unacceptable feelings and thoughts.

I think now that from these two evaluations of the problem of stuttering I have confused causes and consequences. The laboratory studies provided information on the cause of stuttering, while the psychotherapeutic approaches furnished a picture of all the things a stutterer thinks and feels about the trouble. In stuttering a person is isolated, shut off from others, and bereft of expressing the everlasting need to be accepted and loved. And the stutterer conjures up all sorts of reasons why.

Why? Really one lives only in terms of another; one has no way other than through someone else to realize who oneself is. This isolation due to stuttering allows only a dim view of self and results in a variety of awkward and bizarre struggles to see oneself clearly and to have a full being in significant relationships with other people.

Thus, stuttering is not caused by repressed thoughts and feelings expressed on the couch; instead, they are caused by the stuttering, which results from a lack of the two cerebral hemispheres cooperating sufficiently in managing the bilaterally innervated peripheral speech mechanism.

What can we do to help the stutterer speak more understandably? I like the approaches presented by Perkins in the numerous reports of his research over the last dozen years. Essentially the replacement of stuttering with normal speech, as he puts it, is accomplished by DAF-Rate-Control[1] procedures, by breath stream management, by achieving normal prosody, and by establishment of self-confidence. Perkins says that those who wish to speak normally can do so by learning to use the behaviors of normal speech. I think that in general this is not true. Instead, I think that some stutterers, at least, can never speak normally under all conditions of speaking. By this I mean they cannot acquire and maintain compensatory movements of the speech organs to offset stuttering. In my judgment, the treatment for stuttering is to help the individual compensate for an organic defect that currently cannot be directly treated. By psychotherapy and other psychological methods, we can lighten the burden of anxiety, tension, stress, and fear placed upon the stutterer in attempting to speak with a defective mechanism. With successful psychotherapy, the stutterer will be freer to use his maximum capacity to speak with a defective piece of equipment.

---

[1]Delayed auditory feedback slows the speaker's rate of speaking.

Postscript   5

REFERENCES

Travis, L. E. (1931). *Speech pathology.* New York: D. Appleton-Century.

Travis, L. E. (1957). *Handbook of speech pathology.* New York: Appleton-Century-Crofts.

Travis, L. E. (1971). *Handbook of speech pathology and audiology.* New York: Appleton-Century-Crofts.

Travis, L. E. (1978). The cerebral dominance theory of stuttering. *Journal of Speech and Hearing Disorders, 43:3,* 278–281.

A Study of the Onset and Development of Stuttering

Wendell Johnson

Postscript
Semantics and Beliefs

Oliver Bloodstein

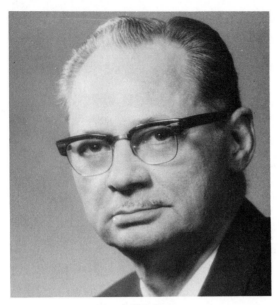

Wendell Johnson

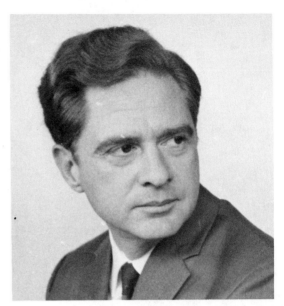

Oliver Bloodstein

Although to our knowledge Bloodstein and Johnson have not published together, in this volume they share a topic that is not as popular as it once was. Johnson's Diagnosogenic Theory was perhaps the most widely accepted theory of stuttering ever espoused. It had its greatest impact on the management of stuttering in children, and is still most popular with practitioners who treat that population, while its application to adults has given way to a number of other approaches. The theory has the appeal of simplicity and optimism and for many of us carries the ring of truth. A critical scrutiny of a theory with such dimensions is difficult to perform, especially when the theorist is a person of the stature, warmth, personability, and sensitivity of Wendell Johnson. It is probably for this reason that it has taken so long for such criticism to emerge. Bloodstein, a student and later colleague of Johnson's, has finally taken on the task of re-evaluating the semantic nature of the onset of stuttering. As a highly productive scholar in his own right, Bloodstein is eminently qualified to reassess the validity of the Diagnosogenic Theory. He does this with the recognition of the impact that Johnson had upon him as he developed his own Anticipatory Struggle Theory.

Against the background of all of the research that came out of Iowa under Johnson's direction, we had surprisingly little difficulty selecting this one article to represent the essence of his point of view. Bloodstein reacted not only to the reasonableness of Johnson's theory, but also to the data and the research strategies designed to test the theory. He points up the obvious drawback of not being able to document the first disfluency of the child that was diagnosed as stuttering. Bloodstein also notes the questionable reliability of judgments about the nondifferentiating features of disfluency between stuttering and non-stuttering children. As a result, he questions the belief that the problem is in the ear of the listener rather than in the speaker.

Bloodstein's own research has attempted to avoid the problems inherent in Johnson's design, pointing up the differences between experimental and anecdotal methods. His contributions to the field of stuttering have been outstanding, and the breadth of his knowledge, exemplified in his *Handbook on stuttering,* puts him among the top authorities in this field. For these reasons we wanted him to contribute to this volume under any circumstances. Additionally, he was there, and had first-hand contact with the man and the theory, which was followed by his own research on the theory. Therefore, we were especially pleased when Oliver Bloodstein agreed to update the classic article of Wendell Johnson.

6

A Study of the Onset and Development of Stuttering

Wendell Johnson, et al.

University of Iowa

INTRODUCTION

This study deals with the general problem of the on-set and early development of stuttering; the specific questions which it considers are implied in the statement of findings. Previous studies and theoretical statements by Bluemel(1),Froeschels (4),Van Riper (7),Johnson (5), Steer (6), Davis (2) and Egland (3) have served in part to indicate the direction of the present investigation. In general, the evidence to date appears to point to the tentative conclusion that at its onset stuttering is different from the disorder into which it usually develops. In fact, the studies and opinions so far published indicate that *on the date of original diagnosis,* stuttering children may speak in a manner that is not always to be clearly differentiated from that of other children of like age who have not been diagnosed as stutterers.

[1]This study was carried out with the collaboration and assitance of Drs. Charles Van Riper, Dorothy Davis, Hartwell Scarbrough, Yuba Hunsley, Frank Bakes, Lee Edward Travis, Miss Susan Dwyer and several others who were serving during the course of the study as assistants in connection with the speech pathology program at the University of Iowa. Three M.D.'s, Drs. Edward Lee Russell, Santa Ana, California; H. F. Shirley, University of Iowa Psychopathic Hospital; and M. L. FLoyd, Department of Pediatrics of the University of Iowa Children's Hospital, assisted with special examinations. Special funds were provided by the Laura Spelman-Rockefeller Foundation through the Iowa Child Welfare Research Station. Dr. George D. Stoddard, Director of the Iowa Child Welfare Research Station, and Dr. Lee Edward Travis, then of the University of Iowa, authorized and supported the investigation. A detailed report of the study is scheduled to be published by the Iowa Child Welfare Research Station.

The present investigation is designed to yield more definite information as to the characteristics of stuttering at its onset, and to explore the problem of the changes that occur as stuttering develops through its early stages into its more advanced phases. It is also designed to throw some light on the problems surrounding the disappearance of stuttering. Several of our cases had regained normal speech by the end of the investigation. We are also concerned with the conditions surrounding the onset, the aggravation, the alleviation and the disappearance of the disorder. Moreover, we are interested in obtaining more adequate information concerning children who develop stuttering and the characteristics which differentiate them from children who do not stutter.

Two groups of subjects were investigated, 46 stuttering children and 46 non-stuttering children. In the stuttering group there were 32 males and 14 females; in the non-stuttering group there were 33 males and 13 females. At time of first interview, the stutterers ranged in age from approximately 2 years, 3 months to 9 years, 3 months with a median of 4 years, 2 months. The non-stutterers ranged in age from approximately 2 years, 3 months to 9 years, 10 months with a median of 4 years, 5 months. The stutterers' I.Q.'s ranged from 80 to 159 with a median of 114. The non-stutterers; I.Q.'s ranged from 95 to 158 with a median of 116. The non-stutterers were drawn from the University of Iowa Preschools and Elementary

Note: From *The Journal of Speech Disorders,* 7, 1942, pp. 251–257. Reprinted with permission of the American Speech-Language-Hearing Association.

School. In general, the socio-economic status of this group is probably slightly higher than that of the stuttering group. About one-fourth of the stutterers were attending or had attended the University Preschool.

The original diagnosis of stuttering was never made by the investigators. In three-fourths of the cases the original diagnoses of stuttering were made by the parents, and in the other cases they were made by teachers or relatives of the children. Only those children were placed in the stuttering group who were referred to the investigators as stutterers; the referral was accompanied in every case by a request for remedial advice and help. A child was accepted as a non-stutterer only if parents, teachers and others associated with the child—and the child—regarded him unquestionably as a non-stutterer. If anyone at all regarded a given child as a stutterer, that child was excluded from the non-stuttering group.

PROCEDURE

In setting up the procedure, several special considerations were emphasized. Since interview and case study techniques were clearly indicated, special care was taken to minimize the usual shortcomings of such techniques. First, an attempt was made to obtain cases in whom stuttering was of recent origin, in order that information might be obtained in relatively great detail concerning the onset of the disorder. The median interval between the date of onset and the date of the first interview was 5 months and 18 days. Second, a fairly long period of observation in each stuttering case studied was desirable. The median period of observation for these cases was 2 years and 4 months. Third, an attempt was made to check the information obtained by carrying out as many interviews as possible and by assigning two or more interviewers to each stuttering case. The number of interviews per stuttering case ranged from 2 to 19 with a median of 4 and the number of interviewers ranged from 2 to 5 with a median of 3. In the study as a whole, 17 different interviewers were involved; all held the M.A. degree in speech pathology or clinical psychology, and 13 now hold the Ph.D. degree. Every stutterer's home was visited by one or more interviewers. The 46 non-stuttering children were investigated by a single interviewer, and only one interview was made in each case. All interviewing was done in the homes, and the information supplied by the parents and by means of the interviewers' ob-

servations was supplemented by data from the files of the Iowa Child Welfare Research Station.

RESULTS

Comparative data for the stutterers and non-stutterers were obtained with regard to birth conditions, general developmental conditions, speech development, diseases and injuries, stuttering and handedness in the family background and handedness and eyedness of the children themselves.

Every indication of a deviation from an entirely normal birth was noted in each case. A careful analysis of these data indicated that the two groups were essentially similar. The one case in whom birth injury was quite definitely serious was that of a stutterer who, however, was no longer stuttering at the close of the present study.

With regard to the age of "standing alone without support," walking, creeping, sitting and teething, the two groups presented almost exactly the same median and quartile values. Data on feeding and dressing self and bladder and bowel control revealed slight developmental differences in favor of the non-stutterers, which seemed to be most adequately accounted for by the fact that the Iowa City parents of the non-stutterers were all in active contact with the Iowa Child Welfare Research Station and its child study program for parents. At least, the other developmental data would hardly support an interpretation in terms of generally retarded development on the part of the stutterers.

The median and quartile values for the ages at which words and sentences, respectively, were first spoken are exactly the same for both groups.

A few more diseases and injuries were reported for the stuttering group. This was to be expected, of course, since the diseases and injuries experienced by the stutterers during the course of the investigation were included in their totals. This means that their illness and injury records covered about 2.5 years more, on the average, than did those of the non-stutterers. No one type of disease was reported by as many as half of either group. There was a higher incidence of tonsilitis and ear infections among the non-stutterers and a higher incidence of whooping cough, measles and influenza among the stutterers. However, examination of the individual case records reveals that in no case was either whooping cough or influenza even fairly closely associated temporally with the onset of stuttering. In fact, in only four cases could any kind of disease condition be mentioned among the factors possibly associated with onset of stuttering; these included one case of "very mild measles," one case of infected tonsils, one case of a cold and sore throat and one case who was thought to have been weakened by pneumonia some time before stuttering began. In each of these cases, however, there was no unmistakable relation between these conditions and the onset of stuttering, and in each case a number of other factors were also temporally associated with the stuttering onset. It is to be concluded that in no case did illness stand out as the only precipitating factor or even as an undoubtedly definite one.

"Significant" injuries were reported for only four non-stutterers and six stutterers, and none of these injuries had left any permanent effects of serious degree. No injury was temporally related to the onset of stuttering. Insofar as there might be a difference between the two groups so far as the incidence of illnesses and injuries is concerned, its significance in relation to the stuttering would appear to lie necessarily in the possible general effects of the illnesses since they were not found to be temporally related in any significant degree to the onset of stuttering.

Data concerning stuttering in the family background showed that for the stutterers one father and two mothers were stutterers and four fathers and three mothers were former stutterers; for the non-stutterers, two fathers were stutterers and one mother was a former stutterer. Fifteen stutterers and

four non-stutterers each had one or more stuttering relatives. Of the 56 speaking siblings of the stutterers, 9 were stutterers and 3 were former stutterers; of the 32 speaking siblings of the non-stutterers, only 1 was reported as a stutterer. Thus, there are more stutterers in the families of the stutterers than in the families of the non-stutterers. Any attempt to interpret this difference must involve a consideration not only of possible hereditary factors but also of family patterns of evaluation.

The parents of the two groups did not differ appreciably as far as handedness was concerned, nor did the siblings of the two groups differ appreciably in this respect. However, 15 of the stutterers and 4 of the non-stutterers had left-handed relatives outside of the immediate family. Handedness and eyedness data concerning the two groups of children were obtained. Judgments of handedness and of changes of handedness were based on detailed interview data and on systematic and casual observation by the examiners. A hand usage questionnaire was filled out for all of the non-stutterers and for 36 of the stutterers. These data were treated with special care because of the controversial nature of the issues involved. The data are summarized in Table 6-1. This table indicates that there is practically no difference between the two groups with respect to eyedness or handedness. It is of special interest that 12 stutterers and 14 non-stutterers were judged to have had their handedness changed. Most of the changes were from a condition of ambidexterity to right-handedness. Two stutterers and one non-stutterer had been

Table 6-1. Handedness and eyedness conditions of the 46 stutterers and 46 non-stutterers.

	Stutterers	Non-stutterers
No. right-handed (present)	36	36
No. left-handed (present)	6	4
No. ambidextrous (present)	4	6
No. originally right-handed	26	24
No. originally left-handed	10	8
No. originally ambidextrous	10	14
No. changed handedness	12	14
Left to right	2	1
Left to ambidextrous	2	2
Ambidextrous to right	8	11
No. right-eyed	22	26
No. left-eyed	16	10
No. amphiocular	0	5

changed from left to right-handedness, and two children from each group had been changed from left-handedness to ambidexterity. Space does not permit a detailed discussion of the procedures used and the principles of interpretation of the data. It can only be said here that the most defensible conclusion appears to be that our two groups of subjects do not differ to any theoretically significant degree with respect to early handedness, handedness at time of interview or handedness changes.

In summarizing all of the comparative data, it is to be pointed out that the similarities between the two groups of subjects appear to be much more significant than the differences. These comparative data do not seem to offer any definite bases on which one might account for the speech condition of the stuttering group.

An attempt was made to obtain detailed information concerning the speech phenomena that were originally diagnosed as stuttering in each case. In over 90 per cent of the cases it was possible to obtain quite adequate descriptive accounts, for in a few cases the parents were unable to recall specific incidents sufficiently to furnish a thoroughly reliable description of the very first phenomena which they had regarded as stuttering. For purposes of this summary report, in which it is not possible to give a full account of the clarifying details, it is sufficient to say that in approximately 92 per cent of the cases the first phenomena that were diagnosed as stuttering were beyond doubt essentially effortless repetitions of words, phrases or the first sounds or syllables of words. In the other cases also, these phenomena were, so far as could be determined, the predominating features, although there is some question as to whether, in these cases, diagnoses of stuttering were made before the child had begun to exhibit some degree of hypertonicity in connection with the repetitions or before the child had begun to exhibit such other reactions as prolongations of sounds, conspicuous pauses, etc. It can definitely be said that the characteristic phenomena originally diagnosed as stuttering in these cases were those involving simple repetition apparently without noticeable strain or tension and apparently without any awareness on the part of the child either that he was repeating or that the repetitions constituted a difficulty or abnormality.

The reactions involving hypertonicity, facial grimaces, holding of the breath, definite blocking and overt evidence of the child's awareness of difficulty,

overt manifestations of embarrassment, annoyances, etc., and apparent devices and attempts to postpone or avoid speech—these reactions, with very few if any exceptions, appeared after the diagnosis had been made. The most reasonable conclusion appears to be that they were consequences of the diagnosis in the sense that the making of a diagnosis appeared to be part of a general parental policy. In turn, it appeared to intensify the parental policy in the direction of increased anxiety and vigilance. We are all familiar with the principle that the way in which one classifies a person largely determines one's general reactions to that person. This principle seems to have operated in these cases in which the parents classified their children as stutterers and then proceeded to react to them largely in terms of the implications of the label. These reactions on the part of parents were not confined to inner states of tension and anxiety or chagrin, but usually also involved overt attempts to influence the child's speech behavior and definite communication to the child of the parental evaluations of his speech.

An example will help to illustrate how this process works out in practice. The father of a three-year-old boy happened to notice one evening that the boy repeated a number of sounds or words. He reported later that there was no apparent tension or self-consciousness involved in the child's behavior and that until that time he had assumed that the child's speech was entirely normal. For some reason, however, he regarded these repetitions as stuttering, and the next day he consulted the family physician. He was advised to instruct the boy to take a deep breath before speaking. Within approximately 48 hours after the boy had received this instruction, he had developed an apparent habit of frequent and serious gasping reactions which the father interpreted as constituting a marked increase in the severity of stuttering. This is a particularly clear-cut example which, however, illustrates the fundamental principle by which one is able to explain in large part the transition from the simple repetitions to the more complicated phenomena which developed following diagnosis in these stuttering children. It is to be noted further that the simple repetitions originally diagnosed as stuttering were found in the speech of the non-stuttering children, where they had not been so diagnosed, and they have been reported by Davis (2) as more or less characteristic of the speech of young children, generally. The question as to why such phenomena are diagnosed as stuttering by some parents and not by others deserves further intensive investigation. There can be little question of the fact that highly similar varieties of speech in young children are thus differently evaluated by different parents, and there can be little question that the way in which they are evaluated plays a determining role in the subsequent speech development of the child. In the present study, there were some striking examples of the diagnosis of stuttering being applied to speech that was undoubtedly quite normal with very serious results.

More highly quantifying procedures would be necessary in order to settle the question as to whether those children who come to be diagnosed as stutterers actually do exhibit a higher frequency of repetitions or of other evidences of non-fluency than do other children before they are diagnosed. Some of them certainly do not. When it is true that they do, they serve to raise the question as to the conditions under which simple repetition would give way to more serious reactions in the absence of a diagnosis of stuttering. From the study by Davis (2) and from the present study, it is obvious that children generally tend to repeat more often in some situations and in certain types of speaking than in others. In homes characterized by conditions particularly conducive to repetition, one would expect children to show more of it and such children might more readily come to be regarded as defective in speech and so suffer the further speech interference consequent to such an evaluation. In some of the homes involved in this study, such conditions appeared to be significantly in evidence, but this was true in varying degrees of the homes for both groups of children. In general, the sheer frequency of speech repetitions did not appear to be as significant as the evaluations placed upon them by the parents.

The severity of stuttering during the course of the disorder in our 46 children was judged by the examiners to be mild in 12 cases, average in 28 and severe in 6. By the end of the study, 25 were judged to be definitely normal, 5 nearly normal, 3 indefinite, 1 mild, 11 average and 1 severe. Thus only 13 out of the 46 were still unquestionably or to any significant degree stuttering when the investigation was closed. In the course of its reduction in severity and disappearance, the stuttering changed not only with respect to the frequency of its occurrence, but also with respect to the degree of hypertonicity and affectivity involved. In general, it went as it came in that it re-

ceded from a complicated strenuous pattern to one of simple effortless repetition. In the majority of cases, the only remedial advice offered the parents was that designed to reverse their evaluations of the child's speech and to insure his being stimulated and responded to on the assumption that he was a normal child capable of normal speech accomplishments. In other words, the diagnoses were challenged and reversed. In some cases, specific recommendations were made with regard to the alteration of certain home and school conditions which seemed to be particularly conducive to non-fluency. In a few cases handedness changes were recommended and some of these were carried out reasonably well while others were not. In very few instances was any attention given directly to the child by way of exercises or drills or even discussion of the problem.

CONCLUSION

This study of the onset and development of stuttering in young children suggests the advisability of intensive investigation of the apparent probability that stuttering in its serious forms develops after the diagnosis rather than before and is a consequence of the diagnosis. While in no way disregarding the importance of other possible factors, this conclusion is intended to focus attention upon a factor that seems to be highly significant and that appears to have been disregarded in previous theoretical approaches to the problem of stuttering.

REFERENCES

1. Bluemel, C. S., Primary and secondary stuttering, **Proceedings of the American Speech Correction Association,** 1932, 91–102.
2. Davis, Dorothy M., The relation of repetitions in the speech of young children to certain measures of language maturity and situational factors: Part I, **Journal of Speech Disorders,** 1939, 4, 303–318.
3. Egland, George O., An analysis of repetition and prolongations in the speech of young children. State University of Iowa, unpublished Master's thesis, 1938.
4. Froeschels, Emil, Beitrage zur Symptomatologie des Stotterns, **Monatschr, f. Ohrenheilk,** 1921, 55.
5. Johnson, W., The role of evaluation in stuttering behavior, **Journal of Speech Disorders,** 1938, 3, 85–89.
6. Steer, M. D., Symptomatologies of young stutterers, **Journal of Speech Disorders,** 1937, 1, 3–13.
7. Van Riper, C., The growth of the stuttering spasm, **Quarterly Journal of Speech,** 1937, 23, 70–73.

Semantics and Beliefs

Oliver Bloodstein

In "A Study of the Onset and Development of Stuttering," Wendell Johnson first made public the theory for which he later coined the word "diagnosogenic." The year was 1942. By the 1950s this had become perhaps the most widely accepted, and certainly the best known, theory of stuttering in the United States. This renown was probably due in large measure to the appealing simplicity of the idea that stuttering is caused by its own diagnosis. In part, the theory's swift rise to popularity was also the result of Johnson's skill and persuasiveness as a writer and his great personal influence as a teacher of teachers of teachers. By the 1980s, most serious seekers of the secret of stuttering had long since begun to grope along other paths, but the diagnosogenic theory still appears to claim a large number of adherents among a generation of workers in the field, and has left its mark on theory, research, and clinical work on stuttering. My aim is to present a brief biography of the theory, and to trace its influence on various aspects of thinking about stuttering today.

ORIGIN OF THE THEORY

Anyone who advances a supposedly new idea about stuttering must be put on notice that someone has probably said it before and that someone else will probably disprove it. Johnson's theory has not yet been disproved, but it did have a notable antecedent. As a student of Johnson's, I once heard him acknowledge a debt to Emil Froeschels when another student asked him how he had arrived at his theory. In the early decades of this century, Froeschels wrote that most normal children exhibit an early pattern of effortless repetitions of initial syllables of words that he called "physiologic stuttering." He believed that some children who become conscious of these repetitions may begin to talk with exceptional effort in order to overcome what they think is a speech difficulty, with the result that the simple repetitions develop into "tonic" blocks. Froeschels put much of the blame for this development on fearful attitudes and faulty advice from persons in the child's environment, although he thought children might often evaluate their speech repetitions negatively on their own (Froeschels, 1915, 1933). The influence on Johnson's thinking is clear. The difference in Johnson's theory, besides the greater emphasis on the perfectionism of the parents, is that in place of "physiologic stuttering" there is merely "normal nonfluency." Accustomed as we are today to the concept of disfluency as a normal feature of children's speech, this may not seem a very difficult step to take, but in the 1930s it took considerable creativity.

A point of view somewhat similar to Froeschels' was expressed by Bluemel (1932), who said that stuttering begins in the form of a "primary" stage of simple repetitions of initial words, sounds, or syllables. He suggested that this first stage may soon develop into the struggle behavior of "secondary" stuttering if the child is punished or scolded for primary stuttering. This is far from the diagnosogenic theory, but it embodies a basic element, the onset of struggle reactions as an effort to avoid simple repetitions. Johnson was certainly familiar with Bluemel's influential paper.

Beyond the immediate antecedents of the diagnosogenic theory, we must note certain broad influences that contributed to it. One summer in the late 1930s, Johnson fell ill with pneumonia. During a lengthy convalescence, he occupied his time by reading "Science and Sanity," the 800-page volume in which Alfred Korzybski developed the discipline that he called "general semantics." Korzybski's central thesis, that many human ills result from identifying words with things, proved to be a turning point in Johnson's thinking about both the nature and treatment of stuttering. The concept is clearly evident, of course, in Johnson's inference that stuttering develops when parents label a child a stutterer and then react to the label instead of to the realities of the child's speech.

Finally, the diagnosogenic theory was a product of the intellectual outlook of its time in the most fundamental sense. By the 1930s a new zeitgeist had developed, one that favored a view of human behavior in which social environment, not heredity, played the preponderant role. Johnson was riding with this tide in rejecting the dominant organic theories of Travis and West and the medical model of stuttering that had long prevailed. In keeping with the fervor of a new movement, this rejection was extreme. To the end of his career, in the face of the very high familial incidence of stuttering, Johnson refused to assign even a small role to heredity in the development of the disorder.

I don't know the exact year that Johnson first conceived of his theory, but it was evidently some time in the late 1930s. He used to tell his students that the idea first came to him in the course of a study of young stutterers and nonstutterers that was carried out as a collaborative effort of the University of Iowa speech clinic. Johnson's role was to examine the speech of the children. The notion that stuttering begins "not in the child's mouth, but in the parent's ear" occurred to him when he found that he could not always tell the stutterers apart from the non-

Postscript 6

stutterers by the way they spoke. Johnson apparently was referring to the investigation he reported in 1942 as "A Study of the Onset and Development of Stuttering."[1]

All of this now has such a strong historical resonance that it is hard for me to believe that when I first came to Iowa City, in the fall of 1941, Johnson's report of the onset study had not yet been published and the diagnosogenic theory was still very new. Having read Travis's *Speech Pathology* shortly before my arrival at the university, I came to Johnson's lectures believing that stuttering is caused by a lack of sufficient cerebral dominance. I soon changed my mind. Johnson's lectures were captivating. We chuckled appreciatively at a string of aphorisms: "A rose by any other name does not smell as sweet." "We don't know much about heredity, and most of what we do know is about the fruit fly." "A stutterer is not a person who can't talk fluently—he's a person who can't talk nonfluently." The ingenious simplicity of the diagnosogenic theory captured our imaginations. Johnson was 36 years old at the time. He was sociable and insisted that we call him "Jack." For good measure, there was that engaging flaw of his—not the conventional scar on the cheek, but the blemish that was evident when he spoke. Who would not be a disciple of such a man?

INFLUENCE ON LATER THEORIES

Johnson's inferences about the development of stuttering were important not only in themselves, but also for what they contributed to other lines of thinking about the disorder.

The next important theoretical development following Johnson's theory was the application of learning theory in the early formulations of Wischner (1950, 1952) and Sheehan (1953), both of whom had studied with Johnson. Although this development drew mainly on the work of the learning psychologists Clark Hull and Neal Miller, it also derived much of its initial impetus from Johnson. It was Johnson who had asserted that stuttering is learned behavior, in opposition to the prevailing theories of the day, and who kept reiterating this in his teaching and writing like a slogan. Furthermore, Johnson had studied the experimental psychology of learning at the University of Iowa, where speech pathology and psychology were closely integrated areas of study, and when he said "learned behavior" he was using the term with all the connotations it had to learning psychologists. In part, Wischner's view of stuttering as an anxiety-motivated instrumental avoidance act was a reformulation, in learning theory terms, of Johnson's assertions about the role of anxiety, anticipation, and avoidance in stuttering be-

---

[1] Johnson published a more detailed version of this report in *Stuttering in children and adults* (Johnson, 1955), where he states in an editor's note that the study was conducted from 1934 to 1939 by himself, Charles Van Riper, Dorothy Davis Tuthill, Yuba Hunsley, Hartwell Scarbrough, Susan Dwyer, and Esther Glaspey Ogdahl, with the assistance of a number of others, under the guidance of Lee Edward Travis. Why it was Johnson who took the initiative in publishing the results is apparently related to the fact that the comparisons of the stutterers and nonstutterers yielded largely negative findings. It was mainly for Johnson that this outcome was significant.

havior. Later, Shames and Sherrick (1963) contributed an interpretation of John-son's concept of the onset and development of stuttering that was based on B. F. Skinner's operant analysis of behavior.

An additional service that the diagnosogenic theory performed was as a ve-hicle for the transmission of the anticipatory struggle hypothesis from workers of the past to those of the present. Theories of stuttering are of two kinds: theories of the etiology of the disorder and hypotheses about the nature of the stuttering block. The theory that stuttering is caused by its diagnosis explained its etiology. When Johnson looked for a conceptual model of the stuttering block that was compatible with the diagnosogenic theory, he found it in the assumption that stuttering is what the stutterer does in the effort to avoid stuttering. This is one way of stating a theory that has been worded in various ways by many writers for more than a hundred years. I have used the term "anticipatory struggle" as a gen-eral name for this model. Johnson called it "anticipatory avoidance." So great was Johnson's influence that it has often been assumed that he originated the antici-patory struggle concept as part of his theory of stuttering, and when similar ideas have been found in earlier writings, they have sometimes been regarded as re-markable "anticipations" of Johnson. In reality, few observations have been more common in the literature of the past than the suggestion that the stutterer's basic problem is the conviction that speech is difficult; or doubt about the ability to speak; or the use of effort to overcome what the stutterer erroneously perceives as a speech obstacle; or an expectancy "neurosis." Such views were held in Eu-rope by Wynecken, Denhardt, Isserlin, Kraepelin, Froeschels, and Freund, among others (see Freund, 1966, pp. 22–43). In the American literature this hypothesis was clearly articulated many years ago by Tompkins (1918), who believed that the stutterer makes "conscious speech efforts" to remedy temporary speech inter-ruptions. "The failure of these misdirected efforts he takes for an inherent speech difficulty; so he continues his efforts, not realizing that they are the difficulty" (p.293).

Johnson, then, did not create the anticipatory struggle hypothesis. But his theory gave it wide currency in the United States at a time when this model of the stuttering block had few exponents in this country, and served to hand it on to a later generation of American workers. My own efforts to understand stuttering have been based on this hypothesis, and others will almost certainly make use of it in the future. Until it is found to be invalid, it is unlikely that a theory that has proved so durable will cease to be so.

INFLUENCE ON RESEARCH

The diagnosogenic theory is extremely difficult to prove or disprove. This is not because, as in the case of a poor theory, it is logically unverifiable, but only be-cause of a technical difficulty. The central assumption of the theory is that at the moment that a child is first diagnosed as a stutterer by a parent, the child's dis-fluencies do not differ from those of ordinary children. Unfortunately, no one has

Postscript 6

found a way to post objective, scientific observers at the right place at the right moment. For this reason, researchers have tried instead to verify more easily testable assumptions that may be deduced from the theory. These attempts have not served to test Johnson's theory conclusively, but they have resulted in a great many findings that are interesting and may be useful from the point of view of any theory.

One deduction that is easily made from the theory is that the average stutterer's social environment in the early years should be marked by anxiety and pressure, especially with regard to speech fluency. This question has prompted a good number of investigations of the attitudes and adjustments of stutterers' parents, as well as some research on the incidence of stuttering on different socioeconomic levels and in various cultures. The findings to date do not tell us much about the parents' standards of fluency, but they suggest that stuttering may have some relationship to generally high aspirations, competitiveness, and pressures toward conformity in the stutterer's environment.

My first research at the beginning of my career at Brooklyn College was a direct attack, in collaboration with two of my students, on the question of the standards of fluency of stutterers' parents (Bloodstein, Jaeger, and Tureen, 1952). We asked parents of young stutterers and nonstutterers to listen to recorded samples of normal children's speech and to identify the children they regarded as stutterers. True to our hypothesis, the stutterers' parents made significantly more diagnoses of stuttering, and we reported this as evidence in support of Johnson's theory. Oddly enough, this was the beginning of my disaffection with regard to the theory. I wasn't aware of it at the time, but I had, I think, been somewhat sobered by the small extent of the difference we found, statistically significant thought it was.

Another inference that may be drawn from Johnson's theory is that listeners may differ with respect to what they define as stuttering blocks. For this reason, many studies have been done on the extent of agreement among listeners on the occurrence of stuttering, on the types of disfluencies that are most likely to be identified as stutterings, and on the kinds of listeners that are most prone to make such identifications. Perhaps the outstanding finding from this research is that agreement among listeners on the occurrence of a stuttering block is considerably lower than most workers prior to Johnson would probably have expected.

Finally, the diagnosogenic theory led naturally to research comparing the disfluencies of young children thought to be stutterers with those of other children. Although numerous investigators have made contributions in this area, the findings of Johnson and his co-workers, published as *The onset of stuttering* (1959), remain the outstanding source of information on the subject. Faced with the difficulty that there is no way to observe the disfluencies of children at the moment of original diagnosis, Johnson adopted two alternatives, each having a serious drawback. One was to study the parents' descriptions of these disfluencies, ignoring the doubtful reliability of memories and the ambiguities of language. The other was to observe the children's disfluencies when they had been brought to the speech clinic, in most cases many weeks or months after the parents had first regarded the children as stutterers. As it turned out, neither method produced results that supported the diagnosogenic theory in a simple, unequivocal way.

The parents of the "alleged" stutterers most often recalled syllable and word repetitions as the earliest stuttering of their children. The parents of a comparable group of nonstutterers most often recalled word and phrase repetitions, pauses, and interjections as their children's earliest disfluencies. Despite this difference, there was also considerable overlapping between the two sets of recollections, and Johnson interpreted this to support his theory that stuttering is largely a "perceptual and evaluative" problem of adult listeners.

The other method, the analysis of the recorded samples of the speech of the children, produced two main findings. One was that the children who were regarded by their parents as stutterers were considerably more disfluent than the nonstutterers, having more repetitions of all kinds, prolonged sounds, and broken words. The other finding was that every form of disfluency was exhibited by both groups of children, and that there was no "natural line of demarcation" that separated one group from the other. What did this mean? Johnson did not go as far as to say that the "alleged" stutterers were really speaking normally. What he did say was that, since there is no feature of their speech that serves to differentiate stutterers from nonstutterers, one could not very well define stuttering in terms of a child's disfluencies. Stuttering must be defined, he said, as a "problem" that arises for a listener (Johnson et al. 1959, pp. 214, 218–220, 232, 262).

I suspect that most readers of *The onset of stuttering* who were not ardent devotees of Johnson found it strange to hear that stuttering could not be defined as a feature of a child's speech. Robert West, who loved to needle me about my old teacher's gaffes, as he considered them, wrote me a note saying, "Honestly, don't you think Johnson spins his ideas to gossamer thinness?" Johnson, however, was attracted to observations that exposed the untrustworthiness of common sense. (He was fond of the quotation, "The rudiments of common sense are not difficult to learn; they are just unusual.") With regard to the development of stuttering, he believed that an adequate understanding required an appreciation of issues that were inherently "subtle," as he put it. It saddened him when he found that I was not up to it.

It seemed to me that there was a simpler interpretation of Johnson's results, one that permitted a definition of stuttering as a feature of a child's speech despite the absence of the natural line of demarcation. It was the rather obvious possibility that the repetitions, prolongations, and broken words of young stutterers belong on a continuum with those of normal speakers, and can be sharply demarcated from them only arbitrarily, as hearing loss is separated from normal hearing, delayed language development from normal language development, mental retardation from normal intelligence, and so on. In other words, I thought it a plausible hypothesis that children commonly perceived as incipient stutterers are doing things that many ordinary children do, and for the same reasons,

Postscript 6

but to such a marked degree that they come to be regarded, first by one and then by another, as defective in speech.

It is important to note that the diagnosogenic way of thinking does not permit this "continuity" hypothesis. A common misconception of beginning students is that Johnson believed stuttering and normal disfluency in young children to be "the same thing." On the contrary, his concept that incipient stuttering is the effort to avoid normal disfluency tends to separate them in an either/or fashion, and Johnson often stated explicitly that we must make a sharp distinction between stuttering and normal disfluency. When he found that there was no sharp distinction between how young stutterers and nonstutterers spoke, he defined stuttering in a manner that allowed him to make such a distinction—that is, in terms of whether or not there was a "problem."

Johnson's reaction to the continuity hypothesis is instructive. When I first broached it, in an article on the development of stuttering in 1961, he wrote me, ". . . it seems to me that you come close to saying that what might possibly be regarded as 'normal nonfluency' is really stuttering . . ." In a sense, that is exactly what I was saying. Johnson's implication that the statement is self-evidently false reveals how implicitly he believed that a "normal-speaking" child can't be "stuttering" because one either is a stutterer or is not. As a result, Johnson never accepted what I believe to be one of the outstanding contributions of his research to our understanding of stuttering—the possibility that there is a continuity between early stuttering and certain kinds of normal childhood disfluency.

INFLUENCE ON THERAPY

The diagnosogenic theory had at least two discernible effects on the attitudes and practices of clinicians. First, the theory made us question how we knew that a child was stuttering, and promoted the belief that we had to determine whether the child was a stutterer or a nonstutterer before we could be of help. We were compelled to realize that we didn't know how to make such a differentiation, and this problem has continued to create doubt and controversy to the present day.

Secondly, the diagnosogenic theory strengthened the conviction of many clinical workers that parent counseling should be the principal method of treating early stuttering. Today, when new prospects for helping incipient stutterers are continually being explored, Johnson is sometimes held responsible for advocating a policy of "ignoring" early stuttering. This criticism is neither just nor accurate. His great concern with parent counseling was, in the first place, something he shared with others, especially Van Riper, whose widely used textbook, *Speech correction: Principles and methods,* warned that "the way to treat a young stutterer in the primary stage is to let him alone, and treat his parents and teachers"(Van Riper, 1939, p. 336), an admonition that clearly shows the influence of Bluemel.

In the second place, both Johnson and Van Riper early on favored certain forms of working "directly" with the child, generally in the guise of play. What they cautioned against was any kind of therapy that would make very young children aware that they were being treated for a defect or disorder, and in this they would almost certainly have the support of most clinicians today.

When all is said and done, however, it is true that Johnson's writing may have been open to the misinterpretation that he advocated completely ignoring early stuttering. This misapprehension is possible because he asserted that young children brought to the clinic with the complaint that they were stuttering should be treated as far as possible on the assumption that they were essentially normal speakers. The goal was not so much remediation, but prevention. To be sure, most of these children had more than the average amount of disfluency in their speech, but why call them stutterers, he thought, when they seemed for the most part to be doing what normal speaking children do, only more so? This message was particularly clear in Johnson's famous "Open letter to the mother of a 'stuttering' child," which miraculously gave parents to understand that they were the cause of their child's stuttering without giving them any offense, or more guilt than was necessary to inspire them to change their behavior. Copies of this letter were probably distributed to parents by the thousands, and did much to influence the thinking of clinicians and students, as well as parents.[2]

Needless to say, I was strongly affected by Johnson's outlook too. When I first arrived at Brooklyn College as a young instructor and clinic supervisor, I tried for about two years to convince a succession of parents of stutterers that their children were not talking very abnormally. On the whole, their reactions to this were much like the helpless reactions of almost anyone who has gone to the doctor with a pain to be told that there is nothing wrong. They often pleaded with me to see that there was something seriously the matter. "You should have heard him on Saturday," they would say. Finally I began to ask myself whether, in all honesty, I could maintain my sanguine clinical attitude if my own child were talking like many of those who were brought to see me. My answer was no. I decided that what most parents needed was not to be told that their child was talking normally, but that I understood their perceptions and feelings and accepted them. So I began to tell most parents, "Yes, your child is showing some stuttering reactions. Many normal children do. It's nothing to be alarmed about, provided we handle it in the proper way." That seemed to work far better, for me.

This experience did little to shake my faith in the assumption that the children had been speaking normally when the parents had originally diagnosed them as stutterers. My serious doubts about the diagnosogenic theory began a few years later, when I was able to look back over a longer series of cases. Then I saw evidence that many parents of stutterers had indeed been concerned about their children's speech before the children had begun to exhibit an abnormal amount of disfluency, but it seemed to me that the concern had usually been about the children's language or articulation rather than about their fluency.

---

[2]Johnson's "Open letter to the mother of a 'stuttering' child" is reproduced in Johnson et al. (1967), pp. 543–554.

Postscript 6

How shall we evaluate the status of the diagnosogenic theory 40 years after the publication of "A Study of the Onset and Development of Stuttering"? It is now an old theory. A truism of our field is that theories of stuttering are seldom abandoned because they have been disproved. Most often we just get tired of them. To some extent, this has probably happened in the case of the diagnosogenic theory. In the absence of clear verification of the theory, we have gone on to other things. Many today believe that organic factors play some part in stuttering. Evidence is increasing that biological inheritance does have some influence. The great majority of present-day writers and researchers do not appear to hold with Johnson that a parent's evaluation of normal disfluency as stuttering is the principal cause of the disorder, or that stuttering is the avoidance of normal disfluency. On a deeper level, Johnson's theory has collided with a new zeitgeist that tends to take more seriously the effect of genes on behavior and to regard the old preoccupation with environment as somewhat excessive.

Yet the theory still has adherents, and what is more remarkable, it continues to impress and fascinate students who hear about it for the first time, even from a teacher who has not been a believer for many years. More importantly, the theory has left a legacy of provocative and fundamental questions. We still do not know whether it is possible to identify stuttering blocks in any meaningful sense independently of the judgments of listeners. We still do not know whether early stuttering bears any relationship to normal childhood disfluency, and if so, what kind of relationship; and we are not agreed on how to differentiate "stuttering" children from those who speak "normally." It may be that workers in our field will continue to ponder such questions long after most of them have forgotten where the questions came from.

In sum, the diagnosogenic theory was an ingenious hypothesis that had exceptional intellectual appeal and enjoyed wide acceptance; the theory has been exceedingly difficult to prove or disprove; it has come into conflict with certain observations, including some of Johnson's own, and has declined in popularity relative to other points of view; but it has engendered thinking and research, and that is perhaps as much as we can ask of any theory.

REFERENCES

Bloodstein, O., Jaeger, W., & Tureen, J. (1952). A study of the diagnosis of stuttering by parents of stutterers and nonstutterers. *Journal of Speech and Hearing Disorders, 17,* 308–315

Bluemel, C. S. (1932). Primary and secondary stammering. *Quarterly Journal of Speech, 18,* 187–200.

Froeschels, E. (1915). Stuttering and nystagmus. *Monatschrift für Ohrenheilkunde, 49,* 161–167.

Froeschels, E. (1933). *Speech therapy.* Boston: Expression Co.

Freund, H. (1966). *Psychopathology and the problems of stuttering.* Springfield, IL: Charles C. Thomas.

Johnson, W. (1955). A study of the onset and development of stuttering. In Johnson, W. (Ed.) *Stuttering in children and adults.* Minneapolis: University of Minnesota Press.

Johnson W. (1967). "An open letter to the mother of a 'stuttering' child," *You and your child,* April, 1941. Reprinted in Johnson et al., *Speech handicapped schoolchildren,* 1967, pp. 543–544

Johnson, W., et al. (1959). *The onset of stuttering.* Minneapolis: University of Minnesota Press.

Johnson, W., Brown, S. F., Curtis, J. F., Edney, C. W., & Keaster, J. (1967). *Speech handicapped school children* (3rd ed.). New York: Harper & Row.

Shames, G. H., & Sherrick, C. E., Jr. (1963). A discussion of nonfluency and stuttering as operant behavior. *Journal of Speech and Hearing Disorders, 28,* 3–18.

Sheehan, J. G. (1953). Theory and treatment of stuttering as an approach-avoidance conflict. *Journal of Psychology, 36,* 27–49.

Tompkins, E. (1918). Perception of stammering. *Quarterly Journal of Speech Education, 4,* 290–295.

Travis, L. E. (1931). *Speech pathology.* New York: D. Appleton-Century.

Van Riper, C. (1939). *Speech correction: Principles and methods.* New York: Prentice-Hall.

Wischner, G. J. (1950). Stuttering behavior and learning: A preliminary theoretical formulation. *Journal of Speech and Hearing Disorders, 15,* 324–335.

Wischner, G. J. (1952). An experimental approach to expectancy and anxiety in stuttering behavior. *Journal of Speech and Hearing Disorders, 17,* 139–154.

7

Two-Factor Behavior Theory and Therapy

Postscript
The Two-Factor Theory

Gene J. Brutten

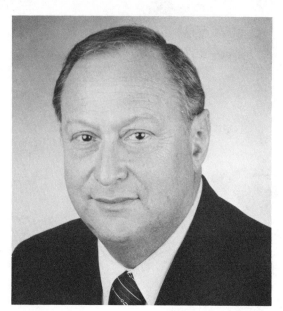

Gene J. Brutten

With the *Modification of stuttering,* which he published with Shoemaker in 1967, Brutten's impact on the field of stuttering became much more clearly defined. In this volume he attempted to integrate the previously dichotomous positions of genetic versus acquired etiologies of stuttering. Brutten's Factor One represents a classically conditioned, genetically based process. Individuals differ genetically in their emotional reactivity, which in stutterers precipitates a breakdown in the motor coordination of speech, giving rise to repetitions and prolongations. Factor Two represents a process of operant conditioning whereby stutterers learn to compensate and to cope with their fluency failures. Brutten's thinking evolved to this position from a background of physiological assessment as an indication of anxiety, and a strong identification with the classical conditioning point of view. While he carefully distinguished between the two types of conditioning, his attempts to integrate them in an analysis of stuttering behavior presaged more recent research in the area of biofeedback, where the distinction between classical and operant conditioning has become blurred.

Two-Factor Theory provides yet another theoretical model to support Wolpe's Systematic Desensitization Therapy for stuttering, which itself is based upon Wolpe's theory of Reciprocal Inhibition. Where Wolpe's theory was a general attempt to deal with the acquisition of neurotic behaviors, Brutten is more directly concerned with the acquisition and maintenance of stuttering. His Factor Two extends the therapeutic implications beyond Systematic Desensitization to operant-based behavior modification strategies.

Brutten reaches out to people with different perspectives. He sees the potential for synthesizing opposing points of view and to understand stuttering as a multidimensional problem. His own sharply honed thinking has not only had a marked influence upon his professional colleagues, who can be easily recognized by their critical alertness, but also has been transmitted to his students. Brutten is an active researcher and has provided a model and standard for bridging the gaps between the experimental research of the laboratory and case management in the clinic.

Two-Factor Behavior Theory and Therapy

Gene J. Brutten

BEHAVIOR THEORY

Life would be much simpler for the therapist if all behaviors were learned and unlearned in the same way. More often than not, however, experience has led learning theorists away from such one-factor explanations. They know that learning can result from two, quite different conditioning procedures—classical conditioning, which is also called respondent conditioning, and instrumental conditioning, which is also called operant conditioning. When a therapist wants to modify a particular behavior, he can do so most efficiently if he can determine whether that behavior was originally learned by classical or by instrumental conditioning. Although some therapeutic techniques are effective on both classical and instrumental responses, most techniques are effective only on the appropriate class of behavior.

Recently, behavioral scientists have focused on instrumental responses, like the word-changing and arm-swinging of stutterers, but they are still fully aware of the classically conditioned responses, such as the emotional reactions seen so often in stutterers. This recent focus on instrumental responses is probably just another example of the pendulum of scientific popularity swinging from one emphasis to the next.

Classical Conditioning

At the turn of the century, Pavlov created a great deal of excitement with his experiments on classical conditioning. Pavlov observed that there were two different types of stimuli. One type of stimulus was always followed by a specific response. For example, if a dog's paw was shocked electrically, the dog would always lift his paw up. Or, if food were presented to a hungry dog, he would salivate. Pavlov called these stimuli *unconditional stimuli* and the reflexive responses that followed them *unconditional responses,* because the relationship between them was unconditionally present, that is, it did not depend on learning. Through a slight mistranslation, they have come to be called unconditioned stimuli and unconditioned responses. The other type of stimulus that Pavlov observed was not associated, like the unconditioned stimulus, with a particular response. Such stimuli as a ringing bell or a red light would usually produce no more than a casual glance from the subject. For obvious reasons, these stimuli have come to be called neutral stimuli. By experimenting with different arrangements of these two types of stimuli, Pavlov found that when the unconditioned stimulus was made consistently contingent on the neutral stimulus, the neutral stimulus would eventually

From "Two Factor Behavior Therapy" by G. Brutten in *Conditioning in Stuttering Therapy,* 1970, Speech Foundation of America #7, pp. 37–56.

come to evoke a response similar to the uncondi-tioned response. This new response was called the conditioned response, and the originally neutral stimulus was called the conditioned stimulus.

In the traditional example of classical condition-ing, a neutral stimulus like a tone is presented, fol-lowed by an unconditioned stimulus, like an intense shock. From previous observation it is known that the intense shock will produce a number of different arousal behaviors. After the shock has been contin-gent on the tone for a number of trials, the subject eventually begins to show some form of arousal or excitation after the tone occurs *but before the shock occurs,* or even if the shock does not occur. Once these arousal behaviors occur before the shock, clas-sical conditioning has taken place. The subject has come to respond to the tone in a way that is similar to his response to the shock. He responds to the tone as if it were a sign of the impending shock. He has learned that when the tone occurs, shock is likely to follow.

Simple as the procedure sounds, classical condi-tioning is not limited to the training of lower animals like dogs, mice, or pigeons. The same results are ob-tained with humans. Furthermore, this procedure is not limited to laboratory stimuli, like a tone or a light. Any stimulus that an organism can see, hear, feel, or taste can be classically conditioned. A person, a word, or an entire stimulus situation may be classi-cally conditioned. This is true of stutterers and non-stutterers alike. All of us, in fact, have experienced a conditioned emotional response to originally neutral stimuli. Bugs, supervisory personnel, heights, water, teachers, and mice are some of the neutral stimuli that can come to arouse us through classical condi-tioning.

Because of our own similar experiences, we should be able to understand the classically condi-tioned emotional response of stutterers. You have un-doubtedly seen many stutterers for whom initially neutral stimuli have come, through experience, to evoke negative emotion—a certain word, a particular sound, words that begin a sentence, or words that are longer than average, are examples. Many stutterers report that particular listeners, their age, sex, or number, the topic of conversation, the specific set-ting, or the feel of a particular articulatory posture or movement, evoke a negative emotional response. These stimuli consistently make them uncomforta-ble, afraid, or anxious. Their hearts pound, their mus-cles are tense, their hands sweat, and their breathing

becomes irregular. Furthermore, the emotional re-sponse is usually associated with fluency failure. Neg-ative emotional responding seems to interfere with the accuracy and continuity of motor performance that is so vital to fluent speech. It's hard to speak fluently—in fact it's hard to perform any fine motor act—when the body is under stress and functioning less than perfectly. The result is a disrupted and dis-organized performance. We have all had this experi-ence. We all remember—perhaps even with some wistfulness—the ungainly way we tripped and sput-tered on our first date, with our first client, or meet-ing our future in-laws. The experiences of stutterers are not unusual. What is unusual is that they are *con-sistently* aroused by specific words and specific speech situations that are not objectively dangerous and that do not concern most people. A stutterer's experiences do not generally diminish the emotional reaction, they often make it worse. The negative emotional reaction to words and situations generally becomes more consistent and so too does the con-sequent stuttering.

Classical conditioning is not limited to a *negative* emotional response. Neutral stimuli may also be con-tingently followed by stimuli that are positive or pleasant. The sounds of mother's speech and the sight of her face may come to elicit a positive emo-tional response in an infant because these neutral stimuli are consistently associated with being fed (unconditioned stimulus). Eventually, the baby has a positive emotional response when he sees his mother approaching the crib. For the stutterer, as for anyone else, many stimuli have come to arouse posi-tive emotional reactions. On certain sounds and words and under certain circumstances they have lit-tle or no difficulty. Many stutterers, even severe ones, are fluent when they are with a girl friend, out with the boys, or reading a passage from a book. Positive emotion facilitates the normal fluency of speech. The successful speech performance, in turn, enhances the positive emotional reaction. We have all had sim-ilar experiences. When we feel confident we are fluent and coordinated—not only in speech but in any motor act, such as holding a cup and saucer at a buffet, deftly hitting a drop shot in tennis, or placing a running bunt in baseball. Apparently, people per-form best when the stimulus circumstances elicit po-sitive emotion.

Of course, not all of the stimuli people experience in their daily lives have been emotionally condi-tioned. Some have been classically conditioned, but in a way that results in only a minimal emotional response. For the most part, then, the speech of both stutterers and nonstutterers is neither facilitated nor disorganized by their reaction to environmental stimuli. In this way the stutterer and the nonstutterer are no different. Like the nonstutterer, the stutterer reacts without great emotion to most of the vast stimulus world that surrounds him, to the words he uses and many of the situations in which he speaks. It should be no surprise, then, that the average stutterer's speech is far more fluent than dysfluent. It is not the absence of fluency, therefore, that sets the stutterer apart from other speakers. It may not even be the quantity of fluency failure that distinguishes a stutterer from a nonstutterer. What seems to set the stutterer apart is that his fluency failures are generally associated with originally neutral situations and words that have been conditioned to elicit negative emotion. Stuttering, then, is the disruption of normal fluency that occurs when specific situations and words (conditioned stimuli) consistently elicit negative emotion (conditioned response). The emotional response elicited by these stimuli interferes with the accurate motor performance that is required for fluent speech, and speech becomes disorganized.

Instrumental Conditioning

Conditioned and unconditioned responses are involuntary, reflexive reactions to stimuli. There are also voluntary responses—ways of adjusting with purpose and direction to environmental stimulation. These adjustive responses are learned from past consequences. For example, certain responses, to certain people, in certain situations, are likely to result in negative or positive stimulation. From experience, we learn to discriminate which adjustive responses will avoid negative consequences and which will bring about positive consequences. In other words, we learn to make those responses that are *instrumental* in reducing negative stimulation or in increasing positive stimulation.

We learn not only *which* response to use, but we learn *when* to use it. We learn which response to use by instrumental conditioning, but we learn when to use it by classical conditioning. Consequently, in the learning of instrumental responses, both classical and instrumental conditioning are involved. Through classical conditioning we learn which situations will result in positive consequences and which situations will result in negative consequences; and through instrumental conditioning we learn which responses to use in order to achieve or avoid the consequences in any given situation. The very same stimulus that is the consequence of a response in instrumental conditioning is also the consequence of the stimulus situation in which it occurred, and when a stimulus is a consequence of another stimulus, we have the arrangement for classical conditioning. The two types of conditioning are practically inseparable. It might be said that this relationship between the two types of conditioning is as follows: We are emotionally motivated by classical conditioning to respond in ways that are instrumental in achieving positive stimulus consequences or in avoiding negative stimulus consequences.

We engage in instrumental responding when we try to get an invitation to an event that we expect to be interesting or pleasant or when we slow down at the sight of a police car. Stutterers do the same thing, trying to please their friends and attain their goals. But in addition, they may attend certain events or become friendly with certain people because there is a better chance of their speaking fluently. In the same way, stutterers may come to feel positively about certain words or phrases. They may be motivated to use them, even if they are not entirely appropriate because they have been associated with fluency and the ability to communicate. The stutterer learns, then, approach responses as well as avoidance responses on the basis of their consequent stimulation.

Since the conditioning histories of stutterers are not exactly alike they will avoid different situations, listeners, and words. There are stutterers who avoid speaking before any group and stutterers who approach such speech situations with eagerness and fluency. Similarly, there are stutterers who are fluent on words that begin with particular vowels or consonants and there are also those who react negatively to the very same sounds and who consistently stutter on them. The commonality among stutterers, then, is not in the particular situations, listeners, or words, to which they react emotionally or in the way that they may approach or avoid these negative stimuli. What stutterers *do* have in common is their negative emotional response to speech-associated stimuli such as these.

Stutterers, like anyone else, will approach stimuli they regard as positive and avoid those they regard as negative. Sometimes negative stimulation is avoided only for an instant, but that is all it takes to *reinforce* a response. On the basis of such momentary reinforcements stutterers can learn to inhale deeply before speaking a feared word, to tap their foot rhythmically while speaking, or to look away from listeners. But these responses are not always successful or instrumental in avoiding negative consequences. Stuttering often occurs anyway, and communication is interfered with or blocked. The stutterer wants to escape from this negative circumstance; he wants to complete the sound or word on which he is blocked by repetition or prolongation. He struggles, adjusts, and varies his responses in an attempt to escape from this negative state of affairs. He may try a great many responses in order to escape; he may, for example, hold his breath, close his eyes, turn his head, swing his arm, stamp his foot, or tighten up his abdominal muscles. Eventually, the fluency failure will end, the sound or word will be completed, and the responses associated with this escape from negative stimulation will be instrumentally conditioned. This reinforcing experience will shape the way he responds. As a result of this experience, he will be more likely to respond in this or in a similar way the next time he tries to escape from negative stimulation. Through repeated experiences he learns a number of different ways of removing negative stimulation. Sometimes he will use one way and sometimes another. Sometimes he will use a combination or sequence of instrumental responses to escape from the negative stimulation that is associated with stuttering. In any event, the stutterer learns, as we all do, to adjust to the environment and the stimulation that emanates from it. The stutterer's instrumental responses, then, are fundamentally like those of the nonstutterer. They differ only in that they are tied specifically to speech and the act of speaking by conditioned negative emotion.

BEHAVIOR THERAPY

From our discussion, we have learned that man reacts both emotionally and adjustively as a result of his individual experiences with his environment. Unfortunately, emotional and adjustive learning are not always adaptive. Some people are afraid of all cars because they were once in an automobile accident. Some people refuse to try to sew, make potato salad, or play bridge because their early attempts were met with strong and consistent negative stimulation. The stutterer is no different. The mere sight of a tele-

phone, an /s/ word, or an audience may send chills through him. Because of his past experiences, he may pretend that he does not know the answer to a teacher's question or that he is severely hard of hearing. In order to avoid or escape negative stimulation he may also have learned to swing his arm, change words, tap his foot, or do any of the things that have been described as secondary symptoms, devices, or associated responses.

How can we modify responses that are inappropriate or maladaptive? We can make these changes by using procedures that alter the stutterer's experience with contingent stimuli. We can provide him with experiences in which he can learn that there is no need to fear the telephone, /s/ words, or specific listeners. We can give him experiences which tell him that these stimuli do not signal the occurrence of negative consequences. Indeed, these experiences can teach him to react positively to speech and the act of speaking. In these ways we can recondition the stutterer so that his classically conditioned emotional responses are more appropriate to the world around him. As far as the instrumental responses are concerned, we can also modify them by manipulating the stimulus consequences of their occurrence. In addition to eliminating these maladaptive avoidance and escape responses, we can shape the stutterer's speech behavior generally in ways that increase the accuracy and acceptability of his speech signals. Behavior modification is therefore not limited to changing maladaptive responses. It includes also the strengthening of appropriate responses already in the stutterer's repertoire.

CLASSICAL CONDITIONING: MODIFICATION PROCEDURES

There are two basic procedures for modifying classically conditioned responses—deconditioning and counterconditioning. Both of these procedures alter the contingent relationship between the conditioned stimulus and the unconditioned stimulus.

Deconditioning

The purpose of deconditioning is to return the conditioned stimulus to its originally neutral status, so that it no longer signals the occurrence of negative stimulation. To accomplish this change, the stutterer must repeatedly experience the conditioned stimulus to which he has come to respond inappropriately. He must do this under conditions that do not permit him to avoid or escape, so that he can find out that the telephone, a specific listener, /s/ words, etc., are not followed by negative stimulation. This is vital. For when a conditioned stimulus is presented repeatedly and in quick succession in the absence of negative consequences it loses its value as a signal of forthcoming danger, and eventually it will fail to arouse the organism. Since there is no longer a consistent relationship between the conditioned and unconditioned stimuli, the classically conditioned relationship between the two stimuli is deconditioned or unlearned. The previously threatening situations, listeners, and words no longer concern the stutterer. He stops being afraid of them because they no longer signal the approach of unpleasant consequences.

Deconditioning can be carried out in many different ways, but the underlying principle is always the same—the conditioned stimulus is no longer contingently followed by the unconditioned stimulus. Speech pathologists have traditionally used this principle to remove the negative emotions of stutterers. They have sent stutterers out to experience those life situations that threaten them but are not objectively dangerous. Stutterers who were frightened by the sight of an audience, who shuddered when a salesgirl approached them, or who dreaded the sound of the phone ringing have been deconditioned when clinicians made arrangements for them to experience these stimuli in the absence of negative consequences. Usually, the stutterers learned from these reality-testing experiences that the stimuli that frightened them were not necessarily followed by or even frequently associated with negative consequences, that the audiences were often polite, that salesgirls can be helpful and friendly, and that a ringing phone is not inherently dangerous.

There are, of course, limits to how useful and efficient such life situation procedures are for deconditioning stutterers. Such procedures *can* lead to behavior change, but they are not always possible to arrange nor are they always therapeutic. Social clubs soon tire of listening to stutterers. A stutterer's first experience with a salesgirl might well be negative, so that conditioning rather than deconditioning might occur. Some experiences are simply impossible to arrange. For these and other reasons, life situation procedures have either been replaced or supplemented by procedures that can be efficiently programmed in

a clinical setting. Situations, listeners, words—experiences of various kinds—are tape recorded, put on slides, or filmed so that they can be repeatedly faced in the absence of negative consequences. These reproductions can either be prepared in advance, so that the clinic has a ready library of commonly feared sounds, words, and situations, or the therapist can record specific stimuli that evoke negative emotional responses in their clients. In either case, these stimuli are presented over and over until they become commonplace, unimportant, and no longer threatening for the stutterer. Because of its repeated presentation in the absence of negative consequences, the stimulus no longer makes the stutterer uneasy. When this point is reached he finds that he can stop the presentation and say the sound or word that previously threatened him. Indeed, he can now record his own fluent production and listen to it over and over again. These experiences are helpful not only in deconditioning the stutterer to fear-inducing stimuli but in maintaining the behavior change. The repeated experience of a sound or word in the absence of negative consequences will outweigh the occasional and random negative experiences of life. Thus, deconditioning can be maintained even if random or noncontingent negative experiences do occasionally occur.

Deconditioning experiences do not require the constant presence of a therapist or even a clinical setting. They can be provided also in a listening laboratory to which stutterers can go at a time that is convenient for them. Thus, at any time of the day it should be possible for them to select the appropriate tapes and listen repeatedly to their feared sounds or words until they become neutral stimuli. This laboratory setting can also be used by the therapist to supervise the practice of a group of stutterers. But practice of this kind need not be limited to a laboratory. Deconditioning can take place at home, on the way to work, or at the office. The readily available and inexpensive cassette tape recorders allow deconditioning to be carried out almost anywhere. Furthermore, the success of the deconditioning procedures can then be tested in the reality of these very same settings.

Deconditioning experiences need not be limited to word and sound fears nor to auditory procedures of presentation. Narrative descriptions of stimulus situations that elicit unobjective negative emotion have been tape recorded so that the stutterer can experience them repeatedly in the absence of negative consequences. Stimuli that evoke negative emotion have also been presented visually. Letters, words, people, and places have been repeatedly presented with a slide projector. Videotapes and film clips have been used to present more dynamic stimulus events. Although the equipment is more expensive, the advantages over a tape recorder or a slide projector are obvious. Anyone who has laughed, cried, or been frightened during a movie knows how real the reaction to motion pictures is. And anyone who has heard a joke lose its ability to provoke laughter when repeatedly told should understand why the repeated presentation of feared stimuli reduces the fear they evoke. To bring about fear deconditioning, videotapes and film clips of common experiences are being used more and more. They simplify the procedure through which the history of conditioned stimuli can be modified from those that signal negative consequences to those that are relatively neutral.

Counterconditioning

Counterconditioning is another procedure for modifying a classically conditioned response to a conditioned stimulus. It differs from deconditioning in that a new response is learned. In counterconditioning, the conditioned stimulus, instead of returning to a neutral status, is conditioned to evoke a new conditioned response as a substitute for the old one. So, counterconditioning involves both the *unlearning* of the old response and the *learning* of a new response to replace it. With stutterers, this procedure is used to replace a negative emotional response with a positive emotional response to the same stimulus. The evocation of a particular conditioned response depends upon a specific relationship between a conditioned and an unconditioned stimulus. If this relationship is changed, the conditioned response will also change. Consequently, when a conditioned stimulus, like a word or situation, is followed by a positive consequence rather than a negative one, the conditioned response will be changed as well as the contingency. The conditioned stimulus remains the same; the response is changed.

The events of real life are more likely to compete with counterconditioning than this simplified description would suggest. The negative consequences of conditioned stimuli are often not completely absent. Unconditioned stimulation can be an occasional consequence of the situations and words a

these determinations must be based on data; clinical reaction to conditioned stimuli can be maintained even though the negative consequences occur only rarely. Because of this, a newly conditioned relationship between stimuli will be in competition with an older and more established one. Whether a conditioned stimulus will evoke a negative or positive emotional reaction depends, then, on which contingent relationship is the more strongly habituated. The therapist's job is to strengthen the new relationship as much as possible through counterconditioning. It can be strengthened until the words and situations are far more likely to evoke positive than negative reactions.

Although counterconditioning is a viable procedure, it is not a miraculous technique. It requires a workmanlike precision. It depends on clinical steps that are often undramatic and laborious and which are highly specific to the individual in therapy. Before counterconditioning begins, the therapist determines: (1) the conditioned stimuli that elicit an unobjective emotional reaction, (2) the way these various stimuli cluster together to form different categories that elicit negative emotion (for example, telephones, girls, specific word classes, parents, teachers, strangers, or audiences), (3) the relative intensity of the emotional reaction to the different conditioned stimuli that make up a category (for example, there may be a mild reaction to telephoning a buddy, a measurably greater one to calling a girl friend, and a strong reaction to talking to a long-distance operator or an employer), and (4) the frequency with which the stutterer would meet each of the categories of emotion-inducing stimuli if he were not to avoid them. In other words, the speech pathologist must determine the conditioned stimuli that are critical to a stutterer, measure and evaluate the intensity of the emotional reaction they elicit, and find out how important behavior change will be to the patient, at least in terms of the frequency with which he is likely to experience the stimuli that evoke negative emotion.

Determinations of the kind we have been discussing are not difficult or beyond the training level of speech therapists. The behavioral terms used may be a bit unfamiliar, but speech therapists have long recognized the need to determine the situational and word stimuli that arouse a stutterer and disrupt his fluency, the severity of the emotional reaction to specific stimuli, and the frequency with which the stimuli occur. Speech therapists have known, too, that stutterer faces. Furthermore, a negative emotional judgments are vital, but hard data about a stutterer's performance are an inestimable aid to the therapist.

An orderly procedure is essential for successful counterconditioning. The conditioned stimuli within an emotion-evoking category as well as the categories themselves should be presented so that the least feared stimuli are experienced first and the rest in order of the negative emotional reaction they are known to evoke. The categories and stimuli that evoke little negative emotion are presented early. Those that are reacted to more strongly are presented later. This data-bound ordering of the stimuli makes it possible to reduce markedly or even eliminate the therapy drop-out that tends to result when clients are asked to face stimuli that are more threatening than they can withstand. The presentation of conditioned stimuli is ordered also because even a small change in the stutterer's everyday responses will help motivate him to continue therapy and to take the steps that successful behavior modification requires.

Once the order of presentation has been determined, the therapist must decide how to present them for counterconditioning. The conditioned stimuli can be presented auditorally, visually, or audiovisually by means of tape recorders, slide projectors, and film clips or video tapes. They can also be presented through imagination, which may or may not be made more vivid with hypnosis. In any event, for counterconditioning to occur, they must be contingently associated with stimulation that is positive or predominantly positive. In this way the conditioned stimuli will come to evoke a positive rather than a negative emotional response. For this reason, the conditioned stimuli are best presented in a setting that has a positive past history and in which positive stimulation can be contingently delivered. For example, a child who is afraid of all dogs because he was once bitten by one will be faced with this fear-evoking stimulus or a weakened version of it (the word *dog*, a still picture, a cute-looking puppy, or a dog seen at a distance) and then receive stimulation that is known to be pleasant to him. After the conditioned stimulus *dog*, or a version of it, is repeatedly followed by an ice cream cone, playing a favorite game, hitting a punching bag, or whatever the child enjoys, it will no longer evoke fear. This is not to say that in the process of counterconditioning the child will not experience some fear reactions. But if the counterconditioning procedure is designed well, the stimu-

lation that follows *dog* will be more positive than negative. As a result, the *net* emotional reaction will be positive. This dominance of positive consequences over negative must be maintained as the dog is brought closer to the child, in an ordered way. In time, because of the counterconditioning that takes place at each step, the dog's presence will signal positive rather than negative consequences. The child will have learned a new relationship in which the conditioned stimulus *dog* signals that positive unconditioned stimulation is likely to follow. Under such circumstances the conditioned emotional reaction is appropriately positive.

The process of counterconditioning is the same for both children and adults. It applies equally to the stutterer's fear of words, telephones, or people, or to anyone's fear of dogs, cars, or bugs. To be sure, the procedure has to be adjusted for the age of the client and the nature of the problem and for any number of other individual differences. There are, however, certain constants around which the therapeutic strategy must be designed. The therapist must determine the critical conditioned stimuli, group them into categories in terms of their thematic similarity, arrange the component stimuli and the categories themselves in an order that is determined by the intensity of the fear reaction they evoke, and present them in order, beginning with those that are least feared, in a clinical setting where the consequences, the contingent stimuli, are positive.

INSTRUMENTAL CONDITIONING: MODIFICATION PROCEDURES

Although deconditioning and counterconditioning will modify speech-associated fear and therefore the involuntary repetitions and prolongations it precipitates, it may not immediately cause any change in the instrumental adjustive responses. Certainly, if negative emotion has been modified so that stuttering has decreased, there are no longer any negative consequences to escape or avoid. Consequently, instrumental responses will occur less often. Nevertheless, some of them may hang on anyway because they have been conditioned to various stimulus compounds or because they have a complex record of reinforcement spanning a number of years.

The instrumental responses stutterers use are not always successful in permitting them to escape or avoid negative stimulation. Consequently, these responses are only reinforced some of the time. Contrary to what you might think, instrumental responses that have been learned by partial reinforcement are more difficult to extinguish than ones that have been reinforced every time they occurred. Also, many of these responses have come to have reinforcing consequences other than the reduction of negative emotion. They may have been conditioned originally because they permitted the stutterer to avoid or escape negative stimulation, but they can be maintained by positive stimulation. The stutterer's parents may pay more attention to him or to his requests when he closes his eyes and inhales before he speaks. His teachers may tell him that his good grade on an oral report or speech is partly a reward for his perseverance in the face of great difficulty. It is for reasons such as these that a stutterer's instrumental responses may not be immediately or totally eliminated when negative emotional reactions to situations or words are modified. A reduction in negative emotion will usually make them occur less often, but they will continue as long as they are instrumental in attaining positive stimulation.

Because classical and instrumental conditioning are not independent of one another the therapist should plan carefully the behavior therapy for changing these two types of responses. First, the speech therapist must consider that listeners may negatively stimulate the instrumental responses of stutterers and that this very same stimulation can create emotional conditioning. Because listener reactions can reinstate the speech-associated emotion that the therapist has worked so hard to remove, it is extremely important to integrate the therapy for instrumentally and classically conditioned responses. It is for this reason that in two-factor therapy we do not work first just on the negative emotional responses and then just on the maladaptive adjustive responses. Instead, we integrate the modification of emotional responses to specific situations or words with the modification of the instrumental responses that are associated with these very same stimuli. Second, speech therapists must choose carefully from among a number of procedures for modifying instrumental responses. These procedures differ both in their efficiency and in their effect. You will recall that instrumental responses are learned because of the positive consequences of their performance, either an increase in positive stimulation or a decrease in negative stimulation. When such consequences no longer

follow an instrumental response, it occurs less and less often. It may also be made to occur less often if it is followed by negative stimulus consequences. The speech therapist therefore has a choice of a number of different methods he can use, singly or in combination, in order to bring about behavior change. He can modify responses through reinforcement, nonreinforcement, and punishment.

Reinforcement

If the consequence of a specific response is positive, the stutterer is informed of its usefulness and will use it more often. The therapist should recognize this relationship so that he can reinforce those speech behaviors that are adaptive. Speech is after all an instrumental response, and much of what the stutterer does when he speaks is adaptive rather than maladaptive. The adaptive speech responses, particularly those that occur infrequently, should be identified and strengthened by positive consequences. Behavior therapy for the stutterer is not, then, simply a matter of making maladaptive responses occur less often. It also includes procedures that make the adaptive ones occur more often. Consequently, the therapist must know the dimensions of adequate speech. He must be able to survey the stutterer's speech responses and tease out those that are relatively adaptive. The performance of these behaviors can then be shaped by the selective use of reinforcement. For example, the therapist can make reinforcement contingent on articulatory accuracy, adequate voice intensity, and an appropriate rate of speaking. Listeners will not then ask the stutterer to repeat what may well have been said fluently just because it was spoken inarticulately, rapidly, or too softly. The therapist may also find it useful to reinforce the at-rest position of the articulators prior to speech, the manner in which speech is initiated, or the rhythm pattern of speech.

Positive consequences can be made contingent on the absence of maladaptive responses as well as on the presence of adaptive ones. You can teach the stutterer what *not* to do as well as what to do. Consequently, the therapist can provide reinforcement when an eye-blink, a lip-purse, or rhythmic foot-tap does not occur. The stutterer will be informed that reinforcement is contingent upon the absence of these behaviors; he learns also that the reinforcement follows a different way of responding. As a result of this information his behavior will be modified so as to bring about more positive consequences.

It is inefficient to wait for the stutterer to discover that when he responds in one way or another he will be rewarded by the therapist. The point of therapy is not to determine the client's intelligence. The stutterer should be told just what responses are going to be reinforced at the beginning. This will quicken the pace of behavior change. Indeed, the stutterer can be told that certain responses will be instrumental in developing a more adequate speech performance— one that is likely to be reinforced and accepted rather than rejected by listeners.

We have been stressing the fact that instructions can increase the efficiency with which the instrumental responses of stutterers are modified. These instructions are not response contingent, they are stimulus contingent. In clinical and real-life settings stutterers can be informed that positive stimulation will follow specific responses that have not yet been made. Through classical conditioning (stimulus-contingent stimulation), then, stutterers can learn to discriminate the responses that will be instrumental in obtaining reinforcement. They need not wait for the instrumental response and its contingent stimulation. Indeed, the instruction will serve as a conditioned stimulus for instrumental responding. This points up again the clinically important interaction between classical and instrumental conditioning.

Nonreinforcement

One of the techniques of nonreinforcement is selective reinforcement. When a therapist selectively reinforces certain responses, he is selectively extinguishing others. If the therapist praises the stutterer for articulating more accurately or talking more loudly, he is at the same time withholding reinforcement from speech that is misarticulated or weakly delivered. Similarly, when the therapist reinforces the stutterer for speaking without blinking his eyes or pursing his lips, reinforcement is being withheld from these maladaptive responses.

In addition to selective reinforcement, the therapist can arrange the speech circumstances so that reinforcement does *not* follow as the consequence of a particular response. If an instrumentally conditioned response occurs repeatedly without reinforcement, the stutterer will come to perform it less and less often. When blinking the eyes, pursing the lips, or

changing words are no longer instrumental in bringing about reinforcement, the stutterer will stop using them. The absence of reinforcement informs the stutterer that these responses are not useful.

Of course, the therapist does not have to wait until the stutterer learns that an instrumental response is no longer followed by reinforcement. Behavior modification can be made much more efficient if the therapist informs him that a specific response will not be reinforced, informs him also each time that response is made, and then gives him a great deal of such experience. When using nonreinforcement, the therapist should make the stutterer immediately aware each time the unwanted response occurs. Unless he is consistently and immediately informed, the unwanted behavior will not be modified efficiently. Telling your client to watch himself in a mirror or listen to a recording of his speech is not enough. These procedures are too vague. They do not tell the stutterer explicitly which response is to be changed. In the absence of this specificity the therapist may well be providing noncontingent stimulation rather than stimulation that is contingent on a specific behavior. Noncontingent stimulation is inconsistent—it brings attention to many different behaviors and information about none. In part, such inconsistent stimulation is a result of a definition of stuttering that lacks specificity. Traditionally, stuttering has been described in all inclusive terms, such as "moments of stuttering," so that the absence of reinforcement could be a consequence of anything—a lip-purse, an /s/—prolongation, a phrase repetition, or a word-change. The inconsistency that results does not serve therapy, it interferes with it.

We may have dealt with stutterers inconsistently because we were concerned that calling attention to "stuttering" would be punishing, that it would increase fear conditioning and consequently increase maladaptive emotional and adjustive responding. This is a very real worry and one that therapists have faced repeatedly. But response-contingent stimulation need not be punishing. Contingent stimuli that are relatively neutral can be informing without being punishing. Any stimulus that the stutterer can discriminate can be used to inform him that a maladaptive response has occurred. A signal light, the word "now," or a tone are examples. Again, the therapist should not wait for awareness to develop. He should call the stutterer's attention to a specific instrumental adjustment and tell him whenever this behavior takes place. Indeed, the therapist should train him to identify accurately the behavior being modified. At first he will make mistakes, but as the target behavior is more precisely identified, the stutterer's awareness will be increased even more than if the therapist continues to apply the contingent reaction.

The speed with which behavior change occurs under nonreinforcement depends partly on the frequency of this experience. The more often the response occurs without reinforcement, the more quickly it will be extinguished. As a result, when the response occurs, the stutterer should make a precisely imitative version of it repeatedly. Through this massed repetition the stutterer experiences an increased number of unreinforced occurrences of the maladaptive response. The massed practice also serves to increase the stutterer's awareness of the unreinforced response; he learns its "feel," and this serves as an informing stimulus that carries over to settings and times outside the clinic.

Massing a nonreinforced response serves another purpose too. When a response is made repeatedly in quick succession, its occurrence can be temporarily inhibited. Thus, if a stutterer repeatedly swings his arm, turns his head, or purses his lips, the response becomes increasingly difficult to make. The time interval between occurrences of the response will become longer and longer. As the same response is repeated over and over again, there will develop what has been called response "fatigue" or reactive inhibition, as a result of which the response is temporarily suppressed. The time period during which this response is not made eventually becomes long enough so that the temporary inability to make the response can be used to produce a conditioned inhibition that has clinical significance. Significant conditioned inhibition will result if, during the rest period when the stutterer is unable to make the instrumental response, the therapist presents a stimulus that previously led to its occurrence. With this technique, the *inability* to make the maladaptive response can be conditioned to stimulus events such as ordering in a restaurant, talking on the phone, or speaking in class. In other words, response inhibition can be conditioned so that events which previously elicited it will now keep it from occurring. Conditioned inhibition of a stimulus-response relationship is not temporary; it does not dissipate with rest like reactive inhibition does. The stimuli presented when the instrumental response cannot be made come to serve as conditioned or learned inhibitors of its occurrence. This is not to say that the response will not

occur in other settings. The conditioned inhibition of an instrumental adjustive response is specific to the stimulus scenes that are presented and to those that are like them. The response will continue to occur in other settings unless these too are made to serve as conditioned inhibitors.

There are then a number of techniques of reinforcement that a therapist can use. None of them needs to be used alone. Often, in fact, the most efficient strategy is for the therapist to use a combination of these techniques to modify an adjustive response. The fundamental principle behind these various techniques is nonreinforcement.

Punishment*

There is much disagreement about the term punishment and it is used by different people in quite different ways. Therefore, it is important that we know what a therapist means when he says that he uses punishment to modify stuttering. What exactly does he *do?*

Punishment may be said to take place when a specified response is consistently followed by a negative stimulus. The negative stimulus need not occur every time the behavior occurs; it may be delivered every fifth or tenth time. It does not even have to be delivered immediately, as long as it is a consequence of the response. The response must be specified. It is not very helpful to say that a negative stimulus is contingent on "stuttering moments" or "secondary behaviors." This is too vague. Stuttering moments include various behaviors. To discuss the effect of punishment meaningfully, it is necessary to specify the behavior that is contingently followed by a negative stimulus.

Punishment, like reinforcement or nonreinforcement, is informative. When a stutterer receives an electric shock or a verbal reprimand as a consequence of a response, he soon becomes aware of the contingent relationship. He may then suppress the response. Despite the fact that behavior change may result, the therapist might be best advised to consider other, less risky, techniques for achieving the same end. Behavior can often be modified at least as efficiently with nonreinforcement and selective reinforcement procedures. Moreover, nonpunishing approaches to behavior modification appear to be

---

*The comments made in this section are based in part on experiments which are listed at the end of this chapter.

more lasting and less likely to have nontherapeutic side effects than punishment. Punishment is not being rejected here for moral reasons (except insofar as risking harm to a client is immoral). If punishment could lead to normal fluency it would be inhumane to withhold it from stutterers. It is being rejected because its use involves a risk that is not commensurate with its limited effectiveness. One of the reasons punishment is risky and other procedures for modifying behavior are preferred is that it cannot be made critically specific to a particular response. The therapist cannot guarantee that the punishing stimulus will be contingent on only a maladaptive response. If the therapist punishes a stutterer for pursing his lips he may also be punishing him for all the other behaviors that are present at the same time. If all of these concomitant behaviors happened to be instrumentally conditioned responses that were maladaptive and that had a similar learning history, the result would probably be beneficial. The punishment would probably lead to the suppression of a number of maladaptive responses. The fact that complex moments of stuttering have occasionally been reduced by punishment may be evidence for this multiple effect. But such an effect is not the only possible one or even the most likely one. The responses that occur at about the same time as the target response may well have learning histories that are different. Punishment does not suppress all responses—there are some that it increases. An increase would not be unanticipated for example if the response being punished had been learned as an adjustment to punishing stimulation. It is noteworthy, in this respect, that many of the responses of stutterers seem to have this history. Another reason for concern is that a negative stimulus that is contingent on one response may also be noncontingent as far as other behaviors are concerned. This is important because noncontingent negative stimulation has been observed to cause certain stuttering behaviors to occur more often. Critical also is the evidence that noncontingent negative stimulation leads not only to an increase in fluency failures but to fluency failures that resist behavior change. The use of punishment is contraindicated for still another reason. The suppressive effect of contingent negative stimulation is most noticeable with instrumental responses. In contrast, it seems to increase the frequency and the magnitude of emotional responding. But even if the therapist were not concerned with the emotional aspects of a stutterer's difficulty—even if he were concerned only with the

speech disruptions—he should know that punishment has not led to any significant decrease in repetitions. The repetitions of stutterers have at best been minimally reduced for short periods of time and at worst increased markedly by punishment. Punishment is not, then, a procedure that is applicable to all behaviors. It is apparently not a powerful tool for modifying the repetitions of stuttering and it may well do harm.

There is more to be considered. Punishment has been known to have undesirable side effects. It has increased the frequency of repetitions, prolongations, and maladaptive adjustments. Punishment has not only had undesirable effects on the contingently stimulated behavior, it also has had undesirable effects on the noncontingently stimulated behaviors that occur at the same time; they have been increased rather than decreased. The lack of a decrease has not been the result of using a punishing stimulus that was too weak. On the contrary, a mildly punishing stimulus seems more likely to decrease contingently stimulated repetitions and less likely to increase noncontingently stimulated repetitions than a strong punisher. That a strong punisher leads to more stuttering repetitions than a mild one is not totally surprising. After all, a mild punisher is less disruptive than one that is very strong. A strong punisher can set off an intense emotional reaction, and this reaction can interfere with normal fluency. At least as much change in instrumental responding has occurred when the contingent stimulus was relatively neutral. What seems necessary is that the stutterer be informed of the occurrence of a maladaptive adjustment. Any stimulus that can be discriminated will serve this purpose. Punishing stimuli need not be used.

SUMMING UP AND LOOKING AHEAD

We have stressed that not all responses are learned in the same way and that the therapist must bear this in mind as he sets about to modify a stutterer's behavior. Consequently, we have focussed our attention on both classical and instrumental conditioning. It may be considered unfortunate that the two-factor approach does not give the therapist one tool that he can use with all behaviors, but by distinguishing between the two types of responses, the two-factor approach provides a more efficient strategy for behavior change. The probability of successfully modifying behavior is much less when we treat all responses as if they were learned the same way. But just because we have distinguished between classically and instrumentally conditioned responses does not mean that the two types are unrelated. We have pointed out their interrelationship and stressed its clinical significance.

Although the two-factor approach has the great advantage of additional efficiency as a result of not oversimplifying stuttering and associated instrumental behavior, it has a disadvantage in not being able to supply any direct technique for modifying classically conditioned responses. Someday, however, this may be possible, and the possibility has great clinical significance. Consequently, we must maintain the more comprehensive two-factor approach and make precise observations and measurements of classically conditioned responses. The measurement of emotional responses may not be as easy as the measurement of instrumental responses, but it is not impossible, even now. Heart rate, palmar sweating, muscular tension, and breathing rate are just a few of the reactions we can currently observe and reliably measure. Technological advancements, like those that led to the current surge of interest in instrumental responding, are sure to increase the attention given to classically conditioned responses. Eventually, we will learn more about the part conditioned emotion plays in disturbing speech and in motivating instrumental adjustments. This technology will also give the speech therapist a much better way of measuring the effectiveness of his therapeutic techniques. He will be able to monitor the effect of his stimulus-contingent as well as his response-contingent procedures for changing the emotional and adjustive responses of stutterers. But we must begin *now* to observe these response classes if we are to learn more about them.

Finally, we have seen that there are a number of issues surrounding therapy for stutterers. These issues have not been fully resolved. Many areas of disagreement remain because behavior theory and therapy is in its infancy. We have not yet arrived at *the way* that is the most efficient for modifying all behaviors. The therapist is best advised, therefore, to re-main flexible so that he can change as new information comes out of the laboratory and clinic.

BIBLIOGRAPHY

Brookshire, R. H., "Effects of Random and Response Contingent Noise upon Disfluencies of Normal Speakers." *Journal of Speech and Hearing Research*, 1969, pp. 126–134.

Brookshire, R. H., and Eveslage, R. E., "Verbal Punishment of Disfluency by Random Delivery of Aversive Stimuli." *Journal of Speech and Hearing Research*, 1969, pp. 383–388.

Frederick, C. J., III, "An Investigation of Learning Theory and Reinforcement as Related to Stuttering Behavior." Unpublished doctoral dissertation, University of California at Los Angeles, 1955.

Martin, R. R., Brookshire, R. H., and Siegel, G. M., "The Effects of Response Contingent Punishment on Various Behaviors Emitted During a 'Moment of Stuttering.'" Unpublished manuscript, University of Minnesota, 1964.

Starkweather, C. W., "The Simple, Main, and Interactive Effects of Contingent and Noncontingent Shock of High and Low Intensity on Stuttering Repetitions." Unpublished doctoral dissertation, Southern Illinois University, 1969.

Rescorla, R. A., "Pavlovian Conditioning and its Proper Control Procedures." *Psychological Review*, 1967, pp. 71–80.

Webster, L. M., "An Audio-Visual Exploration of the Stuttering Moment." Unpublished master's thesis, Southern Illinois University, 1966.

Webster, L. M., "A Cinematic Analysis of the Effects of Contingent Stimulation on Stuttering and Associated Behaviors." Unpublished doctoral dissertation, Southern Illinois University, 1968.

READINGS

Brutten, E. J., and Shoemaker, D. J., *The Modification of Stuttering*. Englewood Cliffs, N.J.: Prentice-Hall, Inc., 1967.

Beecroft, R. S., *Classical Conditioning*. Goleta, Calif.: Psychonomic Press, 1966.

Kimble, G. A., *Foundations of Conditioning and Learning*. New York: Appleton-Century, 1967.

Kimble, G. A., *Conditioning and Learning*. New York: Appleton-Century, 1961.

Wolpe, J., *Psychotherapy by Reciprocal Inhibition*. Stanford, Calif., Stanford University Press, 1958.

Wolpe, J., *The Practice of Behavior Therapy*. New York: Pergamon Press, 1969.

The Two-Factor Theory

Gene J. Brutten

It has now been more than a decade and a half since the theoretical postulates and therapeutic strategies of the two-factor framework were first set forth in an integrated way (Brutten & Shoemaker, 1967). On that occasion, Van Riper appropriately pointed out that this model ". . . like all models will doubtless find revisions in future years. That is what models are for. They help free us from the inertia bred of confusion; they permit us to progress" (Brutten & Shoemaker, 1967, p. v).

Progress has certainly been made during the intervening years. The two-factor model, like other contrasting models, has contributed to this progress by stimulating pure and applied research that tested its premises. The resulting data have lent support to some of the two-factor positions and caused others to be refined or limited. Still other viewpoints have had to be abandoned as experimental results proved them unsupportable. The two-factor model thus has been of service in promulgating data. These data have required changes in the two-factor position. They also have led to modification in the particulars of other models of stuttering.

Though the explanation of *why* certain events take place in the way that they do has always been a concern of scientists, it has not necessarily been the major emphasis of the clinician concerned with stuttering. The therapists' prime interest has been the methods by which behavior can be changed so that interfering or inappropriate responses can be replaced by those that support and maintain speech production that is normally fluent. Therapists are necessarily pragmatic; faced with clients who stutter and who clamor for help, they seek overall strategies and specific behavioral tactics that make fluency the hallmark of their clients' verbal behavior. Therapists are generally put off by theoretical arguments. They are not in a position to wait until all of the pieces of the puzzle fit into place, causal relationships become evident, and the explanation of the pertinent events become clear. They need procedures that, for whatever reason, enable their clients to modify and control fluency-determining behaviors. Because of this, clinicians have come to favor therapy tactics that are specific to observable behaviors rather than ones that are directed at underlying events presumed to affect fluency. Moreover, the emphasis on attaining normal fluency has led them

Postscript   7

away from approaches that involve an acceptance of their disorder and the speech disruptions that are associated with it. Clinicians have rejected the suggestion that once a particular developmental stage has been reached one will inevitably remain a stutterer. Most therapists have also turned away from the previously accepted view that all that they can do is help the client become a more fluent stutterer. Indeed, some clinicians have gone so far as to state that this is an unethical position, that therapy should not be initiated if this is all that the clinician can truly offer. They have contended that more is possible than a mental hygiene approach designed only to help stutterers live with disrupted speech.

Current clinical practice is marked by an emphasis on achieving fluency, on self-actualization through behavioral engineering. Traditional strategies, tactics, and goals have generally been replaced. In their stead, clinicians have increasingly turned to behavior therapy and response management through the use of tactics associated with classical (respondent) or instrumental (operant) conditioning. This change in direction is notable, and follows years in which speech therapists were often berated for being unwisely concerned with stuttering symptoms rather than with the underlying conflicts that supposedly cause speech disruption. But, this change did not take place without some blind alleys and missteps. In the rush to cast aside the unproductive past, some speech therapists, like some behavior therapists concerned with other problem areas, made inordinate claims for particular procedures. Soon, however, clinical experiences and the results of applied laboratory studies made it apparent that the road to fluency had not yet been fully cleared. There was no doubt that therapeutic change had been enhanced by focusing, in behavioral ways, on particular responses. But, with respect to the choice of tactics, speech therapists were advised to avoid inflexibility and to anticipate that:

> . . . further changes as well as additions will be forthcoming. The therapist should not be bound, therefore, by the procedures that are described. Behavior therapy is in its infancy and its application to the modification of stuttering will be served by those therapists who advance our knowledge in the efficient means of achieving extinction. (Brutten & Shoemaker, 1967, p. IX)

This call for clinical wisdom rather than overzealousness was directed at behaviorally oriented therapists, whatever their learning framework and management leanings. It reflected an awareness that the tactics of behavior therapy were likely to change, and that, as a result, clinicians needed to stay current and to avoid a hardened commitment to particular therapy procedures. The importance of remaining flexible in regard to clinical tactics was stressed again, a few years later, when the multidimensional and multimodal approach of two-factor therapy was broadened and updated. At that time, in articles like the one to which this postscript refers, the attention of clinicians was drawn to an array of deconditioning and counterconditioning procedures on the one hand, and to a number of contingency management procedures on the other. The variety of these tactics, designed to affect respectively fluency disruptive respondents and maladaptive operants, reflected the fact that the procedures available to the clinician had increased considerably in the relatively few years since the two-factor position was first proposed. Even some cognitive techniques for modifying speech-associated operant responses were described. These foretold of a clinical emphasis that was to significantly affect behavior therapy in the years that followed. Yet, once again, we stressed that other and often more efficient ways of bringing about behavior change were on the horizon. In a move that seems to have been designed to counter what looked like premature curative claims it was pointed out that "we have not yet arrived at *the way* that is most efficient for modifying all behaviors. The therapist is best advised, therefore, to remain flexible so that he can change as new information comes out of the laboratory and the clinic" (Brutten, 1970, p. 55).

The last few years have been marked by a rush of data that has greatly changed the way therapy for stutterers is conducted. The cautionary notes that were sounded presaged a real and continuing shift in the tactics of therapy. Moreover, the new and sometimes unexpected findings also forced theorists to re-evaluate their thinking. They had to contemplate the data from naturalistic investigations and ponder why the results of experimental studies strained their explanatory frameworks. These findings made them increasingly aware that they did not yet have a full understanding of stuttering and its controlling elements. But, clearly, knowledge had been advanced, and there was every indication that the stage had been set for still more significant discoveries. Evident too was the likelihood that the future held great promise. In part, this was because the new data released theorist and therapists alike from the stranglehold of past thinking. The data forced certain of our long-held premises to be put aside and others previously relegated to the trash bin to be reconsidered, reformulated, or restructured.

TWO-FACTOR BEHAVIOR THEORY

Specific premises underlie all frameworks. These premises, which often differ considerably from model to model, give them shape and direction. The two-factor paradigm does not differ from other frameworks in this regard: it contains viewpoints that characterize it and differentiate it from other explanatory models. These premises were deliberately chosen because they appeared to best fit the data and to suggest predictions that would be theoretically and clinically meaningful.

The premises fundamental to the two-factor position need to be made explicit so that they and the model in which they are imbedded can be evaluated. They need to be made fully evident so that their explanatory and practical value can be assessed.

Interactionism: Nature and Nurture

Basic to the two-factor position is the assumption that genetic and environmental factors interactively determine the behaviors of stutterers. This stance is clearly

Postscript 7

at odds with the purely environmental explanations of stuttering that have dominated the scene until recently. It differs sharply from the positions that look with considerable skepticism at genetic risk, predisposition, and conditionability (Johnson, 1967). It rejects the view that stuttering is a response pattern that is acquired as the result of only environmental consequences (Shames & Sherrick, 1963; Siegel, 1970). In contrast to semantic, Skinner-based, and operant positions, among others, the two-factor position has always maintained that:

> ... both heredity and environment contribute to the determination of behavior (and that) most theorists concerned with stuttering have directed their attention to the environmental influences and have failed to consider the organism in which learning takes place. ... (Brutten & Shoemaker, 1967, p. 49)

The determining influence of heredity, widely disregarded in recent times, has come to the fore again. That stutterers are significantly more likely to have a family pedigree of stuttering than are nonstutterers is no longer seen as the exclusive result of social history. Though environmental events undoubtedly play a role, it is now clear they alone cannot account for the fact that males are more likely to stutter than are females, that if the parent who stutters is female there is a greater risk that a child will stutter than if the stuttering parent is a male, and that a sex-limited polygenic model of inheritance accounts for about 71% of the variance that relates to the risk of being a stutterer (Kidd, 1977; Kidd, Kidd, & Records, 1978). As Van Riper has stated, "It is difficult to believe that environmental factors alone could account for the results" (1982, p. 330).

The sex ratio among stutterers and the risk-factor data have led to the conclusion that there is an inherited threshold that influences the likelihood that one will stutter and that because males have a lower threshold they are more susceptible than females to the triggering created by stressful environmental events. This position, which rests on the current evaluation of demographic information, bears on a number of premises that are basic to the two-factor framework. One such premise is that individuals differ in emotional reactivity and that, as a result, a given amount of environmental stress will elicit different amounts of potentially disruptive arousal. Another tenet is that the sex ratio reflects the presence of "a differential susceptibility to emotionally induced disorganization" (Brutten & Shoemaker, 1967, p. 52).

Few would argue against the existence of individual differences in emotional reactivity and the notion that these differences are, at least in part, genetically determined (Bridger & Birns, 1963; Jost & Sontag, 1944). On the other hand, the suggestion that males have a lower threshold for stress and are therefore more emotionally reactive may not be as easily accepted because the data are sparse and inconclusive. It is circular reasoning to use as supportive evidence the fact that more males stutter. Moreover, it might well be "reaching" to associate reactivity with the fact that the male is generally the weaker organism. But emotionality is considered a learned function of the primary drive of pain, and males seemingly do have a lower pain threshold than females. There is some reason to believe, therefore, that a fundamental sex difference does exist with respect to emotional reactivity. This is not to say that the sex difference in the fluency of speech performance is totally dependent on differences in stress thresholds. As we have indicated, susceptibility to disruption also seems to be an interactive function of differences in an individual's motor coordination for speech. Speech skills are acquired earlier and more easily by girls than boys. Moreover, the early speech performance of girls appears to be more stable and less likely to be disorganized by stress than the speech of boys. This has led to an alternate explanation, one based *only* on inherited differences in the motor coordination of the sexes (Van Riper, 1982). But if fundamental motoric differences do indeed exist among the sexes it would be hard to imagine that they would not be enhanced by stress variables, ones that flood the organism and its various systems. So, once again, we are forced to return to the interactionist position that is basic to the two-factor model. Again we must restate that "the most reasonable solution to stuttering is the recognition that *both* constitutional and environmental factors are involved in its development" (Brutten & Shoemaker, 1967, p. 54). By extension this implies that both factors are involved, too, in the development of fluency.

Response Definition: A Molecular Viewpoint

From its very inception, a primary tenet of the two-factor position has been that the behaviors displayed by those who stutter require precise molecular specification rather than gross molar description. Basic to two-factor theory, therefore, is the rejection of the use of moments, be they of stuttering or fluency.

Moments of stuttering came into use largely as a result of a lack of agreement as to what constitutes the behavioral elements of stuttering. Fluent moments were given little consideration; they were merely instances when stuttering was not present. Moments were a seemingly necessary convenience. They allowed speech pathologists to continue their activities in the face of definitional disagreement. But ultimately the decision to use moments in clinical and experimental determinations was unfortunate. It misdirected our attention. It drew us away from the search for the constituent elements that characterize stuttering and fluency. Moreover, the use of moments fostered imprecision and hampered the gathering of potentially relevant information. It led pathologists away from behavioral specificity and down a perceptual path. As a result, it is only now, many years after the decision to use moments, that researchers are actively investigating the behavioral dimensions of stuttered and fluent performance.

Moments have not yet been abandoned despite their molar and subjective nature. Their use is too firmly rooted in clinical practice. Nevertheless, the clinician needs to be aware that by employing moments, behavioral differences may be masked that are vital to distinguishing stutterers from nonstutterers and both from persons who have other disorders of fluency. This masking of differences is not the only problem that has resulted from the use of moments. Their unspecified character has led some to suggest that all people stutter and others to indicate

Postscript 7

that "stuttering" is a symptom of quite different disorders (e.,g., aphasia, dyspraxia, cerebral palsy, hysteria, or mental retardation). The vagueness that is basic to moments has led still others to view behavior assessment and differential diagnosis as unnecessary. They have maintained that one need only determine the base rates of stuttered or fluent moments prior to initiating therapy. Recently the barrenness of this kind of approach has become generally apparent (Adams, 1980; Brutten, 1975; Haynes, 1978; Kanfer & Phillips, 1970). As a result, the clients' behaviors and their specific clinical needs have once more become the focus of attention.

It is currently recognized by many that through molecular analysis we can sharpen our understanding of stuttering. The molecular approach has come into use because it made it possible to distinguish the particular forms of fluency failure that denote stuttering from the adjustive responses associated with anticipated or ongoing disruption. It also made it possible to study the differential effect of contingent stimulation on these two types of behavior. These are but some of the forces that have given impetus to the rather general increase in molecular analysis. Despite this, the move away from molar moments of stuttering and macro-analysis has not been supported by everyone (Martin & Haroldson, 1981). Yet, the importance of a molecular approach seems clear. Indeed, it has been said that "one of the major contributions of the decade of the seventies was the recognition that it was necessary to specify the exact characteristics of the behaviors generally lumped together under the label of a moment of stuttering" (Van Riper, 1982).

The terms molar and molecular are relative ones. The behaviors that are viewed as stuttering are but the end product of movements that can be described in still more molecular ways. Awareness of this fact has been emphasized by the research findings and theoretical comments of a number of pathologists who were schooled in the two-factor tradition (Adams & Hayden, 1976; Adams & Reis, 1971; Starkweather, Hirschmann & Tannenbaum, 1976; Zimmerman, 1981a, 1981b). They have noted that it is advantageous to take a still more reductionist view and look at the neuromotor events that take place when speech is produced in a stuttered or fluent manner. They have extended molecular analysis and given it additional utility and breadth. In doing so, they have moved attention away from the signal level to the neurologic activities and the motor movements that are basic to speech. They have stressed the need to analyze the specific actions that take place in the respiratory, laryngeal, and oral systems during speech. They have heralded, also, the importance of looking molecularly at the timing of movements and at the presence or absence of coordination within and across the systems involved in speaking. In this way, they have moved us toward a more fundamental understanding of the neuromotor processes that underlie the disfluent and fluent production of stutterers and nonstutterers.

The neuromotor approach to stuttering has received considerable support in recent years. The research that this viewpoint generated has increased our ability to evaluate the two-factor contention that stuttering represents "a disruption of functioning in the organism" (Brutten & Shoemaker, 1967, p. 41). This emphasis also enhanced the study of the two-factor position that fluency failures result when "the accuracy and continuity of motor performance that is so vital to fluent speech" (Brutten, 1970, p. 38) is interfered with. It should lead, moreover, to a fuller assessment of the two-factor position that particular forms of fluency failure are indicative of an *involuntary* breakdown that occurs because "the speaker is engaged in the performance of a motor act that requires fine coordination, and this performance is disrupted" (Brutten & Shoemaker, 1967, p. 30). It should, also, shed light on the contrasting and rather widely held position that stuttering is but a learned set of inappropriate behaviors that are voluntary in nature.

Whether stuttering is indicative of a breakdown in the motor precision necessary for fluency or voluntary behavior that the stutterer has learned and is responsible for requires increased knowledge about the events that are associated with fluent production. Knowledge of this sort is still relatively scarce. To no small extent this resulted because clinical needs drew our attention to stuttering and its modification. There are other reasons, too. We lack knowledge about the constituents of fluent speech performance because we have tended to look at fluency merely as the absence of stuttering. In addition, we were satisfied with molar observations, ones that lacked denotative specificity. As a result, fluency became a virtually empty construct. It was not something that was behaviorally palpable. Fluency did not have reference to particular response events. And so, moments of fluency, like moments of stuttering, served only to cloud the picture. Its use led us all away from the vital observations and needed understandings that are likely to result when the behavioral events associated with fluent motor speech performance are molecularly analyzed.

Currently, as we have seen, researchers are emphasizing the need to observe and analyze the timing and coordination of speech-associated movements. We anticipate that in due time molecular analysis will become even more reductionistic. Our analyses will be extended to include the electrochemical activities that stimulate motor movements that are organized and fluent or disrupted and disfluent. All of this will ultimately set the stage for a cross-level evaluation of the neuromotor processes that generate speech behavior that is or is not fluent. We are not suggesting that fluency or its failure cannot meaningfully be dealt with at any of a number of separate levels. But we do wish to emphasize that the effect that these levels of activity have on each other and on the acoustic end product warrants special consideration. Analyses of this kind will ultimately lead to a fuller understanding of the molecular building blocks that serve to support or disrupt fluent performance.

Fluency, Fluency Failure, and Stuttering

We have considered a number of assumptions about fluency and the failure of its occurrence that are inherent in the two-factor position. Each of them bears importantly on this theoretical framework and on the clinical decisions that flow

Postscript 7

from it. Some of these assumptions have found more support than have others and some appear to have more practical value than do others. But all, in one way or another, serve to provide a way of thinking about fluency and its failure that has an integrative purpose. This is why your attention has been drawn to these premises.

Some other viewpoints have been implied but not directly stated. One of the more important of these is that people are normally fluent when they speak. This critical contention argues against the widely held position that people are *normally* "disfluent". Moreover, the stance that speech is typically fluent carries with it a rejection of the corollaries that (a) "disfluencies," regardless of type, are of no particular significance since they are displayed to some extent by all who speak, and (b) stuttering is the *purposive* attempt to avoid normal speech glitches.

We have discarded the concept that speech is *normally* disfluent because it is inconsistent with the data. It is quite evident that our speech is not characterized by fluency failures (Brutten, 1975; Brutten & Shoemaker, 1967). Fluency failures are *not* normal; that is, they are not typically or generally evidenced during speech. Fluency failures occur rarely. People are generally fluent. Fluency normally characterizes all motor performance and speech performance is no exception. Fluent performance generally typifies our motor actions when, for example, we walk, chew, or write. This is not to say that, on occasion, people do not trip, bite their tongue, or transpose written letters. Occasionally, they also speak *dis*fluently. But, for the average speaker, dysfluencies are atypical (Bloodstein, 1982).

Fluency failures indicate that motor speech performance has been disrupted. However, their presence is not necessarily indicative of a disorder. Stated differently, fluency failures are not always behavioral events that are diagnostically significant. Yet they should not, as they have in the past, be wantonly dismissed as devoid of meaning (Johnson, 1956). Simply because they are sporadically displayed by normal speakers does not indicate that they are either normally occurring events or lacking in possible import. To be sure, some forms of disfluency like interjections, incomplete phrases, and revisions are usually indicative of nothing more than editing. However, other forms, particularly the involuntary glitches like *fast* multiple unit repetitions of sounds and syllables and inappropriate silent and oral prolongations, are an indication that, for one reason or another, the organism has failed to respond in a smooth and adequate way (Adams, 1980; Janssen & Kraaimaat, 1980). These particular failures indicate that the organism's neuromotor functioning has been momentarily and *involuntarily* disorganized.

What is being stressed here is that *certain* fluency failures are not voluntary; they are, to the contrary, the involuntary result of organismic conditions and environmental circumstances that affect motor performance. We restate the two-factor position now because we desire to re-emphasize that these particular disfluencies reflect neuromotor breakdown. Time has not changed the belief that they, unlike other somewhat similar behaviors, are not acquired through re-sponse-contingent reinforcement. We do not mean by this that we cannot learn to repeat or prolong. We may well repeat a word or phrase and we have been known to stretch out the pronunciation of a word. But molecular analysis has made it evident that topographical and behavioral differences exist between these voluntary acts, which often result from a desire to correct or emphasize what has been said, and the involuntary behaviors that are indicative of break-down. This dissimilarity is like the differences between voluntary and involun-tary eyeblinks (Kimble, 1961); the former are relatively slow, complete, and tension-free events, while the latter are characteristically fast, incomplete, and hy-pertensive (Brutten, 1975; Brutten & Shoemaker, 1967, 1971; Janssen & Kraai-maat, 1977; Kraaimaat & Janssen, 1980). These differences, among others, are apparent to stutterers. They have rather consistently made a distinction between their voluntary and involuntary behaviors. Interestingly, this separation is in keep-ing with the fact that the former are readily manipulable by response-contingent stimulation and the latter are not (see Brutten & Shoemaker, 1971 for a review).[1]

The point is that not all of the behaviors that affect the forward flow of speech are indicative of disorganization or disorder. Even the presence of dis-fluencies that are indicative of breakdown are not necessarily evidence of a dis-order. They may merely be the result of a momentary and sporadic lack of the organization that fluent production requires. What needs to be highlighted, also, is that disordered fluency and stuttering are not necessarily one and the same (Brutten, 1975). It is inappropriate to equate disfluencies of all types and patterns with stuttering because various conditions are known to affect the neuromotor accuracy, coordination, and organization that is required to achieve fluency. Dis-fluency is known to be behaviorally symptomatic of alcoholism, apraxia, dys-phonia, mental retardation, and syphilis. They are concomitants of various other disorders, too. Each of these disorders, in their own way, undoubtedly disrupts neuromotor activities. But, to call the resulting speech disruptions stuttering, and, presumably, therefore, to treat these disfluencies as stuttering is to disregard fundamental differences in both their antecedents and their behavioral charac-teristics. This is not to say that some of the same procedures that are effective in modifying the speech of stutterers and in instating fluency might not be useful in modifying disordered fluency that has quite different origins and histories. It is to say, instead, that diagnostic assessment is necessary, because there are real differ-ences among these conditions and they need to be recognized and addressed. It follows that special procedures, ones that are specific to a disorder, may well be needed. If these special clinical tactics are added to those that have been shown to be useful across the various disorders that affect motor competence the

[1]Recently, Costello and Hurst (1981) have presented data that are not consistent with this statement. Brutten (1983) has challenged the internal validity of this study. Costello and Hurst, in their rebuttal, have asked why their findings are different from those that we have alluded to (1983). As was implied in our challenge and dis-cussed elsewhere (Brutten & Shoemaker, 1970), they are likely the result of methodological differences.

Postscript   7

power-efficiency of therapy will be enhanced (Brutten, 1973). What is being emphasized is that though stuttering and other disorders that affect fluency share certain characteristics, this does not mean that they are one and the same condition or that they require the very same forms of therapeutic attention (Brutten, 1975).

Stuttering and Negative Emotion

The relationship between negative emotion and stuttering has been the object of considerable discussion for many years. During these years the pendulum of opinion has swung back and forth. Negative emotion has been seen as the cause of stuttering, a result of stuttering, or as essentially unrelated to its presence or absence. In part, these differences in viewpoint reflect changes in the popularity of particular theories and theoreticians. In part, too, they represent the ebb and flow of the data that bear on the existence of a functional relationship between negative emotion and the behaviors that define stuttering.

Probably the element of the two-factor position that has been most debated by theoreticians and experimenters and the one that is the most prone to thoughtful and provocative evaluation concerns the posited relationship between negative emotion and stuttering. As we have seen, it is the two-factor position that motor speech performance is fundamentally like all other motor performance; its efficiency is interfered with by the presence of excessive negative emotion (Malmo, 1959). For stutterers this interference is said to occur with a consistency that exceeds chance partly because excessive emotionality has become classically conditioned to the speech situation and/or certain elements of speech and the act of speaking. Stated differently, the speech of stutterers is disorganized with a certain regularity in part because specific elements of speech situations have come to occasion negative emotion. As we have seen, a fundamental corollary of this position is that genetic predisposition makes some individuals more susceptible than others to emotionally induced neuromotor breakdown. For these individuals negative emotion is more easily cued-off and motor speech performance is more easily disorganized.

The matter of predisposition, at least as it relates to the risk of becoming a stutterer, has already been addressed. Earlier in this chapter we saw that there is now little question that genetic factors affect the likelihood that one will become a stutterer. Moreover, in another context, it was pointed out that genetic factors are specifically related to individual differences in emotional reactivity, conditionability, and susceptibility to disorganization (Brutten & Shoemaker, 1967). These findings suggest that genetically determined individual differences play a significant role in stuttering.

The full explanatory potential of genetically determined individual differences must await the results of further research. Yet, the renewed interest in organismic factors has made us all keenly aware of genetic influences other than those that relate to emotional reactivity. Specifically, there is now evidence that the neuromotor functioning basic to speech may well differ significantly between stutterers and nonstutterers. Even during the production of speech that listeners perceive to be fluent, stutterers generally appear to differ from nonstutterers. Stutterers tend to show lags in the onset of phonation that may be a result of inadequate and unsteady subglottal pressure, longer movement durations at the onset of phonation, longer delays in achieving peak velocity of the lips and jaw, longer articulatory transition times, greater supraglottal pressure, greater movement variability, and a relative slowness in terminating phonation (Adams, Runyan, & Mallard, 1975; Agnello & Wingate, 1971; Hillman & Gilbert, 1977; Starkweather & Myers, 1978; Zimmerman, 1980b). These findings, ones that are not confounded by the presence of stuttering, suggest that stutterers differ importantly from nonstutterers in terms of neuromotor functioning. Clearly, these are important findings, yet they must be viewed with a degree of caution. The data should not be over-interpreted. It is important to note that *not all* of the stutterers tested in these studies evidenced neuromotor differences that set them apart from nonstutterers. One would be hard pressed, therefore, to support the assertion that differences of this kind are sufficient in themselves to cause stuttering. Furthermore, most of the studies have employed adult subjects. The generalizability (external validity) of the findings can thus be questioned. To be sure, children have been used in some studies, and differences have sometimes been observed. For example, Cross and Luper (1979) found that the *average* voice reaction times of children who stutter differ from those of their nonstuttering peers. However, some other studies have failed to find significant differences among children who do and do not stutter with respect to voice onset, speech timing, and manual reaction times (Cullinan & Springer, 1980; Long & Hand, 1982). What this suggests is that neuromotor capabilities vary among individuals, be they stutterer or nonstutterer, in a way that may affect the likelihood of mistimings and discoordination and the extent to which they occur. The data do not, however, currently permit the conclusion that neuromotor limitations cause stuttering. The lags and mistimings may even be the result of adjustments that some stutterers have learned to make because of their speech difficulty.

Caution also needs to be expressed about the findings that relate to emotional arousal. Speech performance, like other forms of motor performance, has been shown to be disrupted by circumstances that are noxious or stressful (Hill, 1954; Meyer, 1972; Savoye, 1959; Stassi, 1961). Once again, however, this effect was not displayed by all individuals who faced these circumstances. At the stress levels tested, then, negative emotion cannot be seen as a sufficient cause of disfluency. Negative emotion may, however, interact with other variables that are also known to affect fluency. In this respect, it should be noted that if lags and asynchronies do indeed underlie the fluent speech movements of stutterers, " . . . one can see how tension, fear, or communicative stress might magnify them enough so that 'overt' stuttering would emerge" (Van Riper, 1982, p. 397). Conversely, if speech-associated negative emotion is present even when the stutterer's speech is fluent, one can see how neuromotor lags and asynchronies might serve to magnify their potential for disruption. What the preceding two statements imply, of

Postscript   7

course, is that negative emotion and neuromotor abberations can interact in a catalytic fashion (Neale & Liebert, 1980). Though neither of these elements may, at a particular time, be sufficient to disorganize fluency, their conjoint presence may well be disruptive enough to produce fluency failures.

The specific interactive contributions of negative emotion and neuromotor limitations undoubtedly differ from stutterer to stutterer. There is absolutely no reason to view these factors as being constant among those who stutter. This argues for assessment and therapy strategies that incorporate the recognition " . . . that the amount of variance contributed by each of these sets of factors may fluctuate over a wide range from case to case . . . that is, there is not always the same amount of variance contributed by constitutional factors or by experiential factors" (Brutten & Shoemaker, 1967, p. 54). The interactive contribution of each of these factors to the likelihood that speech will be fluent or disfluent is undoubtedly affected also by momentary changes in the neuromotor complexities involved in the act of speaking and by the speaker's emotional reactions to the speech situation and to the words to be spoken. It follows from this that negative emotion is not seen as *the* cause of stuttering. As was stated when the two-factor framework was first set forth: " . . . not everyone commits fluency failure every time he speaks under conditions of negative emotion . . . Quite to the contrary, neither stuttering nor fluency is perfectly predictable, suggesting clearly the operation of several, if not many causative factors" (Brutten & Shoemaker, pp. 42–43).

Stuttering: Definitional Issues

As we have seen, the two-factor position is that stuttering is the disruption of normally fluent speech that results from the interference created by the interaction of speech-associated negative emotional and neuromotor factors in an interplay of genetic and environmental influences. Behaviorally, stuttering is characterized topographically by fast, hypertensive, repetitive runs of simple or compound phones that are oral or silently postured and/or by generally tense and inappropriate prolongations that are silent or oral. These fluency failures are tied to speech situations and/or neuromotor movements that are word- or sound-specific to an extent that exceeds chance. As has been pointed out, stutterers consistently report that these particular repetitions and prolongations are involuntary. With notable regularity, they distinguish these behaviors from grossly similar slow and voluntary rehearsals, "bounces," easy initiations, and sound "stretches," and from the many other voluntary coping responses that are often associated with either the anticipation of stuttering or its occurrence. These coping adjustments, behaviors that are seemingly used to avoid and escape speech difficulties, are not typically considered to be stuttering by those who stutter. However, stutterers fully recognize that they are a significant part of their speech problem. They are attention-getting, debilitating, and emotion-inducing behaviors. Moreover, their presence can reduce the flow of information and interfere with communication.

Like the stutterer, we have limited the term *stuttering* to the involuntary signal static that reflects speech disorganization. We have excluded from our definition of stuttering, though not as we shall see from our clinical endeavors, all of the voluntary coping maneuvers that stutterers tend to display. These adjustments are *secondary to* stuttering and to its anticipated occurrence. They are not representative of the disruptions that characterize stuttering. It has been said with respect to this voluntary-involuntary distinction that there seems to be " . . . no better way of accounting for the more complex speech symptoms and associated body movements" (Andrews et al., 1983). Yet, some have felt that the exclusion of the concomitant responses makes the definition of stuttering unduly restrictive. Possibly so, yet this definitional posture is consistent with the fact that associated responses, ones that we call Factor II behaviors, are not universally displayed by all who stutter. Since this is the case, logic demands that they be omitted from the definition. They are not behaviors that are distinctive of the disorder called stuttering.

Factor II responses are not the only behaviors that are not considered denotative of stuttering. Disfluencies like interjections and revisions that are the result of editing as well as those behaviors that are employed for emphasis are also excluded. Only particular forms of disfluency, those with certain topographic characteristics and antecedents, are considered representative of stuttering. Data and definitional logic aside, one can understand, therefore, why some may see our definition of stuttering as being rather limited.

One alternative to limiting what is to be called stuttering to those behaviors that appear to be distinctive of the disorder is to seek a more general definition. Here the attempt is to search out and include all of the speech and speech-associated behaviors that are displayed by those who, for one reason or another, have been called stutterers or who have viewed themselves as stutterers. We contend that this is an indiscriminate approach that makes stuttering a wastebasket term. It lacks utility because it fails to point up the behaviors that are distinctive of the group to which it refers. Moreover, it produces a diagnostic and clinical Gordian knot. It is no wonder that differential diagnostic procedures for evaluating fluency have developed very slowly over the years and that clients are still accepted for therapy and given treatment procedures that are thought to be specific for stutterers if they declare themselves to be stutterers or if they are considered by some "important other," such as a parent, relative, or teacher, to be a stutterer.

There is no question that the two-factor approach to defining stuttering is restrictive. But its limiting nature is also its strength because the definition includes the particular behaviors that tend to separate stutterers from normally fluent speakers and from those whose fluency failures are characteristic of disorders other than stuttering. Its use thus helps the clinician avoid diagnostic errors. This does not at all mean that the definition does not have its weaknesses. At present, however, there is no definition of stuttering that is free of criticism. One facet or another of every definition has been found wanting, even when theoretical considerations are put aside.

Postscript 7

Determining the distinctive features that are characteristic of stuttering is no simple task. The attempt to isolate the features that define stuttering has led to considerable debate and anything but full agreement (Bloodstein, 1982; Brutten & Hegde, 1983; Floyd & Perkins, 1974; Wingate, 1962). Moreover, on the basis of the data that are now available, there is little reason for optimism that this matter will soon be fully resolved. This is a troublesome circumstance, for only if we know what it is about stuttering that is truly distinctive can we make diagnostic determinations that are valid and therapeutic decisions that are fully useful. Stated differently, the absence of behavioral markers that are known to denote stuttering fosters alpha and beta diagnostic errors and clinical mismanagement.

Some have suggested that the defining characteristics of stuttering have not become evident because it is not truly a disorder. It is, they suggest, nothing more than a problem that is created by listeners. Stuttering, from this point of view, is merely a reflection of listeners' evaluations (Johnson, 1956). Others have pointed out that definition, by its very nature, is nothing more than a judgment (Bloodstein, 1982). What is defined as stuttering, then, is a judgment call. Of course, judgment calls are notoriously subject to disagreement. And, with respect to the definition of stuttering, it is evident that disagreements abound. It does not necessarily follow that stuttering is not a definable disorder, and it does not mean that stuttering cannot be distinguished from the behavioral display that typifies other disorders, or that the search for its distinguishing elements should be abandoned. It means instead that the search for the defining features of stuttering is not over; that it must go on until we know whether or not it is possible to clearly denote its presence. It means, also, that for the time being at least we need to turn to the definitional framework that appears to be the most revealing and seems to have the greatest practical value. Specifically, we need to use the definition of stuttering, and parenthetically the definition of fluency, that is the most illuminating and that best guides our clinical activities.

TWO-FACTOR BEHAVIOR THERAPY

In the preceding portions of this chapter your attention has been drawn to a number of the assumptions and viewpoints that are basic to the two-factor approach to stuttering. Some of the clinical implications of the two-factor viewpoint have also been brought to your attention. What this has undoubtedly made apparent is that there is a direct relationship between this model and the decisions that are basic to clinical practice. It follows that the overall strategy of two-factor therapy and the specific tactics that are employed are not freestanding; they rest on the two-factor explanation of the behaviors evidenced by those who stutter. The framework gives shape and direction to clinical determinations. With respect to the assessments that precede therapy or are associated with ongoing intervention, it suggests where to look and what to look for (Brutten, 1973; 1975). As such, the model helps the clinician pinpoint the targets of therapy. It also guides the observation of behavior change. As it relates to clinical procedures, it provides the clinician with an understanding of the where, when, and how of therapy. The model thus helps the clinician avoid an eclectic approach, one whose hallmark is the use of a variety of procedures whose premises are typically inconsistent with each other. It also makes it possible for the clinician to avoid dependence on those therapy programs that disregard individual and behavioral differences. Programs of this type are undoubtedly convenient, but at their core are the assumptions that stuttering clients do not differ notably or that if differences exist they are not clinically relevant. As a result, the therapist is asked to resort to clinical procedures that are essentially constant. The tactics do not vary from client to client regardless of their differences.

The two-factor approach to behavior change is neither eclectic nor predetermined. The two-factor position is that therapy should involve tactics that are internally consistent from a learning viewpoint, and that the change procedures employed should be tailored to the client's specific needs and strengths (Brutten, 1975). Emphasis is given also to the fact that change tactics differ in power efficiency and in their appropriateness for use with behaviors that are representative of different response classes (Brutten & Shoemaker, 1967, 1971; Rimm & Masters, 1979).

Like other models, the two-factor framework has a clinical function. But models, be they theoretical or atheoretical, are imperfect. They have inherent limitations and weaknesses. They do not serve clients equally well. Therefore, clinicians need to choose wisely among the available models. Moreover, they need to understand that they are not forever wedded to one framework. Clinically relevant models come and go. Their focus is changed or altered. The ultimate test of their worth is how well they serve the client. The power of different models is a matter of debate. But it is being resolved, to some extent, by outcome studies. Though not easy to design or to carry out in ways that make the findings free of challenge, outcome studies are moving us away from dependence on authorities, single case findings, and the publicity that is used to sell particular clinical programs or devices.

The Strategy of Two-Factor Therapy: A Critical Evaluation

A number of interrelated viewpoints give shape to the strategy of therapy that is two-factor. As the name implies, a fundamental tenet of this model is that the behaviors typically displayed by stutterers are not a function of but one form of conditioning and that they should not, therefore, be dealt with in the same way. As this tenet suggests, two-factor strategy is neither unidimensional nor unimodal. It leads to a differential consideration of those behavioral components displayed by the stutterer that are reflective of respondent conditioning and those that are a result of operant conditioning. As a result, specific attention is directed at both the behavioral components that are in part a function of emotional learning (Factor I disruptions) and those that are a direct function of positive and negative reinforcement (Factor II responses). Moreover, the two-factor approach

Postscript 7

concentrates on therapeutic planning that leads to a managed integration of the particular respondent and operant responses that facilitate fluency and support its maintenance. The implications of each of these statements about conditioning and therapy are worthy of reflection. There is no doubt that the conditioning procedures that lead to respondent and operant responses are fundamentally different (Kimble, 1961). However, it is now equally clear that the training procedures contain certain elements that are common to each form of conditioning. The respondent-operant separation is thus not absolute. It is not fully possible to rule out the presence and the influence of these two conditioning types on each other. It follows from this that therapeutic strategies need to accommodate this fact and take advantage of it. This is not to say that respondent or operant tactics should not be employed and should not be directed at particular targets. It is to say, instead, that a therapeutic strategy that is exclusively respondent or singularly operant in nature is not fully viable. These procedures have a limited effect. Therapies designed to deal only with the stutterers' disruptive negative emotional reactions have been successful, on occasion. So, too, have procedures that are purely operant even though the speech-associated concerns of stutterers may have been disregarded. Yet, therapy that is exclusively respondent or operant in nature is often too limited in scope. With respect to respondently based therapies, this has been made apparent by clinical reports and applied studies that have repeatedly shown that some maladaptive Factor II responses may remain in place following one form or another of deconditioning or counterconditioning. These responses often serve as the basis for clinical regression. It is not just that the Factor II responses that remain may draw attention and fuel a reconditioning of negative emotional reactions. It is also that these adjustive responses, and others like them, are the behaviors that clients turn to when they are faced with stress or the momentary emergence of speech disruption. Moreover, respondent procedures do not generally provide the client with skills that are appropriate to these circumstances. They are only designed to desensitize the stutterer so that nonobjective concerns are not elicited. These therapies, then, have a useful but limited purpose.

Contingency management procedures that are designed to modify operant responses or instate specific speech-associated skills have also been found to be limited in clinical scope. Even though significant changes have resulted from consequating specific responses, the resulting improvement has not always been maintained in the face of stress. The results have made it apparent that the skills that promote fluency, for example, may not be maintained unless attention is also directed at the stutterers' self-concepts and speech-associated attitudes, concerns, and emotional reactions (Gronhovd & Zenner, 1982; Perkins, 1979; Shames & Egolf, 1976).

What we have been addressing is the fact that stuttering is a multidimensional problem that involves a mosaic of emotional and adjustive responses that need to be dealt with. It has been pointed out, also, that therapies that are directed at either respondent or operant responses are limited in scope and produce change that is subject to regression. But making therapy more inclusive also carries with it difficulties that are real. Therapies of this type are faced with a wider range of targets and the consideration of both the various stimuli that set the occasion for responses and the stimuli that control response probabilities. Two-factor therapy is a case in point. This approach dictates the targeting of specific respondent and operant behaviors so that they can be instated, enhanced, modified, or limited by procedures that are consistent with their conditioning class. That is to say, they are to be brought under stimulus-contingent or response-contingent stimulus control. This tends to be a readily accomplished feat. Experimental and clinical data alike have rather definitively shown that the behaviors in the two response categories can be brought under control by tactics that are appropriate to their conditioning class. However, the data make it equally apparent that the general effectiveness of therapy is reduced if the array of the behaviors to be dealt is inordinately large. This is not at all surprising. Therapeutic success has long been known to vary with severity. But this begs the issue being considered. What practitioners must face up to is that change appears to be specific to the targeted respondent or operant. Currently, there is no evidence that a therapeutic change in one respondent will necessarily produce a positive effect on a different respondent. For example, it is not likely that the elimination of concern about talking on the phone or saying words that begin with the sound [g] will reduce anxiety about answering a question in class or saying words initiated by [m]. Similarly, bringing about the omission of an instrumental arm swing in no way suggests that the rate or magnitude of any other such response (e.g., foot tic, head turn, word omission) will be concomitantly affected in a positive way. This means that therapy, at least as presently constituted, must proceed in a step-by-step manner to bring about change in the targeted behaviors. Moreover, therapists recognize that the change that occurs must be made a part of, that is, must be chained to, the alterations that have previously taken place. This piecing together of therapeutic gains becomes increasingly demanding and complex as the number of targeted respondents and operants increases in frequency and habit strength. This task must nevertheless be undertaken, because an approach that fails to deal with the various behaviors that are vitally in need of attention usually produces an effect that is at best ameliorative and temporary.

Clearly, clinicians may be faced with a difficult and intricate problem. A step-wise therapy designed to strip away maladaptive respondents and operants and to instate integrative responses of both types is severely stressed when a considerable number of behaviors are necessarily the targets of therapy. What this means, of course, is that a molecular approach to therapy has limitations. It should not be used wantonly. The therapist needs to assess the client's needs and the appropriateness of the clinical plan as it relates to the type and number of the targeted responses.

The recognition that a step-wise approach is not the method of choice for all who stutter added some impetus to the ongoing search for effective techniques that are more general. Toward this end, attention has increasingly been

Postscript 7

directed at clinical strategies that, in one way or another, involve the reinforcement of fluency (Leach, 1969; Ryan, 1970; Shaw & Shrum, 1972). Two-factor therapists saw this as a way of taking advantage of the operant-respondent overlap. They were aware that the reinforcing stimulus would consequate both fluency and the conditional stimuli that are associated with both speech and the speaking situation. They understood that R–S (operant) and S–S (respondent) conditioning that is positive would thus occur at the same time. They recognized that, because of this, there would be an increase in both positive emotion and fluency-enhancing skills. Seen from a different perspective this means that both Factor I and II behaviors should decrease. Molecular analysis has shown that this does indeed happen (Hegde & Brutten, 1977). The disruptions of speech that are associated with negative emotion and the maladaptive adjustments that are an attempt to cope with anticipated or actual speech disruptions both diminish significantly. This finding has been shown to be reliable. It is no wonder, then, that fluency reinforcement has become a favored therapeutic tactic, especially with children (Adams, 1983). Possibly this is because fluency is often more readily available for reinforcement among children than adults. Possibly, also, it is because clinicians are still appropriately hesitant about using punishment procedures with youngsters. Primarily, however, it is because reinforcing fluency generally puts aside the need to work directly on either speech management or maladaptive avoidance responses.

The operant-respondent overlap does not occur only when the consequences are positive. Overlapping occurs, also, when response-contingent negative stimuli (punishment) are delivered. That is why the use of punishment, whether the client is a child or an adult, has been severely questioned. That fact is that the use of punishing consequences carries with it the unnecessary risk of an increase in Factor I behaviors (Brutten & Shoemaker, 1971). Also, the use of aversive stimuli can lead to an increase in certain forms of Factor II responding (Zenner & Webster, 1972). This is especially likely when the stimulus is strongly negative and when its delivery is made contingent on the mixed bag of ever-changing behaviors that is the stuttering moment (Brutten & Shoemaker, 1971; Krych, 1978).

The use of punishment is of less concern when the stimulus is mildly aversive (Starkweather, 1970) and when it is made contingent on a specific Factor II response. Nevertheless, we are more favorably disposed to the use of suppressing consequences that are nonaversive. These stimuli are *informative*; they advise the client when the response targeted for change has occurred. In doing so, they help bring the maladaptive response under stimulus control without the presence of contra-indicating side effects. But the stutterer needs to know more than what not to do. As we have stressed on other occasions, he or she needs to be informed about what to do! The response alternatives that lead to fluency need to be brought to the client's attention, and they need to be reinforced when they occur. This strategy enables the therapist to avoid the potentially dangerous recourse to trial and error adjustments that tends to occur when therapy emphasizes only the negative. Moreover, accenting the positive provides the client with the particular skills that are needed to achieve fluency. But still more, reinforcement has a stabilizing effect because the conditioning overlap serves to increase positive emotion and an approach toward rather than an avoidance of speech and speech situations. This fact is of considerable import as it relates to response transfer and maintenance, matters that are of considerable concern to all behavior therapists (Boberg, 1981; Boberg, Howie & Woods, 1979).

Making positive stimulation contingent on fluency does not greatly enhance the client's knowledge of what to do. Though reinforcing moments of fluency undoubtedly has a salutary effect, it serves merely to inform clients about the times when their speech is appropriately produced. They still must cast about to determine what they did that promoted fluency. Reinforcement of this kind does not, in itself, draw attention to all of the specific motor skills that are basic to the occurrence of normally fluent speech. It follows that fluency reinforcement has a power-efficiency that is limited. This has been made apparent by the fact that not all stutterers are helped by this procedure. Furthermore, those who have been helped seem to evidence improvement that is slowed by the need to discover for themselves the adjustments that support fluency. For these and other reasons, fluency reinforcement has tended to give way to those reinforcement procedures that are more skill-specific.

The advantages that result from reinforcing fluency-dependent operant responses rather than instances of fluency have been apparent for some time. It has been suggested to therapists that they "make reinforcement contingent on articulatory accuracy, adequate voice intensity, and an appropriate rate" (Brutten, 1970, p. 49). At the same time it has been pointed out that they "may also find it useful to reinforce the at-rest position of the articulators prior to speech, the manner in which speech is initiated, the rhythm pattern of speech" (Ibid.). But these are relatively general statements made within the context of a theoretical article. It was not a setting designed to provide the clinician with the definitional boundaries that were necessary for pinpointing either the particular responses that were to be stimulated or the performance level that was the goal of therapy. The terms *manner, adequate, accuracy,* and *appropriate* are conceptual rather than operational. Though clearly they referred to the respiratory, phonatory, and articulatory aspects of speech, they lacked the denotative specificity that therapy requires. They did not carry with them the precision that would allow clinicians to either perform specific manipulations or determine if their clients' fluency-related skills had improved. This exactness was provided by clinicians who were pragmatic and by researchers whose investigations were directed at assessing where in the respiratory, phonatory, and articulatory systems differences or miscoordinations exist that separate stutterers from nonstutterers and stuttered speech from fluent speech. The results were instructive. As we discussed earlier, they indicate that the inspiratory and expiratory portions of adult stutterers' respiratory cycle tend to be shallow and consequently that the subglottal pressures may not be consistently adequate to support and sustain voicing. The findings

Postscript   7

also have made it apparent that adult stutterers generally show a delay in phonation and voice onset time even when their speech production is fluent (Agnello, Wingate & Wendell, 1974). A lag has been found to be present not only at the initiation of phonation but also at its termination. Moreover, adult stutterers have shown a relative slowness both in initiating the articulatory movements required for speech and in the transition from one set of movements to another (Zimmerman, 1980a). These data, and those from an ever-growing list of investigations, suggest that the repetitions and prolongations of stuttering are at least in part the end product of fundamental difficulties in achieving tempero-spatial organization. These disfluencies may, that is, be reflections of the oscillations and fixations that result from "some basic difficulty in motor organization, timing, and control" (Van Riper, 1982, p. 397).

The data have led Zimmerman (1980c) to propose that it would be useful to view stuttering as a disorder of movement. Specifically, he has suggested that it might be unifying to consider stuttering a disorder that involves the respiratory, phonatory, and articulatory systems and the integration among the speech-related movements that occur in these systems. This rationale is consistent with the thrust of many recently developed therapies. The current trend is to provide clients with skills that are specific to these systems and that are presumably needed for the production of fluent speech. Generally, these therapies involve clinical targets like full breath, easy voice onset, continuous voicing, slow transition from one articulatory gesture to another, and a general reduction in rate of speaking (Adams, 1983; Perkins, 1973a, b; Shames & Florance, 1980; Starkweather, 1982; Webster 1975). Clearly, these therapies make evident the skills that are the targets of therapy. Furthermore, reinforcement is provided when the desired skill levels are achieved and orderly steps are taken to stabilize the targeted responses, chain them to each other, and shape them so that the client's speech approximates that of the nonstutterer. Fluency often results, and for a number of people the new pattern of speaking is maintained. Moreover, with time the client's speech seems to become more and more like that of the nonstutterer. Even the speech-associated attitudes ultimately improve (Andrews & Cutler, 1974). For others, however, the improvement is transitory. They are unable to hit their targets while under stress and away from the clinical setting. They begin to use the separate skills that they have been taught as Factor II adjustments. They do not use them in the coordinated way that seems to promote fluency. The fluency failures and the coping responses that were present prior to therapy return in full force. After all, the Factor I and II behaviors were not truly "extinguished"; their response probabilities were merely reduced for a time. The word and situational concerns again become evident. And, still more. The relapse seems to be marked by evidenced frustration and reports of guilt, shame, and depression. These reactions seem to be a function of the fact that the client once more faces failure in the search for fluency. In part, also, it seems to result from the fact that as one aspect of some therapies the clients are advised that if they hit their targets they *will* be fluent, and that if they are not fluent it is because *they* and not the therapy are at fault. This implies that the therapy has a universality. It carries with it a strong suggestive force that is bound to support a precision-oriented therapy. However, as has been intimated, the emotional cost to the client who does not maintain fluency can be staggering.

The fact that therapies designed to enhance fluency, through a changed manner of speaking, have not always been successful should not be seen as a necessary denial of the general approach. It should, instead, lead to a search for ways to improve the strategy and tactics that are employed so that fluency can be both achieved and maintained (Boberg, 1981; Zenner & Gronhovd, 1983). This comment does not bear on fluency-based therapies alone. It has a greater generality. It reflects the still-present need for improvement in the way therapy for stutterers is conducted. This need has been made apparent throughout this discussion. Note has been made that a number of clinical approaches have been shown to have a degree of merit. But, it also has been pointed out that none of them are free of limitations. There is thus no therapeutic program that can presently ensure lasting fluency or improvement for all who seek help.

The fact that we still have a way to go before therapy is routinely successful does not mean that great strides have not been made in the last few years. Undoubtedly they have. We have become increasingly knowledgeable about the comparative power of our clinical procedures (Azrin, Nunn & Frantz, 1979; Ingham, Andrews & Winkler, 1972). Not only do we know that some procedures are generally likely to be more powerful than others, but we know that some lead to speech that is generally more accepted by speakers and listeners than is other speech. (Ingham & Packman, 1978; Mallard & Meyer, 1979; Runyan & Adams, 1979). Moreover, we are now aware that the power-efficiency of our tactics and the acceptability of the speech signal are not the only matters to be considered. This was made evident by the fact that clients on occasion have rejected fluency-enhancing procedures because they involved instruments that were cumbersome, bothersome, or of restricted utility in particular circumstances (Janssen, 1982; Perkins & Curlee, 1969; Van Riper, 1982).

Though much that is clinically important has become apparent in recent years, there are more than a few matters that must be weighed before we can progress toward increasingly powerful ways of achieving fluency that is lasting, normal sounding, free of discomfort, and present in all circumstances. As has been intimated throughout this chapter, to achieve these ends we will need to pay more attention to those variables that play a determinative role in therapy. In addition, we are going to have to pay increasing attention to the clinically relevant variables that limit the degree of improvement and contribute to the likelihood of failure. It is our contention that the limiting effect is partly the result of management variables that contribute to unsystematic or error variance. This conclusion is clinically relevant because the efficiency of all therapies decreases as the error variance associated with their tactics increases. Put another way, the more unsystematic variance inherent in a therapy, the more powerful its tactics must be to produce the desired effect.

Postscript 7

Error variance is present to some degree in all therapies. It undoubtedly acts to limit somewhat the potential of every therapy program. But this fact should not be used as justification for failing to take steps that will serve to reduce its influence. At this time, its undermining affects are needlessly great. Moreover, there is good reason to believe that some relatively simple clinical actions can be taken that will notably reduce the error term that limits the power of our clinical techniques. One such technique involves steps to ensure that those who receive therapy designed for use with stutterers are indeed stutterers and not individuals who display speech disruptions indicative of other problems. Differential diagnosis is needed to reduce client heterogeneity and increase the probability that the clients served and the procedures employed are appropriate to each other.

Unsystematic variance can be reduced, also, by the simple expediency of assessment so that there is a greater congruence between the individual needs of clients and the therapeutic tactics employed. Often times, the importance of individual differences is not seen. Therapy is prepackaged. The behaviors in need of attention are not separated from those that are not. This omission promotes more than inefficiency; it dampens progress. But this does not have to be the case (Brutten, 1975). Fluency-enhancing programs, ones based on the premise that certain gestures must be instated to achieve fluency, can be made to accommodate the real differences in the requirements of clients who stutter (Cooper, 1982). Benefits of various kinds accrue from this accommodation. Greater therapeutic time and attention can be given to those behaviors that interfere with fluency. Skill training can be focused upon. In addition, response measurements that are appropriately specific can be used to determine if particular behaviors are being affected in the way and to the extent required.

Clearly, therapy, for stutterers as for those who display other behavioral problems, requires planning so that the steps taken to bring about change are systematic, precise, and as error-free as possible. Here, as throughout this treatise, a call has been made for a congruence between the strategies and tactics we employ as clinicians and the needs of clients. This call has involved attention to such therapy-related matters as the locus of difficulty, the type of response, the neuromotor system or systems involved, and the power-efficiency of different tactics. We have stressed, also, that a balance needs to be struck between therapeutic considerations that relate to individual differences and those that reflect the fundamental similarities among stutterers. Clinicians must be ever mindful of both the individual and group elements that determine therapeutic success. They must also recognize the limitations that are inherent in both an over-emphasized attention to differences among individuals and the behaviors they display and to the group commonality that obscures the particular individual needs of those who stutter.

The blend of individual- and group-related variables that aids therapy to the greatest extent has not yet been determined. We know that they both deserve consideration but we are not fully aware of the exact contribution that each makes in determining therapeutic success. We do know, however, that certain clinical actions generally heighten the probability of success. One of the more important of these revolves around the need to mass therapy experiences. Massed clinical practice is an aid to learning that cuts across clients and the conditioning class of the targeted responses. No matter which response class is involved, respondent or operant, massing serves to facilitate behavior change. In contrast, therapy that is occasional or sporadic in nature slows down the rate and amount of behavior change. This is so whether one is attempting to instate, modify, or remove a particular response or response pattern (Ingham & Andrews, 1973; Kimble, 1961; Webster, 1979). In part, this is because response variability is increased when therapy is scheduled a few times a week and involves relatively few practice hours. Intermittent therapy of this kind, which is traditional in the public schools and in university clinics, increases the unsystematic error that impedes clinical progress. It follows that clinical programs must either allow more encompassing and consistent practice, or techniques must be developed for bridging the between-session gap so that the interfering effect of error variance is reduced. We have attempted to accomplish this in a number of ways. One has been to schedule therapy so that it is massed in its early stages and distributed later. Another way has been to develop cassette tapes so that the client can experience the required and controlled practice at available times throughout the day. By these means, too, we have embedded distributed practice into the strategy of therapy so that the change promoted by massing will have a better chance of being maintained. For while massing facilitates change, distributed clinical practice supports its maintenance (Kimble, 1961).

The role of distributed practice in maintaining fluency has not been given as much consideration as it clearly warrants (Schwartz & Webster, 1977). This lack of emphasis seems to be especially true for those fluency programs that are of fixed duration (e.g., Webster, 1975). Moreover, attempts to deal with this problem by instructions to continue target-related practice at home after two or three weeks of intensive in-patient treatment does not appear to have proven all that helpful. Possibly this lack of efficacy results because clients tend to carry out their assignments on anything but a regular schedule once they return home. Possibly, also, home practice of this kind tends to fail because it is not directly supervised and so lacks the full precision that is required for maintenance. What these comments suggest is that maintenance, like change, is affected by those factors that are unsystematic and that increase response variability.

Practice that is massed and distributed is known to play a vital role in the learning and maintenance of responses of all kinds. It is also known that the import of practice increases when, as in speech, the behaviors involved are more complex and finer response tuning is required. We must keep in mind, too that in relation to stutterers we are not dealing with speech acquisition at its initial point. We must contend with troublesome aspects of past learning that is respondent and operant in nature. We must overcome an experience history that contains behavioral failures that are consistent beyond chance, the expectation of difficulty, well-learned emotional and coping adjustments that are maladaptive,

Postscript   7

and an organism that may well be limited in the neuromotor requirements that are fundamental to the production of normally fluent speech. These and other factors heighten still further the importance of practice. For the practice must overcome the handicapping past and stabilize the responses that support the presence of fluency. To accomplish these ends, that is to restructure speech so that fluency is normally present in all circumstances, not merely for a short period of time and in settings that are protective, it is clear that therapies are going to have to emphasize practice. Therapists are going to have to resort to overlearning so that the clients can withstand the environmental and organismic stresses that disadvantage them. Only then will the reactions and skills that are so carefully nurtured in therapy maintain themselves. For in the absence of overlearning our clients will continue to experience regressions and failures that are unnecessary. These will occur even though the tactics of today are obviously more powerful than those employed in past years.

EPILOGUE

Theories are explanations of why things happen the way they do. Scientific theories are data-sensitive. They are constantly tested by the findings of the studies they spawn. If a theory's predictions are not supported, the explanatory model must either be refined or abandoned.

Theorists must perforce be tough-minded. They must recognize from the beginning that the explanations they propose are not likely, at least as originally set forth, to withstand the test of time. They must bend with the data, correct their course, be willing to accept change. That does not mean that they serve science well if they respond in a will-of-the-wisp manner to currently popular ideas. For too often what is popular and what stampedes the thinking of the time turns out to be of limited value. Conversely, as we have seen, some ideas that have been rejected or even derided at one time are later seen as having more than a degree of worth. Theorists, then, walk a fine line. No matter how wide-ranging or restricted their explanatory and clinical statements, they must almost constantly decide whether to stand pat or reformulate their position. They must decide whether the evidence is strong enough and reliable enough to warrant a change. They must determine if continued support for a position is indefensible and representative of nothing more than inflexibility.

It is not always easy to divine whether the time has come to change one's stance at any of the many points that are basic to a theoretical position. In part this is because critical studies that truly test a position or set the prediction of one position against that of another are difficult to design (Anderson, 1971). Partly, also, it is because the very same data can be supportive of or explained by frameworks that differ notably. Furthermore, theorists are faced with the fact that many of the studies on which they depend are flawed, involve data that are less than conclusive, or have not been adequately replicated. Theoreticians are, then, in a ticklish decision-making position.

The comments that I have just made reflect the fact that I have worried over many of the points that are critical to the two-factor theory of stuttering. This is nothing new! I am always more than a bit restive when I attempt to organize and integrate the available data. There is always a degree of concern that the obvious may have been overlooked, the data may have been misinterpreted and personal predilections may have seriously colored my thinking. I am aware, too, that I will be held responsible for the statements in this chapter long after I may wish to claim continued responsibility for at least some of them. Times change, facts bring clarification, but the printed word remains. Yet, I dearly love the considered and constructive feedback that typically results from writing such as this. It is stimulating, and it provides direction. It also feeds life's fire.

I am sure that the concerns that I have expressed are shared, to some degree, by all of those who have contributed to this volume of stuttering. All of us must have been intrigued when we looked back at what we said decades ago (Perkins, 1977). We all must have been startled by the understanding occasionally contained in a statement or two. But I suspect that each of us found, as I have, that we did not always have foresight. On more than one occasion, we probably followed the wrong road or did not continue on the right one long enough. This floundering can be seen now that our material has grown cold and can be looked at dispassionately. What this means to me is that undertakings such as this are instructive. They should be periodically engaged in by all who seek to understand stuttering and to help those who stutter.

REFERENCES

Adams, M. R. (1980). The young stutterer: Diagnosis, treatment and assessment of progress. *Seminars in Speech, Language and Hearing, 1,* 289–299.

Adams, M. R. (1983, April). The relationship between stuttering theory, research, and therapy. Paper presented at the meeting of the International Congress of Speech Therapists, Antwerp, Belgium.

Adams, M. R., & Hayden, P. (1976). The ability of stutterers and nonstutterers to initiate and terminate phonation during production of an isolated vowel. *Journal of Speech and Hearing Research, 19,* 290–296.

Adams, M. R., & Ries, R. (1971). The influence of the onset of phonation on the frequency of stuttering. *Journal Speech of Hearing and Research, 14,* 639–644.

Adams, M. R., Runyan, C., & Mallard, A. R. (1975). Air flow characteristics of the speech of stutterers and nonstutterers. *Journal of Fluency Disorders, 1,* 3–12.

Agnello, J. G., & Wingate, M. E. (1971, November). Air pressure and formants of stutterers and nonstutterers. Paper presented at the meeting of the American Speech and Hearing Association, Chicago.

Agnello, J. G., & Wingate, M. E., & Wendell, M. (1974). Voice onset and voice termination times of child and adult stutterers. *Journal of Acoustical Society of America, 56,* 362.

Postscript   7

Anderson, B. F. (1971). *Psychology experiment: An introduction to the scientific method* (2nd ed.). Belmont, CA: Brooks/Cole Publishing Company.

Andrews, G., Craig A., Feyer, A. M., Hoddinott, S., Howie, P., & Neilson, M. (1983). Stuttering: A review of research findings and theories circa 1982. *Journal of Speech and Hearing Disorders, 26,* 226–246.

Andrews, G., & Cutler, J. (1977). Stuttering therapy: The relation between changes in symptom level and attitudes. *Journal of Fluency Disorders, 2,* 217–224.

Azrin, N. H., Nunn, R. G., & Frantz, S. E. (1979). Comparison of regulated breathing versus abbreviated desensitization on reported stuttering episodes. *Journal of Speech and Hearing Disorders, 22,* 331–339.

Bloodstein, O. (1982). *A handbook on stuttering.* Chicago, IL: The National Easter Seal Society.

Boberg, E. (Ed.). (1981). *Maintenance of fluency,* New York: Elsevier.

Boberg, E., Howie, P., & Woods, L. (1979). Maintenance of fluency: A review. *Journal of Fluency Disorders, 4,* 93–116.

Bridger, W. H., & Birns, B. (1963). Neonates' behavioral and autonomic responses to stress during soothing. *Recent Advances in Biological Psychiatry, 5,* 1–6.

Brutten, G. J. (1970). Two-factor theory and therapy. In *Conditioning in stuttering therapy,* (pp. 37–56). Memphis, TN: Speech Foundation of America.

Brutten, G. J. (1973). Behavior assessment and the strategy of therapy. In Y. Lebrun & R. Hoops (Eds.). *Neurolinguistic approaches to stuttering* (pp. 8–17). The Hague; Holland: Mouton.

Brutten, G. J. (1975). Stuttering: Topography, assessment, and behavior change strategies. In J. Eisenson (Ed.). *Stuttering: A Second Symposium,* (pp. 199–262). New York: Harper and Row.

Brutten, G. J. (1983). A reply to Costello and (Roemer) Hurst. *Journal of Speech and Hearing Research, 26,* 155–156.

Brutten, G. J., & Hegde,M. N. (1984). Stuttering: A clinically related overview. In S. Dickson (Ed.), *Communication disorders* (2nd ed.). (pp. 178–239) Glenview, IL: Scott, Foresman, and Company.

Brutten, G. J., & Shoemaker, D. J. (1967). *The modification of stuttering.* Englewood Cliffs, NJ: Prentice-Hall.

Brutten, G. J., & Shoemaker, D. J. (1970). Additional comments on the modification of stuttering. *Journal of Communication Disorders, 3,* 68–75.

Brutten, G. J. & Shoemaker, D. J. (1971). A two-factor learning theory of stuttering. In L. E. Travis (Ed.), *Handbook of speech pathology and audiology.* Englewood Cliffs, NJ: Prentice-Hall.

Cooper, E. B. (1982). A disfluency descriptor digest for clinical use. *Journal of Fluency Disorders, 7,* 355–358.

Costello, J. M., & Hurst, M. R. (1981). An analysis of the relationship among stuttering behaviors. *Journal of Speech and Hearing Research, 23,* 247–256.

Costello, J. M., & Hurst, M. R. (1983). A reply to Brutten. *Journal of Speech and Hearing Research, 26,* 156–159.

Cross, D. E., & Luper, H. L. (1979). Voice reaction time of stuttering and nonstuttering children and adults. *Journal of Fluency Disorders, 4,* 59–77.

Cullinan, W. L., & Springer, M. T. (1980). Voice initiation times in stuttering and nonstuttering children. *Journal of Speech and Hearing Research, 23,* 344–360.

Floyd, S., & Perkins, W. H. (1974). Early syllable dysfluencies in stutterers and nonstutterers: A preliminary report. *Journal of Communication Disorders, 7,* 279–282.

Gronhovd, K. D., & Zenner, A. A. (1982). Anxiety in stutterers: Rationale and procedures for management. *Speech and Language, 8,* 285–311.

Haynes, S. N. (1978). *Principles of behavior assessment.* New York: Gardner Press.

Hegde, M. N., & Brutten, G. J. (1977). Reinforcing fluency in stutterers: An experimental study. *Journal of Fluency Disorders, 2,* 315–328.

Hill, H. E. (1954). An experimental study of disorganization of speech and manual responses in normal subjects. *Journal of Speech and Hearing Disorders, 19,* 295–305.

Hillman, R. E., & Gilbert, H. H. (1977). Voice onset time for voiceless stop consonants in the fluent reading of stutterers and nonstutterers. *Journal of the Acoustical Society of America, 61,* 610–611.

Ingham, R. J., & Andrews, G. (1973). An analyses of a token economy in stuttering therapy. *Journal of Applied Behavior Analysis, 6,* 219–229.

Ingham, R. J., Andrews, G., & Winkler, R. (1972). Stuttering: A comparative evaluation of the short term effectiveness of four treatment techniques. *Journal of Communication Disorders, 5,* 91–117.

Ingham, R. J., & Packman, A. C. (1978). Perceptual assessment of normalcy of speech following stuttering therapy. *Journal of Speech and Hearing Research, 21,* 63–73.

Janssen, P. (1982). De Edinburgh Masker: Een welkom geluid voor de stotteraar? *Logopedie en Foniatrie, 54,* 54–63.

Janssen, P., & Kraaimaat, F. (1978). The relation between stuttering and state anxiety. *Logopedie en Foniatrie, 50,* 8–13.

Johnson, W., Brown, S. F., Curtis, J. F., Edney, C. E., & Keaster, J. (1956). *Speech handicapped school children* (rev. ed.). New York: Harper and Bros.

Jost, H., & Sontag, L. W. (1944). The genetic factor in autonomic nervous system function. *Psychosomatic Medicine, 6,* 308–310.

Kanfer, F. H., & Phillips, J. S. (1970). *Learning foundations of behavior therapy.* New York: John Wiley and Sons.

Kidd, K. K. (1977). A genetic perspective on stuttering. *Journal of Fluency Disorders, 2,* 259–269.

Kidd, K. K., Kidd, J. R., & Records, M. A. (1978). The possible causes of the sex ratio in stuttering and its implications. *Journal of Fluency Disorders, 3,* 13–23.

Kimble, G. (1961). *Conditioning and learning* (2nd ed.). New York: Appleton.

Kraaimaat, F., & Janssen, P. (1980). Relation between specific types of dysfluencies and autonomic and cognitive indices of anxiety in stuttering and nonstuttering adolescents. In B. J. Urban (Ed.), *The proceedings of the 18th congress of the IALP.* Rockville, MD: American-Speech-Language-Hearing Association.

Krych, D. (1978). *An audio-visual analysis of behavioral sequences evidenced during moments of stuttering.* Unpublished master's thesis, Southern Illinois University.

Leach, E. (1969). Stuttering: Clinical applications of response-contingent procedures. In B. B. Gray and G. England (Eds.), *Stuttering and the conditioning therapies* (pp. 115–125). Monterey, CA: Monterey Institute for Speech and Hearing.

Postscript 7

Long, K. M. & Hand, C. R. (1982, November). Manual reaction time to linguistic stimuli in stutterers and nonstutterers. Paper presented at the meeting of the American Speech and Hearing Association, Chicago.

Mallard, A. R., & Meyer, L. A. (1979). Listener preference for stuttering and syllable-timed speech production. *Journal of Fluency Disorders, 4,* 117–121.

Malmo, R. B. (1959). Activation: A neuro-physiological dimension. *Psychological Review, 66,* 367–386.

Martin, R. R., & Haroldson, S. K. (1981). Stuttering identification: Standard definition and moment of stuttering. *Journal of Speech and Hearing Research, 24,* 59–63.

Meyer, W. H. (1972). *The effects of contingent and noncontingent shock, presented in a neutral and negative environment, on phonemic repetitions of adult normal speakers.* Unpublished Ph.D. dissertation, Southern Illinois University.

Neale, J. M., & Liebert, R. M. (1980). *Science and behavior* (2nd ed.). Englewood Cliffs, NJ: Prentice-Hall.

Perkins, W. H. (1973a). Replacement of stuttering with normal speech: I. Rationale. *Journal of Speech and Hearing Disorders, 38,* 283–294.

Perkins, W. H. (1973b). Replacement of stuttering with normal speech: II. Clinical Procedures. *Journal of Speech and Hearing Disorders, 38,* 295–303.

Perkins, W. H. (1979). From psychoanalysis to discoordination. In H. Gregory (Ed.), *Controversies about stuttering therapy* (pp. 97–127). Baltimore, MD: University Park Press.

Perkins, W. H., & Curlee, R. F. (1969). Clinical impressions of portable masking unit effects in stuttering. *Journal of Speech and Hearing Disorders, 34,* 360–362.

Rimm, D. C., & Masters, J. C. (1979). *Behavior Therapy* (2nd ed.). New York: Academic Press.

Runyan, C. M., & Adams, M. R. (1979). Unsophisticated judges' perceptual evaluations of the speech of "successfully treated" stutterers. *Journal of Fluency Disorders, 4,* 29–38.

Ryan, B. P. (1970). An illustration of operant conditioning therapy for stuttering. In *Conditioning in stuttering therapy.* Memphis, TN: Speech Foundation of America.

Savoye, A. (1959). *The effect of the Skinner-Estes operant conditioning punishment paradigm upon the production of non-fluencies in normal speakers.* Unpublished master's thesis, University of Pittsburgh.

Schwartz, D., & Webster, L. M. (1977). More on the efficacy of a protracted precision fluency shaping program. *Journal of Fluency Disorders, 2,* 205–215.

Shames, G. H., & Egolf, D. B. (1976). *Operant conditioning and the management of stuttering.* Englewood Cliffs, NJ: Prentice-Hall.

Shames, G. H., & Florance, C. L. (1980). *Stutter-free speech: A goal for therapy.* Columbus, OH: Charles E. Merrill.

Shames, G. H., & Sherrick, C. E., Jr. (1963). A discussion of nonfluency and stuttering as operant behavior. *Journal of Speech and Hearing Disorders, 28,* 3–18.

Shaw, C. K., & Shrum, W. F. (1972). The effects of response-contingent reward on the connected speech of children who stutter. *Journal of Speech and Hearing Disorders, 37,* 75–88.

Siegel, G. M. (1970). Punishment, stuttering, and disfluency. *Journal of Speech and Hearing Research, 13,* 677–714.

Starkweather, C. W. (1970). *The simple, main, and interactive effects of contingent and non-contingent shock of high and low intensities on stuttering repetitions.* Unpublished Ph.D. dissertation, Southern Illinois University.

Starkweather, C. W. (1982). *Speech and language.* Englewood Cliffs, NJ: Prentice-Hall.

Starkweather, C. W., Hirschman, P., & Tannenbaum, R. S. (1976). Latency of vocalization onset: Stutterers versus nonstutterers. *Journal of Speech and Hearing Research, 19,* 491–492.

Starkweather, C. W., & Myers, N. (1978, November). The intervocalic interval in stutterers and nonstutterers: A close analysis. Paper presented at the meeting of the American Speech and Hearing Association.

Stassi, E. J. (1961). Disfluency of normal speakers and reinforcement. *Journal of Speech and Hearing Research, 4,* 358–361.

Van Riper, C. (1982). *The nature of stuttering* (2nd ed.). Englewood Cliffs, NJ: Prentice-Hall.

Webster, R. L. (1975). *Precision fluency shaping program.* Roanoke, VA: University Publications.

Webster, R. L. (1979). Empirical considerations regarding stuttering therapy. In H. H. Gregory (Ed.), *Controversies about stuttering therapy* (pp. 209–239). Baltimore, MD: University Park Press.

Wingate, M. E. (1964). A standard definition of stuttering. *Journal of Speech and Hearing Disorders, 29,* 484–489.

Zenner, A. A., & Webster, L. M. (1972, April). The molar and molecular effects of contingently stimulating the stuttering moment. Paper presented at the meeting of the Southern Speech Communication Association, San Antonio, TX

Zimmerman, G. (1980a). Articulatory behaviors associated with stuttering: A cinefluorographic analysis. *Journal of Speech and Hearing Research, 23,* 108–121.

Zimmerman, G. (1980b). Articulatory dynamics of fluent utterances of stutterers and nonstutterers. *Journal of Speech and Hearing Research, 23,* 95–107.

Zimmerman, G. (1980). Stuttering: A disorder of movement. *Journal of Speech and Hearing Research, 23,* 122–136.

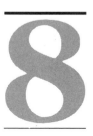

8

Theory and Treatment of Stuttering as an Approach–Avoidance Conflict

Joseph G. Sheehan

Postscript
Approach-Avoidance and Anxiety Reduction

Vivian M. Sheehan

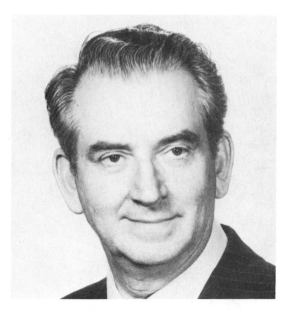

Joseph G. Sheehan

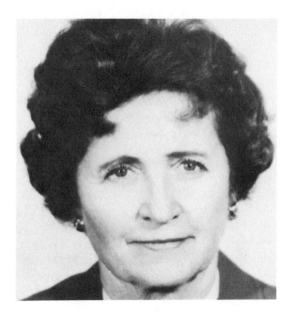

Vivian M. Sheehan

Joe Sheehan's Approach-Avoidance concept stems from Experimental Psychology and Learning Theory (Dollard & Miller, 1950) where a subject's ambivalence in the face of two bivalently varied stimuli had long been studied in the laboratory. The aversiveness of stuttering has been documented by stutterers for ages but what, in particular, they were avoiding in the act of speaking was not as clear as what they were approaching: the business of communicating, of saying what they had to say. In the laboratory, the parameters are always simpler: the attraction of a reinforcer, usually guaranteed by a controlled preceding period of deprivation, and the aversiveness of a noxious stimulus, shock or noise or the like. If stuttering is the noxious stimulus the stutterer avoids, then the avoidance behaviors themselves (the hesitations, prolongations, circumlocutions, etc.) have to go by some other name than stuttering. Both Bloodstein and Brutten, elsewhere in this volume, have addressed the same issue. Sheehan, in fact, saw the moment of stuttering as the point of convergence where the two drives of approach and avoidance were equal. Relating the professional, applied field of speech pathology to the more basic psychological sciences was a signif-

icant contribution for Sheehan. Although subsequent research took him in the direction of psychoanalytic theory and therapy, his classical contribution remains Approach-Avoidance conflict. His identification of five different levels of conflict provided direct attention and guidance for clinical management, both of a behavioral and psychotherapeutic nature. His facility with analogies made the most complex of concepts understandable. Sheehan's premature death interrupted his work on this book, and we were most fortunate to receive the cooperation of Vivian M. Sheehan, a professional speech pathologist in her own right, in updating the contribution of her late husband and colleague. She has helped us to keep sight of Joe Sheehan's other important concerns like the imagery associated with the moments preceding and following the stuttering block, documenting both anxiety and anxiety-reduction components of the behavior, as Wischner had also done, and also the issue of ultimate cures or outgrowings of stuttering later in adult life. We have in this chapter, then, a rich assortment of themes and issues alongside the classical treatment of Approach-Avoidance anxiety.

8

Theory and Treatment of Stuttering as an Approach-Avoidance Conflict*[1]

Joseph G. Sheehan[2]

THE PROBLEM

Seldom is the rôle of conflict, so important in every problem of adjustment, so clearly portrayed as in the disorder of stuttering. Stuttering behavior is essentially a hesitancy, an interruption in the forward flow of speech, a holding back in a situation which calls for going ahead. In the author's view, this hesitant or avoidant aspect of stuttering reflects the fundamental nature of the disorder:

> Stuttering is a result of approach-avoidance conflict, of opposed urges to speak and to hold back from speaking. The "holding back" may be due either to learned avoidances or to unconscious motives; the approach-avoidance formulation fits both (45).

This is, briefly stated, the theory to be presented in this paper. It seeks to integrate advances in speech pathology, psychopathology, and learning theory into a systematic theory of stuttering.

In recent years Miller (40) and Dollard and Miller (10) have formulated in systematic terms the nature of conflicts, especially those involving simultaneous

approach and avoidance tendencies. Lewin (36) analyzed conflicts between driving and restraining forces in relation to positive and negative valences. Travis, (53, 54) Glauber (24), and Fenichel (16) have developed psychoanalytic theories of stuttering based in part on conflict between conscious and unconscious wishes. Johnson (17, 30), Bryngelson (8), Van Riper (60, 61), and speech pathologists of the Iowa tradition have evolved, under different theoretical banners, systems of treatment which stressed non-avoidance and reduction of fears.

Aspects of conflict in stuttering have been noted by a number of investigators. More than 80 years ago the German writer Wyneken called the stutterer a *Sprachzweifler,* a "speech-doubter," comparing his plight to that of one seized with uncertainty at the moment of attempting a leap (63). In 1936 Johnson and Knott (32) defined stuttering as the manifestation of a conflict between the communicative drive or impulse and the impulse to inhibit expected stuttering. Knott and Johnson noted " . . . an experimental conflict . . . marked by the attempt of the stutterer to perform two mutually opposed tasks simultaneously; one is to talk, the other not to stutter (34).

As part of his analytically oriented theory, Travis held stuttering to be "a compromise between 'letting out' and 'holding in' (54) . . . The stutterer wishes to express himself, and at the same time fears doing so" (53). Fenichel stated: "The symptom of stuttering reveals a conflict between antagonistic tendencies; the patient shows us that he wishes to say something and

*Accepted for publication by Roy M. Dorcus of the Editorial Board, received in the Editorial Office on January 22, 1953, and published immediately at Provincetown, Massachusetts. Copyright by The Journal Press.

[1]Based on papers delivered at the meetings of the Western Psychological Association, April, 1950, and the American Speech and Hearing Association, November, 1950.

[2]The author wishes to express his indebtedness to his teachers, Drs. C. Van Riper and Wendell Johnson, whose influence is apparent beyond their many acknowledgments throughout the paper.

Note: From *The Journal of Psychology, 36,* 1953, pp. 27–49. Reprinted with permission of Journal Press.

yet does not wish to" (16, p. 311). Closely related observations of conflict in stuttering may be found in Blanton and Blanton (3), Bluemel (5,6), Dunlap (11), Fletcher (18, pp. 231-232), Froeschels, (22, 23), Glauber (24), Hill (26), Johnson (29, 30, 32), Solomon (51, 52), Van Riper (57, 60, pp. 269, 277, 287, 321-322, 61, pp. 19-20), Wischner (62, p. 330), and Wyneken (63).

Wide divergence has appeared among various writers as to the nature of the conflict and its relation to the stuttering. For some it has been a conflict over gratification of instincts, for others a conscious interference with an automatic process, for still others a rivalry between cortical hemispheres. Many apparently competing theories attack the problem at different levels and do not necessarily contradict one another. In like manner, the approach-avoidance conflict theory presented here involves only its own level of analysis and is sufficiently broad to be compatible with many other interpretations of stuttering.

Two Essential Questions

If we reduce stuttering behavior to the simplest possible terms, we find that it is a *momentary blocking*. Almost mysteriously the stutterer is stuck on a word, and then, for reasons just as baffling, he is able to continue. An explanation of stuttering must account for these twin features of the stutterer's behavior.

Most theories of stuttering have focused on the hesitancy, on what produces the blocking. But from the standpoint of systematic theory as well as therapy, it is just as important to explain termination of the block as the block itself. This problem has been considered in an earlier study: "What seems to determine the moment of release, the moment at which the stutterer can finally say the word?" (44, p. 69).

Two questions then become essential in the explanation of the stutterer's behavior: (1) What makes him stop? (2) What enables him to continue? To answer them fully, with support for the answers, requires the complete spelling out of the theory portion of this paper.

The two central hypotheses, however, may be stated quite briefly:

1. *The Conflict Hypothesis.* The stutterer stops whenever conflicting approach and avoidance tendencies reach an equilibrium.
2. *The Fear-Reduction Hypothesis.* The occurrence of stuttering reduces the fear which elicited it, so that *during* the block there is sufficient reduction

in fear-motivated avoidance to resolve the conflict, permitting release of the blocked word.

The discussion that follows will take up each of these in turn.

THE CONFLICT HYPOTHESIS

Statement

If stuttering occurs whenever approach and avoidance tendencies reach an equilibrium, we should be able to analyze the process in terms of relative strengths of gradients of each. Miller (40, 41) and Dollard and Miller (10) have provided us with an excellent theoretical model for such an analysis (Figure 8–1).

For the stutterer, the speaking of a difficult word involves a goal, that of communication, but also a fear, that of inability to communicate. The stutterer thus has a "feared goal" in Miller's sense. Conflicting tendencies in the stutterer to approach and to avoid are represented by solid and broken lines respectively. From the fact that the fear-motivated avoidance gradient is steeper than the reward-motivated approach gradient, it can be seen that an organism put in an approach-avoidance conflict situation will *go part-way and then stop*, or oscillate helplessly in the zone where the gradients cross. This is exactly the behavior the stutterer shows in attempting a *feared word*, or upon entering a *feared situation*. He says "K-K-K-Katy" or blocks silently after having begun the word. He freezes at the instant of picking up the phone, or halts on the threshold of a strange office.

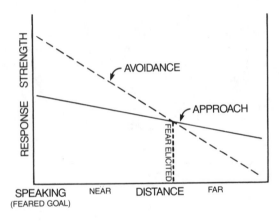

Figure 8–1.

If this formulation is essentially correct, we are in a position to answer the first question. The stutterer stops after advancing part-way because he is in a conflict situation, and the moment of his stopping is determined by the relative strengths of approach and avoidance gradients. Stuttering behavior itself has a hesitant character because it is the result of a conflict. Such an interpretation of stuttering accords well with Freud's classic view of the nature of neurotic conflict:

"... neurotic symptoms ... are the result of a conflict. The two powers which have entered into opposition meet together again in the symptom and become reconciled by means of the *compromise* contained in the symptom-formation" (19, p.313).

In the compromise, i.e., the symptom of stuttering, the conflict is neatly externalized.

Many of the secondary symptoms of stuttering, as analyzed by Van Riper (57), may be interpreted as compensatory efforts to overcome avoidance, to go forward in the face of fear. Others, as he has pointed out, are just reactions to fear, directly expressed avoidance. Among the compensatory measures to overcome avoidance are the devices of starting, antiexpectancy, and release. These are, in effect, attempts to reach the goal by a roundabout route, a characteristic of conflict behavior noted by Lewin (37, p. 263). Devices of avoidance and postponement, on the other hand, are essentially reactions to fear, direct expressions of the approach-avoidance conflict.

The primary symptoms of stuttering can equally be attributed to approach-avoidance conflict. Repetition and prolongation may represent oscillating and stopping, respectively, near the point where the gradients cross, at the point of equilibrium in the conflict. Both Johnson and Van Riper have pointed out that syllable repetition and other forms of nonfluency in children characteristically appear in the midst of many conflicting speech pressures, e.g., vocabulary acquisition, phrase choices, and sentence building. Adults similarly tend to speak hesitantly in pressure situations.

Speech is a sequence of movements, and stuttering is a breakdown in the sequence. Whatever the involvements of the disorder, the point at which the breakdown occurs must bear a relation to these involvements. The breakdown occurs early in the sequence, but seldom prevents initiation of the sequence. Stuttering is, in other words, chiefly a disorder of *release*, of going partway and then stopping.

Froeschels (22) has called repetition and prolongation ("clonus and tonus") the only symptoms common to all stutterers, an observation supported by the author's findings (44, p. 62). The stopping and oscillation which these symptoms may express are the features common to approach-avoidance behavior.

For clarity in presentation, this discussion has centered on stuttering as simple approach-avoidance conflict. Speaking has been the approach response; not speaking the avoidance response. But at times there are approach and avoidance tendencies to the act of speaking itself as well as to the act of not speaking. This involves some additional assumptions[3] and a further analysis, in terms of Miller's double approach avoidance conflict (Figures 8–2 and 8–3), which may account better for certain occurrences of stuttering.

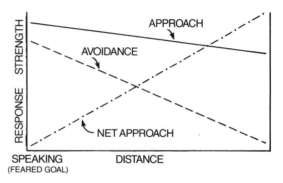

Figure 8–2.

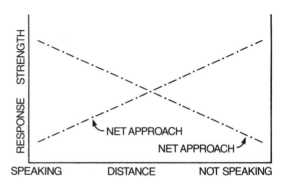

Figure 8–3.

---

[3]The writer is indebted to Dr. Irving Maltzman for portions of this analysis.

The conflict on speaking is as follows: There is an approach tendency for speaking, since it is socially demanded. But since speaking entails the danger of stuttering, there is an avoidance tendency based on the fear elicited by this danger. This is the type of conflict which Johnson and Knott (32) held responsible for stuttering.

The conflict on not speaking is as follows: There is an approach tendency for not speaking, because silence becomes an attractive alternative to the danger situation of speaking. But this alternative also is to be feared.

In a situation which calls for speech, not speaking or not being able to speak in itself involves a threat. Many stutterers show a *fear of silence,* and any dead stop in their communication spurs panicky efforts to release the block. Many of the irrelevant and apparently unintelligent symptoms of the stutterer can be understood as a filibustering, a measure taken against the fear of silence.

Consequently, there is an avoidance tendency for not speaking as well as an approach tendency for not speaking. Movement toward either feared goal elicits more fear, so that the net approach tendency will be greater toward the more distant goal. As this is approached, e.g., as the stutterer gets closer to the speech attempt or as he gets further away from it, the alternative goal becomes more distant, hence less dangerous and more attractive. The stutterer will then turn and approach the other goal until it becomes too feared. Dollard and Miller's prediction for this type of situation is "one of stable equilibrium like that of the pendulum" (10, pp. 366-367). Such behavior toward feared words and situations is characteristic of the stutterer.

The paradoxical increase in "fear elicited" as lowered avoidance permits a closer approach to the feared goal is equally true of simple approach-avoidance conflict (1).

Evidence

What predictions flow from conflict theory, and what evidence can be brought to bear on these predictions? If stuttering is a form of conflict, a resultant of competing urges to approach and avoid, then it should vary systematically as follows: Stuttering should be increased by (a) a heightening of the avoidance drive through an increase in the penalty upon which fear and avoidance are based; (b) by a lowering of the approach drive. Stuttering should be decreased by (a) a reduction in the avoidance drive (fear, penalty); (b) by an increase in the approach drive.

What are the findings? The effect of penalty upon stuttering was shown in an important early study by Van Riper (58), who found that frequency of stuttering is increased by expectation of electric shock to be administered according to the number of blocks. Trial shocks only were administered, so that Van Riper's procedure was essentially a shock threat situation, a neat experimental paradigm for the relationship between stuttering and fear. Recently these results have been repeated by Frick as part of a comprehensive investigation of the relationship between punishment and stuttering. In other portions of his experiment, Frick administered shock for each stuttered word, in one condition at the end of the passage and in another immediately after the block. In each case the added penalty resulted in greater frequency of stuttering (21). Porter found that the frequency of stuttering is increased by greater social penalty, as measured by the number of persons in the audience (43). On the other hand, the frequency of stuttering is decreased by a reduction in penalty as measured by the meaningfulness of the material (Eisenson and Horowitz, 13), and by degree of communicative responsibility (Eisenson and Wells, 14). Bloodstein (4, p. 296) has suggested that the adaptation effect, the reduction in frequency of stuttering with repeated readings of the same passage, may be explained on the basis of a reduction in propositionality. As in the Eisenson studies, this involves a reduction in penalty. These findings accord well with the predictions of the approach-avoidance theory.

So much for penalty, and increases or decreases in the avoidance drive. What about the approach drive? The evidence on this is sparse. That which we do have, mostly clinical observation, supports our formulation. Stutterers, like people generally, show markedly more hesitancy when dealing with material they are reluctant to reveal. Literature is full of descriptions of small boys stammering their excuses and of the hesitant speech of marriage proposals. Stuttering has been known to start from a parental demand of an oral confession of guilt. The reduction of communicatory drive in such a situation is fairly obvious. On the other hand, increases in the approach drive brought about through hypnosis, suggestion (4) or speaking under strong or unusual stimulation (4) brings increased fluency. Stutterers sometimes surprise themselves and their associates by speaking normally in a crisis situation. Anger or sudden stress may produce a spectacular fluency.

Such events point to the effect of a temporary increase in the approach drive.

A recently completed study bears directly on the strengthening of approach behavior in stutterers. Twenty adult stutterers read two 200-word passages five consecutive times under different conditions. The control condition was a standard adaptation situation, in which the subject simply read the passage each time as naturally as possible. Under the experimental condition, the subject repeated each stuttered word until he had attacked it once successfully. This technique led to more normal speech and less stuttering ($P = .02$). Under the assumptions stated in the study, the approach response of speaking was thereby strengthened while the avoidant response of stuttering was moved futher away from the point of reinforcement and correspondingly weakened (46).

Levels of Conflict

In order to present the conflict hypothesis directly and simply, more thorough analysis of the different levels at which conflict may occur in stuttering has been reserved for separate presentation. Five distinct levels emerge: word-level; situation-level; emotional content level; relationship level, and ego-protective level.

At the *word level* the conflict is between the urge to speak the word and the urge not to speak the word. For example, the stutterer wants to say "hello," i.e., he approaches this word, but fear holds him back, because "h" sounds have through past experience acquired cue value.

At the *situation level* there is a parallel conflict between entering and not entering a feared situation. The stutterer's behavior toward using the telephone, reciting in classes, or introducing himself to strangers illustrates this conflict. Many situations which demand speech hold enough threat to produce a competing drive to hold back.

These two levels are based upon Van Riper's distinction between specific expectancy, or word-fear, as contrasted with general expectancy or situation fear (57, 60). Such fears are usually based on past speech experiences and involve directly learned avoidance. How conflict based on word fear and situation fear can lead to blocking has been illustrated briefly by our diagram, Figure 8-1, and analyzed in detail elsewhere (46).

Conflict due to the *emotional content* of words, apart from their phonetic properties, such as has been described by Travis (53, p. 202), involved unconscious motivation for avoidance. This is illustrated by the stutterer whose speech grows worse in describing a traumatic experience, or upon giving information he is reluctant to divulge. It is the emotional and verbal content that is involved, not the situation or the words in themselves. Dunlap (11) said of the stutterer: "Sometimes he is in constant fear lest he inadvertently reveal something he would rather his elders did not hear." The inhibition of emotional content, especially hostile feeling, is a common denominator in many instances of stuttering (1).

At a closely related level of conflict, the occurrence of stuttering is in part a function of the *relationship* between the stutterer and his listener. Some stutterers experience no fear when they play a dominant rôle. One may give a fluent public address but stutter to individuals in the audience before and afterward. A child may block severely before one parent but speak easily to the other. An army enlisted man could never say "sergeant" until he became one. The fact that many stutterers can act in plays seems to show the effect of changed rôle. Several of the conditions listed by Bloodstein (4) as involving the behavior of the listener may equally be interpreted in terms of relationship. Pointing out that the stutterer can usually talk well when alone, Adler concludes, "... I can only interpret his stammer as the expression of his attitude toward others" (2, p. 63). Fletcher (18), Travis (53), Fenichel (16, pp. 311-314), Abbot (1), and many others have stated in one way or another the importance of the relationship between the stutterer and his listener.

Since stuttering may be termed a compromise between speech and silence, we should consider the symbolic significance of all three in analyzing what is expressed toward the listener. Depending upon our initial reference points, we may get widely differing results (a) stuttering may be considered an act of aggression against the listener; fluency then would be nonaggressive or friendly behavior; (b) speech may be considered an aggressive, competitive, phallic (in psychoanalytic terms) act; silence here is presumably neutral; (c) silence in itself may be viewed as hostile. Noting that in dreams to be mute is a symbol of death, Fenichel (16, pp. 311–313) likened stuttering to a partial mutism resulting from a turning inward against the stutterer's own ego of hostile urges originally directed against the listener. From his discussion it is possible to infer all three of the above meanings. Perhaps it should be concluded simply that either stuttering or speech or silence can be used to express hostility or more positive feelings at various times, but that no constant or universal meaning can be offered. Whatever the behavior through which the feeling is expressed, the occurrence of stuttering will in part be determined by degree of conflict at the relationship level.

At the *ego-protective level,* stuttering serves as a lifelong defense mechanism keeping its possessor out of dangerous competition. Through the stuttering, certain aspirations may be abandoned which might involve threat of failure, or threat of success.

Although our formulation of the ego-protective level stresses life aspirations and goals, the concept is sufficiently broad to include any defensive function of stuttering. Travis' excellent formulation more nearly represents the classic Freudian view of symptoms as defenses against forbidden impulses:

> " . . . stuttering is a defense created with extraordinary skill and designed to prevent anxiety from developing when certain impulses of which the stutterer dares not become aware, threaten to expose themselves" (53, p. 193).

That stutterers do tend significantly to avoid threat of failure is shown by their behavior in an experimental level of aspiration situation. Compared to normal controls, stutterers set less exacting (though more realistic) goals for themselves, predicted more modest performances, and showed in general a lower level of aspiration (49).

Any particular moment of stuttering may be understood in terms of the interplay of conflicting forces at these levels. Whatever the level of conflict, the overt conflict is experienced at the word-level. Conflict at the ego-protective level, for example, might explain a stutterer's resistance in therapy. It would not explain his blocking on a word, except through the mediation of word-fear. In like manner, the pressure of the situation, emotionality of the utterance, or nature of the interpersonal relation must ultimately be expressed at the word-level. It is in this fundamental sense that stuttering is a conflict between speaking and not speaking.

THE FEAR REDUCTION HYPOTHESIS

Statement

If stuttering results from a conflict, how is the conflict resolved? According to the conflict hypothesis, the stutterer stops when approach and avoidance tendencies reach an equilibrium. Why then doesn't the stutterer remain permanently in a conflict situation? How is he able to obtain release from the block?

At the beginning of a block the stutterer is stuck. He cannot get the word out. By the end of the block some change has taken place, so that he can now utter the word. What has happened between these points? If the stutterer cannot say the word for a time, why is he able to say it at all? To account for this, the hypothesis is advanced that the occurrence of stuttering brings about a reduction of the fear which elicited it.

During the moment of stuttering, there must be sufficient reduction of fear, avoidance tendency and conflict to "release" the blocked word. Were it not for this fact, once the stutterer became stuck on a word, he would remain stuck indefinitely.

How can the occurrence of stuttering reduce the fear that elicits it? Why should the stutterer be in any better position to speak the word at the end of a block than at the beginning? After all, the symptoms of stuttering frequently bear little relevance to the actual speaking of the word (57, 44).

The occurrence of stuttering may effect a reduction of fear in several ways:

First, since the stutterer's fear is tied up with his avoidance and is an effort to hide the disapproved symptoms, once the stuttering begins to occur it can no longer be hidden. The stuttering block itself forces the stutterer to "face" his stuttering to a certain extent. This reduces the conflict. The thing the stutterer feared has now occurred. He can no longer avoid it completely, and this partially reduces the fear. On the other hand, successful avoidance builds up tension.

Second, once the stuttering block begins to occur it is a known entity. As the stutterer begins to approach a block, he has a vague dread, a generalized expectancy. As he nears the actual moment of stuttering, he recognizes more familiar landmarks (initial sound, length of word, cf. Brown, 7) and is even able to predict the duration of the block with some precision (study by Milisen and Van Riper, 39). Hence, he gets some feeling of control, the fear is now more specific and there is less fear of the unknown, and there is a reduction of the element of fear from a sense of helplessness (study by Mowrer and Viek, 42).

Third, to the extent that stuttering can be interpreted as an aggressive act directed against the listener (Fenichel, 16) the stuttering relieves the aggression (frustration-aggression hypothesis), hence reduces the inhibition to aggression, hence reduces the approach-avoidance conflict of the stuttering.

To test these corollary hypotheses is obviously beyond the scope of this paper. They are stated here for the completeness of the theory and as problems for future research.

Evidence

Among studies which may be interpreted as revealing the effect of stuttering on fear are the following:

1. The study by Meissner (38) in which voluntary non-fluency reduced stuttering.

2. The studies of Johnson and Knott (33), Johnson and Inness (31), Shulman (50), and other studies showing the adaptation effect. From the fear-reduction hypothesis, we may infer that the occurrence of stuttering in the first reading dissipates sufficient anxiety so that there is less stuttering in the second reading, etc. Such an interpretation of adaptation is in agreement with and in large part contained in Johnson's current published view:

   The adaptation effect would appear to be a particularly clean-cut example of the effect of improved adjustment to the reading situation, lowered anxiety about stuttering resulting from "doing the thing feared" and discovering on the spot that the dreaded consequences turn out to be less dreadful than expected (30, p. 210).

3. The study by Brown (7) showing that stutterers tend to stutter more on the first word in a sentence. According to our hypothesis, the stuttering which occurs on the first word will, through generalization, make subsequent words in that sentence easier.

4. The effectiveness of the technique of negative practice as reported by Dunlap (11, 12), Case (9), and Fishman (17). Duplicating the stuttered performance voluntarily should "satisfy" the fear, lower the avoidance drive, and diminish the conflict causing the stuttering.

5. Van Riper's study of thoracic breathing (56) in which stutterers show a rehearsal of the block during an expectancy period. The rehearsal behavior is here interpreted as an effort to reduce the fear by stuttering subvocally first.

6. The finding of Travis, Tuttle, and Cowan (55) that during tonic stuttering block, heart rate becomes progressively slower.

7. Van Riper's study showing the relation of tremors to perpetuation of and release from the stuttering block (59). Results showed a tendency toward decrease in the rate and amplitude of jaw tremors during the block.

8. In an effort to verify Van Riper's result, and as a specific test of the fear-reduction hypothesis presented here, the author and Mr. Robert Voas of U.C.L.A. carried out a study of physiological tension patterns of 15 stutterers during the moment of stuttering (47, 48). Masseter muscle action currents and other measures showed a rise in amplitude (tension) at the beginning of the block followed by a dropping off to the moment of release. Upon the speaking of the word—the reaching of the goal—the resolving of the conflict—a marked reduction in tension occurred as the muscle group returned to the resting state. It should be pointed out that this type of tension reduction occurs normally with the speaking of a word whether stuttered or not. The theoretically important feature is that sufficient fear reduction occurs *during* the stuttering block to permit release of the blocked word. Van Riper has analyzed some of the ways in which stuttering brings about fear-reduction:

   "The relationship of fear to stuttering is so great that stutterers often feel that, if they could destroy the fear of approaching words, they would be able to say them without any difficulty (60, p. 298). . . . Fear of a word brings an automatic reaction of the oft-practiced tricks previously used to reduce or counteract that fear" (60, p. 286).

   The results of the study just described support this interpretation as well as Van Riper's unpublished findings in the tremor study.

9. Two other findings may be cited in support of the fear-reduction hypothesis. First, in applying a non-reinforcement procedure to a group of stutterers, it was possible to obtain a normal speaking of the word simply by asking the subject to repeat the word, i.e., to stutter on it until all fear present was "satisfied." That the subjects were able to do this, that they could speak the word more easily the second, third, and fourth attempt, is in itself strong evidence for a mechanism of fear reduction resulting from stuttering (46). In another study, (44, p. 25) a tendency was noted toward stuttering with succeedingly larger portions of the word, e.g., "th-thir-thirty." From our hypothesis, the

stuttering which occurred on the first attempt reduced fear and avoidance sufficiently so that succeeding points of stoppage occurred closer to the goal, i.e., nearer the speaking of the word.

Implications

These results have interesting ramifications. Van Riper states that successful avoidance increases the stutterer's fear and causes more trouble in the long run (60, pp. 284-285). The concept of stuttering as a fear-reducer clarifies this relationship. When the stutterer is able to avoid stuttering he does not dissipate the anxiety, the tension builds up and even though he may continue to be fluent, he is building up future trouble through the avoidance. On the other hand, when he stutters or pretends to stutter, he is reducing his fears and building toward greater fluency later on. Hence we have a paradoxical relation—the stuttering produces the fluency and the fluency produces the stuttering. This is a possible explanation of something frequently observed, namely, that stuttering tends to occur in waves.

We could thus view stuttering as having a function similar to that of tics, asthma, and many neurotic symptoms, that it "binds" the anxiety and has the property of reducing it. We would have a parallel here to compulsive acts. When the person cannot stutter or successfully does not, the fear builds up. Stuttering may be thus viewed as an expression of accumulated anxiety. When the behavior occurs, the anxiety erupts and is let out. This concept may go a long way toward explaining the apparently paradoxical fact that we can build up a stutterer's tension by asking him to be fluent and we can reduce his fear by encouraging him to engage freely in the expression of the symptom.

On the concept of anxiety binding, Freud gives us one view, " ... all symptom formation would be brought about solely to avoid anxiety. The symptoms bind the psychic energy which would otherwise be discharged as anxiety... if a compulsion neurotic is prevented from washing his hands after touching something, he becomes a prey to almost insupportable anxiety" (20, p.85).

In the same context, the concepts of the stuttering symptom as a defense against anxiety has long been stressed by Travis (53, 54, p. 35).

It is as though each stutterer carries around with him a "stutter potential," a *reservoir of fear* which is tapped from time to time by the occurrence of stuttering. Such a concept, while more figurative than real, may help us understand the seemingly neurotic stutterer who suffers agonies in anticipation of stuttering that never quite happens. It is precisely because the individual never stutters that he never obtains relief. His need for stuttering, as Travis aptly put it, becomes acute. In a psychological sense he is much worse off than the individual who can express his conflict, and reduce his fear, through outward stuttering behavior. Such a concept has interesting possibilities: not only does it provide theoretical support for procedures used by Johnson and Van Riper with stutterers, but it suggests potentialities for *symptom expression* as a psychotherapeutic technique with any problem based on fear.

Theoretical Relationships

A paradoxical effect of fear-reduction during the block may be inferred from the nature of the conflict. By the lowering of the avoidance gradient, the stutterer is brought closer to the feared goal and hence may experience a paradoxical increase in "fear elicited." Thus a reduction in fear shifts the equilibrium of the forces in conflict and brings the stutterer closer to the speaking of the word, but simultaneously he is experiencing more fear as he nears the goal.

From the basic diagram of approach-avoidance conflict (our Figure 8–1), Dollard and Miller state their assumption that *fear elicited* is fixed by the height of the intersection of the two gradients, and proceed with the following analysis:

> ... When the avoidance is strong relative to the approach, the two gradients intersect far from the goal. ... At this distance the approach tendency is so weak that the subject is not strongly tempted to do frightening things. ... Extinguishing the fear of the goal or making it seem less dangerous ... will lower the entire gradient of avoidance ... this will produce a paradoxical effect ... as the apparent danger is reduced the subject will be more strongly tempted to do things which frighten him. Stronger fear and conflict will therefore be elicited (10).

At this point the situation must sound discouraging, but Dollard and Miller further point out:

> This deduction holds only for the range within which the gradients of approach and avoidance intersect. If the gradient of avoidance is weakened so much that it no longer intersects the gradient of approach, the subject will advance to the goal and further decreases in the gradient of avoidance will decrease the amount of fear and conflict (10).

This discussion may help us distinguish between the fear reduction *during* the block which permits release and that which results from the release, because the goal of speaking the word is reached. The fear reduction which determines the release may be obscured somewhat by a simultaneous increase in fear, conflict, and avoidance strength with the nearing of the feared goal.

Two shifts are occurring at once. For a given amount of fear and avoidance tendency, the point at which the stutterer initially stops is determined in part by the strength of the approach drive, which is in turn a function of his need to communicate and ability to tolerate anxiety. When he reaches the point of stoppage the stuttering begins to occur, reducing the fear which elicited it and lowering the avoidance gradient so that he moves closer to the goal. Thus the amount of fear subjectively experienced may remain relatively constant throughout the block. If the stutterer does not complete the block, but leaves the field or engages in some instrumental escape response, or if by using a device or trick he successfully reaches the goal in a roundabout manner, he does not "satisfy the fear" present and may continue to experience tension after the block. The unsatisfied fear may transfer over to a subsequent word and be dissipated on that word. When the opposite happens and there is rehearsal or sub-vocal satisfying of the fear first, there may be a stuttering on the word preceding the word originally feared, an observation made by Hill (26). Since fear-reduction reinforces the instrumental acts which bring it about, and reinforced responses tend to move up in the response sequence, (25, pp. 212-215) the stuttering tends to become anticipatory. Van Riper has shown that the actual form of the block may be rehearsed in breathing patterns prior to speech attempt. Through secondary reinforcement such rehearsal behavior will be fear-reducing, which indeed appears to be its function. Proprioceptive feedback from this rehearsal behavior enables the stutterer to anticipate his blocks, even to predicting their duration with some accuracy (39).

Thus there are indications of fear-reduction occurring during at least the first two of the three stages of the stuttering process as analyzed by Johnson: pre-spasm, spasm, and post-spasm (28). From fear-reduction occurring before and during the block and at the moment of release, the symptom is reinforced and maintained, the anxiety is "bound" within it, and a vicious circle is perpetuated.

TREATMENT

If stuttering is basically an approach-avoidance conflict, then the fundamental goal of treatment becomes the elimination of all tendency to avoidance, whatever the source. Since the avoidance is based on fear, stuttering is to be treated as a fear problem. Successful treatment then requires gaining a mastery over fear and finding expression of whatever needs, feelings, and tendencies have been locked up in the symptom. The approach-avoidance conflict theory of stuttering thus gives strong theoretical support to therapeutic procedures employed by Van Riper, Johnson, Bryngelson, Travis and others of the "Iowa School" of stuttering therapy.

Since approach-avoidance conflict theory was implicit in non-avoidance training and other techniques of the "Iowa School," the therapeutic approach presented here springs largely from this school. Two specific values of the approach-avoidance formulation should be mentioned: *(a)* Approach-avoidance theory relates fear, avoidance and conflict to stuttering, and theory to treatment in a systematic way. The paramount importance of reducing fears and avoidances becomes clearly apparent from the theory itself. *(b)* The analysis of levels of conflict and the distinction between learned avoidances and unconscious motives for avoidance provides for an integration of psychotherapy and speech therapy not always apparent in the writings of psychologists and speech pathologists.

The relative utilization of speech therapy and psychotherapy in present-day clinical work offers many contrasts. On one hand a few stragglers still use a purely symptomatic treatment which tries to ignore fears, prevent blocks, and build fluency directly through "confidence" measures. These people neglect all psychotherapy, and in a modern sense, speech therapy as well. At the opposite pole are many able clinicians, often psychoanalytically oriented, who insist that we must "ignore the symptom" and work toward the original cause, presumably something in the stutterer's past. For these people the speech pathologist could offer the stutterer nothing except in terms of whatever general psychotherapeutic abilities he might possess.

However, when stuttering is treated as a form of conflict, speech therapy and psychotherapy are not in competition, but have a common goal; the reduction of all tendencies to avoidance and of the fears which motivate them.

Although the stutterer's need for psychotherapy is now widely accepted, many of those who see this need most clearly continue to ask, "Why work on the speech at all?" To answer this question, and to defend the rôle that speech pathologists have come to assume in helping stutterers, we list the following points:

First, if we are really justified in viewing stuttering as an externalized conflict, should we now avail ourselves of this ready avenue to other levels? Conflict at the relationship level, for example, is mediated through situation and word-fear; why then not begin where the stuttering occurs and work back to the stutterer's relationships? The stutterer's blocks and his reactions to them mirror his self-concepts, attitudes toward others, mechanisms for handling conflicts, and many other aspects of his personality. Each time the stutterer has a block he is reliving in a small way one of the most significant experiences of his life.

Second, if we accept the hypothesis that stuttering reduces to some degree the fear that elicits it, possibilities suggest themselves for planned use of stuttering behavior as a tension reducer or outlet for fear. The "negative practice" techniques employed by Dunlap (12) probably owed some of their efficacy to this effect, though he advocated their use on different grounds. Such Iowa School methods as a voluntary repetition of "bounce," smooth prolongation or "slide," and duplication of the true pattern have been used successfully for years to reduce the stutterer's anxiety. Some of the best successes have been obtained with cases who had little outward stuttering to begin with and who underwent no discernible speech changes. But through such speech therapy, with very little conventional psychotherapy, they have been freed from the taxing strain of anticipation.

Third, profound personality changes can result from successful speech therapy. Teaching a stutterer how to handle his fears and his blocks, helping him develop healthier attitudes toward his problem, toward himself, and toward others—these things are not mere symptom treatment. Encouraging the stutterer to attack feared and difficult situations may support him strongly in something he really has wanted to do. Many stutterers relate that they get tired of running away; it is a deeply moving experience to master situations from which they have always retreated.

Fourth, a certain amount of direct speech therapy is necessary to deal with the maintaining causes of stuttering. Van Riper states, "Stuttering is peculiarly able to maintain itself once it gets started (60, p. 276)... in the secondary stage... the disorder has become 'chronic' or self-perpetuating... a vicious circle" (60, p. 239). Johnson observes: "Stuttering is something like our fear of thunder—there is no inherent or rational necessity for it, but once started it tends to be maintained, generation after generation" (30, p. 194). Both these authorities, as well as Dunlap (11, p. 199), Case (9), Wischner (62, pp. 330-331), and others, have pointed out how stuttering may perpetuate itself on a learned behavior, or habit level. Wischner considers stuttering as learned behavior which seems to resemble responses set up by instrumental avoidance training (62, p. 327), hence difficult to extinguish (62, p. 332).

An experiment by the author has shown that when reinforcement of the stuttering can be prevented, modified or decreased, stuttering is reduced. In this way the vicious circle may be broken (46, pp. 61-62). Van Riper's method of "cancellation," as well as a host of other techniques of the Iowa School, are directed toward the same result (60, pp. 348-371). With such techniques available, it is unnecessary to let the stutterer struggle helplessly with his blocks for an indefinite period while searching for buried complexes. And in long-range terms, if the therapist disdains all direct work on speech, he offers the stutterer only a purely verbal system for coping with long-reinforced habitual responses that are permitted to remain intact.

Treatment may begin at the topmost level of conflict and work downward. Conflicts due to immediate word fear and situation fear are dealt with through that specialized portion of the therapeutic process known as speech therapy. The speech therapy techniques appropriate to a conflict interpretation of stuttering have been so thoroughly developed in publications of Van Riper, Bryngelson, Johnson, and Travis as to require no repeating here. Conflicts at deeper levels are straight problems in psychotherapy, which may be handled concurrently. To the extent that such conflicts express themselves through outward stuttering behavior, they may be reached via the speech therapy. The stutterer's reaction to speech therapy frequently reveals the nature and extent of his resistances.

At the beginning the stutterer is caught in a vicious circle. He doesn't have the tools with which to work. Increasing his motivation at that point only increases the penalty on stuttering, therefore fear, conflict, and number of blocks. Speech therapy of the non-avoidance type can serve two important functions: first, for those whose stuttering has become self-maintaining or functionally autonomous, reducing drives toward avoidance may be sufficient to break up the "vicious circle" and free the stutterer; second, speech therapy gives the stutterer tools for dealing with word and situation fears he had not formerly possessed. When a stutterer rejects this opportunity he provides a focal point for the analysis and understanding of his own resistances. Such analysis is considered an essential first step in therapy by Fenichel (15, p. 46), who recommends that analysis of resistance precede analysis of content. This leads to the problem of dealing with unconscious sources of avoidance and conflict, i.e., psychotherapy for the stutterer.

Since the emotionality of the utterance is so frequently a source of conflict in the stutterer, an important goal in psychotherapy is *release of feeling*. Pentup feelings or repressed emotional material responsible for producing blockings in speech require free expression and adequate outlet. Such goals are common in psychotherapy, and numerous techniques to achieve them are familiar terms in its literature: release of feeling, clarification of feeling, catharsis, abreaction, working through, play therapy, psychodrama, and others. It is interesting that one of the few modern therapists reporting fair success with stutterers is David Levy (35, pp. 77-79), whose "release therapy" is aimed primarily at the expression of feeling.

Many of the speech therapy techniques of the "Iowa School" may be interpreted as exercises in the expression of aggression. The stutterer who changes his mind about "faking" to a clerk because, "He seemed so nice, I couldn't do it to him," may illustrate a common underlying attitude. A "spluttering" or choking up of speech, behavior which at least superficially resembles stuttering, is a cultural caricature for inexpressible aggression. If stuttering may be viewed this way, in accord with Fenichel, then such techniques as negative practice and "bouncing" not only provide a means of abreaction but reduce the need to be aggressive. Such needs on the stutterer's part may be reduced in two ways: through the use of stuttering behavior itself, and through release of feelings behind it.

All maladjustments are in a sense due to a lack of satisfactory *relationships* in early life. People are neurotic to the extent that they lack good interpersonal relations. Psychotherapy, as the undoing process of maladjustment, must be directed toward establishing that which has been lacking—warm and satisfying relationships. In the beginning phases the therapist himself supplies the relationship. Later on, as treatment begins to be effective, the individual's improved adjustment is reflected in more congenial relations outside therapy.

Stuttering not only expresses the nature of the stutterer's relationships but is in part determined by them. When there is considerable conflict at this level, the working through of certain crucial relationships becomes essential to success. Fletcher showed awareness of this in regarding stuttering as a "social morbidity" (18, pp. 222-240), symptomatic of the victim's attitude toward all society. Recognition of the stutterer's need for better relationships has undoubtedly stimulated the development of group therapy methods with stutterers.

Dollard and Miller's analysis of the nature of approach-avoidance conflict may serve as a warning against bringing the stutterer too quickly into new and dangerous rôles. They point out that because of the paradoxical effect of a lowering of avoidance tendencies in eliciting greater fear, it is necessary to "dose anxiety" or to pace the individual so that he will not experience too much conflict at once and drop out of therapy (10, pp. 400-403). A further danger of reducing avoidance too quickly, and in all attempts at sudden cures, emerges from the ego-protective level of conflict.

At some point in the treatment of a stutterer it is necessary to consider the effect of the handicap, and possible recovery from it, upon goals and aspirations, upon what the individual has planned to do with his life. Specially constructed sentence completion test items, or open-ended questions, may elicit revealing projective material in this area. Examples: "What kind of a person would you be if you didn't stutter?" or "If your stuttering suddenly disappeared, what difference would it make in your life?" or "If I could get over stuttering, I would. . . . "

Frequently such questions make the stutterer anxious. Because the defeat may have become a peg upon which to hang all his shortcomings, or perhaps because of the capacity of the human organism to adapt itself to disturbance, the stutterer is likely to feel a little strange without his symptom. The individual may have lived with his stuttering so long that functioning without it involves a radical change in self-concept which must be gradual. To put it in another way, fluency may have become ego-alien. In the later stages of treatment the stutterer must learn to accept his new rôle with its fluency, just as in the early stages he needed to accept his old rôle with its stuttering.

As changes during treatment begin to occur, there should be a certain amount of *preparation for recovery.* Such preparation should include a careful psychotherapeutic exploration of the adaptiveness of the stutterer's goals, and the relation of these to the disorder. If the stutterer has enslaved himself to a striving toward unattainables, the therapist should help him find freedom. If the stutterer's level of aspiration is lower than his capabilities warrant, the therapist may help him realize the new possiblities opening up before him. All these have the effect of reducing avoidance and conflict due to ego-protective functions of the symptom.

From the foregoing, it may be seen that therapy is carried out at all five of the levels at which conflict occurs in stuttering—word and situation, feeling, relationship, and ego-protective. Psychotherapy and speech therapy are twin avenues to the common goal of reducing fear and avoidance. In the course of treatment, as well as in theory, the problem of stuttering may be handled and understood in terms of approach-avoidance conflict.

6. In this way the symptom is reinforced and maintained, the anxiety is "bound" within it, and a vicious circle is perpetuated.

7. Conflict is directly expressed in primary symptoms of repetition and prolongation, which reflect a breakdown in the sequence of movements necessary to speech.

8. Secondary symptoms involve learned behavior representing compensatory efforts to overcome avoidance or to reach the goal by a roundabout route.

9. Conflict may occur at several levels—word, situation, emotional content, relationship, and ego-protective levels; any particular moment of stuttering is determined by interplay of forces at these levels.

10. Approach-avoidance theory relates fear, avoidance, and conflict to stuttering in a systematic way, so that goals of treatment become apparent from the theory itself.

11. Treatment proceeds through an integrated psychotherapy and speech therapy, aimed at attacking feared words and situations, releasing feelings, improving relationships, and freeing the individual from unadaptive goals, thereby achieving a total reduction of the fear and avoidance tendency responsible for the stutterer's conflict.

SUMMARY

1. Stuttering is a resultant of approach-avoidance conflict, of opposed urges to speak and to hold back from speaking.

2. The "holding back" may be due either to learned avoidances or to unconscious motives.

3. Principal hypotheses concerning stuttering behavior spring from two fundamental questions: *(a)* What produces blocking? *(b)* What determines release?

4. The Conflict Hypotheses: The stutterer blocks or stops whenever conflicting approach and avoidance tendencies reach an equilibrium.

5. The Fear-Reduction Hypothesis: The occurrence of stuttering reduces the fear which elicits it sufficiently to permit release of the blocked word, resolving the conflict momentarily and enabling the stutterer to continue.

REFERENCES

1. Abbott, J. A. Repressed hostility as a factor in adult stuttering. *J. Speech Disor.,* 1947, **12,** 428–430.

2. Adler, A. Problems of Neurosis. London: Kegan Paul, Trench, Trubner, 1929.

3. Blanton, M. G., & Blanton, S. Speech Training for Children. New York: Century, 1924.

4. Bloodstein, O. N. Conditions under which stuttering is reduced or absent: A review of literature. *J. Speech Disor.,* 1949, **14,** 295–302.

5. Bluemel, C. S. Stammering and Allied Disorders. New York: Macmillan, 1935.

6. Bluemel, C. S. Stammering and inhibition. *J. Speech Disor.,* 1940, **5** 305–308.

7. Brown, S. F. The loci of stutterings in the speech sequence. *J. Speech Disor.,* 1945, **10,** 182–192.

8. Bryngelson, B., Chapman, M. E., & Hansen, O. K. Know Yourself: A Workbook for Those Who Stutter. Minneapolis: Burgess, 1950.

9. Case, H. M. Stuttering and speech blocking: A comparative study of maladjustment. Ph.D. dissertation, University of California at Los Angeles, 1940. Pp. 78.

10. Dollard, J., & Miller, N. E. Personality and Psychotherapy. New York: McGraw-Hill, 1950.

11. Dunlap, K. Habits: Their Making and Unmaking. New York: Liveright, 1932.

12. Dunlap, K. Stammering: Its nature, etiology and therapy. *J. Comp. Psychol.,* 1944, **37**, 187–202.

13. Eisenson, J., & Horowitz, E. The influence of propositionality on stuttering. *J. Speech Disor.,* 1945, **10**, 193–197.

14. Eisenson, J., & Wells, C. A study of the influence of communicative responsibility in a choral speech situation for stutterers. *J. Speech Disor.,* 1942, **7**, 259–262.

15. Fenichel, O. Problems of Psychoanalytic Technique. Albany: Psychoanalytic Quarterly, 1939.

16. Fenichel, O. The Psychoanalytic Theory of Neurosis. New York: Norton, 1945.

17. Fishman, H. C. A study of the efficacy of negative practice as a corrective for stammering. *J. Speech Disor.,* 1937, **2**, 67–72.

18. Fletcher, J. M. The Problem of Stuttering. New York: Longmans. Green, 1928.

19. Freud, S. A General Introduction to Psychoanalysis. New York: Garden City Publ., 1943.

20. Freud, S. The Problem of Anxiety. New York: Norton, 1936.

21. Frick, J. V. An exploratory study of the effect of punishment (electric shock) upon stuttering behavior. Ph.D. dissertation, State University of Iowa, Feb. 1951.

22. Froeschels, E. Stuttering and nystagmus. *Monatschr. f. Ohrenh.,* 1915, **49**, 161–167.

23. Froeschels, E. Uber des Wesen des stotterns. *Wien, Med. Schnschr.,* 1914, **64**, 1067–1076.

24. Glauber, I. P. Psychoanalytic concepts of the stutterer. *Nerv. Child,* 1943, **2**, 172–180.

25. Hilgard, E. R., & Marquis, D. G. Conditioning and Learning. New York: Appleton-Century, 1940.

26. Hill, H. An interbehavioral analysis of several aspects of stuttering. *J. Gen. Psychol.,* 1945, **32**, 289–316.

27. Johnson, W. People in Quandaries. New York: Harper, 1946.

28. Johnson, W. An interpretation of stuttering. *Q. J. Speech,* 1933, **19**, 70–76.

29. Johnson, W. (and others) A study of the onset and development of stuttering. *J. Speech Disor.,* 1942, **7**, 251–257.

30. Johnson, W., & Brown, S. F., Curtis, J. F., Edney, C. W., & Keaster, J. Speech Handicapped School CHildren. New York: Harper, 1948.

31. Johnson, W., & Inness, M. Studies in the psychology of stuttering: XIII. A statistical analysis of the adaptation and consistency effects in relation to stuttering. *J. Speech Disor.,* 1939, **4**, 79–86.

32. Johnson, W., & Knott, J. R. The moment of stuttering. *J. Genet. Psychol.,* 1936, **48**, 475–480.

33. Johnson, W., & Knott, J. R. Studies in the psychology of stuttering: I. The distribution of moments of stuttering in successive readings of same material. *J. Speech Disor.,* 1937, **2**, 17–19.

34. Knott, J. R., & Johnson, W. An interpretive demonstration of ten observable facts about stuttering. In *Proceedings of the American Speech Correction Association.* Madison: College Typing Company, 1936, **6**, 150–154.

35. Levy, D. Release therapy. In Tomkins, S. S. (Ed.), *Contemporary Psychopathology.* Cambridge: Harvard Univ., 1947.

36. Lewin, K. Dynamic Theory of Personality. New York: McGraw-Hill, 1935.

37. Lewin, K. Field Theory in Social Science. New York: Harper, 1951.

38. Meissner, J. H. The relationship between voluntary non-fluency and stuttering. *J. Speech Disor.,* 1946, **11**, 13–23.

39. Milisen, R., & Van Riper, C. A study of the predicted duration of the stutterer's blocks as related to their actual duration. *J. Speech Disor.,* 1939, **4**, 339–345.

40. Miller, N. E. Experimental studies of conflict. In Hunt, J. McV. (*Ed.*), *Personality and the Behavior Disorders.* New York: Ronald Press, 1944. (Vol. I, pp. 431–465).

41. Miller, N. E. Comments on theoretical models illustrated by the development of a theory of conflict. *J. Personal.,* 1951, **20**, 82–100.

42. Mowrer, O. H., & Viek, P. An experimental analogue of fear from a sense of helplessness. *J. Abn. & Soc. Psychol.,* 1948, **43**, 193–200.

43. Porter, H. v. K. Studies in the psychology of stuttering: XIV, Stuttering phenomena in relation to size and personnel of audience. *J. Speech Disor.,* 1939, **4**, 323–333.

44. Sheehan, J. G. A study of the phenomena of stuttering. M.A. thesis, Univeristy of Michigan, 1946.

45. Sheehan, J. G. A theory of stuttering as approach-avoidance conflict. *Amer. Psychol.,* 1950, **5**, 469.

46. Sheehan, J. G. The modification of stuttering through non-reinforcement. *J. Abn. & Soc. Psychol.,* 1951, **46**, 51–63.

47. Sheehan, J. G. Fear-reduction during stuttering in relation to conflict, "anxiety-binding" and reinforcement. *Amer. Psychol.,* 1952, **7**, 530 (Abstract).

48. Sheehan, J. G., & Voas, R. Tension patterns during stuttering in relation to conflict, fear-reduction, and reinforcement. *Speech Monog.,* (in press).

49. Sheehan, J. G., & Zelen, S. A level of aspiration study of stutterers. *Amer. Psychol.,* 1951, **6**, 500 (Abstract).

50. Shulman, E. A study of certain factors influencing the variability of stuttering. Ph.D. dissertation, State University of Iowa, 1944.

51. Solomon, M. Stuttering as an emotional disorder, *Proc. Amer. Speech* Correct. Assoc., 1932, **2**, 118–121.

52. Solomon, M. Stuttering as an emotional and personality disorder. *J. Speech Disor.,* 1939, **4**, 347–357.

53. Travis, L. E. The need for stuttering. *J. Speech Disor.,* 1940, **5**, 193–202.

54. Travis, L. E. My present views on stuttering. *Western Speech,* 1946, **10,** 3–5.

55. Travis, L. E. Tuttle, W. W., & Cowan, D. W. A study of the heart rate during stuttering. *J. Speech Disor.,* 1936, **1,** 21–26.

56. Van Riper, C. A study of the thoracic breathing of stutterers during expectancy and occurrence of stuttering spasm. *J. Speech Disor.,* 1936, **1,** 61–72.

57. Van Riper, C. Effect of devices for minimizing stuttering on the creation of symptoms. *J. Abn. & Soc. Psychol.,* 1937, **32,** 185–192.

58. Van Riper, C. The effect of penalty upon frequency of stuttering. *J. Genet. Psychol.,* 1937, **50,** 193–195.

59. Van Riper, C. The relation of tremors to perpetuation and release from the stuttering spasm. Unpublished paper read at 1939 meeting of the American Speech Correction Association, Chicago, Ill. See A.S.C.A. Program, *J. Speech Disor.,* 1939. 336.

60. Van Riper, C. Speech Correction; Principles and Methods. (2nd ed.) New York: Prentice-Hall, 1947.

61. Van Riper, C. Stuttering. Chicago: National Society for Crippled Children and Adults, 1949.

62. Wischner, G. J. Stuttering behavior and learning: A preliminary theoretical formulation. *J. Speech & Hear. Disor.,* 1950, **15,** 324–335.

63. Wyneken, C. Ueber das Stottern und dessen Heilung. (Concerning stuttering and its cure.) *Zeitschrift für Rationelle Medicin,* 1868, **31,** 1–29.

Approach-Avoidance and Anxiety Reduction

Vivian M. Sheehan

Approach-avoidance conflict has been so closely associated with Sheehan as to be almost a trademark—and rightly so. He devoted his professional career of 35 years of research and clinical work to its study, development, and testing.

THE RESEARCH ODYSSEY

While the preceding article represents the major statement of the approach-avoidance hypothesis, the first explanation came in the publication "The modification of stuttering through non-reinforcement" (Sheehan, 1951). Steeped in learning theory, Sheehan was concerned primarily at this time with the reinforcement aspect of stuttering, and secondarily with its conflict aspect. He felt that the persistence of stuttering was one of its principal mysteries, and that the utilization of such non-reinforcement techniques was one of the greatest needs of stuttering therapy. Thus he anticipated to a remarkable degree the present interest in modifying stuttering behavior through reinforcement methods. However, even though he was a forerunner in the application of operant conditioning to stuttering, he became one of its severest critics in its present form.

The next two years saw an increasing emphasis on the development of the two conflict hypotheses arising from two issues: What makes the stutterer stop, and what enables him to continue again? Thus came the development of approach-avoidance conflict with great stress on learning theory and the habitual aspect, but also with the inclusion of the role of fear, guilt, anxiety, tension, and self-concept as a part of the psychotherapy aspect.

It was natural, then, that the next stop was a complete integration of psychotherapy and speech therapy as seen in 1954, a more complete exposition of the idea that treatment of stuttering must be treatment of the stutterer—the whole person. This expansion of the work on approach-avoidance conflict at the same time made clear the psychotherapeutic nature of speech therapy itself. The therapy of the day had come under criticism as being only symptomatic, superficial, and problem-oriented. Sheehan pointed out that the role of speech therapy is to deal with the basic struggle and conflict, with the fear and desires and feel-

Postscript   8

ings (all externalized in the block) and with the stutterer's guilt over punishing others. All of these symptoms can be effectively treated through a permissive attitude toward stuttering, which encourages the expression of the symptom without social penalty, thus leading to acceptance of the role of stutterer. This therapeutic framework provides an opportunity to the stutterer for profound personality changes, for a mastery of hitherto feared situations, and, through direct speech therapy, for a mode of handling problems that is relatively independent of the way he feels at the moment.

Sheehan always expressed a compelling interest in the treatment of stuttering as psychotherapeutic, with the therapist as accepting and permissive, leading the stutterer through the conflicts by experiencing the stuttering in a new way: by approach rather than retreat. This tactic meant confronting and mastering the fear, by learning a new, easier, less socially punishing form of stuttering, which in turn would lead to a mastery of the handicap and to the eventual enjoyment of "normal" speech with normal "bobbles" or disfluencies.

When in recent years the "new" therapies offered impersonal, unaccepting, harsh, sometimes punishing treatment of stuttering, Sheehan became outspoken in his denial of the techniques, whether the therapies sought to reach the same personality changes that he outlined or completely ignored their existence. Those therapies subjected the stutterer to the very same avoidance of stuttering and pressure for fluency that he had always experienced in his lifetime as a stutterer, but in larger doses in a marathon race for fluency.

During the ensuing years Sheehan investigated ways of increasing approach and lessening avoidance. One significant piece of research (Sheehan & Voas, 1957) was a comparison of techniques involving increasing the approach gradient: imitation of the stuttering block (advocated by Knight Dunlap), the bounce pattern of voluntary stuttering used by the Iowa school, and the prolongation pattern of voluntary stuttering, often called the "slide." Their efficacy was studied in relation to the adaptation effect. The results suggested that voluntary stuttering techniques are likely to strengthen the approach behavior, with the slide bringing the greatest improvement when used prior to the difficult or feared word. This finding gave additional support to Sheehan's theory and his belief that the way out of a stuttering handicap is through stuttering openly, not through avoidance or holding back.

Always interested in the relation of conflict and frustration to the feelings of the stutterer, Sheehan investigated the dimensions of guilt, shame, tension, and dejection (Sheehan, Cortese, & Hadley, 1962) and concluded that two different groups of stutterers may exist; those who find relief when the stuttering block is ended, and those who show increased tension, shame, and dejection, as well as guilt in that situation. This research suggested that stuttering is not a unitary disorder, and that the nature of reinforcement may also differ. Some stuttering seems to operate on a reward basis and some on a frustration basis.

Further studies analyzed clinically observed factors that appear to increase avoidance. One was the effect of silence (Sheehan & Gould, 1967) since the fear of silence, of breaking silence with speech, is one manifestation of stuttering. Silence was shown to have many meanings, and the most ambiguous created the greatest fear and elicited the greatest frequency of stuttering.

The study of the impact of authority (Sheehan, Hadley & Gould, 1967) provided support for the "status gap" hypothesis that an authority figure typically becomes a more threatening punisher than does a peer figure, resulting in increased avoidance and subsequently increased stuttering.

Another intriguing area of research (Sheehan & Martyn, 1966) was derived from a hitherto unexplored population of those who had spontaneously recovered from stuttering. These studies provided further support for the theory of approach-avoidance, for it became apparent that the 80% who recover, virtually unaided, attribute their success to their determination to confront and approach stuttering, to accept the role of stutterer, and to building up self-esteem. This research also provided clear-cut support for the therapy Sheehan had derived from his theory.

During his research odyssey Sheehan became interested in role theory and expressed the conflict levels of the approach-avoidance theory in role theory terms (Sheehan, 1968). He called stuttering a self-role conflict and a false role disorder. This theory led to his developing the concept that stuttering is not a speech problem per se, but an interpersonal communication disorder. And as an approach-avoidance conflict it involves two factors: the self-variable and the role variable.

The occurrence of stuttering is a function of how the stutterer feels about himself and especially about himself as a speaker. In other words, it is role-specific behavior. In behavioral terms the stutterer is a stutterer only when talking. This fact is the self-variable factor.

The second factor is the role variable—with stuttering dependent on how the stutterer feels about the listener. Stuttering is an interpersonal disorder, which explains why most stutterers are fluent when alone. Sheehan's earlier study of the impact of authority had shown the importance of the position of the listener in the eyes of the stutterer.

Sheehan was concerned by the burgeoning literature on behavior modification and the claims of cures, or reduction of stuttering, resulting from a noxious stimulus contingent upon stuttering. In 1969, he and Biggs (Sheehan & Biggs, 1969) replicated the 1958 study by Flanagan, Goldiamond, and Azrin (1958) with dramatically different results. By using a control condition, Sheehan found that the stimulus was merely a distraction device, and worked as well randomly as contingently, but which had no permanent or real effect in either case. Despite this highly significant finding, however, the article, entitled "Punishment or Distraction? Operant Conditioning Revisited," has never once been confronted or even alluded to by any operant conditioner.[1] And, unfortunately, contingent distractions continue to be applied in the effort to decrease stuttering.

Sheehan continued his interest in the true nature of the nonreinforcement of stuttering. He undertook (Sheehan, 1972) a mini-replication of his original 1954 study. This second study led to his reaffirmation of the view that stuttering

[1]See Flanagan, p. 221, for a discussion of this issue.

Postscript 8

may be modified by reinforcement principles and reduced by systematic nonreinforcement. But it also led to the following warning:

"Perhaps asking a stutterer to repeat the stuttered word until he has spoken it once fluently involves a kind of behavioral suppression that leads to future trouble. . . . Perhaps the path toward response suppression leads but to the experience of grave later consequences. Perhaps there is an artificiality in some 'reinforcement' techniques that is inconsistent with the ongoing conceptions of the self. Perhaps we have here a false-role enactment which pays the price of later difficulty. . . . We would still counsel against the procedure of having Johnny 'say it over and say it right,' not only because it may serve as a penalty, but because the ultimate effects may be the opposite of those immediately obtained. Perhaps all behavior therapies involve some possibility of some immediate 'dramatic improvement' at the cost of ultimate exacerbation of the problem" (pp. 464-65).

In retrospect this last discussion contained the seed of the final hypothesis Sheehan advanced just prior to his death in 1983. This theory was presented in a paper at the IALP meeting in Edinburgh in September 1983 (Sheehan, 1983) and subsequently was published in the "Stuttering Disorders" volume of a series on communication disorders (Sheehan & Sheehan, 1984). The chapter is entitled "Avoidance-reduction therapy: A response-suppression hypothesis."

Related in Sheehan's own words, the hypothesis states "Stuttering is perpetuated by successful avoidance, by the successful suppression of outward stuttering behavior and the substitution of false fluency, or by inner patterns of stuttering" (p. 147).

This response-suppression hypothesis differs from the explanation of perpetuation of stuttering from frustration or the successful use of tricks and crutches. It changes the previous concept or theory that stuttering results from the unsuccessful attempt to avoid expected stuttering and thus also differs from the anticipatory-struggle hypothesis of Bloodstein. In the words of Sheehan, "It is not the struggle but the successful avoidance of struggle that perpetuates stuttering. . . . through successful learning of a suppressive mechanism."

The response-suppression hypothesis is still an outgrowth of the approach-avoidance conflict theory and simply carries it one step further. It explains the difficulties of the stutterer who is fluent most of the time and who has great difficulty ever overcoming infrequent but severe stuttering moments. Such a stutterer holds onto a fragile but apparently successful fluency gained through suppression of stuttering. And like the little girl with a curl, when he is bad he is horrid. The stutterer is an extreme avoider, never accepting that he is a stutterer. The stutterer is not really open, is full of denial and full of fears of stuttering that may never occur. When frequency counts are made the stuttering is mild; he hides so successfully from all but himself—at a price. And therapy for him is very difficult.

The response-suppression hypothesis also explains the "cures" of many operant approaches that pressure for perfect fluency. It is a fact long known that stutterers have the ability to suppress their stuttering for a time, by some subtle techniques not yet understood. Rewarding the false fluency can increase this successful suppression for a time, but the consequences are disastrous; relapse is inevitable and the final cure further out of reach than before.

We have observed clinically that when stutterers who have been taught to avoid stuttering and to practice fluency do relapse, they regress back beyond their degree of severity at the time therapy began. Recovery is thus enormously more difficult.

We have had occasion to work with some of these people, but rarely could overcome their need to suppress stuttering and maintain fluency; they had been too successful as avoiders to relinquish the pattern though it failed in important or critical moments. They had been encouraged by the false hope that suppressing stuttering and practicing fluency would beget stutter-free speech.

Avoidance-reduction therapies have their cases of relapses, too, but we have never seen one regress even as far back as the initial severity. All have improved some, and often can continue to improve again at a faster rate and with lasting change. Actually we encourage relapse as a part of the learning process. And we try to prevent a too-early departure from therapy; overlearning and a consolidation of gains while still in therapy appear to be desirable.

ANALYSIS OF THERAPY TECHNIQUES

Approach-avoidance conflict theory, including the new hypothesis of response-suppression, provides a consistent framework for keeping the focus of the therapy on nonavoidance. When applied carefully to analysis of techniques, it can help to determine whether they encourage fluency to make the stutterer sound better for the moment, or whether they really aim to eliminate avoidant behavior and lead to fluency as a by-product.

Frequency counts, for example, while necessary for research data, are a disaster for stuttering therapy. They imply that stuttering is bad and should be eliminated, and that the therapist would like to hear less stuttering and more fluent speech. Instead, deliberately encouraging openness and allowing stuttering to be heard, temporarily increasing frequency, is the proper pathway toward recovery. The therapist must learn to accept the stuttering as much as the stutterer must. He must resist the temptation to praise the appearance of fluency, for early on in therapy it is usually not earned, but based upon suppression of stuttering. To greet such fluency with joy is a trap into which the therapist, like the stutterer, may readily fall. The stutterer has lived a life of avoidance, of trying to please, of struggling to prevent moments of stuttering. The stutterer needs the support of a therapist who can tolerate and be comfortable with the sound of stuttering.

The work on stuttering cannot focus on lowering the frequency of stuttering; it must focus on the gradual change of the form of stuttering, thus reducing the social penalty and the fear attached to it. A temporary increase in frequency is actually a healthy sign when it is a result of decreasing suppression, of overcoming the use of substitutions, and of openly accepting the role of stutterer. In the

Postscript   8

long run these practices will lead, as a by-product, to lessened frequency and to the ultimate good of normal fluency.

Relaxation is a technique that therapists are tempted to use because it seems so harmless and because it appears so obvious that if the stutterer can just relax the stuttering will cease. But this is not the case. Avoidance-reduction theory makes it apparent that relaxation should not be part of the arsenal of the therapist.

The intent of relaxation is to prevent, to stop the stuttering. It represents an avoidance of the occurrence of stuttering. It implies a possibility, which reality has long denied, that somehow, if only he practices hard enough, the stutterer can learn directly to be relaxed even in a crisis. However, unless the stutterer knows what to do when stuttering, unless he admits the problem and tolerates the normal disfluency, he cannot be relaxed, no matter how many rituals or meditations are performed prior to a critical speaking situation. Practiced relaxation offers no real help. Relaxed speaking is a logical ultimate goal, of course, and can be achieved as a result of nonavoidance. But practiced relaxation is counterproductive when used as a technique to encourage fluency.

Techniques designed to *control stuttering,* when seen in the light of approach-avoidance theory, are totally unacceptable. Anything, any trick, any tool that makes the stutterer sound better for a given moment may give false hope and cheat him in the long run. We have learned that control of stuttering is a continuation of the myth of cure by avoiding the outward appearance of stuttering. We no longer permit even the use of the word *control* as a part of our therapy. Part of the reason is that in the literature on stuttering the word *control* inevitably implies a way to avoid, to suppress stuttering, to provide immediate fluency. In a sense, all work on stuttering involves a certain amount of control of one's self to carry out any assignments, to even submit to the undertaking of therapy. But it is different; it is not control designed to stop stuttering. It can better be labelled effort to improve by nonavoidance and openness. The language one uses affects attitude and performance, and that is important in avoidance reduction. Stuttering is something the stutterer does, not something which happens to him; it is changed by what the stutterer does, and indirectly by what his attitudes and values are.

Mechanical devices, such as maskers, delayed feedback gadgets, and metronomes, are aimed toward providing immediate fluency to permit the stutterer to get by for the moment. They are not cures and offer no real improvement for the stuttering. The same can be said of *drugs,* which hide symptoms on a temporary basis and may cause devastating side-effects with prolonged usage. Such devices and drugs, giving temporary relief, may indeed retard progress or even completely prevent it as the stutterer becomes addicted.

Voluntary stuttering, not faking, (role-taking, not role-playing) is a tool consistent with avoidance-reduction therapy. It allows the stutterer to touch the moment of stuttering without struggle. It lets the stutterer learn to tolerate imperfections in fluency, as the normal speaker does. It teaches an easier way to meet fear head-on, resisting temptation to flee and avoid. It provides an opportunity to work on the moment of stuttering during fluency, when the fear is at its lowest level. The stutterer who waits for involuntary moments to happen finds that they have gone by too rapidly to be experienced in any way but with the old panic. This situation is especially true for the implicit or internalized stutterer, the one who shows little stuttering but feels an inordinate amount of fear over the possibility of stuttering. Later in the therapy voluntary stuttering provides a tool for cancellation of failures, the real second chance the stutterer needs. It helps the stutterer learn what he needs to know: how to stutter. The stutterer already knows how to be fluent, and that has not increased self-confidence about speaking. Only when stutterers know how to stutter will they be relaxed and comfortable as speakers.

OTHER CLINICAL CONTRIBUTIONS FROM THE THEORY

Over the years, while in the process of expressing and revising the approach-avoidance conflict theory and putting it to practical use in therapy, Sheehan developed colorful, expressive conceptualizations that help both the stutterer and the therapist to understand the problem of stuttering and its psychological impact.

One of these is the *iceberg* concept: stuttering is like an iceberg with its greatest portion lying beneath the surface. What is seen and heard is the smaller portion; what is hidden from view is far greater and more dangerous and destructive, experienced as fear, guilt, and shame. The way to deal with this iceberg is to bring it out in the open, to get rid of hiding, suppression, and avoidance. This bringing-out is likened to taking the iceberg out into the sunlight to melt away. Sheehan himself thoroughly enjoyed the iceberg analogy. He produced a film called "The Iceberg of Stuttering," and later edited a shortened version that he dubbed "The Ice Cube of Stuttering."

Another concept is the *giant-in-chains* effect. The stutterer feels stuttering is the cause of all personal problems—if only he did not stutter he could be successful. Often the stutterer cannot give up this excuse for failure and resists change. Stutterers may begin to overcome their stuttering, only to fall back in order not to face other problems. When stutterers face their fear of stuttering and are open about it, its ego-protective function is removed and they find they are no longer giants in chains. They must now be helped to face the fear of fluency. This second adjustment may be more overwhelming than the first. The therapist must understand this possibility and help stutterers accept their human frailties, which have been obscured by the stuttering. In some instances it may even be more fitting to refer stutterers for help with the greater problems. In any case, this concept indicates another need for focus on the person, not on merely observable speech symptoms.

In another analogy Sheehan showed how the effort by the stutterer to keep from stuttering is similar to *walking a plank*. It is easy to walk across a 2" by 4" plank laid on the floor, but when it is placed between two high buildings the task becomes overwhelming. The consequences of failure are so great and the fear so

Postscript 8

debilitating that the effort to walk becomes enormously difficult. Similarly, the extra effort to avoid the consequence of stuttering actually creates the difficulty. For the stutterer, as Sheehan has often indicated, the fear of falling off the fluency plank merely increases avoidance and stuttering. Only by reducing the perceived penalties on stuttering and the resulting fear and avoidance can the attempt to speak become effortless.

As avoidance increases, so do crutches, tricks, and devices employed by the stutterer to conceal stuttering or provide distraction. The result is an accumulation of these unproductive behaviors or their residues which Sheehan aptly called a *walking museum* (or talking museum) of everything the stutterer has ever tried. They are false behaviors, a totally unnecessary collection whose dismantling is a major goal of nonavoidant therapy.

RECENT DEVELOPMENTS

Recently, at the Second Banff International Conference on Stuttering (1984), many therapists (most of whom were operant conditioners) who felt they had reduced stuttering with their therapies, and in effect "cured" most stutterers, expressed one great concern. Although the frequency of stuttering had been reduced, the stutterers' speech did not sound normal, and the therapists could not make it sound normal. The therapists still felt confident, however, that they had a cure for stuttering. But it is surely no cure when the frequency of stuttering has been reduced by the substitution of drawled, robot-like, stilted, or taut delivery of speech that neither feels normal to the stutterer nor sounds normal to the listener. These speech abnormalities are evidence that the fluency obtained under these therapies is false, merely the result of the suppression of stuttering. The problem of achieving normal-sounding speech, which so disturbed the Banff participants, is one that is entirely created by the nature of their therapies. Surely, though, Sheehan would have quipped, to reassure them not to be so concerned about this new problem, "It will go away on its own when the relapse to stuttering occurs."

The real problem is how to prevent false fluency and the suppression of stuttering. Nonavoidant therapies teach the stutterer how to stutter more easily and thus reduce the fear and avoidance. The stutterer is prepared for easy, normal speech and the tolerance of imperfections of that normal speech. When fluency is achieved honestly through nonavoidant therapy, there is no problem in creating normal-sounding speech, for the abnormalities, which are a result of suppression, have simply never developed. Rather, the stutterer has earned fluency and is comfortable with it.

At this same Banff conference, an interesting development occurred. Two of the most outspoken proponents of the "work-only-with-the-observable-behaviors" school of therapy admitted that maybe the stutterer and the stutterer's personal feelings and attitudes have been overlooked. This breakthrough may be a small triumph for the ideas Sheehan long espoused. But, a word of caution: At best, such therapy probably will continue as before, with the addition of new attention to attitudes and feelings but without a real understanding that the ultimate therapy depends on complete acceptance of self as a stutterer and an about-face on avoidance and suppression.

Although techniques and methods may vary, the theory and framework for therapy must remain rooted in nonavoidance, and the problem of stuttering must be recognized and treated as the problem of the person.

CONCLUSION

Although there have been many gradual changes and some shifting of emphasis over the years, approach-avoidance conflict theory has retained its major point of view. This chapter has not attempted to cover all the research efforts and results derived from the theory. Rather, it has sought to review briefly the most significant developments and contributions.

Sheehan's illness and death prevented him from testing his response-suppression hypothesis, and that task remains for those of us who carry on his work. All that we can do is to present the ideas and explain their relevance to approach-avoidance conflict theory, as well as their impact on therapy. We hope, as in the past, that this final challenge from Sheehan will encourage others to look at stuttering in a different way and will stir further controversy about the methods used in its treatment. This challenge may be his final contribution, lasting evidence of the dedication of so much of his life, love, time, effort, and knowledge to the world of the stutterer.

REFERENCES

Biggs, B.E., & Sheehan, J. G. (1969). Punishment or distraction? Operant stuttering revisited. *Journal of Abnormal Psychology, 74,* 256–262.

Flanagan, B., Goldiamond, I., & Azrin, N. (1958). Operant stuttering: The control of stuttering behavior through response contingent consequences. *Journal of the Experimental Analysis of Behavior, 1,* 173–177.

Gould, E., & Sheehan, J. G. (1967). Effect of silence on stuttering. *Journal of Abnormal Psychology, 72,* 441–44.

Sheehan, J. G. (1951). The modification of stuttering through non-reinforcement. *Journal of Abnormal and Social Psychology, 46,* 51–63.

Sheehan, J. G. (1954). An integration of psychotherapy and speech therapy through a conflict theory of stuttering. *Journal of Speech and Hearing Disorders, 19,* 474–482.

Sheehan, J. G. (1968). Stuttering as a self-role conflict. In H. Gregory (Ed.), *Learning theory and stuttering therapy* (pp. 72–83). Chicago: University Press.

Sheehan, J. G. (1972). A new venture into the nonreinforcement of stuttering. In E. Trapp & P. Himelstein (Eds.), *Readings on the exceptional child* (pp. 495–465). New York: Appleton-Century-Crofts.

Postscript 8

Sheehan, J. G. (1983, August). *Suppressive control as a barrier to recovery from stuttering.* Paper presented at the XIX Congress of the International Association of Logopaedics and Phoniatrics, Edinburgh, Scotland, U.K.

Sheehan, J. G. (1984). Avoidance-reduction therapy: A response-suppression hypothesis. Method of Joseph G. Sheehan and Vivian M. Sheehan. In W. H. Perkins (Ed.), *Stuttering disorders. Current therapy of communication disorders* (pp. 147–151). New York: Thieme-Stratton, Inc.

Sheehan, J. G., Cortese, P., & Hadley, R. (1962). Guilt, shame and tension in graphic projections of stuttering. *Journal of Speech and Hearing Disorders, 6,* 249–254.

Sheehan, J. G., Hadley, R., & Gould, E. (1967). Impact of authority on stuttering. *Journal of Abnormal Psychology, 72,* 390–293.

Sheehan, J. G., & Martyn, M. M. (1966). Spontaneous recovery from stuttering. *Journal of Speech and Hearing Research, 9,* 121–135.

Sheehan, J. G., & Voas, R. B. (1957). Comparison of therapy techniques involving approach and avoidance. *Journal of Speech and Hearing Disorders, 22,* 714–723.

9

Operant Stuttering: The Control of Stuttering Behavior Through Response-Contingent Consequences

Bruce Flanagan, Israel Goldiamond, and Nathan Azrin

Postscript
Operant Stuttering Update

Bruce Flanagan

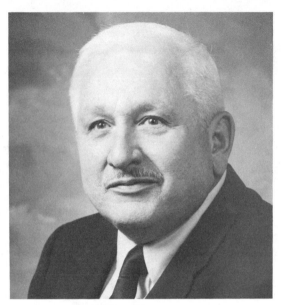

Bruce Flanagan

If there are benchmark publications in the field of communication disorders, the article by Flanagan, Goldiamond, and Azrin on stuttering as operant behavior ranks among the top. Aside from its impact on the subject of stuttering, this single publication of a series of experiments on stuttering forced our attention to viewing processes of communication and its disorders as behavior. With this operant conditioning perspective came the rigor of its laboratory heritage. The importance of concepts of base rates, controls, schedules, and description of experimental procedures came to the forefront. Mentalistic constructs such as drives and habit strength and concepts such as anxiety reduction and approach-avoidance conflict, each of which enjoyed a legitimate place in learning theory (in reinforcement theory in particular), were viewed as unnecessary mediating hypotheses that attempted to explain behavior, but neither described behavior nor described those procedures or operations required for changing behavior. If the event was not "ostensible," could not be available to our sensorium, could not be observed and quantified, it was something less than, or perhaps more than, behavior. The data from this perspective were observable frequencies, and the motivations for

behavioral change were operations external to the person emanating from a person's environment. Such ideas were laden with controversy because they attacked the notions of independence and free will, rejected the internal states of the human as a motivating force, and often ignored covert events such as thinking and feeling. When applied to the problem of stuttering, operant conditioning added more fuel to the controversy by demonstrating in the laboratory that the frequency of stuttering could be reduced through procedures of punishment. This particular piece of information rankled because it flew in the face of the most popular theory of the onset of stuttering; that is, that punishing disfluency or calling attention to or doing anything aversive following instances of it aggravates the problem.

However, even as these ideas generated controversy and became a target, sometimes due to the enthusiasms of its proponents and perhaps because of the controversies, there was a general "call for data," short-term and long-term, that began to echo throughout the field. As the behaviorists made claims for their clinical successes, they were asked to "show their data" and describe what they did. This openness became infectious to the point where these same demands were being made of all therapies for stuttering and across the field of communication disorders in general. Whether the principles of operant conditioning adequately explain the acquisition, maintenance, and dynamics of stuttering we have yet to learn. At this point, a major contribution of the Flanagan, et al. work has been its impact on the accountability, openness and descriptiveness, and sharing of ideas within the field as a whole, a most healthy development.

Flanagan, in his chapter, questions some of his earlier work on the clinical viability of punishment. He strongly suggests that we need paradigms of positive reinforcement for alternative responses by the stutterer in therapy. Although he still feels that principles of operant conditioning are helpful in explaining and clinically managing stuttering, and strongly defends the results of his punishment studies, he appears to reject punishment as a preventive or therapeutic tactic unless it is combined with other tactics that reinforce responses that compete with stuttering.

The earlier article was a pioneering effort and we are indeed fortunate in having the man from the laboratory to share his views with us.

9

Operant Stuttering: The Control of Stuttering Behavior Through Response-Contingent Consequences[1]

Bruce Flanagan, Israel Goldiamond, *Southern Illinois University*

Nathan Azrin, *Anna State Hospital*

The attempt to understand and control stuttering has received considerable attention in both clinic and laboratory. The concept of anxiety has played a major role in formulations in both areas; stuttering is considered "an anxiety-motivated avoidant response that becomes 'conditioned' to the cues or stimuli associated with its occurrence" (5).

This study reports a preliminary investigation designed to explore the extent to which stuttering can be brought under operant control.

Three male stutterers from the speech clinic, ages 15, 22, and 37, served as S's. The S read from loose printed pages; every time he stuttered, E pressed a microswitch which activated an Esterline-Angus recorder. A check was run by turning the microswitch over to another E, who had not been informed of the nature of the experiment, and instructing him to press upon each moment of stuttering. The E observed S through a one-way mirror in a room adjoining the experimental room, and heard him through a sound-amplification system.

When a curve of stuttering frequency considered smooth was obtained, E turned a switch which initiated a 30-minute period of response-contingent stimuli. After this period, S was observed for another 30 minutes without such stimuli following each press of the microswitch. No specific S^D's were introduced

to differentiate periods. A constant noise level of 60 decibels was present throughout the experiment.

Response-contingent periods were of two kinds. During the *aversive period,* every depression of the microswitch which activated the recorder also produced a 1-second blast of a 6000-cycle tone at 105 decibels in S's earphones. During the *escape period,* such a blast was constantly present; every depression of the microswitch shut off the tone for 5 seconds. Such use of noise as an aversive stimulus which was contingent upon responding or which could be escaped by responding followed a procedure used by Azrin (1).

Each S was run on two consecutive days. For S-1, the escape period was presented on the first day, and the aversive on the following day. For S-2 and S-3, the order was aversive-escape.

Record was kept not only of stuttering frequency, but also of elapsed time and number of pages of copy read. Data are presented in the accompanying figures. For all S's, the ordinate is cumulative words stuttered. For S-1, the abscissa is time, producing rate curves. For S-2 and S-3, however, the abscissa is number of pages read, and the curves depict stutters per page read.

Curves for sessions containing escape periods are presented in Fig. 9-1. For all S's, stuttering increases when escape from the tone is made contingent upon stuttering. When the tone is turned off, stuttering is no longer followed by such consequences, and the

[1]The authors wish to express their appreciation to Dr. Chester J. Atkinson, of Southern Illinois University, for his assistance with equipment problems and active interest during the course of the study.

Note: From Journal of the Experimental Analysis of Behavior, *I,* No. 2, 1958, pp. 173–177. Copyright 1958 by the Society for the Experimental Analysis of Behavior, Inc.

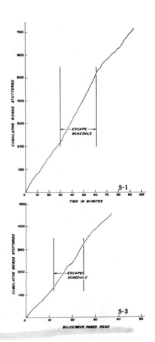

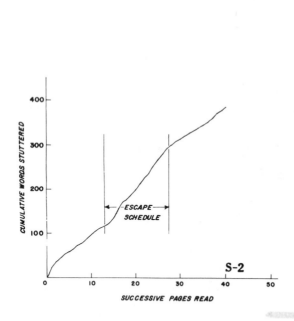

Figure 9-1.   Escape Periods.

rate drops. All *S*'s display short interludes of diminished rate, characterized by irregularities in the curves. All sessions open with a high-burst stuttering activity. This concurs with findings of "adaptation" studies in stuttering (7).

Curves for sessions containing aversive periods for *S-1* and *S-3* are presented in Fig. 9-2. Making presentation of a blast contingent upon stuttering tends to depress the rate of stuttering during such a period in a marked manner; *S-1* seems to have been moving toward an asymptote of complete suppression. The compensatory rise previously noted (2,8) following cessation of aversive consequences is pronounced in both *S*'s. The adaptation burst is again present.

The aversive-period session for *S-2* is presented in Fig. 9-3, which depicts total suppression of stuttering during the aversive period, and beyond. The period during which definition of stuttering was turned over to another *E* is designated under the heading, Control *E*.[2] There is no discernable effect on response rate, arguing for the validity of the major *E*'s judgment of stuttering. The adaptation burst is again present.

Comparisons of the various figures tend to indicate that number of pages read can apparently be

equated with time as a component of rate. Such an equation would follow if rate of reading itself, that is, pages per unit of time, were constant. For *S-2* and *S-3*, the mean reading times in minutes per page are [Table 9-1]:

The only safe conclusion seems to be that *S-3* reads more slowly than *S-2*; the apparent randomness of the data suggests constancy in reading rate.

The data presented suggest that the stuttering response is an operant which occurs in the context of another operant, namely, verbal behavior. Although one cannot stutter without talking, neither can one limp without walking, and limping can be controlled separately from walking. Reading rate was apparently not systematically affected by the response-contingent stimuli which controlled stuttering, hence the two are separable responses. The operant nature of reading has been discussed elsewhere (9); the way in which stuttering responses reacted to operant controls in this study can not be distinguished from reactions of other operant behaviors, and suggests that they are in this class of behaviors.

When termination of a noxious stimulus was made contingent upon stuttering, response rate rose. When onset of a noxious stimulus was made contingent upon stuttering, response suppression occurred, displaying compensation upon cessation of

---

[2]Both *E*'s are speech therapists. The major *E* is a stutterer who has had 7 years of experience as a speech therapist specializing in stuttering.

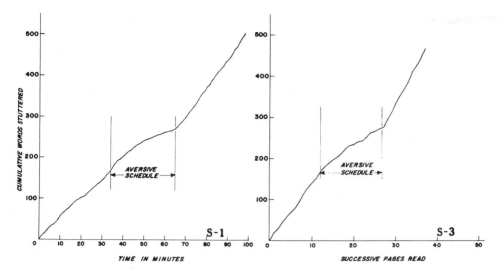

Figure 9-2.   Aversive periods for S-1 and S-3.

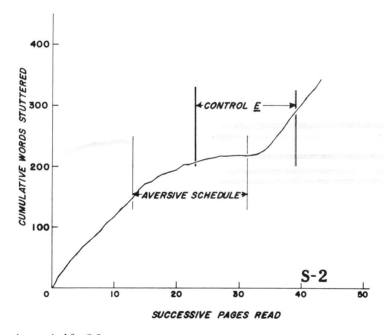

Figure 9-3.   Aversive period for S-2.

Table 9-1.

	Base line	Escape	Final	Base line	Aversive	Final
S-2	2.20	2.12	2.07	2.28	2.10	2.30
S-3	2.48	2.30	2.42	2.50	2.65	2.75

such consequences. For one *S*, the response was completely suppressed, and this suppression continued beyond the termination of the aversive contingency. Where *S* avoids certain consequences by suppressing a response, the suppression will be maintained by absence of the consequences. Accordingly, elimination of the consequences by *E* will tend to maintain the suppression. The adaptation effects reported in the speech literature were found here. These consist of an initial burst of stuttering, which then "adapts out," that is, drops to a base-line rate. These curves have been considered similar to respondent extinction curves (10), although classical extinction is not obtained (cf. 7). Consideration of conditions related to the establishment of an operant base line would involve a stuttering response being occasioned by S^D's. Placing a stutterer in a speech clinic with instructions to speak is not a procedure calculated to diminish generalization of the S^D's to new stimuli present in the experimental session. The response rate should rise. As the experiment progresses, and no new consequences are applied to responses occasioned by the new S^D's, we are establishing conditions for discrimination of new from old S^D's; the new stimuli lose their control; the situation is "perceived as familiar," or "perceived as non-threatening." Operant discrimination involves *operant* extinction of responses to *S*, the new S^D's.

Concerning the relationship of stuttering to anxiety, presumably of a respondent type, anxiety is associated with the suppression of operant behavior (3); stuttering behavior was both suppressed and intensified, and these changes are explainable on an operant basis. Since the stuttering response can be isolated from regular speech as a unit of response, we might speculate that such isolation would come about through differential consequences applied to breaks in speech, and smooth speech. Such differentiation might relate to the anxiety of the parent (rather than the child) upon hearing a stuttering response. She may reinforce the behavior by becoming attentive, and should she later decide to extinguish by ignoring, the usual burst of increased stuttering behavior during onset of extinction (4,6) might increase *her* anxiety, lead to remorse, reinstatement of reinforcement—and the establishment of a variable-interval schedule making extinction all the more difficult.

If further research supports the operant analysis presented here, then it would seem that controlled alteration of such behavior, that is, therapy, would involve application of procedures from the experimental analysis of operant behavior, notably of responses reinforced on a variable-interval schedule.

REFERENCES

1. Azrin, N. Noise and human behavior. *J. exp. anal. Behav.,* 1958, 2, 183–200.
2. Estes, W. K. An experimental study of punishment. *Psychol. Monogr.,* 1944, 57, No. 263.
3. Estes, W. K., and Skinner, B. F. Some quantitative properties of anxiety. *J. exp. Psychol.,* 1941, 29, 290–400.
4. Ferster, C. B. Withdrawal of positive reinforcement as punishment. *Science,* 1957, 126, 509.
5. Johnson, W. J. *Stuttering in children and adults.* Minneapolis: University of Minnesota, 1955.
6. Keller, F. S., and Schoenfeld, W. N. *Principles of psychology.* New York: Appleton-Century-Crofts, 1950.
7. Rousey, C. L. Stuttering severity during prolonged spontaneous speech. *J. speech and hearing Res.,* 1958, 1, 40–47.
8. Skinner, B. F. *The behavior of organisms.* New York: Appleton Century Co., 1938.
9. Skinner, B. F. *Verbal behavior.* New York: Appleton-Century-Crofts, 1958.
10. Wischner, G. J. Stuttering behavior and learning: a preliminary theoretical formulation. *J. speech and hearing Dis.,* 1950, 15, 324–325.

Operant Stuttering Update

Bruce Flanagan

In 1958 Israel Goldiamond, Nathan Azrin, and I joined in an endeavor to empirically evaluate the question: Is stuttering amenable to operant control? Based on the systematic observation of three adult stutterers, the answer was yes. When the consequences for stuttering were changed the frequency of stuttering changed.

Today if one were to submit a report that addressed altering the frequency of stuttering by manipulating the consequences of the stuttering behavior to a journal associated with the Association for Behavior Analysis[1] the editor would probably question the uniqueness of the contribution. In 1958, however, the editors treated the report on operant analysis of stuttering with interest. This project was one of the first to apply the principles (Ferster & Culbertson, 1982) and methods (Sidman, 1960; Johnston & Pennypacker, 1981) of behavior analysis to human behavior.

ZEITGEIST

Prior to the 1950s, empirical scientists working in the discipline of behavior analysis had concerned themselves mainly with the laboratory study of lower-order phylogenetic species. However, change was in the air. In 1953, Skinner argued the case for invoking the scientific attitudes of empiricism, determinism, parsimony, and experimental manipulation in the study of human behavior. He then put forth a set of ideas about how the principles of behavior developed in the operant animal laboratories might apply to humans.

Subsequently, Skinner (1957) extended his position on the scientific analysis of human behavior to include verbal behavior. He included talking, reading, writing, and thinking in his definition of verbal behavior. In this analytic paradigm, speech is assumed to be an operant, the frequency and topography of which are controlled by consequences provided by the listener. As in other kinds

---

[1]*Journal of Applied Behavior Analysis, Journal of the Experimental Analysis of Behavior, Journal of Precision Teaching,* and *The Behavior Analyst.*

Postscript   9

of operant behavior the actual form of the behavior (its topography) is not as critical as its consequences on the environment. In the case of verbal behavior, this environmental change occurs in the reactivity of the listener to the speaker.

Operant speech is viewed as a complex integration of muscle movements of the chest, diaphragm, larynx, pharynx, jaw, tongue, and lips. These movements are reinforced by the patterns and magnitudes of the acoustic wave forms that prompt the listener to provide reinforcement. However, reinforcement of the speaker's behavior would be unacceptably delayed if the initial consequence was in fact the reinforcement provided by the outside listener. The auditory stimuli produced by the vocal muscles is the only reinforcer that could produce such diverse forms of vocal behavior. It is because the speaker and listener are within the same skin that the listener can provide necessary reinforcement for the highly differentiated, high-rate behavior of speech. The vocal utterance of a word or phrase can be parsimoniously viewed as a response chain (Skinner, 1938) where each microresponse of the utterance serves as the auditory discriminative stimulus for the next response component. The vocal stimulus response chain is terminated and reinforced when the speaker hears the utterance completed with point-to-point correspondence to the controlling verbal stimulus. We have only to observe the disruption that occurs when one attempts to speak under conditions of delayed auditory feedback to appreciate how the sounds of speech control the speaking performance. The deterioration of speech caused by anatomical damage to the hearing mechanism provides another example of the control exerted by the auditory stimuli produced by the speech mechanisms.

External control of speech is provided by the reactivity of the outside listener to the speaker's vocal response chain. For example, a child asking a parent for a cookie is a simple interaction where the vocal response chain produced by the speaker is reinforced by the behavior prompted in the outside listener. After hearing the child's request, the parent may walk to the cookie jar, pick up a cookie, and hand it to the child. The parent's movements serve as secondary reinforcers to the child's request. Eating the cookie is the primary reinforcer. This episode is minimally verbal because the reinforcer maintaining the child's verbal activity depends on food deprivation. The essential properties of most verbal behavior involve reinforcement by a change in the verbal behavior of the listener rather than the practical result, like the cookie in this example. In his behavior analysis of the teaching process, Skinner (1968) provided a plethora of examples of how the verbal behavior of the student is controlled by the verbal behavior of the teacher.

While behavior analysis of how speech and stuttering develops has merit, its relevance to this update of the operant nature of chronic adult stuttering is limited. It should be emphasized, however, that in Skinner's 1957 work he noted that verbal behavior may be followed by the kind of consequences called punishment. Further, he noted that punishment does not maintain operant behavior, but must be included among special effects that modify behavior already established through positive reinforcement. Punishment was defined (Ferster & Skinner,

1957) as an operation in which an aversive stimulus[2] is made contingent upon a response. Stuttering along with slowed and hesitant speech were cited as examples of the special effects or by-products of punished speech. Given Skinner's paradigm, stuttering is viewed as behavior that occurs in the context of the various classes of operant speech. Further, punishment of the vocal speech chains should lead to an increase in disfluency and other hesitancy-related phenomena.

Skinner's position appeared to be in harmony with the speech pathology literature of the 1950s, which held that listener evaluation of disfluency caused stuttering (Johnson, 1955) or, at a minimum, aggravated the problem (Van Riper, 1937; Frick, 1951). However, the cancellation procedure advocated by Van Riper (1957) to ameliorate stuttering appeared to be functionally similar to a punishment procedure that involves the systematic withdrawal of positive reinforcement (Ferster, 1957). The original operant stuttering research in 1958 was approached to seek data relevant to the apparent inconsistency concerning the effect of punishment on stuttering.[3]

Some of the first studies that successfully and systematically manipulated the operant behavior of humans were: Lindsley (1956), who conditioned chronic psychotic patients to pull a plunger for a variety of tangible reinforcers (candy, cigarettes, etc.); Holland (1957), who controlled the frequency and topography of vigilance behavior in Navy enlisted men using signal detections as the reinforcing contingency; Ferster and Sapon (1958), who taught college students German using immediate feedback of correct performance for reinforcement; and Azrin (1958), who evaluated the contingency properties of high-intensity noise on the performance of soldiers. Azrin's work was of particular importance to the operant stuttering research because it provided a framework for evaluating the effects of negative reinforcement and punishment on behavior maintained by a human reinforcement system. Azrin replicated the vigilance research to obtain baseline data and then imposed several contingency schedules of noise on the observing response while holding other aspects of Holland's experimental procedure constant. The intent of Azrin's research was to determine whether intense noise would function as known aversive stimuli.

1958 REVISITED

The purpose of the 1958 operant stuttering study was to evaluate the effects of response-contingent aversive stimulation on the frequency of stuttering from the theoretical and methodological viewpoint of behavior analysis. What would be the effect of an escape condition on stuttering frequency, where each moment of stuttering eliminated aversive stimulation? Would a response-contingent aversive

[2]An aversive stimulus was defined as a stimulus that when removed increases the frequency of a response through negative reinforcement (Ferster & Skinner, 1957)

[3]The inconsistency to which Flanagan refers is the expected suppression of a response (i.e., stuttering) following punishment, on the one hand, and the position that disfluency will increase when a vocal chain is punished, on the other.

Postscript 9

stimulus increase or decrease the frequency of stuttering in chronic adult stutterers? And, would the rate of speech be systematically affected by either of the contingency schedules?

The subjects were instructed to read orally from printed pages. After a stable rate of stuttering was observed either an escape or a punishment contingency schedule was instated for 30 minutes, followed by a comparable period during which the contingency schedule was not operative. On the following day the alternative contingency schedule was employed using a counterbalanced treatment order among subjects. The stimulus used was a 105 dB (re: ASA-1951) 6000 Hz noise delivered to the subject's earphones. The intensity was at the approximate level Azrin (1958) had found to be an effective aversive stimulus. The experimenter recorded moments of stuttering and pages read by pressing microswitches. During the contingency-schedule periods the microswitch that recorded instances of stuttering also programmed the presentation (punishment schedule) or withdrawal (escape schedule) of the noise.

Azrin's research on the aversive properties of noise suggested the noise employed in the 1958 stuttering research could function as an aversive stimulus. At that time it did not seem reasonable to argue that button pressing by soldiers for signal-detection reinforcement was comparable to the stuttering behavior of chronic stutterers that occurred during instruction-controlled emission of vocal textual responses. The selected alternative was to assess directly the aversive properties of the selected noise stimulus on the frequency of stuttering that occurred during the escape condition. According to Ferster and Skinner's definition of aversive stimuli and punishment, the finding that the noise-escape schedule resulted in an increase in the frequency of stuttering for each subject permitted us to define the selected noise (105 dB, 6000 Hz) as an aversive stimulus and the presentation of that stimulus in a response-contingent manner as punishment.

Analysis of the data of the effect of punishment in the form of response-contingent noise on the frequency of stuttering indicated punishment decreased stuttering in each subject. When the punishment schedule was terminated the frequency of stuttering rapidly returned to the baseline rate. These data indicated the effect of punishment on stuttering was to suppress that behavior. As was indicated previously, when stuttering was negatively reinforced by terminating an aversive stimulus the frequency of stuttering increased. Furthermore, the rate of oral reading was not systematically affected by either the escape- or punishment-contingency schedule. The failure of the contingency schedules to influence speaking rate indirectly suggested that stuttering was an ontogenetic response class (Skinner, 1969). If stuttering and fluent speech had existed as an undifferentiated response class prior to the contingency schedules one would expect the frequency of fluent speech to increase and decrease according to the schedule in effect while the response differentiation process occurred. Taken as a whole, these data suggested that the stuttering behavior of these chronic adult stutterers was a separate class of operantly defined verbal behavior that could be parsimoniously viewed like other verbal operants.

REPLICATIONS

In 1959, Felty (cited in Bijou & Baer, 1966) replicated and extended the 1958 findings on operant stuttering to children as young as 12 years. The subjects read from material considered easy and interesting for their age level to supply an ongoing operant level of speech and stuttering. As in the 1958 study, the reinforcement and punishment schedule produced the expected strengthening or suppression of the stuttering behavior independent of overall reading rate.

Biggs and Sheehan (1969) reported a replication of the 1958 operant stuttering project with six adult stutterers as subjects. Their experimental conditions consisted of escape, punishment, and random treatments. A 108 dB (re: ISO-1964, ANSI-1969) 4000 Hz noise was used for an aversive stimulus. They reported a decrease in the frequency of stuttering during the punishment condition but failed to find an increase in the frequency of stuttering during the escape condition. The decrease in stuttering observed during the punishment condition was attributed to "distraction effects" by the authors. Biggs and Sheehan (1969) also offered a variety of mentalistic arguments to advance the idea that the noise used in their study was more aversive than the noise used in the 1958 operant stuttering research. There are four factors that cause concern about the validity of this replication.

First, the escape condition, as Biggs and Sheehan point out, failed to cause an increase in the frequency of stuttering, which raises questions concerning the aversive properties of their noise stimulus. Recall that Ferster and Skinner defined an aversive stimulus as one that has the power to negatively reinforce a behavior. Punishment was defined as presenting such an aversive stimulus to a response class in a contingent manner. Respecting this definition, Biggs and Sheehan did not punish stuttering during their punishment condition.

Second, despite the arguments over why the selected noise was more aversive than the one employed in the 1958 study, converting both stimulus intensities to a common reference of SPL (re: .00002 N/m^2) the replication study's stimulus intensity was 117 dB and the original study's stimulus intensity was 123 dB (Industrial Noise Manual, 1975).

Third, in the 1958 study the subjects were instructed to read orally from ongoing printed pages. In the replication the subjects were instructed to repetitively re-read the same passage. At the minimum one would expect different ontogenetic histories from these tasks within the same subject.

Fourth, inspection of the baseline data for the two subjects presented in the replication report failed to persuade this author that a stable baseline rate had been achieved before instatement of the experimental conditions. This inspection suggested that stuttering frequency was exhibiting the characteristics of deceleration throughout the baseline condition.

Martin, St. Louis, Haroldson, and Hasbrouck (1975) also reported a study of the effects of negative reinforcement and punishment on the frequency of stuttering of five adult stutterers. An electric shock was used in place of noise as the

Postscript   9

aversive stimulus. These authors reported the escape schedule increased the frequency of stuttering in two subjects but had little effect on the other three subjects. With respect to the punishment schedule, they reported the relative frequency of stuttered words increased for two subjects, decreased for two subjects and was unchanged for one subject. The authors reported this study provided equivocal support for the position that stuttering is an operant response class. They concluded that when "stuttering subjects are run under similar experimental procedures for long periods of time, there emerge as many distinct patterns of behavior as there are subjects." (p. 489). Some of the factors that were apparent in the Biggs and Sheehan replication are also a cause for concern in this study. Again there is a question about the properties of the stimulus designated as the aversive stimulus. Inspection of the charts of the individual subjects for evidence of stimulus control provided only one or possibly two subjects who exhibited reactivity to the designated "aversive" stimulus. This finding suggests the shock was an effective negative reinforcer for a minority of the subjects. Regarding the physical properties of electric shock, a general rule in the behavior analysis laboratories is that 1.25 mA of current is required to provide consistent reactivity to electric shock across subjects and species. To obtain an estimate of how the shock used by Martin et al. compared to this benchmark value, the electrical resistance between the index and third fingers of five adult males' left hands was measured. The lowest resistance reading obtained was 200k ohms. The value was divided into the highest available voltage reported by the study. This calculation yielded a value of 0.5 mA, which is less current than that regarded as necessary to provide consistent stimulus control. In the light of these observations it is not surprising that Martin et al. found equivocal results.

RELATED RESEARCH

Goldiamond and Flanagan (1959) and Goldiamond (1960) reported the effects of delayed auditory feedback presented to chronic adult stutterers using escape-avoidance and punishment procedures. The punishment procedure suppressed stuttering frequency for each subject. Stuttering frequency increased during the following control periods, but did not return to the original baseline level. The escape-avoidance procedure increased the frequency of stuttering in two subjects but the effect was not durable. The overriding long-term effect of the escape-avoidance procedure when using delayed auditory feedback as the consequence was to decrease the frequency of stuttering. Speaking under conditions of continuous delayed auditory feedback over a number of days also resulted in a decrease in stuttering frequency. Extended observation of post-baseline control conditions failed to provide data to suggest reinstatement of the pre-baseline frequency of stuttering. Taking these data as a set, it was difficult to conclude that response-contingent delayed auditory feedback possesses the functional properties of known aversive stimuli such as electric shock or intense noise. According to Sidman (1960), it is difficult to assess the true effect of an independent variable if the trailing control condition does not recapture the original baseline rate of the behavior. It appeared that the effect of delayed auditory-feedback was to reduce the frequency of stuttering independent of the contingency schedule.

As an aside, Goldiamond, Atkinson, and Bilger (1962) pursued the idea that delayed auditory feedback was altering the microresponses of the speech chain, which in turn led to a decrease in the rate of stuttering. Later, Goldiamond (1965) presented a training program in which the stutters substituted a new, fluent, response pattern of speech for their previous nonfluent speaking pattern. Although Goldiamond's theoretical orientation and methodology was radically different from the traditional speech pathology orientation, his objectives appeared similar to Van Riper's (1958) goals for therapy.

A number of studies reported in the speech pathology literature have investigated the effects of response-contingent presentation of a variety of stimuli on the frequency of stuttering. There appears to be unanimous agreement from these reports that the immediate response-contingent presentation of an external event results in decreased frequency of stuttering. Some of the investigators who studied chronic adult stutterers include: Martin and Siegel (1966a, 1966b), who used shock as their contingent stimulus; Quist and Martin (1967), who presented the verbal stimulus "wrong"; Cooper, Cady, and Robbins (1970), who compared the effects of the verbal stimuli of "wrong," "right," and "tree"; and Reed and Lingwall (1980), who presented recorded laughter as the response-contingent stimulus. Daly and Kimbarow (1978) replicated Cooper, Cady, and Robbins's study with school-aged children. This author agrees with Bloodstein (1981, p.278) who stated, "research findings point to the conclusion that response-contingent stimuli have a broad potential for reducing the frequency of stuttering. The reason for this reduction, however, is far from clear." Various mentalistic terms have been offered to explain this phenomenon, including "distraction," "highlighting," and "punishment." Such naming activity contributes little but suggestive fictional names for the observed effects (Skinner, 1953).

In summary, punishment is defined in terms of presenting an aversive stimulus in a response-contingent manner to a behavior under the control of positive reinforcement (Ferster & Skinner, 1957; Ferster, Culbertson & Boren 1975; Ferster & Culbertson, 1982). Several of the cited speech pathology studies provided scant empirical evidence to support the notion that they employed an operantly defined punishment procedure. It is probable that there are effective conditioned aversive stimuli for verbal behaviors that are not necessarily physically aversive. Skinner's discussion of verbal behavior and punishment (Skinner, 1958) appears to support this point of view. It may be that any stimulus, even very mild, which consistently follows stuttering would be reacted to by stutterers as aversive because of its generalization or association with more severe aversive stimuli in the ontogenetic history (Felty, 1959). One could also argue the position that it is aversive to be interrupted by an external stimulus before completing a verbal response chain, thereby accounting for the suppression of stuttering, but this

Postscript 9

position would require supporting data. It could also be argued that the decrease in stuttering frequency was a function of external inhibition (Flanagan & Webb, 1964) of the stuttering component of the operant verbal chain. Again, an empirical demonstration would be required.

There appears to be confusion concerning punishment that may relate in part to the *working* definition of punishment provided by Azrin and Holz (1966). They stated "... punishment is a reduction of the future probability of a specific response as a result of the immediate delivery of a stimulus for that response" (p. 381). Michael (1975) and Van Houten (1983) have amplified and supported this alternative definition of punishment. In a review of the effects of punishment on stuttering and disfluency, Siegel (1970) took note of Azrin and Holz's position. This definition may have been taken too literally by Cooper et al. (1970) and Daly and Kimbarow (1978). D. M. Baer (personal communication, December 1984) suggested that Azrin and Holz's *working* definition of punishment is as functional as Ferster and Skinner's definition, but it places an additional burden on the investigator to demonstrate the durability and generality of the effects of their punishment procedure. The research methods employed by Goldiamond (1965) and the Minnesota studies (Martin & Siegel; 1966a, 1966b) demonstrated cognizance of the need to show the durability and generality of their contingency procedures.

PUNISHMENT

Confusion about the effects of punishment on stuttering may also relate to the complexity of the punishment literature. The definition of punishment, like positive reinforcement and negative reinforcement, refers to a procedure. Punishment involves the behavioral control that results when a response is followed by an aversive event. The procedure of punishment is simple, but its effects are complicated because a number of behavioral processes interact. The behavior must occur with some frequency before it can be punished. And the aversive event may be either the presentation of a negative reinforcer, called *positive punishment*, or the removal of a positive reinforcer, called *negative punishment*. In this update the discussion of the effects of punishment on stuttering has been limited to positive punishment. The following discussion is a general discourse on positive punishment, followed by a brief discussion of the clinically relevant procedures of positive reinforcement and negative punishment.

Positive Punishment

Skinner (1938) reported that the effect of a mild punishment was to decrease the frequency of a response during the initial stages of an extinction period. However, when compared to those of a control group, an equivalent number of responses were emitted before the extinction process was completed. Although the punishment procedure initially depressed the rate of responding, it did so only temporarily. Skinner suggested that the effect of punishment may be described as suppression of behavior, and that only extinction can decrease the frequency of a behavior in the sense of removing the response class from the organism's repertoire.

Solomon and Wynne (1953), Azrin (1960), and Appel (1961) reported data that indicated that severe punishment can eliminate a response for long periods of time. However, a report by Waters and Grusec (1977) suggested such prolonged disruptions may not contradict the opinion that punishment suppresses the response. It is possible, given a free operant environment, that the "elimination effect" may be that avoidance behaviors do not permit the aversive stimuli to appear.

A behavior analysis of positive punishment (Azrin & Holz, 1966) indicates that the effects of a punishing stimulus depend so much on the conditions under which the punishment was administered that without a careful specification of these conditions it is impossible to make general statements about the effect of the aversive stimulus. Some of the conditions pertinent to applying positive punishment in a treatment or educational setting are detailed here.

Tolerance for punishment.   Azrin, Holz, and Hake (1963) found that the manner in which punishment was introduced was critical to whether a given stimulus would suppress a response maintained by positive reinforcement. Control animals were administered a brief, intense punishment each time they responded on a fixed ratio schedule of reinforcement. This punishment successfully suppressed the responding. The experimental animals were initially administered a low-intensity punishment that was gradually increased over the sessions. The experimental animals continued to respond, even when they were receiving nearly twice the punishment received by the control animals. If the observer did not know the history of the experimental animals it would be easy to conclude that the punishment procedure was not effective.

Positive punishment as discriminative stimuli for positive reinforcement.   A response-produced aversive stimulus can be paired with positive reinforcement and become a discriminative stimulus for that reinforcement. Holz and Azrin (1961) reinforced animals with food on a 2-minute variable interval schedule and subsequently punished the animals for each response. Response rates were half of what they were during the nonpunishment periods. Later, they alternated periods of reinforcement–punishment with periods of no-reinforcement–no-punishment (traditional discrimination training). After several weeks, the animals continued to respond at a steady rate throughout the reinforcement–punishment condition, while responding during the no-reinforcement–no-punishment condition was nearly eliminated.

Later in the experiment, sessions were run in which punishment was presented for responses during one 10-minute period of each session, and *no responses were ever reinforced during the entire session.* During the time when responses produced punishment, response rates accelerated to the level that was

Postscript   9

present during earlier sessions when the reinforcement–punishment condition was in effect. Response rates continued to be low during the periods when responses did not produce punishment. The animals responded more when being punished than when not being punished, and yet it is clear that the stimulus possessed aversive properties. This result demonstrated that an aversive stimulus, functioning as a punisher to reduce response rates, can concurrently have an additional function. The positive punishment may also be a discriminative stimulus for positive reinforcement, and may actually raise the rate of responding under certain conditions. In the light of this finding it is tempting to speculate about the ontogenetic history of the chronic stutterer whose rate of stuttering is increased by positive punishment.

Positive punishment and training.   Thorndike's (1935) initial *Law of Effect* ("satisfiers" stamp in behavior; "annoyers" stamp out behavior) was later revised as a result of his research with humans. Thorndike reported that the word *wrong*, provided after an incorrect choice emitted in a multiple-choice context, was not effective in altering the subject's choice on subsequent trials. Thus, he concluded that punishment did not weaken behavior. Consider a learning situation with ten possible alternative responses, one correct. If the training punishes for an incorrect response, the organism now has nine possible alternatives. There is very little potential that learning has occurred. However, if the alternative responses are limited to two, the probability of the next response being correct is high. Given a situation where there are many possible responses and few correct alternatives, using positive punishment procedures for training is at best inefficient.

The 1958 investigation into the operant nature of stuttering used positive punishment because of its relevance to the theoretical issue being studied. The use of positive punishment in the educational or clinical setting is not indicated because of problems related to the factors mentioned previously and the possibility of undesirable by-products. (Hutchinson, 1977) When intense positive punishers are used, the potential for respondent (classical) conditioning is increased, such as increased heart rate, blood pressure, or GSR. Or simply stated, the organism becomes prepared for "fight or flight." It has also been documented (Ulrich & Azrin, 1962) that the use of positive punishers increases the probability of aggressive behaviors including biting, assault, etc., towards the other organisms in the environment. The fact that positive punishment will suppress stuttering is not sufficient justification to rely on such procedures for its treatment. Positive punishment has a place only in well-reasoned experimentation designed specifically to increase the understanding of its role in the nature of stuttering.

Negative Punishment

In general, negative punishment procedures are viewed by the public as more acceptable than positive. Ferster's (1957, 1958) studies established that withdrawing the conditions for positive reinforcement suppressed responses which led to the loss of reinforcement. He also found that organisms would respond to avoid the loss of the conditions for positive reinforcement. These findings validate the procedure of withdrawing of conditions of positive reinforcement as an aversive event, and the response contingent withdrawal of these conditions as punishment. Ferster and Skinner (1957) called this procedure "time out" (TO). The procedure of TO is *intended* to provide a less reinforcing environment contingent upon emission of a specified behavior. Release from TO may be specified in terms of a predetermined time period, the emission of a selected behavior, or both. The reinstatement of conditions of positive reinforcement will probably reinforce whatever behavior is occurring at that time.

The wide use of TO in applied research began with several studies, most notably that of Wolf, Risley, and Mees (1964). They used a TO procedure with a preschool child who had serious physical and behavioral difficulties including tantrums and self-destruction. In addition, the child threw off his eyeglasses, which were needed to prevent permanent eye damage. The authors used what they described as "a combination of a mild punishment and extinction" (p. 306) in a hospital setting. After each incident of "tantruming" or throwing the eyeglasses, the child was put in his TO room for 10 minutes. Suppression of both behaviors was achieved with this procedure, and a reversal design demonstrated its effectiveness. A later study with the same child (Wolf, Risley, Johnston, Harris, & Allen, 1967) provided follow-up information. The child's tantrum behavior increased and he was placed in TO again for "tantruming." In the hospital setting approximately 100 trips to his TO room had been necessary to reduce the rate of tantrums. In the preschool setting however, only three trips were required to eliminate the behavior. For this child, the selected TO procedure was effective across settings, and generalization was relatively easy to attain.

Baer (1962) controlled thumb sucking of a 5-year-old boy by introducing cartoons, and then withdrawing the cartoons contingent on the boy's thumb sucking. During alternate periods of uninterrupted cartoons, the boy's thumb sucking increased. A second procedure, using two other 5-year-old boys, compared contingent with noncontingent cartoon viewing. The results showed that the boy whose thumb sucking caused withdrawal of the cartoons emitted that behavior less frequently, and the boy who was treated to random cartoon withdrawal showed no systematic changes in the frequency of his thumb sucking, thus establishing the effectiveness of the cartoon contingency.

Risley and Wolf (1967) used a TO from positive reinforcement procedure while developing functional speech with echolalic children. The experimenter used food and social praise for appropriate responding during individual sessions. Contingent upon mild disruptive behaviors in the therapy situation, the experimenter would simply look away from the child, thus removing positive reinforcement for those behaviors. For temper tantrums, the child was isolated in a room and allowed to leave following 30 seconds of silence. Both procedures resulted in a decline or cessation of the inappropriate behaviors.

Postscript   9

Time Out and Stuttering.   A number of studies in the speech pathology literature have reported TO to be an effective procedure for suppressing stuttering.
Haroldson, Martin, and Starr (1968), Martin and Haroldson (1969), Egolf, Shames,
and Seltzer (1971), and James (1976) reported significant reduction in stuttering
for adults using this procedure. Similar results have been reported for adolescents (Costello, 1975) and for children (Martin & Berndt, 1970; Martin, Kuhl, &
Haoldson, 1972). In each of these studies the experimenter either signaled the
stutterer to stop speaking or withdrew the audience when a stuttering response
occurred, and reinstated the discriminative stimulus for speech after a period of
time had lapsed. In studies which used an ABA reversal design, stuttering frequency was higher in the trailing baseline[4] than in the treatment condition. However, the post-baseline frequency was less than the stuttering rate observed in the
pre-baseline condition, making it difficult to conclude that TO was the only cause
of the decreased stuttering. As noted earlier, when a neutral external stimulus
consistently follows the moment of stuttering, a decrease in stuttering frequency
is frequently observed. Perhaps a further study is needed that pairs a neutral stimulus (such as noticeable change in the illumination of the room) with each stuttering response throughout the reversal conditions to clarify the relative
contribution of these variables.

James (1981) investigated the effects of self-initiated TO from speaking contingent upon self-hearing of stuttering with an 18-year-old male stutterer. Both
the experimenter-initiated and the self-initiated TO procedures decreased the
frequency of stuttering to comparable rates in monologue and conversation settings. As with the previously cited studies of the effects of TO on stuttering, the
trailing baseline rate of stuttering was greater than the rate during the experimental conditions but less than the rate during the initial baseline condition.
After the trailing baseline was completed, an additional punishment procedure,
response cost (Azrin & Holz, 1966), was initiated. The purpose was to control the
subject's failure to self-initiate TO for approximately 50% of his stuttering responses. During the response cost procedure the ratio of stuttered responses
timed out by the subject increased to 70% and the overall rate of stuttering decreased to less than 1% of syllables emitted in monologue, conversation, and community settings. The durability and generality of the effects of these procedures
was assessed 6 and 12 months after termination of the experiment. The author
provided data and anecdotal reports which indicated that the frequency of stuttering remained at an extremely low level during follow-up probe session.

In the past 20 years, the punishment literature using the techniques of TO,
social reprimands, response cost, and overcorrection has grown. Research
within the natural environment using these techniques has typically provided
demonstrations of the effectiveness of the selected punishment technique, and
largely neglected an analysis of how the technique may be reduced to basic behavioral processes such as reinforcement, extinction, deprivation, or stimulus

[4]That baseline that follows the experimental condition.

control. Ferster and Culbertson (1982) stated that while the punishment procedure appears simple, its effects are so complicated that even when the basic behavioral processes have been identified, their interaction makes it necessary to
analyze their effects on behavior case by case. While sufficient data are not available at this time to make a definitive statement, there is no apparent reason to expect the interactions with negative punishment to be less complex than those in
positive punishment. In contrast to growth in the body of other applied punishment literature, the literature on the use of self-punishment has remained scant.
J. G. Holland (personal communication, May 1985) considers the use of self-punishment from the vantage point of radical behaviorism as being illogical. These
observations cause me to consider the validity of Skinner's (1953) notion that
punishment is more reinforcing to the donor than to the recipient. From the foregoing discussion, it should be evident that the use of punishment in the applied
setting is complex, and the risk of misapplication is high because of the possible
interaction with other behavioral processes.

Skinner and Punishment

Skinner (1953, 1971) has consistently advocated the use of positive reinforcement rather than punishment to control behavior. He opposes the use of punishment for several reasons. Punishment suppresses rather than eliminates
undesired behaviors; i.e., the undesired behavior reappears when the punishing
agent is absent or the aversiveness associated with the punishing agent extin-
guishes. Emotional by-products such as fear or hostility are frequently associated
with punishment and may interfere with learning in applied settings. When punishment is used to eliminate undesired behaviors, the recipient has no opportunity to learn appropriate behaviors. And, finally, Skinner cautions that using
punishment may be reinforcing to the controlling agent.

As alternatives to using punishment to control behavior, Skinner suggests
the use of extinction[5] and reinforcement of incompatible behaviors. He allows
that extinction, or the procedure of ignoring undesirable behaviors, is time con-
suming, may increase the undesired behavior temporarily, is difficult to apply, and
may produce emotional reactions in the recipient. Despite the difficulties extinction presents, its effects are more permanent than those of punishment. To supplement extinction and help the individual learn more appropriate behaviors to
replace the undesirable behaviors, Skinner strongly recommends that behaviors
that are incompatible with the undesired behavior be reinforced. In the control
of stuttering, reinforcement for "easy stuttering" (Van Riper, 1974) or overlearning specific control techniques would be examples. Goldiamond (1965), Shames
(1980), and Webster (1980) have focused their treatments for stuttering on
strengthening and reinforcing behaviors that are incompatible with uncontrolled
stuttering. Also, for the practitioner who is influenced by the philosophy of radi-

---

[5]One case of extinction, the withdrawal of positive reinforcement, has been employed as a punishment
procedure.

Postscript   9

---

cal behaviorism, Skinner presents compelling arguments advocating alternatives to using punishment to control behavior (Nye, 1979).

Empirically, Skinner's argument for not using punishment in the control of behavior rests on the position that punishment does not eliminate behavior but only suppresses it. Others, (Azrin & Holz, 1966; Van Houten, 1983) have indicated that punishment has suppressed behavior for extremely long periods of time, and advance the position for using punishment procedures when appropriate. It is beyond the scope of this report to deal with this issue.

Implications of Stuttering as an Operant

Research has shown the operant nature of stuttering and indicates that stuttering is a verbal operant like speaking, gesturing, writing, or thinking. Stuttering is thus amenable to control as a function of its consequences. Behavior has as its source three classes of independent variables: phylogenetic factors, ontogenetic factors, and the current environmental variables. From the viewpoint of radical behaviorism, these three variables determine behavior. Following this point of view, it is necessary for the scientist to study the variables that are associated with the increase, decrease, or maintenance of stuttering.

Frequently the question is asked, "What is the reinforcement for stuttering?" In the simplest sense, stuttering, along with other components of the verbal utterance, is reinforced by the reaction of the listener. However, the speaker may react to stuttering as a pre-aversive stimulus and learn to engage in behaviors to escape or avoid the anticipated aversiveness of the listener's reaction. When the speaker uses escape or avoidance strategies and the listener reinforces the utterance, these behaviors are also reinforced.

Stutterers need to be viewed as unique individuals with differing phylogenetic and ontogenetic histories who are currently operating in environments that may be supporting diverse behaviors. Thus, it may be counterproductive to treat adult stutterers as a set. What is needed is to maximize the reinforcers that support fluent speech in each individual's environment. It may be that what stutterers share in common is the culture's aversive reactivity to stuttering.

The compelling issue in the experimental analysis of behavior in 1958 was whether or not human behavior could be controlled by the independent variables identified in the operant laboratories. Perhaps it would have been more appropriate to target some other aspect of speaking, rather than stuttering, for the original demonstration. However, this did not occur. The intended suggestion for application from the 1958 article was that operant theory and methodology could be used to increase the frequency of positive reinforcement in the treatment of stuttering. For some this suggestion was apparently translated as meaning that stutterers should be reinforced for not stuttering and punished when they did. This is unfortunate.

Knowledge of the basic processes of behavior and their application to stuttering therapy provides a powerful base for understanding and controlling stuttering. This knowledge also enables the practitioner to recognize aversive control and to avoid its use in stuttering therapy. The analysis of behavior also offers the practitioner a methodology for collecting data to validate the presence or absence of change in the stutterer's speech.

Given that stuttering is an operant, perhaps it is time for the interests of the professional community to focus on stuttering as an individual's problem within the context of verbal behavior as an interaction between members of our society.

REFERENCES

Appel, J. B. (1961). Punishment in the squirrel monkey *Saimiri sciruea. Science, 133,* 36.

Azrin, N. H. (1958). Some effects of noise on human behavior. *Journal of the Experimental Analysis of Behavior, 1,* 183–200.

Azrin, N. H. (1960). Effects of punishment intensity during variable-interval reinforcement. *Journal of the Experimental Analysis of Behavior, 3,* 123–142.

Azrin, N. H., Holz, W. C., & Hake, D. (1963). Fixed-ratio punishment. *Journal of the Experimental Analysis of Behavior, 6,* 141–148.

Azrin, N. H. & Holz, W. C. (1966). Punishment. In W. K. Honig (Ed.). *Operant behavior: Areas of research and application.* New York: Appleton-Century-Crofts.

Baer, D. M. (1962). Laboratory control of thumbsucking by withdrawal and re-presentation of reinforcement. *Journal of the Experimental Analysis of Behavior, 5,* 525–528.

Biggs, B. & Sheehan, J. (1969). Punishment or distraction? Operant stuttering revised. *Journal of Abnormal Psychology, 74,* 256–262.

Bijou, S. W. & Baer, D. M. (1966). Operant methods in child behavior and development. In W. K. Honig (Ed.). *Operant behavior: Areas of research and application.* New York: Appleton-Century-Crofts.

Bloodstein, O. (1981). *A handbook on stuttering.* (3rd ed.). Chicago, IL: National Easter Seal Society.

Cooper, E. B., Cady, B. & Robbins, J. (1970). The effects of the verbal stimulus words *wrong, right,* and *tree* on the disfluency rates of stutterers and nonstutterers. *Journal of Speech and Hearing Research, 13,* 240–244.

Costello, J. (1975). The establishment of fluency with time-out procedures. *Journal of Speech and Hearing Disorders, 40,* 216–231.

Daly, D. A. & Kimbarow, M. L. (1978). Stuttering as operant behavior: Effects of the verbal stimuli *wrong, right,* and *tree* on the disfluency rates of school-age stutterers and nonstuttererers. *Journal of Speech and Hearing Research, 21,* 589–597.

Egolf, D. B., Shames, G. H., & Seltzer, H. (1971). The effects of time-out on the fluency of stutterers in group therapy. *Journal of Communication Disorders, 4,* 111–118.

Ferster, C. B. (1957). Withdrawal of positive reinforcement as punishment. *Science, 126,* 509.

Ferster, C. B. (1958). Control of behavior in chimpanzees and pigeons by time out from positive reinforcement. *Psychological Monographs, 72,* (8, Whole No. 461).

Ferster, C. B. & Culbertson, S. A. (1982). *Behavior principles* (3rd ed.). Englewood Cliffs, NJ: Prentice-Hall.

Postscript 9

Ferster, C. B. & Sapon, S. M. (1958). An application of recent developments in psychology to the teaching of German. *Harvard Educational Review, 28,* 58-69.

Ferster, C. B. & Skinner, B. F. (1957). *Schedules of reinforcement.* New York: Appleton-Century-Crofts.

Ferster, C. B., Culbertson, S., & Boren, M. C. P. (1975). *Behavior Principles* (2nd ed.). Englewood Cliffs, NJ: Prentice-Hall.

Flanagan, B., Goldiamond, I., & Azrin, N. (1958). Operant stuttering: The control of stuttering behavior through response-contingent consequences. *Journal of the Experimental Analysis of Behavior, 1,* 173–177.

Flanagan, B. & Webb, W. B. (1964). Disinhibition and external inhibition in fixed interval operant conditioning. *Psychonomic Science, 1,* 123–124.

Frick, J. A. (1951). *An exploratory study of the effect of punishment (electric shock) upon stuttering.* Unpublished doctoral dissertation, State University of Iowa.

Goldiamond, I. (1960). Effects of delayed feedback upon the temporal development of fluent and blocked speech communication. (AFCCDD, *T. R.* 60–38). Bedford, MA: Air Force Cambridge Research Center.

Goldiamond, I. (1965). Stuttering and fluency as a manipulatable operant response class. In L. Krasner and L. Ullman (Eds.). *Research in Behavior Modification.* New York: Holt, Rinehart and Winston.

Goldiamond, I. (1970). Human control over human behavior. In M. Wertheimer (Ed.). *Confrontation, psychology and the problems of today.* Glenview, IL: Scott Foresman & Co.

Goldiamond, I. & Flanagan, B. (1959). *The use of delayed auditory feedback as an aversive stimulus in the operant control of stuttering.* Paper presented at the meeting of the American Speech and Hearing Association, Cleveland, OH.

Goldiamond, I., Atkinson, G. J. & Bilger, R. C. (1962). Stabilization of behavior and prolonged exposure to delayed auditory feedback. *Science, 35,* 437–438.

Haroldson, S. K., Martin, R. R., & Starr, C. D. (1968). Time-out as punishment for stuttering. *Journal of Speech and Hearing Research, 11,* 560–566.

Holland, J. G. (1957). Technique for behavior analysis of human observing. *Science, 125,* 348–350.

Holz, W. C. & Azrin, N. H. (1961). Discriminative properties of punishment. *Journal of the Experimental Analysis of Behavior, 4,* 225–232.

Hutchinson, R. (1977). By-products of aversive control. In W. Honig & J. Staddon (Eds.). *Handbook of operant behavior.* Englewood Cliffs, NJ: Prentice-Hall.

Industrial Noise Manual (3rd ed.). (1975). Akron OH: American Industrial Hygiene Association.

James, J. E. (1976). The influence of duration on the effects of time-out from speaking. *Journal of Speech and Hearing Research, 19,* 206–215.

James, J. E. (1981). Self-control of stuttering using time-out. *Journal of Applied Behavior Analysis, 14,* 25–37.

Johnson, W. J. (1955). *Stuttering in children and adults.* Minneapolis, MN: University of Minnesota.

Johnston, J. M. & Pennypacker, H. S. (1981). *Strategies and tactics of human behavioral research.* Hillsdale, NJ: Lawrence Erlbaum Associates.

Lindsley, O. R. (1956). Operant conditioning methods applied to research in chronic schizophrenia. *Psychiatric Research Reports, 5,* 118–139.

Martin, R. R. & Berndt, L. A. (1970). The effects of time-out on stuttering in a 12-year-old boy. *Exceptional Children, 37,* 303–304.

Martin, R. R. & Haroldson, S. K. (1969). The effects of two treatment procedures on stuttering. *Journal of Communication Disorders, 2,* 115–125.

Martin, R. R. & Siegel, G. M. (1966a). The effects of response contingent shock on stuttering. *Journal of Speech and Hearing Research, 9,* 340–352.

Martin, R. R. & Siegel, G. M. (1966b). The effects of simultaneously punishing stuttering and rewarding fluency. *Journal of Speech and Hearing Research, 9,* 466–475.

Martin, R. R., Kuhl, P., & Haroldson, S. (1972). An experimental treatment with two preschool stuttering children. *Journal of Speech and Hearing Research, 15,* 743–752.

Martin, R., St. Louis, K., Haroldson, S., & Hasbrouck, J. (1975). Punishment and negative reinforcement of stuttering using electric shock. *Journal of Speech and Hearing Research, 18,* 478–490.

Michael, J. (1975). Positive and negative reinforcement, a distinction that is no longer necessary, or a better way to talk about bad things. In E. Ramp & G. Semb (Eds.). *Behavior analysis: Areas of research and application.* Englewood Cliffs, NJ: Prentice-Hall.

Nye, R. D. (1979). *What is B. F. Skinner really saying?* Englewood Cliffs, NJ: Prentice-Hall.

Quist, R. W. & Martin, R. R. (1967) The effects of response-contingent verbal punishment on stuttering. *Journal of Speech and Hearing Research, 10,* 795–800.

Reed, C. G. & Lingwall, J. B. (1980). Conditioned stimulus effects on stuttering and GSRs. *Journal of Speech and Hearing Research, 23,* 336–343.

Risley, T. R. & Wolf, M. (1967). Establishing functional speech in echolalic children. *Behavior Research and Therapy, 5,* 73–88.

Sidman, M. (1960). *Tactics of scientific research.* New York: Basic Books.

Siegel, G. M., (1970). Punishment, stuttering, and disfluency. *Journal of Speech and Hearing Research, 13,* 677–714.

Shames, G. & Florance, C. (1980). *Stutter-free speech.* Columbus, OH: Charles E. Merrill Publishing.

Skinner, B. F. (1938). *Behavior of organisms.* New York: Appleton-Century-Crofts.

Skinner, B. F. (1953). *Science and human behavior.* New York: The Macmillan Co.

Skinner, B. F. (1957). *Verbal behavior.* New York: Appleton-Century-Crofts.

Skinner, B. F. (1968). *Technology of teaching.* New York: Appleton-Century-Croft.

Skinner, B. F. (1971). *Beyond freedom and dignity.* New York: Alfred A. Knopf.

Skinner, B. F. (1974). *About behaviorism.* New York: Alfred A. Knopf.

Solomon, R. L. & Wynne, L. C. (1953). Traumatic avoidance learning: Acquisition in dogs. *Psychological Monographs* 67: No. 354.

Thorndike, E. L. (1935). *The psychology of wants, interests and attitudes.* New York: Appleton-Century-Crofts.

Ulrich, R. E. & Azrin, N. H. (1962). Reflexive fighting in response to aversive stimulation. *Journal of the Experimental Analysis of Behavior, 5,* 511–520.

Postscript   9

Van Riper, C. (1937). The effects of penalty upon the frequency of stuttering spasms. *Pedagogical Seminary and Journal of Genetic Psychology, 50,* 193–197.

Van Riper, C. (1957). Symptomatic therapy for stuttering. In L. Travis (Ed.). *Handbook of speech pathology.* New York: Appleton-Century-Crofts.

Van Riper, C. (1958). Experiments in stuttering. In J. Eisenson (Ed.). *Stuttering symposium.* New York: Harper & Row, Publisher.

Van Riper, C. (1974). Modifying stuttering behavior. In *Therapy for stutterers. Publication No. 10.* Memphis, TN: Speech Foundation of America.

Van Houten, R. (1983). Punishment: From the animal laboratory to the applied setting. In S. Axelrod & J. Apsche (Eds.). *The effects of punishment on human behavior.* New York: Academic Press.

Waters, G. C. & Grusec, J. E. (1977). *Punishment.* San Fransisco: W. H. Freeman.

Webster, R. (1980). Precision fluency shaping. *Journal of Fluency Disorders, 2,* 303–320.

Wolf, M., Risley, T., Johnston, M., Harris, F., & Allen, E. (1967). Application of operant conditioning procedures to the behavior problems of an autistic child: A follow-up and extension. *Behavior Research and Therapy, 4,* 103–111.

Wolf, M. M., Risley, T. R. & Mees, H. L. (1964). Application of operant conditioning procedures to the behavior problems of an autistic child. *Behavior Research and Therapy, 1,* 305–312.

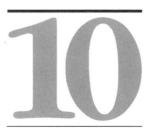

A Discussion of Nonfluency and Stuttering as Operant Behavior

George H. Shames and Carl E. Sherrick, Jr.

Postscript
An Operant Perspective

George H. Shames

10

A Discussion of Nonfluency and Stuttering as Operant Behavior

George H. Shames and Carl E. Sherrick, Jr.

Within the broad purview of verbal behavior, the phenomenon of stuttering has often been singled out for special attention. Stuttering has for some time been of interest to experimental psychology as a vehicle for studying the function of anxiety in the acquisition of behavior. It has also been of interest to cultural anthropology, semantics, psychoanalysis, and clinical psychology as behavior which can be explained by and structurally embedded within their respective theoretical languages. In addition to these disciplines, there is an increasing number of theorists, researchers, and clinicians who are seeking to resolve and understand stuttering as a clinical problem.

It is the purpose of this paper to discuss procedures for the further study of stuttering as a clinical problem within the framework of operant conditioning. As a procedure for categorizing behavior, operant analysis resembles the procedures of any theory of stuttering by which events are placed in relation to one another. However, operant analysis requires minimal assumptions and inferences regarding the

George H. Shames (Ph.D., University of Pittsburgh, 1952) is Associate Professor of Speech and Psychology and Associate Director of the Speech Clinic, University of Pittsburgh. Carl E. Sherrick, Jr. (Ph.D., University of Virginia, 1952) is Research Psychologist, Department of Psychology, Princeton University. This paper was written while the authors were Research Associates at Central Institute for the Deaf, Dr. Shames as a Special Fellow in Research for the National Institute of Neurological Diseases and Blindness, and Dr. Sherrick working with the support of National Institute of Neurological Diseases and Blindness Grant B-1718 to Central Institute for the Deaf.

events which are observed and the principles underlying these events. It is hoped that an improved behavioral analysis of stuttering will eventually provide a better definition of the events grouped under this term. Well-defined and precise observations of individual stuttering histories and of the events before, during, and after specific episodes of current stuttering should help us to arrive at effective methods for experimentally controlling this behavior and, ultimately, to develop techniques for clinical application.

THE SYSTEM OF OPERANT ANALYSIS

Skinner has developed a system of behavioral analysis (*15,* pp. 59–90 which has been demonstrated by Goldiamond (*7, 8*) to apply to the problem of stuttering. Operant behavior may be characterized as that behavior by means of which the organism does something to his external environment. The criterion for deciding whether or not behavior is operant is mainly that its properties may be modified by the effects that result from its appearance. Fundamentally, the system is supposed to stem from a definite pattern of laboratory practices. The subject is trained to behave under certain specified conditions. When the experimenter manipulates these conditions, observations are made of changes in behavior. The events during these controlled observations are categorized

Note: From the *Journal of Speech and Hearing Disorders, 28,* 1963, pp. 3–18. Reprinted with permission of the American Speech-Language-Hearing Association.

into broad classes of stimuli and responses. Some unique relations have been perceived among these classes of stimuli and classes of responses. One such relation is manifest when a given class of responses appears more frequently when followed by one of a set of stimulus classes. These stimuli which appear to increase the frequency of a class of responses that they follow are called positive reinforcers, provided also that their removal reduces the frequency of the response. The weakening or extinction of a response is brought about by removal of the reinforcer. Another relation perceived among responses, and stimuli which follow them, are those stimuli which tend to interrupt or depress responses. This is sometimes referred to as punishment. These stimuli are often thought to be aversive since the subject may increase in frequency those responses which tend to reduce or remove these stimuli. This relation between responses and the termination of ongoing aversive stimuli has been termed negative reinforcement. Both positive and negative reinforcement imply an increased frequency of responses while extinction and punishment imply a weakening of responses.

It has also been observed that certain stimulus events lead to particular responses. Such events do not appear to reinforce behavior; they seem to evoke it. These stimuli come to control responses because they have been discriminated as part of the total stimulus occasion when a response has been reinforced. Skinner has designated these as discriminative stimuli. Thus we have Skinner's basic three-term paradigm of $S^D \rightarrow R \rightarrow Rf$ representing the contingency of discriminative stimulus, response, and reinforcement.

In selecting from the literature and from past experience the events of stuttering to be viewed through operant analysis, we shall employ many of the dimensions of observation that have proved useful to speech pathology. For convenience, we shall trace with the terms of operant behavior a rough progression of conditioning, beginning with the events associated with nonfluency, through the onset and development of early stuttering, to the events observed in advanced stuttering. These include conditioning with positive reinforcement, with negative reinforcement, or with punishment. By placing our observations of nonfluency and stuttering within these paradigms, we can hypothesize more specifically that stuttering responses are under the control of specific discriminative stimuli, aversive stimuli, or other reinforcing contingencies. Past clinical observation and experience directs and restricts the selection to a limited number of stimuli and contingencies that will be discussed in this paper. The ultimate relevance of these stimuli to the responses classed as stuttering can be determined only through experimentation and observation. It is felt that as experimental analyses proceed, many other contingencies will emerge that may have more subtle application to both clinical and theoretical aspects of stuttering. These, of course, are beyond the scope of the present paper.

NONFLUENCY

Studies by Davis (4, 5, 6) and Winitz (18) have suggested that speech nonfluencies in such diverse forms as repetitions, prolongations, interjections, and pauses have a high operant level in children. Repetition has been the most frequently observed form as the repetition of codified speech is a part of the child's repertoire by the age of two.

The conditions surrounding the original emission and early development of nonfluencies in the speech of infants are still quite obscure and in need of detailed observation. It is possible that the repetitions observed in later speech may be related to the vocal behavior emitted by infants during their early speech development (babbling and chaining of syllables). Winitz (18) offers data which can be interpreted to support such a hypothesis. It is also possible that nonfluency in speech is a characteristic of the human organism because of its physiological limitations. Speech is an adjunctive function of organs having basically biological functions. As such, speech appears within the limitations of these other functions; we must, for example, pause and hesitate if only to inhale.

In addition to the possibility of such biological origins, many observations of the modification of nonfluency suggest several hypotheses regarding the conditioning of nonfluency that should also be submitted to analysis. It has been observed that the verbal behavior of a speaker varies due to relatively simple acts by his listener. Many of these acts are such signs of attention as looking, nodding, smiling, or speaking. We infer that these listener activities are positive reinforcers because we observe that the speaker continues to speak as long as these activities continue. Moreover, the speaker's behavior may diminish in strength when these listener activities are no longer forthcoming. Such positive reinforcements not only maintain verbal behavior; they are a part of the basis for conditioning verbal behavior.

It is possible to view the repetition response as a class of verbal responses with a history of complex schedules of reinforcement. The initial appearance of repetition may have a basis that is entirely foreign to its development as nonfluency. For example, we frequently repeat to make sure that a listener has heard us correctly. On several occasions of a repetition having this basis, the speaker is reinforced by the listener for repetitions and not for single utterances. On future occasions the likelihood of repetitions may then become greater than that of single utterances.

States of Deprivation and Aversive Stimuli

The studies of Davis (4, 5, 6), in addition to suggesting the relation of age to the strength and forms of nonfluent speech, have also suggested the occasions for their emission in specific situations. She observed that repetitions, which were the commonest form of nonfluency, seemed to be related to getting attention, directing someone else's activities, trying to gain an object, coercion, seeking status, giving and seeking information, criticizing, seeking a privilege, and trying to obtain social acceptance.

It is interesting to note that nearly all of these occasions involve a type of verbal behavior which Skinner calls 'manding' (16, p. 35). This type of verbal behavior is often in the interrogative or imperative mood and is controlled by the listener's positive reinforcements on the occasion of an aversive stimulus or a specific state of deprivation in the speaker. Typically the listener does something for the speaker or gives something to the speaker. The listener's behavior can have the effect of increasing the likelihood of a particular form of verbal behavior by the speaker on future occasions of similar aversive stimuli or deprivations. An example would be the young child who says, 'Teacher, look!' followed by the teacher giving her attention to the child by 'looking.' The child in essence has indicated to the teacher the form of reinforcement for his utterance, 'Teacher, look!' In the future, if the child wants the teacher's attention, he may emit the same form of verbal behavior.

Davis's observations suggest that a relation between repetition responses and occasions of aversive stimuli or states of deprivation should be studied.

Such manding behavior by the child is on a haphazard schedule of reinforcement; the demands of the child are not always reinforced by parents and peers. If repetitions are frequently connected with the variable reinforcement of these demands, the repetition will then appear in greater strength, since they are being reinforced on the same schedule as the child's manding. An example might be the parent who delays reinforcement of a child's first utterance because of the inconvenience of providing the reinforcement. The child may then repeat the utterance several times, until the repetition becomes undesirable to the parent. The parent finally provides positive reinforcement for the child's demands, perhaps unaware that he is not only doing something for his child but is also *teaching him to repeat.* If we extend this example to consider some future behavior of the parent, we may eventually see some etiological relations among (a) the inconvenience of reinforcing his child's manding, (b) a connection between the child's repetition and this inconvenience, resulting in the repetition's becoming an aversive stimulus event, and (c) the later punishing behavior of the parent in attempting to terminate this aversive 'nagging' behavior of the child. These relations are often seen in the development of stuttering (early positive reinforcement for child's repetitions, later punishment for child's repetitions, and negative reinforcement for parent's behavior). In this sense, the child and the parent may be conditioning one another, since each provides occasioning and reinforcing stimuli for their respective responses.

In addition to the development of repetition under such haphazard schedules of reinforcement, any one occasion for the repetition response may come under the control of other contingencies. These would include discriminative stimuli associated with different listeners, situations, and types of verbal behavior, each of which may provide a unique schedule of reinforcement that interacts with the others. The child may soon discriminate those occasions for which single utterances are reinforced and those occasions for which repeated utterances are reinforced.

A different type of contingency for the repetition response may be found in relation to aversive stimuli. It has been observed in animals and humans that initially neutral conditions, when paired with painful or unpleasant events, acquire control over the individual's behavior. Because of past experiences, the organism may respond to these stimuli as signals of undesirable things to come, and so leave the field of action (avoidance), or it may show a depression in strength of already ongoing operant behavior ('anxiety'). The complexity of the behavior produced in such situations is increased if aversive or conditioned aversive events (punishment) appear following certain behavior patterns of the organism. A child may show avoidance of certain unpleasant conditions by his verbal behavior. The repetition response may be emitted to postpone or avoid aversive conditions associated with a later portion of a verbal response. Thus, if a child is confronted with the necessity for making a verbal response which may have aversive consequences, such as those which occur in lying or in admitting his responsibility in an accident, he may be observed to postpone or avoid his response by repeating a word or a phrase prior to that crucial aversive portion of his statement.

Conversational Pauses, Interruptions, and Silence

Repetition may also arise from early training to speak in a specified pattern established in polite conversation with a listener. Children typically seem to be conditioned quite early (perhaps through a combination of mild positive reinforcement and mild punishment) that two people in conversation do not talk at exactly the same time. There is a conversational sequence to be maintained in polite society such that first one person talks and then the other. The silence of the conversational partner may serve as the occasion for one's emission of speech, while the sound of the partner's voice can serve as the occasion for silence (and presumably listening) in oneself. Significant deviations from this pattern can result in mild punishment.

Sometimes the conversational partner's silence is only a short pause while he is composing his response, and is not meant to be the occasion for speech in the child. If the child speaks on this occasion, it is probably that the first speaker will interrupt him (perhaps irritably) and continue with the remainder of his response. This will result in the child's silence since his partner's voice has become the occasion for his silence. If this happens frequently enough, repetitions and long pauses may become a recurring pattern in the child's speech. A complex process of differential reinforcement, involving possibly both positive reinforcement and punishment,

may strengthen the discriminative properties of silence in the speaking partner. It almost seems as though the child tests the situation under these circumstances in learning to discriminate whether his conversational partner's silence is or is not an occasion for his emission of speech. His partner's silence was heretofore the occasion for the child's utterance. This in turn was the occasion for his partner's silence. These events are not occurring in the accustomed sequence when the partner's silence is merely a pause and the child's utterance is the occasion for an interruption by his conversational partner.

If the speech patterns of the partner are persistently of the sort described, the child may frequently emit the first sound and wait briefly for the interruption. If the interruption is not forthcoming, he repeats the first sound as part of the originally intended message unit and continues with the remainder of his utterances. This repetition pattern in the child's speech may be maintained in great strength under such circumstances. The early conditioning of silence as an occasion for talking is a specified sequence with the later problem of stuttering. This analysis may represent in behavioral terms what clinically is referred to as 'competition for talking time.' It seems possible to study not only the early development of repetitions in relation to alternate silent and vocal periods as discriminative stimuli, but also the reinforcing contingencies, such as punishment for deviations from this sequence and social approval and social interaction as forms of positive reinforcement.

Self-Editing and Correction

It is recognized that speakers very often 'compose' and 'edit' and 'prompt' themselves for their verbal behavior even as they are currently emitting verbal responses (16, pp. 255–258, 344–383). Verbal behavior is emitted in rather discrete, staccato units of varying sizes and dimensions. It is punctuated by pauses during which we assume that the processes of composition and editing go on. The speaker's emission of speech and its editing and composition are almost simultaneous activities. As he hears and feels himself talk, the speaker monitors what he hears. Occasionally he changes and corrects various aspects of his utterances such as his articulation, his pitch, his rhythm or his combination of phonemes. Such changes and corrections are expressed in the forms of short repetitions of sounds or words. Under these circumstances the speaker, as his own listener, is providing positive and negative self-reinforcements for his speech behavior. However, this composing process also may be in part under the control of the 'attending' of the listener. As long as 'attending' is forthcoming, composition and speech emission continue. When 'attending' is withdrawn, speech (and presumably composition) diminishes. It is possible that the repetition response may serve to hold this attention of the listener during composition. Therefore, it is also possible that while a child is composing his response and is making available those portions of his verbal behavior that are weak, he emits repetitions. Furthermore, such repetitions may also serve to fill the silence produced by the pauses for composition, and therefore prevent the listener from responding to those silences by speaking.

STUTTERING

Three basic propositions are offered regarding stuttering:

a. Continuities exist between nonfluency and stuttering.

b. An operant definition of stuttering should include the environmental circumstances associated with specific forms of stuttering responses and their processes of change and deterioration.

c. There is no single, simple contingency for stuttering. It is maintained by positive and negative reinforcements on complex, multiple schedules.

These propositions are contained in the discussion which follows, suggesting specific contingencies and hypotheses for study.

Continuities Between Nonfluency and Stuttering

Much attention has been given to the separation of those speech responses classed as nonfluency from those classed as stuttering. If instead of these two covering terms, we employed behavioral dimensions of description, we might observe many similarities and perhaps even a continuity of the forms of these response classes as well as of their controlling contingencies.

There may be some etiological relations between the early conditioning paradigms of nonfluency and the later conditioning paradigms that may be associated with stuttering. It is likely that conditions aversive for the child surrounding the presence of the parent during the emission of nonfluency responses will persist or even increase in strength when or if stuttering develops. By the same token, any conditions aversive for the parent concomitant with the child's nonfluency may generalize to the nonfluency and thus set the stage for a parental response which attempts to terminate the nonfluency through punishment. The parent may be conditioned to punish the child's nonfluency through negative reinforcement, since the parents' interruptions and corrections seem to terminate, momentarily, the aversive nonfluency.

The conditioning of parental responses of nonfluency may be an antecedent to parental responses associated with stuttering. The postponement of aversive consequences achieved by nonfluency repetition responses is also achieved by stuttering, perhaps in even more subtle ways. Finally, the early conditioning of silence and its functions as both a response and the occasion for a response already described for nonfluency, may have an antecedent relation to its functions in stuttering.

Contingencies for Changing Forms of Speech Responses

Studies by Johnson 9, 10) and by Bloodstein (1, 2, 3) have suggested ways in which nonfluency responses may change in form as stuttering develops. These changes in form of response reportedly occur in situations in which nonfluency is punished. The act of changing the form of the response may be the stuttering itself, made as an avoidance response. Further, their findings suggest that the auditory feedback of the vocal utterance to the stutterer has taken on aversive stimulus properties. These observations reflect not only the operant nature of stuttering behavior, but also suggest many specific variables and contingencies which should be submitted to investigation.

Paradigms and contingencies for study, which might reflect the acquisition and maintenance of stuttering responses, appear in Table 10–1. These paradigms may be descriptive of events which occur a number of times and in a number of settings and are only representative outlines for study. They are presented here to delineate classes of events which should be investigated. While they all suggest the descriptive contingencies which might be encountered in stuttering the first four are suggestive of a developmental sequence.

Number 1 in Table 10–1 shows the most frequently encountered event for children who do not later develop stuttering, that is, no differential reinforcement for the nonfluency. In this contingency, positive reinforcements are provided by listeners for the child's verbal behavior in general. If nonfluencies are emitted, they are usually followed by the positively reinforcing stimuli provided for the other properties of verbal behavior. The important feature is that nonfluency is not differentially reinforced as a class of responses. Nonfluency does not become a discriminative stimulus for differential listener activity. An interesting analysis would be that of tracing the decrement of nonfluency—especially when we recognize that nonfluency responses can be maintained by their connections to reinforcement schedules for other behavior. An analysis of these connections may in part reveal the dynamics of current nonfluencies commonly observed in the speech of nonstutterers.

Number 2 suggests that a child's nonfluent responses were punished. It has been suggested earlier that in studying this class of events, attention must be given to the mutual conditioning of the child and the parent—that is, the occasioning and reinforcing stimuli which control the forms of speech responses emitted by the child, and the occasioning and reinforcing stimuli which control the 'punishment' responses of a parent. This necessarily involves an historical and developmental analysis as well as an analysis of the current status of these variables.

Numbers 3 and 4 suggest that the punisher (listener) has become a conditioned aversive stimulus. As such, this listener may generate an 'emotional situation' and the child emits verbal responses (different forms of stuttering) which both terminate ongoing aversive stimuli emanating from the listener (frowns and grimaces) and attempt to avoid aversive consequences of the original nonfluency response (admonitions and corrections by listener). It can be observed that the original form of the nonfluency response is changed. In fact there may be several cycles of change in response form until a dynamic equilibrium evolves in which the positive reinforcements (listener's attention and social interaction) for a particular pattern of responses are more potent than

Table 10-1. Representative paradigms in stuttering.

Stimulus	Response	Consequence
1. Listener	Nonfluency	No differential reinforcement
2. Listener	Nonfluency	Punishment
3. Aversive listener (threat of punishment)	Changes nonfluency (struggle or silence)	(a) Avoids aversive stimuli of nonfluency and/or (b) Punishment for new response
4. Threatening audience	Changes response i.e., repetition to silence to prolonging, etc.	(a) Terminates ongoing aversive stimuli of punishing audience and/or (b) Punishment for new response
5. Sound of own voice (auditory feedback to stutterer)	Changes response	Terminates preceding aversive response form
6. Listener	Changes response	Positive reinforcement for changing response
7. Other S^D occasions (child may want something)	Stuttering	Positive reinforcement (gains attention) (given desired object)

either their aversive consequences or the reinforcements for changing the response form. Thus, clinically, we see the original, effortless repetition pattern degenerate into response forms that are characterized by muscular tension, bizarre articulatory postures and movements, facial grimaces, unusual phonation and respiratory patterns, and prolonged periods of silence.

Accompanying these behaviors may be other 'secondary' behaviors somewhat remote from the vocal mechanism, such as closing the eyes, stamping the foot, pounding the fist, or violently shaking the head. If these behaviors happened to be emitted when reinforcement was provided for the verbal response, they too may become a part of the stutterer's recurring repertoire.

Number 5 in Table 10–1 suggests that the stutterer is responding as his own listener to his aversive speech forms. By changing the form of his stuttering, from moment to moment, he is also terminating each preceding form. We see operating in these instances the contingencies of punishment and of negative reinforcement.

Numbers 6 and 7 suggest contingencies of positive reinforcement for maintaining stuttering. The possibility that stuttering is maintained by situations in which both positive and negative reinforcements appear has been suggested often in clinical reports. There is the feeling that the stutterer gains attention (positive reinforcement), develops an excuse for failure (negative reinforcement), and in general shifts the responsibilities for his inadequacies from himself to his stuttering and society. He has available a reason for his academic, social, and occupational failures. Williams (17) has very aptly described this shifting of responsibility by a further step. His discussion of the mystical 'it,' inside the stutterer, suggests that the stutterer is trying to relieve himself of any responsibility for emitting the undesirable behavior.

A very important, but as yet undefined, variable in these paradigms is the schedules of punishment and negative and positive reinforcements which are necessary to stabilize a stuttering response. We must know whether the stutterer's responses are reinforced each time they are emitted; whether reinforcements are provided in some uniform ratio system in terms of a given number of responses, or a given passage of time; or whether the scheduling of reinforcements is variable. Such information is important when the issues of extinction and control are considered. However, this information can become available only through appropriately designed studies.

Specific Occasioning, Aversive, and Reinforcing Stimuli

In a detailed analysis of stuttering, many contingencies suggest themselves as being worthy of study, e.g., 'silence,' both as a response and as a stimulus, 'sensory feedback' to the stutterer, and specific reinforcers and models of behavior provided by the listening community.

Silence. First, there is the silence in the stutterer's audience, which can constitute an occasion for the stutterer to start talking. This would be directly related to the earlier conditioning of talking in a specified sequence. However, for a person with a past history of stuttering, the silence of the listener may also have aversive stimulus properties. The silence of the listener has sometimes been an occasion on which his speech responses were punished.

Second, there is the silence of the stutterer. As a response his silence may delay or avoid punishment by his listeners (including himself) which has occasionally followed his utterances. However, stutterers have reported that during their silences they are often quite actively engaged in various types of covert behavior. They may rehearse their response, select and reject words they cannot say, wait for the listener to begin talking again, or make an effort at articulating without phonating. Therefore, in addition to being an avoidance response by stutterers, their silence can serve as a discriminative stimulus for the emission of these covert responses. It is possible that the positive and aversive properties of the listener's silence combine with the positive and aversive properties of the stutterer's silence to provide a complex occasion for the stutterer to emit various types of responses, overt, covert, verbal and nonverbal. The result may be a complicated vacillating response, depending in part on the current deprivations operating for the stutterer and in part on the reinforcing contingencies.

The previous paragraphs attempted to describe how some properties of silent periods during conversations may apply to the problem of stuttering. We suggest that the general properties of the silent periods in conversations are no different for stutterers than they are for people with no speech problem. However, there is a difference in frequency of occurrence or magnitude of strength of these properties of silence as a function of the history of reinforcement and punishment for the stutterer.

Multiple Reinforcement of Responses to Sensory Feedback. The nexus of stimulus conditions that surround the hearing of one's own utterances is common to both stutterer and nonstutterer. Again the difference is one of frequency of occurrence and magnitude.

When a speaker emits an utterance, he responds as his own listener to many properties of the speech sounds he has emitted, e.g., the content, the tempo, the pitch, and the relations of these to the preceding conversational content. He responds also to private stimuli such as tactual-kinesthetic sensations including articulatory and breathing movements. He responds to certain public stimuli such as facial expressions of listeners, their interjected utterances, and their general postural dispositions, including eye contact.

In considering the advanced stutterer as an observer of these public and private stimuli, we may examine some typical clinical reports. One stutterer has reported, 'If I pause for a comma, I'm lost,' indicating he is vaguely aware that his silence is related to his stuttering, as well as some heightened sensitivities to the feedback of his utterances. Another stutterer reports that he gets a tight feeling in his throat or feels out of breath. This stutterer has indicated a response to his tactual and kinesthetic sensations in emitting his utterance. Still other stutterers have reported they cannot say the first sound of a particular word, such as their name, indicating their response to a specific stimulus and reinforcement history.

These reports indicate that such individuals have in the past been taught by the controlling community to be more sensitive to these properties. Such admonitions as 'stop and start again,' 'think, before you talk,' 'take a deep breath and relax,' or 'if you can't say that word, say another one,' are all common examples of efforts of the community to correct the condition. A by-product of such efforts is a heightening of the stutterer's awareness of these concomitants of his speech.

The pairing of these public and private stimuli with these corrective admonitions may set the stage for very complex conditioning. For example, a particular stimulus, such as a sensation of articulatory movement, may become aversive because of its connections with community admonitions. The stut-

terer may then emit a response (some form of stuttering) which terminates these aversive articulatory sensations, thus maintaining his stuttering through negative reinforcement.

Paradoxically, the positive reinforcements provided by the community for attending to one's articulation and breathing, for stopping and starting and repeating utterances, and for circumlocutions may also partially account for the maintenance of these behaviors in stuttering. By providing positive reinforcement for these behaviors, the community actually teaches the stutterer to stutter in certain specific ways. However, the positive reinforcements provided by listeners for each single response form may also increase the frequency of *changing the response form* as well as the frequency of emission of one particular class of response. The agents of positive reinforcement for a particular form of response may unknowingly be strengthening the behavior of shifting rapidly from one class of responses to another, thus further endangering fluency.

It is possible that the very same behaviors described above could be emitted because they terminate the aversive conditions associated with immediately preceding forms of stuttering. The stutterer may rapidly change his forms of stuttering responses (in an almost ritualistic pattern) because each succeeding response form (prolonging, repeating, silence, etc.) terminates the immediately preceding aversive form. These responses may also be emitted to terminate aversive stimuli emanating from his listener, such as 'tense waiting,' or 'empathic mouthing' of the word.

There is the likelihood that positive reinforcement and negative reinforcement coexist in maintaining stuttering responses. The contrapuntal operation of these two reinforcement paradigms may exert a multiple control over stuttering. Their multiple strength is quite different from the controls exerted by each of these contingencies individually or in summated series. An analysis of these two different conditioning paradigms in series may reveal the variables controlling the stutterer's detailed alternation of speech responses, i.e., silence, rapid repetition of first sound, silence, prolonging. etc.

Self-Reinforcement

Thus far we have limited our discussion to the community as the agent of positive and negative reinforcement. However, just as a stutterer may reinforce another speaker, he may reinforce himself. We observe in the early development of speech in infants that single utterances appear sometimes to act as self-reinforcers. That is, a child may repeat sequences of similar sounds, or similar phrases or similar sentences, following the first emission. Such self-reinforcement appears to be interrupted easily, However, at a later age such self-reinforcement is more obvious. At the age of three to four years, before the child has learned to conceal his verbal behavior and while he is still playing alone, we may observe him borrowing from the parent expressions that imply positive or negative reinforcement or punishment. He may be talking aloud and using such terms as 'that's a good boy,' 'no, no, you can't,' 'wait till Daddy comes home,' or inflections which parrot adult vocal patterns. We may observe this same behavior in adults when they 'think out loud' or begin to talk to themselves during prolonged periods of isolation. We may infer from these observations that such self-reinforcement for verbal behavior goes on covertly for all speakers, including stutterers.

Because of its subtlety as a controlling variable, the covert reinforcing or aversive event is of special interest for the problem of stuttering. Quite often during clinical interviews, stutterers have been heard to report that as long as they hear themselves talking, they feel that they can go on emitting speech. Frequently their emissions of speech are short, rapid bursts of perseverative utterances which serve to 'keep their motor running.' Such reports suggest that stutterers reinforce themselves in emitting a chain of verbal responses. On the other hand, stutterers have reported the accumulation of 'anticipation' and 'dread' of stuttering and that they covertly verbalize these ideas. The result is often a long period of silence which sometimes terminates such covert verbalizing. On other occasions they emit speech 'to get it over with,' suggesting that their utterance terminates their aversive 'anticipation.'

Sometimes the stutterer's repetitions and prolongations of the first sounds of words seem to postpone or avoid more aversive forms of stuttering characterized by extreme muscular tension and silence. As the stutterer emits his verbal responses containing pauses and repetitions of fragments of words he may be: (a) positively reinforced by the sound of his voice, or (b) threatened by the accumulation of aversive effects of his stuttering response. The positive and negative self-reinforcing characteristics of his own voice may also exert control over his emissions of alternating forms of verbal responses.

Respondent Conditioning

Certain classes of responses that covary with stuttering are as yet poorly understood and therefore of indeterminate importance. These classes may be roughly defined as autonomic or visceral reactions such as flushing, perspiring, tremors, and changes in respiratory depth and rate. It appears that these responses can be elicited by initially neutral stimulus patterns through the process of classical conditioning. The appearance of such autonomic accompaniments to operant behavior is common in situations involving punishment or avoidance conditioning. This has been observed in both human and animal experiments. The precise relationship between operant and classical conditioning has not been defined experimentally. Skinner has implied that there is an antecedent-consequent relationship between respondent conditioning and operant conditioning such as in avoidance, escape, and punishment (*15,* pp. 160–193). It would not serve our purpose to go into the details of what is called respondent-operant overlap conditioning except to suggest that this may be one model for future investigation of the interaction of positive and negative reinforcement in maintaining stuttering.

IMPLICATIONS FOR RESEARCH ON THERAPY

Because these formulations are in a very early stage, and because experimentation to support these ideas has yet to be done, the application of principles of operant behavior to therapy must be approached with an attitude of skepticism. Goldiamond has already demonstrated that stuttering can be manipulated through operant conditioning techniques (*7, 8),* and that it may therefore be viewed as operant behavior under some conditions. The variables he selected to use as reinforcing and (or) discriminative stimuli seemed to be easily available for laboratory manipulation, and were directly related to the demonstrative nature of his projects.

However, clinicians have also been demonstrating the operant nature of stuttering and of their clinical transactions for some time. These 'clinical demonstrations' of operant conditioning, although not based specifically on laboratory-derived principles, show a great deal of similarity to the procedures and data of the laboratory. Both the clinician and the experimenter are empirical in their attitude. Both introduce independent variables and analyze the occasions for responses. Both attempt to shape behavior and both observe relations between the stutterer's responses and consequent reactions in the stutterer's listening community. Therefore, it is felt that in addition to studies like Goldiamond's, attempts should be made to examine those variables encountered in the clinical problem of stuttering. The study of variables which are relevant (in content) to the clinical problem for the stutterer and for the clinician as reinforcing or discriminative stimuli may provide significant content for later application to therapeutic procedures. It seems reasonable to extend the techniques for such study to include the clinical interview as a basic experimental vehicle. As such, the principles of operant behavioral analysis and manipulation can be brought closer to the problem of stuttering as it is encountered by clinician and stutterer.

Perhaps as clinicians we should immediately come to peace with ourselves as men of good will by acknowledging that all therapy is a form of controlling behavior. Recent research evidence supporting this statement has been summarized and presented by Kanfer *(11, 12)*, Krasner *(13)*, and Salzinger and Pisoni *(14)*. It has been demonstrated that the content of verbal behavior of individuals in a variety of interview, therapeutic, and conversational situations can be controlled by the verbal responses emitted by their interviewers. Such seemingly nondirective comments as 'yes' or 'uh-huh' by the interviewer have been shown to be powerful reinforcing stimuli. It is no longer an issue of control versus no control by the clinician. It is now an issue of what form the controls take, whether they are valid and well founded in principle, and whether they are compatible with the ethical values of our culture.

When contingencies such as those already described have been identified in the behavior of the stutterer, we have available the raw materials for therapeutic manipulation. Such manipulations in general consist of attempts by the clinician to control the stutterer's environment. The clinician can make available to him or withhold from him those specific occasions and reinforcing contingencies which are related to the emission and extinction of his stuttering responses. In a sense, the clinician may recreate for the stutterer a small sample of his life situation in terms of controlling variables. The clinician himself becomes a part of that life situation by becoming the chief source of occasions and reinforcements for speech. The scope of this controlled environment cannot now be defined.

It is possible that experimentation on this particular topic may reveal the efficacy of total control and reconditioning in an isolated environment where all variables are systematically introduced. The technique of removing the stutterer from the complexities of a punishing society for purposes of gradual reconditioning is not too different from those procedures employed in hospitalizing patients with medical and psychiatric disorders. The advantages and disadvantages of such a technique, of course, remain to be determined through research.

The clinician has available discriminative stimuli and reinforcing stimuli only to the extent that his analysis of the history and current behavior of the stutterer is both accurate and exhaustive. Such analysis must include the practices of those members of the community who commonly reinforce the stutterer's speech behavior, e.g., parents, friends, teachers. These reinforcing practices of listeners (including the stutterer) must not be regarded as fixed controlling techniques. They are behavior patterns that have been acquired and that may therefore be amenable to re-education also. We must determine how the responses of these listeners are acquired and maintained, and how they can be modified. One major issue here is whether our direct modification of the stutterer's forms of stuttering have any effect on the listener's reinforcing practices. In many cases, the clinician may find it more profitable to deal with the stutterer's listening community than with the stutterer.

If we retain the viewpoint that the behavior of the stutterer represents only a part of the total set of transactions between him and his community, and if we can identify the functions of the community (including clinicians) in these transactions, our experimental analyses will contribute to the understanding of social behavior as well as to the problem of stuttering.

SUMMARY

Nonfluency and stuttering are examined in the framework of operant conditioning. Relations are hypothesized between repetitions in speech and the following variables:

a.   Listeners' 'attending' behavior.

b.   Coincidental reinforcements for other behavior.

c.   States of deprivation.

d.   Avoidance of aversive stimuli.

e.   Conversational pauses, interruptions, and silence.

f.   Self-editing and correcting.

With regard to stuttering the following propositions are offered:

a.   A continuity exists between stuttering and non-fluency.

b.   An operant definition of stuttering includes the stimulus and reinforcement history of specific forms of responses.

c.   Stuttering is maintained by positive and negative reinforcements on complex, multiple schedules.

Events relevant to stuttering include:

a.   Antecedent conditioning during nonfluency.

b.   Aversive stimuli from listeners.

c.   Changes in the form of stuttering.

d.   'Silence' as a stimulus and as a response.

e.   Sensory feedback to the stutterer.

f.   Reinforcers and models of behavior provided by the community.

The clinical interview may provide an opportunity for experiments in operant conditioning to test these interpretations of stuttering.

REFERENCES

1. Bloodstein, O., The development of stuttering: I. Changes in nine basic features. *J. Speech Hearing Dis.,* 25, 1960, 219–237.

2. Bloodstein, O., The development of stuttering: II. Developmental phases. *J. Speech Hearing Dis.,* 25, 1960, 366–376.

3. Bloodstein, O., The development of stuttering: III. Theoretical and clinical implications. *J. Speech Hearing Dis.,* 26, 1961, 67–82.

4. Davis, Dorothy M., The relation of repetitions in the speech of young children to certain measures of language maturity and situational factors. Part I. *J. Speech Dis.,* 4, 1939, 303–318.

5. Davis, Dorothy M., The relation of repetitions in the speech of young children to certain measures of language maturity and situational factors. Part II. *J. Speech Dis.,* 5, 1940, 235–241.

6. Davis, Dorothy M., The relation of repetitions in the speech of young children to certain measures of language maturity and situational factors. Part III. *J. Speech Dis.,* 5, 1940, 242–246.

7. Goldiamond, I., Blocked speech communication and delayed feed-back: An experimental design. Technical Report No. 1, Progress Report, February, 1960. Operational Applications Laboratory, Air Force Cambridge Research Center, Bedford, Massachusetts.

8. Goldiamond, I., The temporal development of fluent and blocked speech communication. Final Report and Technical Report Nos. 2, 3, 4. September, 1960. Operational Applications Laboratory, Air Force Cambridge Research Center, Bedford Massachusetts.

9. Johnson, W., The role of evaluation in stuttering behavior. *J. Speech Dis.,* 3, 1938, 85–89.

10. Johnson, W., A study of the onset and development of stuttering. *J. Speech Dis.,* 7, 1942, 251–257.

11. Kanfer, F. H., Verbal rate, content, and adjustment ratings in experimentally structured interviews. *J. abnorm (soc.) Psychol.,* 58, 1959, 305–311.

12. Kanfer, F., Phillips, J., Matarazzo, J., and Saslow, G., Experimental modification of interviewer content in standardized interviews. *J. cons. Psychol.,* 24, 1960, 528–536.

13. Krasner, L., Studies of the conditioning of verbal behavior. *Psychol. Bull.,* 55, 1958, 148–170.

14. Salzinger, K., and Pisoni, S., Reinforcement of verbal affect responses of normal subjects during the interview. *J. abnorm. (soc.)Psychol.,* 60, 1960, 127–130.

15. Skinner, B. F., *Science and Human Behavior.* New York: Macmillan, 1953.

16. Skinner, B. F., *Verbal Behavior.* New York: Appleton-Century-Crofts, Inc., 1957.

17. Williams, D. E., A point of view about 'Stuttering.' *J. Speech Hearing Dis.,* 22, 1957, 390–397.

18. Winitz, H., Repetitions in the vocalizations and speech of children in the first two years of life. *J. Speech Hearing Dis.,* Monog. Supplement No. 7, 1961, 55–62.

An Operant Perspective

George H. Shames

Looking back on something that I said or wrote or identified with some 20 years ago becomes a very personal encounter with myself, as it must be for many of the other contributors in this book. As I do so I find myself recapturing some essences of that time. If necessity is considered the mother of invention, then frustration should be considered the grandparent, insofar as my understandings of speech pathology, speech therapy, and stuttering in particular were concerned. I was reared, professionally speaking, with the ideas and concepts about stuttering of Johnson, Van Riper, Travis, Bryngelson, and numerous others who were researching, writing, and sharing their ideas. These were the models of the era. It was a time when the mysteries of therapy were not being frequently shared or openly scrutinized. Persuasive rhetoric and faith in authority were dominant, perhaps as they still are in guiding us in our thinking. It was a time when the etiology of stuttering was receiving a lot of research attention; when therapy for young children was enjoying a lot of success (as it still does); but alas, when the outcome of therapy for the more advanced stages of the problem was generally poor. When adult stutterers were successful in modifying their stuttering we were uncertain whether it was because of the specific validity of the therapeutic tactic; because of the novelty of the therapy; because of the readiness, motivation, and persistence of the stutterer to take on the problem; because of the stutterer's supportive environment and family; or because of the charisma and commitment of the therapist. As both an educator and a clinician this was a period of discomfort.

The 1963 paper with Dr. Sherrick was itself a serendipitous happening. I was on a two-year leave of absence from the University of Pittsburgh, learning about operant conditioning by working in an animal laboratory. My task was to apply that perspective to gaining an understanding of a specific therapy for language problems in aphasic children. As these animal laboratory experiences started to blend with my background as a clinician in both psychology and speech pathology, I began a mental exercise of translating back and forth between the principles of operant conditioning and our more traditional and clinical views of the problem of stuttering. This mental exercise was shared with my office mate, Carl Sherrick, and eventually resulted in our paper published in the *Journal of*

Speech and Hearing Disorders in 1963 titled "A discussion of nonfluency and stuttering as operant behavior."

During this period there were numerous controversies over the application of operant conditioning principles and tactics to the problem of stuttering. These controversies focused on certain general aspects of behaviorism, such as dealing only with overt behavior (when as clinicians we knew that there were many covert aspects to stuttering); questioning the pertinence of the construct of anxiety in reducing stuttering frequency (when as theorists and clinicians we had adopted anxiety as a theoretical cornerstone and foundation for the problem of stuttering); using contingent aversive stimulation (punishment) to demonstrate that stuttering could be reduced by such tactics (when as clinicians and theorists we felt that punishment generated rather than reduced the problem); and the use of a DAF machine, or delayed auditory feedback device (which often was interpreted as nothing more than a distraction technique).

As I approached this review task, I asked myself if I would say the same things today. I, therefore, scrutinized the paper, idea by idea, and now provide these reactions.

The idea that behavior is strengthened or weakened as a function of the consequence generated by that behavior is not, never was, and never was meant to be questioned by that paper. The basic questions addressed whether it is of value to view normal disfluencies and stuttering as no more than behavior.

Generally, the years have demonstrated that such a premise does indeed have value, not necessarily because of its validity, but because of the thinking and research that it may have generated. In retrospect it appears to have been a provocative notion.

The ideas in the 1963 paper were the impetus for three major research programs at the University of Pittsburgh. One was a program that focused on therapy for adult stutterers from 1966 to 1971. That research primarily demonstrated that principles of operant conditioning could be clinically operationalized and were useful in changing the content of what stutterers talked about during clinical interviews. That research also demonstrated that the frequency of stuttering decreased in association with these changes. In a sense it was a program of research that clinically implemented Johnson's semantic theory of stuttering. By addressing stutterers' beliefs as evidenced through their overt utterances during interviews through operant conditioning tactics, we accomplished at least two things and possibly a third. One was a demonstration that the content of what people spoke about could be manipulated through operant conditioning tactics. The second was providing some support for Johnson's ideas about the semantic aspects of the problem, and the third was a possible prototype for counseling stutterers in this fashion. Another series of projects applied operant conditioning tactics to Van Riper's cancellation therapy. The results of these studies showed that such tactics resulted in dramatic reductions in the overt frequency of stuttering to the point that cancellation procedures became inoperative. This finding was interpreted generally as an instrumental punishment process.

Postscript 10

The second major research program from 1972 to 1975 addressed therapy for children. These projects looked at the nature of the verbal interactions between parents and their stuttering children. In these projects the experimental clinician would "mirror image" that interaction and do just the opposite of what was observed during the parent-child interaction. This technique was based on the hypothesis that the child's stuttering was being maintained by that interaction and that a reversal of that interaction would reduce the child's stuttering. The hypothesis was proven to be true, and the therapy did result in reductions in stuttering by the children. The parents were then trained in these new interactions for carry-over into the child's home.

Finally, this initial thinking led to the conceptualization, research into, and development of a therapy program that has come to be known as Stutter-Free Speech. This therapy is composed of five overlapping sequences or phases. Each phase has as its underlying base various principles of operant conditioning and behavior modification. The first phase of Volitional Control, when it employs the DAF machine, is based on a paradigm of negative reinforcement. The second phase, Self Responsibility, is based on tactics of self reinforcement. The third phase, Environmental Transfer, is based on behavioral contracting and positive reinforcement. The fourth phase of Training in Unmonitored Speech is based on processes of generalization and positive reinforcement. The fifth phase involves follow-up studies to determine the long-term durability and impact of changes observed during therapy. From a purely heuristic standpoint this particular publication seems to have had some significant impact on our own research and clinical applications. Generally the ideas and hypotheses stated in the 1963 paper still stand, with an apparent need for revision.

The original ideas about the contingencies operating in normal disfluency still appear to be valid and open to investigation. Except for the need to pause for respiratory purposes, many forms of disfluency ("normal" or "nonnormal") appear to have a conditioning component. Whether it is totally operant or partially classical conditioning is yet to be determined.

It was hypothesized at the time (1963) that early babbling, the repetitive chain of syllable utterances observed in infants, may represent one of the origins of what later is termed disfluency in speech. It was felt that these and later repetitions could persist and be conditioned under certain circumstances of deprivation and aversive stimulation. There have been strong suggestions that the burden of acquiring normal language skills and facility could also be a factor in persistent disfluency (even as it might be observed in adults who are learning a new foreign language). The processes of editing and composing our utterances are closely related to this contingency and are also the occasions for normal disfluency. It was also suggested that conversational pauses, interruptions, and silence are occasions for disfluency.

At this writing I offer an additional hypothesis that expands and impacts on these possible origins of disfluency. However, this is a hypothesis about fluency rather than disfluency. There is a question in my mind as to whether we might be dealing with two classes of responses (disfluency and fluency) that may have different origins, that may co-exist in our repertoires but are incompatible in terms of simultaneous emission. If you emit a disfluency (a repetition, interjection, or any disruption of the smooth flow of a speech utterance) you cannot at the same time emit a fluent utterance. However, fluent utterances are not merely the passive results of the absence of disfluencies in utterances. Likewise, disfluent utterances are not merely the passive result of the absence of fluent utterances. The question is whether we are dealing with one class of responses or two classes of responses, each with a different origin and conditioning history. Just as it was suggested in 1963 that the early repetitive babbling of infants may have been one of the origins of disfluency, it is now being suggested that "fluency" (the smooth, uninterrupted forward flow of a speech utterance) may have some of its origins in the early "jargon" activities of children around 18 months of age. Jargon is a normal phase of speech development. It sounds like "speech play," almost like a rehearsal phase for fluent speech. It is characterized by smooth emissions of different syllables, containing adult-like inflections, stress, and melody. It sounds like a chain of nonsense syllables. But it also sounds like adult phrases and conversation in terms of stress and accent and variations in loudness. It is fluent, melodic, and usually humorous and beguiling. As adults we usually say that it has no meaning, but we do not really know what these variations of stress and loudness mean to the child. Perhaps it means nothing, but perhaps it means a great deal in terms of emotion and feelings. It certainly generates feelings in the adults who hear it. I hypothesize here that fluency may have a history of reinforcement with origins in jargoning by parents that may be quite different from the conditioning history of disfluencies, which may be associated with repetitive babbling. Each is prelinguistic, and each may have positive (and occasionally negative) feelings associated with it. Long-term observations of babbling and jargon and their relationships to fluency and disfluency during later linguistic development could shed some light on the relative contributions of each to the later development of disfluent and stuttered speech.

Perhaps the most controversial aspect of the 1963 Shames and Sherrick paper focuses on the operant nature of stuttering. The hypotheses and contingencies offered in 1963 still seem valid. However, there is a need to discuss more broadly and in greater depth events antecedent to stuttering, and the role of feelings and emotions in the problem. We can identify focal points of this controversy rather easily. There were at least three points of view about the nature of conditioning in stuttering. One is that stuttering is originally classically conditioned, much like Pavlovian conditioning. An instance of speech is conditioned to an emotional negative stimulus, and speech breaks down. A second view is the purely instrumental and/or operant view wherein the effect of a previously conditioned disfluency maintains the disfluency. These are illustrated in the work of Wischner (1958) on anxiety reduction, Seigel (1970) on punishment, Flanagan,

Postscript 10

et al. (1958), and Shames and Sherrick (1963). The third view is characterized by the Brutten and Shoemaker (1967) two-factor theory wherein the primary speech characteristics of stuttering (repetitions, pauses, etc.) are viewed as being classically conditioned through negative emotionality, and the secondary behaviors (forcing, facial gestures, etc.) are viewed as being operantly conditioned as a function of the effects of these secondary behaviors. I would like to expand on one paragraph in the 1963 paper that refers to the operant-respondent overlap. The basic questions for me are: Do feelings and emotions (given the difficulty in measuring and quantifying them) influence behavior, either positively or negatively? Can we ignore feelings when we deal with behavior? Do feelings mobilize a person to behave in certain ways? Can we ever separate antecedent feelings and consequent effects from behavior in general and in dealing with stuttering in particular? It is my feeling that behavior involves both an emotional component and an effect component, and trying to isolate or weight these factors in relation to behavior distorts the total process. Attempts to separate respondent conditioning from operant conditioning may provide an incomplete portrayal of human behavior. Miller (1969), Kimmel (1967), and Katkin and Murray (1968) amply demonstrated that visceral and autonomic responses that had been thought of only as conditionable through classical conditioning could be instrumentally conditioned. From the field of biofeedback we are learning that the distinctions between classical and instrumental conditioning break down, and that we may have a chain of antecedent and consequent events that provide a broader, more cohesive, and interactive account of the dynamics of conditioning. As an explanation for viewing stuttering we need a broader perspective that embraces both classical and instrumental conditioning as part of a unified process.

Skinner (1953) discusses the role of emotions in understanding behavior by talking about "emotional operations." He points out that it is more productive to talk about emotional states as descriptive events that are antecedent to behavior rather than as an internal attribute of the behaving organism. It is in this direction of describing antecedent events that the original Shames and Sherrick paper should be expanded, as a way of making the emotional component more prominent and functional in the operant paradigm of viewing stuttering.

Skinner's discussion goes back to the original James-Lange theory that characterized the behavior, the emotion, and an external event as three links of a causal chain. This theory defined feeling as something physiological that we become aware of, such as the responses of smooth muscles and glands in blushing, weeping, sweating, salivating, and goose bumps. However, he goes on to point out that these responses (and feelings) are difficult to physiologically distinguish from one another in terms of different categories of emotions, and often also occur in nonemotional circumstances such as after heavy exercise or in a chilly wind. It has not been possible to specify a given set of physiological responses or expressive responses (laughing, growling, crying, etc.) as characteristic of particular emotions. In some instances these operations appear to relate directly to "emotional behavior." For example, restraint or deprivation may interrupt a sequence of behaviors that has a strong history of emission and reinforcement (i.e., expecting to open with your key a door that has been bolted results in frustration or rage; the loneliness of a heretofore sociable and amiable man who is alone with strangers).

Skinner goes on to talk about emotion as a predisposition to behave in certain ways. That is, we can categorize (adjectively) the emotions and predict with some degree of probability that a person will behave in a certain way (fear leads to avoidance; love leads to caresses and approach; anger leads to striking out). These behaviors, in turn, may be reinforced by their consequences or effects. However, there is significant variability in what behaviors will be expressed under the same circumstances, even for the same person.

Skinner's conclusion is that we do not advance the practical technology of emotion by conceiving of it as an inner state of human beings. A problem is not solved by saying that some feature of one's behavior is due to frustration or anxiety. We also need to be told how the anxiety has been induced and how it may be altered. "We find ourselves dealing with two events—the emotional behavior and the manipulable conditions of which that behavior is a function." He, of course, is referring to the descriptive antecedent events and the consequent, reinforcing events of the behavior. This conceptualization can be extended to the problem of stuttering.

It appears that many of the antecedent events occurring in the development and maintenance of stuttering are aversive (parental scolding, correction of speech, embarrassment of parents, etc.). Originally neutral events that become conditioned aversive stimuli (see Brutten's chapter) set up negative reinforcement as a powerful paradigm in stuttering. Children learn to avoid or escape from the aversive condition. Much of stuttering behavior may be viewed in this way. However, the chain of events does not terminate merely with stimulus substitution. We must also look at the effects of the behavior that the conditioned aversive stimulus evokes. The child who "says it again" to avoid his parents' admonitions not only avoided the aversive stimulus (effect number one) but also may be lavished with praise for doing so (effect number two).

Stimulus substitution and classical conditioning (as viewed by the Brutten and Shoemaker two-factor theory) may be an important process in the onset, development, and maintenance of stuttering. However, the recent research in the technology of stress management and biofeedback suggests that classical conditioning isn't the only way to affect the responses of the autonomic nervous system. But this research notwithstanding, this phase of the conditioning paradigm, which focuses on events antecedent to the behavior, cannot be isolated as the sole explanation of the stutterer's primary and secondary behaviors. The effects of the behavior are there as part of a chain of events. The speakers and listeners hear and react to the stuttered speech, and provide a contingent consequence that is a critical part of the chain of events.

Postscript   10

The speaker himself may provide antecedent events as well as consequences. Antecedent events, for stutterers as well as for all of us, are not simply external events such as bolted doors that can be physically unlocked or people who can be avoided. As human beings, our thoughts and anticipations and goals (our cognition) constitute powerful events that are antecedent to our behaviors, including stuttering behaviors. For stutterers some antecedent events are followed by fluent speech, while other antecedent events are followed by stuttered speech. Some of these events are external, such as a person, or place, or social circumstance. Some are covert in the form of thoughts and expectations and are not easily observed. Our task, in part, is to describe both the external events and the covert events (sensations, thoughts, feelings) as part of a chain of events that are in turn followed by speech behaviors (stuttered or fluent) that in turn generate consequences (overt and covert) which affect their appearance. Stutterers and researchers alike may need to be trained in such observations to determine the consistency of their linkages. For example, is there a consistent linkage among:

> *Antecedent Events.* The presence of a stutterer's father; the thought by the stutterer that he will stutter.
>
> *Behavior.* An emission of stuttered speech by the stutterer.
>
> *Consequence.* Embarrassment by the father by looking away and shaking his head; cessation of talking by the stutterer

In this example, we can focus on manipulating the antecedent behaviors (avoid the father; substitute other thoughts) and/or the consequent events (have the father maintain eye contact; have the stutterer continue talking) in trying to influence the emission of stuttering. We can also teach the stutterer to emit behaviors that are incompatible with stuttering, which in turn generates other consequences that weaken the strength of the antecedent events to seemingly evoke the stuttering behavior. Such behavioral substitutions can have powerful effects on the stutterer's expectations and anticipations (covert antecedent events or overt if trained in self-reporting) in the presence of these other conditioned antecedent events (the father's presence). Probing for self reports and changes in self reports prior to emitting the substituted behavior and positive verbal reinforcement from a clinician for such verbal reporting by the stutterer may form the basis for "counseling." However, the counseling in this case has a focus on "fluent speaking" rather than on stuttering, its aversive antecedents, and its aversive consequences. Through self-reporting the stutterer can make available to himself some of those emotional antecedents of his talking behavior, which then become manipulable by arranging positive and negative contingencies for their emission. In these cases, the verbal antecedent event becomes verbal behavior about feelings that generates consequences that may weaken or strengthen them and at the least render them more understandable. It is this total chain of events, not a segmentation of its parts, that may eventually account for the conditioning of stuttering. The answers may lie in the detailed descriptions of those events that precede and follow the speech behaviors that we wish to study. Appropriate experimental procedures to study their unique effects will then verify their role in this problem.

REFERENCES

Brutten, E. J., & Shoemaker, D. J. (1960). The modification of stuttering. Englewood Cliffs, NJ: Prentice-Hall.

Flanagan, B., Goldiamond, I., & Azrin, N. (1958). Operant stuttering: The control of stuttering behavior through response-contingent consequences. *Journal of Experimental Analytical Behavior, 1,* 173–77.

Kimmel, H. D. (1967). Instrumental conditioning of automatically mediated behavior. *Psychological Bulletin, 67,* 337–45.

Miller, N. E. (1969). Learning of viseral and glandular responses, *Science, 163,* 434–435.

Seigel, G. M. (1970). Punishment, stuttering and disfluency. *Journal of Speech and Hearing Research, 13,* 677–714.

Shames, G. H., & Sherrick, C. E. (1963). A discussion of nonfluency and stuttering as operant behavior. *Journal of Speech and Hearing Disorders, 28,* No. 1, 3–18.

Skinner, B. F. (1953). Science and human behavior. New York: MacMillan.

Wischner, G. (1958). Stuttering behavior and learning: A preliminary theoretical formulation. *Journal of Speech and Hearing Disorders, 15,* 324–335.

PART THREE

CLINICAL MANAGEMENT

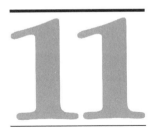

Overview to Part Three: The Roles of the Client and the Clinician during Therapy

George H. Shames and Herbert Rubin

Overview to Part Three: The Roles of the Client and the Clinician during Therapy

George H. Shames and Herbert Rubin

Therapy is a temporary or finite process in which clients come for support and guidance as they contemplate changing about themselves something they don't like. It is unlike any other interpersonal relationship they may have experienced in that both members of the dyad concern themselves primarily with one member. It is the needs, feelings, thoughts, attitudes, and actions of the client that predominate. For the client, therapy means always being in the hot seat; for the therapist it means always responding in terms of the client.

CLIENT'S EXPECTATIONS

Each participant in the therapeutic relationship brings to that relationship a set of individual expectations regarding the other member(s), the process, and the outcome. Depending on the client's history with stuttering and with prior therapy, he may enter the relationship with a mixture of skepticism and hope. The skepticism may be the expression of both fear of failure and fear of success. Although the fear of failure may be self-evident, the fear of success reflects more deeply embedded issues that will be discussed in greater detail at the end of this section. While clients vary, each has more or less specific expectations of where their clinician falls on each of a number of continua: competence, supportiveness, trustworthiness, honesty, concern (caring), authoritativeness, and respectfulness. To what extent is it important for the clinician to address these expectations explicitly in terms of their validity and of the needs of the client? Some of these expectations maintain the defensive and coping strategies of the client and, therefore, serve to perpetuate the problem, while others are more conducive to the therapeutic process. In addition to expecting the clinician to be a certain kind of person, the client has expectations regarding the process of therapy. They expect it to be briefer than it usually is; they expect to be treated more as a passive than an active participant (very often this reduces to a "You tell me and I'll do it" attitude); they expect more instruction and less counseling;

they expect more focus on behavior than on attitude. They expect a consistent progression of tangible evidence of improvement. In a sense these expectations place the responsibility for the success or failure of the therapy directly at the feet of the clinician. Whatever the way clinicians choose to deal with these expectations it is incumbent upon them to recognize and to respect the feelings and perceptions of the client about to enter therapy.

Just as clients come with expectations, therapy may present for them a number of experiences they did not expect that can affect the process or the therapeutic relationship profoundly. Some of these experiences may be pleasant for the client, while others may be aversive; either may be frightening. However, all of them may have therapeutic value. When people work together closely toward a common goal the initial ambiguity with which they perceive each other is likely to give way to a partnership of well-defined roles. The interdependency of the therapeutic relationship commonly results in bonds of mutual affection. What we mean by this is that two people working together toward a common goal are likely to come to care about one another. In the context of this caring the stutterer can become more comfortable in assuming greater responsibility for the conduct of therapy, rather than relinquishing that responsibility to the clinician.

One of the positive consequences of assuming responsibility is a feeling of control, a generally unfamiliar feeling for a stutterer who has been shy, withdrawn, tentative about speaking, quick to avoid both words and situations, and approaching the world from a posture of weakness and apology. By contrast, as he begins to explore and to accept his responsibilities, he will do so in one or more of a number of ways, all of which represent salutary changes in lifestyle. Some of these changes include assertiveness, humor, spontaneity, access to and expression of feeling, dealing with hostility, socialization, and sense of self-worth. Let us now consider each of these changes for which the stutterer may be unprepared.

Many stutterers have suffered in silence, inhibited expressing what they have to say, convinced that their passivity will protect them from rejection. While demonstrated fluency can facilitate assertiveness it is also true that speaking one's mind can facilitate fluency.

Stuttering can narrow one's perspective so that most of a stutterer's life experiences are perceived in terms of that problem. As a result, the light side of life cannot be appreciated or enjoyed. Humor is a great coping mechanism, as Norman Cousins demonstrated in *Anatomy of an Illness* (1981) and reflects one of the unexpected benefits of a shift in perspective.

A very real sense of freedom emerges as the stutterer moves from constant vigilance of his behavior and the perceived effects on others to a more spontaneous way of relating. Both the quantity and quality of socializing improves as the stutterer expands his interpersonal network. He finds himself talking more and enjoying it more.

Our experience has been that stutterers commonly defend against and deny their feelings, both positive and negative. When asked how they feel about a report of being teased, for example, they often say "I don't care," or "I'm used to it," as though it were too painful to face. Perhaps even more threatening than experiencing the feeling is what might happen if they express it; the injury they might inflict, the possible retaliation, the consequence of rejection if they expressed a positive feeling. When the clinician is sensitive to and reflects the feelings of the stutterer, thereby communicating his or her acceptance of the feeling, the stutterer can become freer first to acknowledge both positive and negative affect and then to understand it and to explore ways of expressing it.

Hostility deserves a special consideration in this context since it has been hypothesized that the behavior of stuttering is an indirect expression of hostility (Abbott, 1947). Travis (1957) suggests that the act of stuttering inhibits the awareness and expression of such unacceptable feelings. Conversely, when stutterers do express their anger in words they are invariably fluent, testifying to the close relationship between stuttering and the inhibition of hostility.

Speech is primarily a social behavior, and therefore any increase in the amount or the fluency of speech can be expected to enhance a stutterer's social network. Different therapists approach the goal of increased socialization in different ways: directly, via contract or assignment; or indirectly, as an outgrowth of the client's spontaneous social interactions. Although traditionally we look at the "real world" as that outside of the clinical session, it is possible alternatively to view the relationship between client and clinician as the more real in the sense that it is immediate, the here and now. Therapy can be viewed as a social interaction. It is a special case of social interaction in that the clinician provides what others cannot be relied upon to give: honesty, support, well-defined availability, and persistence. The stutterer can then take from this special therapeutic relationship the honesty, persistence, and generally healthy attitudes into his nontherapeutic social network. We have talked so far about social reality. However, there is also a personal reality, our sense of self and of self-worth, which is profoundly related to the more public world. Stutterers generally approach therapy with rather low self-esteem and a sense of social inadequacy, and emerge from a successful therapeutic experience valuing themselves, as they have been valued by their therapists.

CHANGES IN ATTITUDES AND BEHAVIOR

One of the long-term ongoing controversies among clinicians has been the significance of attitude change and the extent to which it relates to behavioral change in fluency. While we find differences of opinion regarding the significance of attitude change in therapy, no one denies that attitudes do change. The controversy can be broken down into five major categories: (1) Whether attitude change is ever necessary or desirable, (2) Whether most stutterers present the same attitudes as they enter therapy, (3) Whether attitude must be worked on directly in therapy, (4) Which comes first, attitude or behavior change, and finally (5) Do different therapies identify the same goals of attitude change?

Behaviorists traditionally work only with what they can manipulate and measure directly. This means that their basic data are the overt frequencies of behavior that are a function of experimentally controllable events. Goldiamond (1965) and Siegel and Martin (1968) have demonstrated in the laboratory that the overt frequency of stuttering can be reduced without direct attention to attitudes and feelings. We will see later in this section how this perspective has been extended into the clinical context by Ryan (operant-based therapy) and Webster (precision fluency shaping), whose therapies focus solely on behavioral management. The implication of their work is that changing the speech behavior of the stutterer is all that is necessary. Conversely, contributors like Rogers (client-centered counseling), Travis (psychoanalysis), and Wolpe (behavior therapy) feel that attitude and affective change is all that is necessary. It is possible to view both camps as unidimensional with respect to therapy for stuttering. Still a third position, however, emphasizes change in both attitude and behavior as a formal part of therapy. Acknowledging differences in emphasis, all of the other contributors to this volume fall into this middle position.

An interesting question that is seldom addressed is "Do stutterers constitute a homogeneous population?" Since they do not seem to differ from the nonstuttering population with respect to personality or physiology the answer would seem to be no. However, it is conceivable that stutterers differ along some dimension in comparison with a nonstuttering population, but still differ among themselves along that same dimension (e.g., frequency or form of disfluency).

While it is tempting to look for a common denominator in any population bearing the same label, i.e., stuttering, it is equally reasonable to assume that variations in personality and family dynamics overshadow their commonality. In spite of this logic the belief persists that stutterers share more than merely their label. The theoretical construct of anxiety has been a cornerstone of the writings of Johnson (1938), Wolpe (1958), Wischner (1950), Sheehan (1953), and Travis (1957). Therefore, by definition, all stutterers have been viewed as anxious. In addition to anxiety the most common presenting attitudes of stutterers seem to be feelings of helplessness, victimization, low self-esteem, and that what they have to say, in addition to how they say it, especially with regard to feelings, is neither of interest nor of value to their listeners. However, we must be cautious about stereotyping individuals with regard to any of these attitudes that have not been specifically observed in a particular client. For example, some stutterers enter therapy reacting to their problems with overt expressions of aggression, while others present a helpless attitude. To ignore these differences and assume that these two types of stutterers have the same presenting attitudes, and should therefore be treated in the same way, would be a mistake.

A client who enters therapy defiantly may well resist therapies that focus on increased assertiveness. Furthermore, if such a client is treated from a purely behavioral, nonattitudinal perspective, the defiance can also result in increased resistance to change.

It is clear that we feel that attitudes are a part of the problem and must be taken into account by the therapist at some time. This is not to say that attitude must be worked on directly. One of the more interesting questions is: If a change in attitude is important to the resolution of the problem of stuttering, how does such a change in attitude come about?

Most psychologists and speech pathologists recognize that attitude change accompanies behavior change. However, behaviorally oriented clinicians claim that attitude change is a consequence of behavior change, whereas attitudinally oriented clinicians think that attitude change can be effected by discussion, and in turn facilitates behavioral change. They may both be right. Nothing in the arguments presented precludes simultaneous work on attitude and behavior.

Where attitude change is a specific goal of therapy it is often a function of the particular theory and strategies involved. Let us arbitrarily divide therapies into three groups with respect to outcome: controlled stuttering, monitored fluency, and normal fluency. Whether or not the clinician communicates as much to the client, there are three very different attitudes associated with these three different outcomes. In the first case the client remains a stutterer and prepares himself to react to future instances of stuttering in adaptive ways. In the second case the client also remains a stutterer but with the conviction that fluency can always, but only, be purchased at the price of vigilance. Only in the third case is the client likely to be freed from the self-concept of stuttering. This is especially true for young children who may not even remember that they once stuttered. Adults, however, even if they view themselves as normal speakers, will always remember.

Clinician's Expectations

At the beginning of this chapter we discussed the client's expectations regarding therapy. Let us now explore the subject of expectations from the clinician's perspective. As with the client, we may not be aware of some of the attitudes we bring to the therapeutic relationship. Many of these expectations are a function of what we have been trained to look for. As a matter of fact, just as the client goes through a process of selecting a therapeutic strategy (and a clinician), so does the clinician select clients and a therapeutic strategy on the basis of his or her expectations. Unless clinician-client pairs are assigned administratively, some personal selective strategy is likely to occur, based on perceived motivation, intelligence, ability to change, compatibility of personalities, and perhaps even financial commitment. How many different therapeutic strategies is a clinician likely to consider? Is it possible for a clinician to commit to several strategies that differ with respect to theory, goals, and tactics? These questions explore the degree of the clinician's commitment to a particular philosophy of therapy. However, this is not to suggest that commitment should result in a rigidity that prevents us from reacting to the individual problems that different stutterers present and that may require changing therapeutic strategies. We will talk more about this subject shortly as we deal with the therapeutic process.

What are the self-expectations of the clinician entering into a new therapeutic relationship? Does the clinician see himself or herself as an authority, instructor, counselor, reinforcing agent, model, partner, or any combination of these roles at various times within a particular therapeutic relationship? Each of these roles carries with it a set of obligatory strategies and tactics.

We move in and out of these different roles in response to three different therapeutic variables: our view of the needs of the client at any particular point in therapy, the comfort of the clinician with respect to a particular role, and a predetermined logical sequence that relates to the client's moving from a dependent position in therapy to a position of greater responsibility. Shifting, however, is not always easy for the clinician because some of these roles (e.g., authority vs. partner) appear to be oppositional. Such shifting of roles is part of the larger issue of flexibility, with which every clinician must come to grips. The behavior of each client challenges the clinician to abandon stereotypes about age, the disorder, the attainability of long-term goals, the duration of therapy, criteria for termination, and people in general.

Another parameter affecting the expectations of a clinician embarking on a new case is the history of success and failure with previous stutterers. If the record is positive our tactics tend to be reinforced by the progress of our clients. Then we run the risk of getting locked into a limited repertoire of clinical tactics. This is not to say that such tactics will not again be successful, but the reinforcement history can limit our clinical flexibility. On the other hand, if the record is unsuccessful, we may enter a new clinical relationship with a negative attitude and an expectation of failure. It is all too easy in such a situation to project onto the client our own expectation, which in turn does influence his motivation and expectation for outcome. In both examples the previous history of the clinician interferes with our ability to respond to the unique circumstances that each client presents.

There are two other assumptions that clinicians often make: one is that speech is important enough to the client for him to work intensively on it at the expense of other priorities in his life; the second is that the clinician can be a change agent with the power to effect significant control of, and impact upon, the client after he leaves the clinic. Even in intensive therapy, the number of hours and experiences the client shares with the clinician is overshadowed by the necessarily nonclinical life of the client. Given this reality we must acknowledge that while we do have clinical impact, that impact is mitigated by other forces in the client's environment.

Even in programs where stutterers are temporarily removed from their normal environments into intensive residential treatment centers, ultimately they must leave the controlled clinical environment and face the same reduced schedule of contact that the client does who is in less intensive therapy. This fact could account for the observation that ultimately residential programs are not much more successful than conventional ones.

The second assumption, that the clinician can be an influential force in the life of a client in spite of a relatively disproportionate amount of contact, appears grandiose and, in fact, can only be valid if the first assumption regarding the client's motivation is also valid. If speech is not the top priority of a client, no amount of clinical time or skill will be effective.

Having briefly explored the self-expectations of the clinician, let us now look at what the clinician expects from the client. We already referred to motivation as a prerequisite to successful therapy, and as a reasonable assumption by the clinician based on the client's initiatives. However, it may not be such a reasonable assumption, even though the client has appeared for therapy, and especially if the client is a child, for whom a parent has made the arrangements. Overt expressions of commitment and motivation do not preclude ambivalence or resistance to change on the part of the client. Motivation may well be a function of the consequences that the stuttering behavior generates, both positive and negative. While it is easy for stutterers to focus on the negative consequences of their stuttering, there are payoffs such as anxiety reduction, an excuse for failure, securing attention, reinforcing helplessness, and expression of hostility that confound his motivation to change. Even with overt expressions of motivation to eliminate stuttering, stuttering is maintained by consequences about which we know very little and to which we pay insufficient attention. When we really look at what therapy is about, our hope is that we are helping the stutterer to generate consequences for himself that will override the consequences that have maintained the stuttering. When looked at in this way motivation becomes a problem that we can deal with rather than a naive assumption about either the client's commitment or the clinician's limitations. Motivation is not simply a private problem for the client to resolve independently.

Let us now explore the clinician's expectations about the significant people in the stutterer's environment. For children it is reasonable to expect the parents to participate and cooperate in the clinical management of the problem, which is in fact a family problem. It is in the context of the family that the problem has developed. The family creates the atmosphere, the models, and the consequences of talking. It defines the rules for social interaction including timing, pace, and appropriateness. Therefore, it is incumbent upon the clinician to help the family to examine its role in the problem's development, maintenance, and resolution. It will not have been enough merely to bring the child in for treatment. When the clinician enters the picture he or she as well as the client and the family become members of the problem with common goals, in spite of their individual contributions to the process. Just as we cannot assume motivation on the part of the child, we cannot assume motivation on the part of the family, and we may have to work at it. In fact, some members of the family may require as much attention as the stutterer to help to create a supportive environment.

In the case of the adult client, just because he is not living with his parents does not mean that there is no need for a supportive environment. Initially the clinician provides that support. Too often in therapy the clinic becomes the extent of that supportive environment, and the client is left to his own devices outside. What might be the functions of a supportive environment for the adult client? People provide the occasions for talking and positive consequences for fluency, ideally in the form of responding to the content rather than the manner of speech, and they also prevent the occurrence of stuttering or, failing that, withhold the payoffs for stuttering. This can only be accomplished both with the cooperation of the client and by the training of those people who are willing to function in this way.

Having examined the clinician's expectations about the role of the therapist and the client's support system, let us now look at expectations about the process of therapy. Speech clinicians seem to approach this experience with an air of optimism. Intuitively we expect to be successful; it is rare that we say no to a client. How many of us, in fact, establish a formal prognosis based on the information the client provides and the behavior the client demonstrates during the evaluation? Ideally, the clinician's expectations regarding outcome should relate to a particular therapeutic regime as well as the goals associated with that regime. It is obvious that formal prognoses must take into account the processes particular to a therapeutic approach and the clinician's prediction of the client's responses to those processes. Expectations about outcome are directly related to the clinician's expectations about the processes that will occur in therapy. These processes might be arbitrarily categorized as those which emphasize how the person talks as differentiated from what the person talks about. The relative significance of these two categories for the clinician could well determine his expectations for how he functions as counselor, teacher, model, provider of feedback and reinforcement, etc. When the emphasis of therapy is on how the person talks, the motor mechanics of speech, especially at the outset of therapy the schedule of contact reflects this emphasis. For example, those initially intensive schedules of therapy such as those of Shames and Webster attempt to change the speaking behavior as soon as possible, and thereby create a positive reinforcement environment for a new set of behaviors. Once the new speaking behaviors have been established the schedule of the initially intensive therapies becomes more intermittent, reflecting a change in the balance of emphasis in the direction of what the client is talking about. Whether the therapy is initially intensive or intermittent, the first phase of changing the manner of speaking is relatively shorter than the next phase, which emphasizes what the client is talking about. What he is talking about can include his thoughts and feelings as well as reports of his experiences between therapy sessions. The clinician's expectation about the duration of the entire therapeutic experience directly relates to how he sees the significance of changing the client's thoughts and feelings. Where the sole emphasis is on changing the manner of speech, the clinician reasonably expects therapy to be brief. He may then act on that expectation by terminating therapy under criteria of success and failure that directly reflect that emphasis. On the other hand, those therapies that place greater emphasis on what the stutterer thinks and feels confronts the clinician with expectations that are less well-defined with respect to duration and complexity. The clinician doesn't really know how long the therapy will take, nor does he anticipate what cognitive and affective issues may emerge. Criteria for success may vary with the client and always involve more than specifying outcome in terms of speech behaviors in the clinic. The clinician may then have to deal with criteria that embrace the client's perceptions of happiness, feelings of self-adequacy, attitudes about talking, and speech behaviors outside the clinic. As the feeling component becomes more prominent in therapy, the clinician should expect to make a decision about how far the therapy goes beyond the issues of stuttering, and if or when to refer to another professional. This decision will reflect the clinician's self-expectations for dealing with the psychological aspects of therapy.

With regard to the clinician's expectations about outcome, we wish to pose four questions: (1) Do you expect success? (2) How do you define success? (3) Do you communicate your expectation to the stutterer? and (4) Does your definition include the possibility of regression? It is difficult to conceive of any clinician entering therapy without an expectation of success. The issue behind this question is the definition of success. Relative to the way the stutterer talks we can think about outcome as we indicated earlier in terms of (a) the client becoming a controlled stutterer, (b) the client becoming a controlled stutter-free speaker, or (c) the client becoming a normal speaker (i.e., not exercising constant control). Relative to the way the stutterer thinks and feels, the clinician's expectations are directly tied to one of these three outcomes for speech. Each of them carries with it a different self-concept and related attitudes. For example, it is reasonable to expect a controlled stutterer to still think of himself as a stutterer, and it is not reasonable to expect a controlled stutter-free speaker to see himself as a normal speaker. These goals, however, may be revised during therapy on the basis of unexpected progress or lack of progress. The reason we ask the question, "Do you communicate your expectation (of success) to the stutterer?" is that his expectation also must be taken into account. At the same time we recognize that we may want to influence the stutterer's expectation. The clinician's attitude about success may have a direct bearing upon the client's motivation and commitment to therapy. The therapist's commitment is predicated upon a belief in the effectiveness of therapy, and ideally is communicated persuasively to the client. With the current emphasis in the literature on technology and replicability we sometimes lose sight of the subjective attributes of enthusiasm and warmth of the clinician as a major influence upon the client. At more formal levels we discuss outcome in terms of attributes of the therapy, attributes of the client, and attributes of the client's environment. Relatively little attention is given to discussing outcome in terms of the attributes of the clinician. In this sense our understanding and expectations about outcome may be naive and limited. The effectiveness of therapy cannot be assessed independently of what the clinician brings to the encounter. Perhaps the first problem in discussing these categories of attributes is agreement about what they are. Most researchers are reluctant to identify any variables that cannot be objectively measured, and therefore they do not deal with issues like client's motivation, family's involvement, and clinician's conviction. Even where such variables have been isolated they tend to vary from therapy to therapy. A third problem is that these variables affect one another, and to our knowledge no study has attempted to measure these interactive effects. Outcome is not a function of the client's motivation alone; it is not a function of the client's environment alone; it is not a function of the clinician's commitment alone. Rather, it is how these things work together. Given the complexity of these issues and the adaptive nature of the problem of stuttering it is reasonable for us to expect stutterers to regress periodically during therapy and after. We use the term "regression" generically to refer to a client's moving backward after having made progress against the problem. Regression can be evidenced not only in the stutterer's speech behavior but also in his attitudes and feelings, his social relationships, and his relationship with the clinician. "Relapse" is a medical term that has several alternative meanings: regression to a pretreatment condition, or the appearance of a new symptom of the underlying disorder. Because of its limitations this medical term may be inappropriate for characterizing regression in stuttering. How much of this expectation do we communicate to the stutterer, and when? The issue is the effect of this kind of communication upon the client's motivation and commitment versus the possible devastating effects of not being forewarned. While Van Riper's and Luper's chapter is predicated upon the inevitability of regression, only Boberg's chapter in this section deals explicitly with the issue.

CONCLUSION

We have suggested a number of issues and questions for the reader to keep in mind while examining the following chapters, which deal with specific approaches to therapy. Recognizing that we have a necessary diversity of ideas and perspectives, to say nothing of styles and the lapses in time between the original publication and the update, we have tried to provide a way of comparing therapies and integrating their diversity. Each therapy appears to have its own logic and grammar, its own set of underlying principles. Given the uniqueness of each therapy, there may be some commonalities running across therapeutic perspectives. While we have emphasized the role of the clinician, some of these authors have not. However, most of them do arrange, by accident or by design, to slow the speech of their clients, at least to establish fluency. They also seem to place a value on increasing the amount of talking their clients do. We think that the differences among the therapies seem to far outnumber their common elements. If this is indeed the case, two very profound questions emerge: why do so many different therapies have some record of success, and why is no single one successful for everyone.

We must keep in mind as we read this section that each chapter represents a unique conceptualization about therapy and what the author sees as most significant in the problem of stuttering. They do not all address the same issues. They are companions to publications that were written at various times for different purposes. However, we now have the opportunity and the challenge to integrate these separate contributions as components of a multi-dimensional problem.

REFERENCES

Abbott, J. (1947). Repressed hostility as a factor in adult stuttering. *Journal of Speech Disabilities, 12,* 428–430.

Cousins, N. (1981). *Anatomy of an illness.* New York: Bantam.

Goldiamond, I. (1965). Stuttering and fluency as manipulatable operant response classes. In *Research in behavior modification.* L. Krasner and L. Ullmann (Eds.), New York: Holt, Rinehart and Winston.

Johnson, W. (1938). The role of evaluation in stuttering behavior. *Journal of Speech and Hearing Disabilities, 3,* 85–89.

Sheehan, J. (1953). Theory and treatment of stuttering as an approach-avoidance conflict. *Journal of Psychology, 36,* 27–49.

Siegel, G., & Martin, R. (1968). Effects of verbal stimuli on disfluencies during spontaneous speech. *Journal of Speech and Hearing Research, 11,* 358–364.

Travis, L. (1957). The unspeakable feelings of people with special reference to stuttering. In L. Travis (Ed.), *Handbook of speech pathology.* New York: Appleton-Century-Crofts.

Wischner, G. (1950). Stuttering behavior and learning: A preliminary theoretical formulation. *Journal of Speech and Hearing Disabilities, 15,* 324–335.

Wolpe, J. (1958). *Psychotherapy by reciprocal inhibition.* Stanford, CA: Stanford University Press.

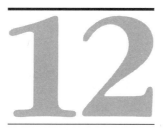

Environmental Manipulation and Family Counseling

Hugo H. Gregory

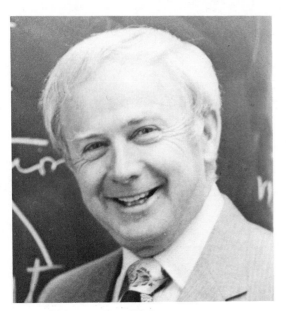

Hugo H. Gregory

Environmental manipulation and family counseling has been a cornerstone in the treatment of the early stages of stuttering quite independently of the management approaches to more advanced stages of the problem. For this reason there is probably more agreement among speech pathologists about the importance of looking at the child's environment than about managing the speech behaviors themselves.

Another way of viewing the issue is to describe the speech behaviors as variables dependent on events in the child's environment that can be directly manipulated in therapy. Although there are alternative approaches to the management of disfluency in young children, such as time out, parent-child interaction, and desensitization procedures, environmental manipulation and family counseling have consistently, and over the long term, enjoyed the greatest success. If the family can be enjoined and mobilized to give a child's disfluency problems a high priority, and if the pertinent variables in the environment can be identified and appropriately managed, success is almost assured. Even with a family history of stuttering, we have seen the permanent effectiveness of this type of therapy.

To discuss this type of therapy, Hugo Gregory agreed to write a new, original chapter. One might think that a therapy that has enjoyed such a long history of success does not require an update. Gregory, however, from his own long professional history and interest in stuttering problems in children, shows us a fine-tuning and sophistication in developing types and combinations of environmental manipulation and family counseling, based on tactics of differential diagnosis and differential responsiveness to treatment programs.

His historical introduction provides the research and clinical literature base for the new directions in which he is moving. Gregory certainly and significantly improves on an already successful approach.

Environmental Manipulation and Family Counseling

Hugo H. Gregory

> Treatment of the young primary stutterer consists primarily of prevention . . . This prevention is accomplished chiefly through the education and cooperation of the parents and teachers. (Van Riper, 1947, p. 321)
>
> The problem arises originally in the listener . . . and only subsequently in the awareness and behavior of the child . . . For the child the modifications must occur primarily in the evaluations of his most important listeners. (Johnson, 1956, p. 69–70)
>
> Parents (of stuttering children) needed help in these areas: (1) better handling of the child's expressions of feelings; (2) better family relationships; and (3) better communication with the child. (Wyatt, 1969, p. 169)
>
> Our concerns should include those factors that appear to evoke stuttering as well as those factors that appear to . . . maintain stuttering . . . This is not a problem merely of dealing with the speaker . . ., but also of dealing with the people and events that affect the stutterer. (Shames & Egolf, 1976, p. 14–15)

As I began writing this chapter, I had just finished looking through over 20 books on stuttering dating back to the 1930s. All of these books hold environmental influences as important in the development and maintenance of stuttering as well as effective prevention and therapy. I have decided that the most useful approach to this broad topic is to (a) analyze the principal points of view and research information about environmental intervention, (b) discuss current evaluation procedures, and (c) outline treatment procedures and their evaluation in light of our current knowledge about the problem of stuttering.

POINTS OF VIEW

Historically, parent counseling, including understanding how parents perceive the child, providing information, and altering the interaction between parents and child, has been deemed necessary by most clinicians. However, specific approaches have differed depending on the clinician's conceptualization of stuttering and clinical experience.

Van Riper (1973), whose ideas are based on the belief that stuttering develops out of an interaction between characteristics of the child and the environment, sums up his many years of clinical work with preschool children on a very optimistic note. He describes how he begins by showing parents that he wants to understand their thoughts and feelings. Subsequently, on the basis of this understanding, he proceeds to give information about speech development, and then describes changes the parents must make in their communication and other interaction with the child. These modifications are aimed toward parental behaviors that are precipitating or maintaining stuttering. When therapy includes the child, Van Riper first works with the child alone; next the parents observe, then participate in therapy, and finally the parents interact with the child as the clinician observes. Results are illustrated this way:

> . . . the same mother, who prior to counseling seemed unable to simplify her own speech or even listen to the child with equanimity, now seems to be able to do it easily. Fathers begin to play with the boy again: they do things together. The daily tempo of living slows down; it becomes more organized. Parents are less demanding, more tolerant—and consistent in their management. There is more evidence of love and consideration in the home . . . Standards are less rigid, more relaxed. The child stops stuttering. (1973, p. 420)

Although most stuttering theorists, even those such as Van Riper who referred to the possibility of constitutional factors in the onset of stuttering, have considered environmental influences as important, it was Johnson (1946, 1956) who stressed that the crucial differences between a child who becomes a stutterer and one who does not is found in the parents' and others' reactions. In some of his last writing, Johnson (1959) hypothesized that stuttering was the result of a general interaction among three major factors: (1) the listener's sensitivity to the child's disfluency, (2) the child's degree of disfluency, and (3) the child's sensitivity to his listener's evaluations. Johnson (1946, 1967) discussed the importance of not reacting differentially to the child's disfluency. In parental counseling, he focused on reducing factors that disrupt the child's fluency such as speaking in a competitive situation, speaking to unresponsive listeners, and speaking in a situation of conflict or when attempting to express an idea for which adequate language is not readily available.

In one of the first books focusing on therapy for children who stutter, Luper and Mulder (1964) dealt with many of the issues that arise in counseling the parents of children showing incipient and transitorial stuttering. For one, the parents may feel responsible for the child's stuttering problem and have guilt feelings. Secondly, a child's stuttering is a public event, not something the family can cope with in the privacy of the home. The parents receive advice, both tactful and otherwise. Thirdly, most parents have feelings of insecurity about child-rearing practices, and both these activities and their anxieties are usually related in one way or another to the child's speech. Finally, there is the issue of what to do if the child mentions "stuttering" with reference to speech. General counseling principles described by Luper and Mulder in responding to these issues are: (a) Be a good listener; help parents to express their feelings about the child and their own behavior, (b) Provide information and give reassurance, not only that "your child will be all right," but also that the parents have come to a knowledgeable, understanding speech-language pathologist who has experience and knows how to help, and (c) Deal carefully with the specific issues involved. For example, if the child says he stutters, " . . . calm acquiescence and an attitude of unconcerned acceptance will do much to put the behavior in a proper perspective" (p. 71). In other words, do not be concerned about the label. It is very hard to know what it means to the child. The clinician or the parents must not project their meaning onto a child.

Those such as Murphy and Fitzsimons (1960), Glasner, (1970) and Sheehan (1970, 1975) who emphasize the interpersonal psychodynamic aspect of the development of stuttering have advocated family-centered therapy. During the 1960s, when behavioral counseling was ascending, Murphy, who was a speaker at many conferences, stressed a more psychodynamic frame of reference. In their book, *Stuttering and personality dynamics* (1960), Murphy and Fitzsimons give this definition:

> Stuttering is a learned, non-integrative, self-defensive reaction to anxiety or fear of threatening circumstances with which the person feels incapable of coping. (p. 145)

They view a child's interpersonal relationships and verbal or nonverbal developmental events during early socialization as the roots of stuttering. Therefore, therapy including parent counseling is directed toward enhancing the child's self-concept, thereby reducing the need for stuttering.

Glasner (1970) also views stuttering in a child as a symptom of anxiety and hypersensitivity caused by parental pressures. In brief, the prognosis for the child's improvement is good if the parents can adjust their standards and if the clinician can establish a relationship in which the child feels the presence of an adult who is not restrictive and who allows expression of feelings. Sheehan (1970) believed that "With a young child still in the family circle, direct speech therapy should more often be a last resort rather than a starting point" (1970, p. 303). Instead, Sheehan recommended parent counseling based on behavioral assignments in which parents explore their behavior and feelings in situations in which the child has particularly great difficulty. Therapy then aims to modify behavior and associated beliefs and feelings of the parent. He concluded: "The child stutterer remains a stutterer because his parents will not permit their pressure on him to subside" (p. 307).

Another psychodynamic description of the onset of stuttering is proposed by Wyatt. She interprets stuttering in children as a loss of parental love, corrective feedback, or modeling of appropriate language forms during the development of language through the presymbolic (babbling), symbolic (naming, words) and relational (phrases, sentences) stages. The loss of corrective feedback is most detrimental when the child is developing from one stage to the next, resulting in compulsive repetition of an earlier developmental form; for example, initial sounds and syllables that are least characteristic of later normal development but that do characterize early speech development. In short, Wyatt says that therapy during the early stage consists of helping the mother establish or reestablish a close relationship and reciprocal identification with the child. Based on the following quote, I have termed my friend Dr. Wyatt's approach "hugging therapy":

This can best be done through the stressing of mutually enjoyed body closeness between mother and child and through the common usage of language on the child's developmental level: The mother is "feeding" the child short phrases which do not go beyond the earliest forms of grammatical speech used by the young child. (1956, p. 163)

Procedures derived from an orientation similar to Glasner's and Sheehan's, but involving more definitive observations and recommendations derived from these observations of stimulus events in the environment and response consequences, are those of Shames and Egolf (1976). In their approach, the clinician observes the child's interaction with the parents to discover disequilibriums in the relationship assumed to occasion increased disfluency or stuttering. An example given is a mother who was authoritative and demanding. She asked her stuttering child questions and gave little time for replies. The clinician's strategy, in this example, was to assume a role opposite to that of the mother in which the initiation of conversational topics by the child was reinforced and time for more lengthy utterances was provided. They also point out that if the stuttering gains attention, and this point may be important in some cases, then the positive reinforcement can increase the behavior. Shames and Egolf recommended that the clinician model desirable behavioral changes for the parents. They concluded: "We can say without hesitation that when parents react to their child in more positive ways the tendency is for fluency to emerge. Appropriate large-scale research may reveal that such positive verbal interactions early in life may function as a prevention for stuttering." (1976, p. 100)

Bloodstein (1975) stresses the role of environmental pressures in the development of stuttering and recommends that the following points be considered in counseling parents:

1. Any effort to change some of the parents' behavior must start with the removal of guilt about the child's stuttering. (p. 58)
2. We must insist on the removal of all speech pressures. (p. 59)
3. When necessary, the parents should be helped to understand in what respects they might be less restrictive and demanding in their attitudes toward the child's behavior as a whole. (p. 60)
4. In a certain number of cases psychotherapy may offer the only practical hope of reducing parental pressures. (p. 61)

I have always been fascinated by a report on therapy with two stuttering children (ages 4 and 9) reported by Wahler, et al. in 1970. Based on the operant conditioning model, they presented punishing consequences following secondary problems such as aggression and shifts of attention. When these behaviors decreased, the children's stuttering behavior was reduced. The researchers were satisfied that the stuttering behavior was not reduced because the secondary problems and stuttering behavior shared common stimulus control variables or because differential attention was given fluent and stuttered speech. They concluded that "control of the stuttering was most clearly related to specific aspects of the child's own behavior—namely changes in their secondary problems" (p. 427). In other words, this is an example of responses being conditional one to the other, or response-response conditioning. Without doubt, this phenomenon does occur in behavior development and functions in behavior modification.

In several publications (Gregory, 1973b, 1984; Gregory & Hill, 1980) I have employed a differential evaluation–differential therapy model in which stuttering in a child may be related to environmental factors alone or in combination with developmental characteristics. In any event, environmental factors, representing either broader cultural patterns (Lemert, 1953, 1962; Morgenstein, 1956; Stewart, 1960) or the attitudes and reactions of individual parents—or perhaps a combination of the two—are considered to be significant determinants of stuttering.

Rustin (1983) describes the way in which a child's speech environment is subjected to a careful functional analysis to ferret out characteristics of the child and the environment that may be related to increased disfluency or stuttering. Therapy with the parents and the child is based on hypotheses derived from this functional analysis and usually includes both communicative and other interpersonal factors.

In recent years, Cooper (1979) has speculated with reference to findings on "spontaneous recoveries" from stuttering that parents, through their early and active intervention procedures with their abnormally disfluent children, may be primarily responsible for improving their children's speech. Parents telling the child to slow down, take a breath, or say it more easily, may acknowledge to the child that there is a degree of trouble speaking and give advice that is beneficial. Cooper believes we have been prone to assume that parental intervention is detrimental. However, he suggests that parental intervention is often successful, accounting in part for the findings, based on retrospective research, that about two out of three children who are considered to have a stuttering problem at one time regain normally fluent speech. The following quotation provides insight into Cooper's counseling of parents whose child is in therapy designed to facilitate fluency:

> Knowing the attitudes and knowledge that the parents have of fluency problems, the clinician can stress information that may correct any inaccurate perceptions the parents hold in the hope that intervention-facilitating parental attitudes may result. It is hoped that parents will not be frightened by words themselves and be fearful of using terms like "stuttering" in front of their children . . . In addition to being comfortable in using words that describe fluency problems, it is hoped that parents will feel comfortable in discussing fluency failures with their children and in offering suggestions to the children in how they might use their vocal mechanisms in a fluency-facilitating manner. If the parents are able to communicate to their children that their concern and their suggestions for altering speech motor patterns are positive expressions of assistance rather than punishments for "bad" behavior, the young child may adopt the kinds of attitudes and behaviors that lead to increased fluency. (Cooper, 1979, p. 73)

EVALUATION PROCEDURES

With environmental factors in mind, clinicians have for many years included in the case history an informant's statement of the problem and an investigation of environmental conditions. It has been considered valuable to know how the parents and others perceive the problem in comparison with the clinician's observations and even the evaluation of the child himself. As we have seen in the previous review, most points of view about the development of stuttering in a child support obtaining a careful description of environmental factors thought to be related to speech development, the onset of stuttering, or the growth of the stuttering problem. More recently, these environmental factors have been categorized as communicative and interpersonal stress (Gregory, 1984). Communicative stress refers to the way in which the parents or others talk to the child, and interpersonal stress refers to the general interaction among family members.

In taking the case history, the speech-language pathologist realizes that in these initial interactions the parents are deciding how they feel about the examiner as a person and how comfortable they are in communicating with the clinician. How successful all treatment and counseling will be may hinge on these early impressions. Therefore, clinicians should not proceed like data gatherers, but in a calm, unhurried conversational fashion in which they come across as persons with a genuine interest in understanding the child and the parents as unique individuals.

The history covers many other areas of the child's development (Gregory, 1973; Hood, 1978; Williams, 1978), but the focus here is on environmental influences. Information about the environment is integrated with other historical information and findings from the clinical evaluation. The evaluation of a child includes a careful assessment of the conditions that elicit stuttering, or as operant conditioners would say, the stimuli that control the behavior (Shames & Sherrick, 1963). What conditions disturb speech? What conditions relax speech? Being definitive, does "Father" or just "Father getting angry" occasion more disfluency or stuttering? Are there environmental conditions that reinforce stuttering responses, such as the child finally getting the parents' attention as he stutters in some situation? Are such things as sibling rivalry or discipline practices causing conflict related to the stuttering? Are the parents in disagreement about certain aspects of the "speech problem?" Do the parents feel guilty about how they have reacted to the child's speech? A parent may have too high a level of expectation for speech development or for behavior in general such as table manners and neatness. The parents may be demanding too much and providing too little support, what Sheehan (1970, 1975) has called an unfavorable demand/support ratio. Other factors, such as hectic or inconsistent family routine or an unhappy marital situation can be discovered through an interview.

When I wrote *Stuttering: Differential evaluation and therapy* in 1973, I depended mostly on the case history and subsequent parent counseling for information about environmental reactions. Since that time, procedures for investigating parent-child interactive behaviors have been studied and are now in use in several clinics. This work was begun by Kasprisin (1970) and Kasprisin-Burrelli, Egolf, and Shames (1972), who trained observers to reliably identify parents' positive and negative child-directed behaviors. Observation indicated that parents of stuttering children exhibited more negative verbal profiles than parents of nonstuttering children. They also reported that the negative profiles of parents talking to stuttering children became less negative following treatment in which the parents participated. Mordecai (1979) conducted a study in which parent-child triads (mother, father, child) were videotaped during a prescribed activity period designed to provide opportunities for parents to instruct, compete, converse, and play with their preschool children. Parents of children evaluated as beginning to stutter were found to allow inadequate opportunities for their child to respond to questions before asking another question or making another statement. Parents of nonstuttering children were found to comment more frequently on the content of their child's preceding utterance, this being generally regarded as a positive behavior.

Gregory and Hill (1980) have observed the following interactive behaviors as important in the development and maintenance of stuttering: interrupting, filling in words, finishing the child's statement, guessing what the child is about to say, asking multiple questions at once, constantly correcting the child's verbal and nonverbal behavior, and modeling rapidly paced speech that includes few pauses and quickly changing topics.

In addition to information from the case history, and in some situations a parent-child interaction analysis, clinics often use procedures such as Cooper's Parent Attitudes Toward Stuttering Checklist (Cooper, 1976) and Zwitman's Child Management Questionnaires and Checklists (Zwitman, 1978). Cooper's checklist is designed to identify attitudes that the clinician may wish to explore with the parents or to modify. Zwitman's questionnaires and checklists are intended to help the parents make observations about features of the child's disfluency and characteristics of the home environment. These instruments are then used in parent counseling and in making environmental modifications.

In many clinics, psychological consultation is routine; in others, referrals are made as the need is recognized. Oftentimes, clinical psychologists, social workers, or school counselors can be of assistance in our study of the child's environment (parental adjustment, parental attitudes, etc.) or in understanding subtle attitudes in stuttering children that the speech-language pathologists may miss. Some of these other professionals, including psychiatrists, are often interested in speech problems. Speech-language pathologists should seek out those with whom they can work best and cultivate a cooperative relationship.

When psychological insecurities and conflicts not so directly related to the child's stuttering problem are expressed, we should be calm and understanding. However, we begin to consider the possibility of a referral. The need for referral may be confirmed or not considered necessary depending on what we learn as a therapy program gets underway. In my own recent experience a parent of a 4-year-old child expressed bewilderment over the responsibility of caring for her children, including concern about appropriate discipline. In another case, a mother in discussing her child's home environment revealed that her married life had been unsatisfactory for several years. In the first case, I made an effective referral to a social worker who has a special interest in child-rearing practices; in the second, a referral was made to a marriage counselor. Without going into detail, both of these referrals and the subsequent cooperative professional relationships has led to successful treatment of the child's problems and the beginning of progress with the more general problems that were discovered.

ENVIRONMENTAL CHANGES

In the first section of this chapter, I reviewed representative historical points of view about the role of environmental influences in the development and maintenance of stuttering and recommended environmental changes based on these ideas. I recognize that there are differences in beliefs about the nature of stuttering and that clinicians have had somewhat different experiences in therapy. In my own experience as a clinician, I have attempted to filter these differing ideas through my own experiences and keep myself in the process of learning. The following discussion is much closer to being an expression of my own beliefs as I have been involved in the process of environmental intervention, working with children and their parents and observing the work of my colleagues. As I do this I will refer to the historical perspective and to the evaluation procedures that have been described previously. I will emphasize therapy for preschool children.

Understanding the Parents' Concern and Feelings about the Child

All of the contributors we have discussed emphasize that in one way or another, parents come to the therapy situation with feelings of insecurity, doubt, and frustration. As Luper and Mulder mentioned, parents have probably been given well-intentioned advice by friends and possibly even some brief advice by the family physician. But in all probability, a knowledgeable professional has not yet dedicated time to understanding their unique feelings, beliefs, and experiences. Considerable parental anxiety generated by their disorganized thoughts begins to become more structured as they find a situation in which another person is sincerely attempting to understand. Beginning clinicians may view listening and attempting to understand as being indecisive and uncertain. Even some professional speech-language pathologists seem to feel more secure providing information and direction.

Previously (Gregory, 1982), I have given three reasons why it is preferable to attempt to understand the parent before we give information and make recommendations. First, parents appreciate the interest we show. It is rare that someone has really tried to understand what they have experienced and their perception of it. Expressing feelings about seeing their child having difficulty communicating, about the frustration they assume is involved, and about wanting to be a good parent help parents begin the process of reducing anxiety. Most important, though, is that we will be able to relate the information we give and modifications we suggest to the *parents' unique experience*. We should not enter these interviews with the parents, whether during the initial evaluation or later, with preconceived notions. Openness is not easy. Our own egos tend to get in the way. However, like the ad says, I can say; "Try it, you'll like it." Recently, I went to a physician who questioned me about my condition. He did not listen carefully to my information and in fact guessed at my answers before I could reply. I did not have much confidence in his diagnosis, which by the way was not correct!

Second, what we do early in therapy establishes some of the basic conditions of the therapeutic relationship. If the clinician gives too much information or becomes too directive at the beginning of therapy, the parents may perceive the relationship chiefly as one in which the clinician knows the answers and will point the way. In this case, we are less likely to get to know some important parental attitudes. It appears easier to move from being more permissive and understanding to more educational and directive as it is appropriate than vice versa. In addition, how else can the clinician make appropriate judgments and decisions without first comprehending the problem adequately?

Finally, as implied earlier, the process of talking, of attempting to describe and explain, will initiate in the client a process of self-education and reorganization of thinking that will open the way for receiving new information and direction. Suggestions by the clinician are related to ideas and experiences previously shared by the parents. Furthermore, there is the possibility that the clinician's accepting and understanding attitude serves as a model for the parents' self-acceptance of their present attitudes and behaviors—a prerequisite, I believe, to constructive change. Sheehan (1970, 1975) always emphasized that the client, parent or adult stutterer, has to accept the reality of the present before he can make realistic change. Sheehan cautioned the clinician to begin where the client is, not where the clinician is.

In parent counseling we listen and ask for further information or clarification. We reward the parents for sharing their perceptions and feelings with us. In what is being suggested for the early stages of the clinician-parent relationship, we have learned a great deal from the writings of Carl Rogers (1951) and the recordings and movies illustrating his client-centered counseling. Over the years, my students and I have concluded that client-centered counseling as taught by Rogers cannot meet all of the needs of stutterers or parents of stuttering children, but that the principles and procedures of client-centered counseling can be integrated into our work in stuttering therapy. Shames and Florance (1980) have described this integration in a discussion of the therapeutic relationship aspect of therapy for stutterers.

Being Empathic, Supportive, and Genuine

The relationship between the clinician and the client that I have been describing includes the clinician emitting certain verbal responses designated as warm, interested, empathic, supportive, accepting, congruent, etc. (Rogers, 1957; Murphy & Fitzsimons, 1960; Cooper, 1965, 1968, 1976; Gregory, 1968; Sheehan, 1970a; Van Riper, 1973, 1975; and Murphy, 1974, 1977). Viewing therapy this way, the clinician can have general goals that become more specific as the clinical relationship develops, but as previously stated, still remain open to the uniqueness of parent attitudes and parent-child interactions. Some clinicians who consider themselves as adhering to more of a behavioral orientation may wish to be specific in analyzing the parent-child interaction in terms of stimulus events and response consequences; however, I see no reason not to approach the task with some of the same attitudes described here. In fact, a number of clinicians emphasize the affective nature of client-clinician relationships but also use specific behavior modification techniques considered appropriate to the situation (Gregory, 1968; Sheehan, 1970a; Van Riper, 1973; Emerick & Hood, 1974; Cooper, 1976, 1979; Shames & Florance, 1980).

In responding empathetically, the clinician is identifying as best as possible with the feelings or affective reactions the client is experiencing and communicating this understanding to the client. The clinician presumably recalls some past experience similar to the client's and to some degree re-experiences the event by covertly verbalizing cues to evoke the feeling. In other words, if clinicians have been sensitive about some attribute of their own behaviors, they can identify with the stutterer's sensitivity about speech fluency. If you have experienced the feeling of seeing a child in your family seem frustrated when trying to do a task, and you didn't know for certain what to do, you can perhaps experience some of the feelings a mother has when she sees her child "beginning to stutter." In the latter case, when the clinician expresses understanding of the mother, the clinician's empathy is reinforcing to the mother and should increase her willingness to explore her attitudes about her child. The clinician is saying to the mother, "I accept your emotional reactions and you can too! Don't be afraid of your feelings." At the same time the clinician is seeing that some personal feelings can be expressed.

A clinician who does not reveal some honest feelings is probably not being genuine. On many occasions, I have said to parents, "I have never had a parent report this particular feeling (or experience) before and I need to think about it." Clients respond better, I believe, to clinicians who seem to be honest about their present limitations. Clinicians need to be knowledgeable about the nature of stuttering and child development, but they don't need to wear a false face of perfection. They should allow their own personality to come through. Just as the client is an interesting individual to the clinician, the clinician can be an interesting person to the client. However, care should be taken to not express feelings that could intrude on meeting the client's need or be aimed more toward meeting the clinician's need. For example, as a parent experiencing frustrations with my own children, I have at times felt a considerable need when counseling parents to talk about my family situation. While I have considered it appropriate to mention that my wife and I experienced somewhat similar difficulties as those discussed with the parents of a stuttering child, I have never allowed the discussion to focus on the specific content of my problems.

The clinician must see the parents' need for support when they come for help, begin to face their problem, explore their attitudes, and seek insight and direction. If a mother is describing the helplessness she felt when she perceived her child as stuttering or when her husband wanted to tell the child to slow down his speech (what he had done to "overcome his stuttering"), recognize that it takes courage to express her feelings, and tell her so! For example, you might say, "I can see that you felt uncertain and anxious about what to do. Your telling me this helps in understanding your feelings. Talking about this kind of thing is not easy."

Providing Information to Parents

A review of the literature indicates that practically all clinicians, whatever their precise belief about stuttering may be, provide information to parents about speech development and the influences of psychosocial factors. I have recommended that giving information be de-emphasized during the early stages of the therapeutic relationship. However, from the beginning of therapy parents expect some information, and it should be given in a way that helps them to clarify what they are describing to the clinician. For example, the clinician may describe different types of disfluencies as the parents are talking about what they observed in their child's speech.

As we counsel parents, parents begin to believe that we have a rather good understanding of their thoughts, feelings, and behavior related to the child's speech and the child's development in general. Gradually, we provide more information. We ordinarily give information about speech development from the babbling stage to first words to conversational speech, giving attention to what is considered normal disfluency. We may talk about factors that precipitate increased disfluency and stuttering. I have found it helpful to discuss several options of how stuttering may begin. In brief, in counseling I may say, "Some children show more of the types of disfluency, sound and syllable repetitions and sound prolongations, the types of disfluency that occur less frequently in most children. Some children are more sensitive about disfluency in their own speech, and some parents are particularly sensitive about their child's fluency. Some combinations of these factors could contribute to the development of stuttering." If there are more questions about the cause of stuttering, I tell the parents that we know a great deal about the factors that contribute to increasing disfluency in a child. From experience we know that dealing with these developmental characteristics of the child (language, articulation, etc.) together with environmental factors does result in a decrease of stuttering and in consequently normal speech development. Frequently, we have parents read sections on speech interaction or nonverbal communication in *If your child stutters: A guide for parents* (Ainsworth & Guess, 1981) and *Between parent and child* (Ginott, 1969).

At this point in our relationship with the parents we have gained insight into the child's communicative and general interpersonal situation. We hope that after giving parents the opportunity to express their thoughts and feelings and after providing appropriate information, we can expect constructive changes on the parents' part and their active support of therapeutic objectives. Such discussions continue, but therapy with the parents becomes more action-oriented. Expressing it another way, our counseling takes a more behavioral orientation, without neglecting the cognitive or feeling aspects. In the final analysis, effective therapy directed toward environmental change should integrate cognitive, affective, and behavioral changes in the parents.

Treatment Strategies

Gregory and Hill (1980) have described three treatment strategies for working with preschool children and their parents. They, like others such as Riley and Riley (1979, 1983) view differential therapy as based on differential evaluation. That the degree of environmental change necessary and the extent of the child's involvement in therapy is different is illustrated by these possible cases: (a) Treatment Strategy I. Preventive Parent Counseling. The parents are seen for four counseling sessions, even though it is judged that the parents are expressing concern about disfluency that seems to be within normal limits. (b) Treatment Strategy II. Prescriptive Parent Counseling. The parents and the child are seen for four to eight sessions on a weekly basis if the child is showing borderline atypical disfluencies (the "problem" has existed for less than a year, and there appears to be no significant complicating speech, language, or behavioral characteristics). (c) Treatment Strategy III. The child is seen two to four times a week and the parents have two counseling sessions a week if the child is demonstrating borderline atypically disfluent or stuttering speech that has been present for a year or longer with or without complicating speech, language, or behavioral factors. The reader should see Gregory and Hill (1980) and Gregory (1984) for a specific discussion of environmental modification associated with these strategies. The point to be made in comparing these strategies is that parent counseling does differ depending on need, and that need is related to the status of the problem as described in the definition of these strategies. The remainder of this section will address general concepts and procedures for environmental changes aimed to prevent stuttering or manage early developmental stages of it.

Charting Situations Related to Increased or Decreased Disfluency

Following up on information gained in the initial evaluation (case history and parent-child interaction analysis), clinicians such as Gregory and Hill (1980), Johnson (1980), and Nelson (1984) have described methods for having the parents observe and chart episodes of increased disfluency and increased fluency in terms of situation, communicative intent, nature of speech fluency, and listener reaction. This procedure helps the parents become more objective. On occasion, the parents observe how much more fluent the child is compared to the amount of disfluency. Parents bring these charts to counseling sessions, either individual counseling with a mother and father or in a group of parents. A parent may report that a child showed increased syllable and one-syllable-word repetition of irregular rhythm when trying to gain the parent's attention while the parent was busy preparing dinner. This example may represent a pattern of parent-child interaction in which the parents do not take time to talk with the child when they are not busy; in general, they are not responsive listeners. This situation can be discussed, and it can be recommended that the mother have a "talking time—attention time" with the child before she begins such tasks as meal preparation. Once this pattern is established, the parent may ask the child to wait a few minutes until attention can be given. It is important that the parent remember to carry through on the commitment to talk.

The Clinician as a Model

During my 30 years as a speech-language pathologist, I have counseled many parents and led many parent groups. We have discussed how parents talk with the child (the parents' speech rate, the number and ways in which they ask questions, the level of vocabulary they use, and the length of their sentences, etc.) and the way they interact with the child (the daily routine, disciplinary practices, pressure put on the child, how they play with the child, etc.). We have described the goals of therapy and how they could help.

Toward the end of the 1960s I began to read about concepts of modeling, especially the work of Bandura (1969). The idea of learning by observing has always been used in speech therapy and we had certainly realized that children acquire much of their behavior in this way. At about this time, I and several other contributors in speech-language pathology began to discuss the possibility of more specifically applying modeling procedures (Gregory, 1973a; Van Riper, 1973; Shames & Egolf, 1976) in modifying the speech of children and adults and in modifying communicative interactions between parents and children. I recall some of my first comments to our staff, such as "We will teach the parents everything we teach the child so that they can be better models for the child." "We will not talk to the parents so much about what we suggest that they do; we will have them observe our interaction with their children and then modify their behavior in terms of our model." "We will not expect our client (child, adult, or parent) to do anything that we cannot model for them." We still did our verbal intraction counseling with parents, but we added the concrete aspect of teaching by example better communicative and interpersonal interaction between parent and child.

For example, if we conclude from the parent-child interaction analysis and the charting of speaking situations just described that the parents' speech rate is too rapid, that they ask too many questions too fast, and that they do not take time to listen to and respond to the content of the child's speech, then we proceed in our work with the child and the parents to countercondition these behaviors through the following sequence. The clinician talks to the child using a slower rate and more relaxed manner. The clinician expresses interest in what the child talks about and asks questions that are relatively easy ones for the child. Turn-taking in conversation is modeled for the child. Once progress is being made, the parents watch the client-clinician interaction from behind an observation mirror for several sessions, and then one or both parents may sit in the therapy room for a session or two. Gradually, the parents take part in therapy, participating at first for short periods (one or more activities) and then later for an entire session. In this example, discussions with the parents center on the parents learning the interactive behaviors modeled by the clinician. The parents are assigned a home activity once the clinician believes it is being performed appropriately in the clinic. Parents understand that the progression is from observation of the clinician to participation in the clinic to activity at home.

We may teach the parents relaxation procedures as well as more easy relaxed speech with smooth movements beginning at the word level and working up to longer utterances, just as we have done with the child. The child knows that the parents are learning what they are learning. As home assignments are given, the parents and the child are experiencing generalization and transfer.

We have found that parents respond positively to this counseling behavior-modification approach. They gain confidence in seeing that they are doing what the clinician is doing and that these actions are contributing to change in the child toward the development of normally fluent speech. In my opinion, the adding of these more specific modeling procedures has greatly enhanced the success of our parent counseling and the general success of our early intervention procedures. The reader should recall that this more direct work with the parents follows a period of counseling in which the clinician has established an open, understanding, supportive relationship with the parents; that relationship continues as the clinician provides information and models different behavior for the parents. The decisions about change in the environment, both communicative and interpersonal situations, should result, insofar as possible, from agreements between the parents and the clinician. The process I have described usually leads to that.

Success of Counseling

Success is relative. All families are different, and the factors we deal with in each case are different. With reference to the three treatment strategies described previously, Preventive Parent Counseling (Treatment Strategy I) and Prescriptive Parent Counseling with Limited Involvement of the Child (Treatment Strategy II) are most often successful after four to eight sessions on a weekly basis. When the parents and the child are seen in the Comprehensive Therapy Program (Treatment Strategy III), 75% of the children we see develop normal fluency that is maintained with 9 to 18 months. With the others, factors interfering with the maintenance of normal fluency are identified and appropriate recommendations are made, such as referring the child for more extensive psychological evaluation or the parents for more specific counseling related to child-rearing practices. In some few cases the parents have entered psychotherapy. There are also parents who refuse to follow our recommendations.

Maintenance

Maintenance consists of telephone checks with the parents and rechecks of the child at six-month intervals at the clinic or in the home. We must stay in contact with the parents until we are satisfied that speech is developing normally. In our program this is usually 18 to 24 months following dismissal.

CONCLUSION

With reference to the historical review at the beginning of this chapter, some contributors to the literature have advocated a more psychodynamic approach and others a more behavior-analysis-modification approach to altering the environment of children who stutter or who may be developing the problem. Still, very few clinicians have been *strict* adherents to one or the other points of view. The surge of work in behavior modification during the last 20 years influenced clinicians to define variables more precisely by generating such procedures as parent-child interaction analyses. Yet, most clinicians acknowledge that beliefs and feelings should be examined using interview-type verbal interactions with parents and children, procedures in which factors discussed are not defined as precisely. The relationship between clinician and client has been viewed as very important. For example, parents need to view the speech-language pathologist as a unique person who wants to understand and help. On the other hand, many clinicians who considered themselves more psychodynamically oriented have responded positively to the need to define parent-child interaction factors more definitively when possible and to use behavioral principles such as modeling to help parents and children modify their behavior. The approach to evaluation and treatment as presented in the latter part of the chapter represents the *consolidation* of procedures that most nearly characterizes contemporary approaches to environmental change. The following brief case descriptions are illustrations of this approach with two children, one requiring only very short-term help and the other requiring two years.*

CASE ILLUSTRATION—JERRY

Jerry was 36 months of age when we first saw him. He was an active, fast-moving, fast-talking little boy who was full of energy and mischief. He loved an audience to talk to, to boast to, and to direct to his bidding. In the previous few months he had become difficult for his mother to manage. She described her son as acting "like he is overloaded."

Evaluation revealed that Jerry's articulation and language development were within normal limits. His speech was characterized by a high frequency of irregular-syllable and one-syllable word repetitions and a few prolongations of sounds. In general, his disfluencies were what we consider as borderline atypical ones (Gregory & Hill, 1980). Jerry did not seem to have any awareness of difficulty talking. In a short period of trial therapy, he was able to imitate models of slower, more easy, relaxed speech.

A 15-minute parent-child interaction revealed that both parents spoke rapidly, changing the topic of conversation often. They asked many direct questions, often not allowing time for Jerry to answer before asking a follow-up or new question. There were several instances of the parents interrupting each other or Jerry. They often praised him and obviously enjoyed interacting with their son. Discussion with the parents pinpointed several environmental factors that could have been significant in maintaining Jerry's atypically disfluent speech pattern. The mother indicated that she and Jerry were always "on the go." She also mentioned that she felt overwhelmed by difficulty in managing her son at times, particularly in dressing him and helping him follow through with daily routines. She described the battle of wills that resulted and said she ended up losing her patience and screaming, which only made matters worse.

Child factors significant in maintaining disfluent speech may have been Jerry's rapid rate of talking, his need to talk a great deal and be in the spotlight, and stress and tension related to his desire to have his own way.

The treatment strategy recommended to this family was enrollment in our comprehensive preschool therapy program beginning in six weeks. Due to the time delay we worked with Jerry and the parents in a program we have termed prescriptive parent counseling with limited involvement of the child. The parents were helped to modify their style of interacting with Jerry by talking more slowly,

*Mrs. Diane Hill, Supervisor of the Primary Stuttering Program, Northwestern University, prepared these case descriptions.

asking fewer questions and commenting more, and gearing down the pace of living. The mother began to see the value in staying home more and not packing too much into a day. This change allowed more of a routine, and both mother and child were happier and had fewer conflicts. Both parents successfully learned to model slower speech, and Jerry in turn picked up on that style of speaking. After four sessions with the parents, in which they first observed and then participated with the clinician and their son, the parents were able to carry on by working with Jerry on their own. By the time the new program was ready to begin, Jerry's fluency was within a normal range and the parents felt comfortable about it.

With the birth of a baby brother six months later there was a reoccurrence of increased disfluency. The parents and Jerry were seen again for four weekly sessions. Fluency returned to normal and was maintained.

CASE ILLUSTRATION—JENNY

Jenny first came to our clinic about a month after her stuttering was first observed by her parents at age 36 months. Her mother was particularly alarmed by her daughter's struggling to speak, her awareness of difficulty, and her verbalizing "I can't talk" when she had obvious trouble. Jenny often put her hand over her mouth when she stuttered, expressed frustration, and threw temper tantrums in response to speech difficulty. Jenny's disfluency was characterized by prolongations; sound, syllable and word repetitions; interjections; hesitations; and combinations of these disfluency types. A moderate degree of tension was observed in the lips, tongue, or jaw in more than half of the disfluencies noted. Jenny also had a hoarse vocal quality and often shouted in play. There was a definite reason to be concerned about her speech.

In the course of evaluation, several child factors were identified as very likely contributing to the maintenance of Jenny's stuttering. These included: (a) her own learned responses to disfluent speech, (b) unhappiness with herself when her performance was what she considered as less than perfect, (c) sibling rivalry with her older sister intensified by her mother's frequent comparison of her to Jenny, and (d) difficult adjustment to other learning environments, including nursery school and the clinic. In the clinical setting, Jenny demonstrated discomfort in being asked to respond to verbal instructions and often resisted the clinician. In sum, she was an anxious little girl.

Environmental factors revolved around the mother's unrealistic expectations for Jenny, which stemmed from her need for perfection and control over her own life, as well as the life of the child. Jenny's articulation "errors" had often been corrected between ages two and three, and she shared her mother's pleasure at achieving production, saying "See, I can finally say it, Mom." In addition she was expected to set the table and vacuum under the table after meals. The mother kept charts for good performance posted in the kitchen.

A combination of therapy approaches was ultimately responsible for a positive outcome. Jenny was enrolled in an intensive therapy program including two hours of individual therapy and a half hour of group therapy, and the mother attended a weekly parent discussion group. Although the mother was cooperative and communicative, she had difficulty discovering the relationship between her needs for control and Jenny's stuttering problem. In this case, the services of both the clinician and consultant social worker were needed. It took about a year for the mother to realize that Jenny's speech problem could not be improved by working harder with her, being more orderly with charts, and more compulsive about carrying out suggestions. She found it difficult to relax and break down her need for rigid control.

Work with Jenny and her parents was fairly long term—almost two years—and was based on the complex effect of Jenny's learned responses to parental expectations, which took considerable time to modify and replace with more adaptive attitudes and behaviors. Therapy included changing speech behavior using a modified programmed learning format to establish an easy, relaxed speech pattern, but it also required work on attitudes and feelings interfering with progress. Jenny gradually learned to be more flexible, to relax and speak in an easy manner, to be more accepting of "mistakes," and to be more willing to venture forth and try new things. She learned to be comfortable without being in control, to compete, and to handle defeat!

The parents' attitudes and behavior were changed by verbal counseling with the speech-language pathologist and a social worker and by the clinician modeling for the parents more relaxed, less perfectionistic behavior, and also more relaxed speech. Jenny is now a normal-speaking teenager.

REFERENCES

Ainsworth,S., & Gruss, J. (1981). *If your child stutters: A guide for parents.* Memphis, TN: Speech Foundation of America.

Bandura, A. (1969). *Principles of behavior modification.* New York: Holt, Rinehart, and Winston.

Bloodstein, O. (1975). Stuttering as tension and fragmentation. In J. Eisenson (Ed.), *Stuttering: A second symposium.* New York: Harper and Row.

Cooper, E. B. (1965). Structured therapy for therapist and child. *Journal of Speech and Hearing Disorders, 30,* 75–78.

Cooper, E. B. (1968). A therapy process for the adult stutterer. *Journal of Speech and Hearing Disorders, 33,* 246–260.

Cooper, E. B. (1976). *Personalized fluency control therapy: An integrated behavior and relationship therapy for stutterers.* Austin, TX: Learning Concepts.

Cooper, E. B. (1979). Intervention procedures for the young stutterer. In H. Gregory (Ed.), *Controversies about stuttering therapy.* Baltimore, MD: University Park Press.

Emerick, L. L., & Hood, S. B. (Eds.). (1974). *The client-clinician relationship.* Springfield, IL: Charles C. Thomas.

Ginott, H. G. (1965). *Between parent and child.* New York: MacMillan.

Glasner, H. G. (1970). Developmental view. In J. Sheehan (Ed.), *Stuttering: Research and therapy.* New York: Harper and Row.

Gregory, H. (1968). Applications of learning theory concepts in the management of stuttering. In H. Gregory, (Ed.), *Learning theory and stuttering therapy.* Evanston, IL: Northwestern University Press.

Gregory, H. (1973). Modeling procedure in the treatment of elementary school age children who stutter. *Journal of Fluency Disorders, 1,* 58–63. (a)

Gregory, H. (1973). *Stuttering: Differential evaluation and therapy.* Indianapolis, IN: Bobbs-Merrill. (b)

Gregory, H. (1984). Prevention of stuttering and the management of early developmental stages. In R. Curlee & W. Perkins (Eds.), *Nature and treatment of stuttering.* San Diego, CA: College Hill Press.

Gregory H., & Hill, D. (1980). Stuttering therapy for children. In W. Perkins (Ed.), *Strategies in stuttering therapy.* New York: Thieme-Stratton.

Hood, S. (1978). The assessment of fluency disorders. In S. Singh & J. Lynch (Eds.), *Diagnostic procedures in hearing, language and speech.* Baltimore, MD: University Park Press.

Johnson, L. (1980). Facilitating parental involvement in therapy of the disfluent child. In W. Perkins (Ed.), *Strategies in stuttering therapy.* New York: Thieme-Stratton.

Johnson, W. (1946). *People in quandaries.* New York: Harper and Row.

Johnson, W. Wendell Johnson. (1956). In E. Hahn (Ed.), *Stuttering: Significant theories and therapies.* Stanford, CA: Stanford University Press.

Johnson, W., et al. (1959). *The onset of stuttering.* Minneapolis, MN: University of Minnesota Press.

Johnson, W. (1967). Stuttering. In W. Johnson, et al. (Eds), *Speech handicapped school children.* New York: Harper and Row.

Kasprisin, A. (1970, November). *Implications of parental verbal behavior for stuttering therapy with children.* Paper presented at the American Speech and Hearing Association Convention, New York.

Kasprisin-Burrelli, A., Egolf, D., & Shames, G. (1972). A comparison of parental verbal behavior with stuttering and nonstuttering children. *Journal of Communication Disorders, 5,* 335–346.

Luper, H. L., & Mulder, R. (1964). *Stuttering: Therapy for children.* Englewood Cliffs, NJ: Prentice-Hall.

Mordecai, D. (1979). *An investigation of the communicative styles of mothers and fathers of stuttering versus nonstuttering preschool children during a triadic interaction.* Unpublished doctoral dissertation, Northwestern University, Evanston, Illinois.

Murphy, A. (1974). Feelings and attitudes. In W. Starkweather (Ed.), *Therapy for stutterers.* Memphis, TN: Speech Foundation of America.

Murphy, A. (1977). Authenticity and creativity in stuttering theory and therapy. *Journal of Communicative Disorders, 10,* 25–36.

Murphy, A., & Fitzsimons, R. M. (1960). *Stuttering and personality dynamics.* New York: Ronald Press.

Nelson, L. (1984). Language formulation related to disfluency and stuttering. In H. Gregory (Ed.), *Evaluation of disfluency, prevention of stuttering, and intervention with children.* Memphis, TN: Speech Foundation of America.

Riley, G. & Riley, J. (1979). A component model for diagnosing and treating children who stutter. *Journal of Fluency Disorders, 4,* 279–294.

Riley, G. & Riley, J. (1983). Evaluation as a basis for intervention. In D. Prins and R. Ingham (Eds.), *Treatment of stuttering in early childhood: Methods and issues.* San Diego: College-Hill Press.

Rogers, C. (1951). *Client-centered therapy.* Boston, MA: Houghton-Mifflin.

Rogers, C. (1957). The necessary and sufficient conditions of therapeutic personality change. *Journal of Consultant Psychology, 21,* 95–103.

Rustin, L. & Cook, F. (1983). Intervention procedures for the disfluent child. In P. Dalton (Ed.), *Approaches to the treatment of stuttering.* Beckenham, Kent, England: Croom Helm, Ltd.

Shames, G., & Egolf, D. (1976). *Operant conditioning and the management of stuttering.* Englewood Cliffs, NJ: Prentice-Hall.

Shames, G. & Florance, C. (1980). *Stutter free speech.* Columbus, OH: Charles E. Merrill.

Shames, G., & Sherrick, C. E. (1963). A discussion of nonfluency and stuttering as operant behavior. *Journal of Speech and Hearing Disorders, 28,* 3–18.

Sheehan, J. (1970). *Stuttering: Research and therapy.* New York: Harper and Row.

Sheehan, J. (1975). Conflict theory and avoidance reduction therapy. In J. Eisenson (Ed.), *Stuttering: A second symposium.* New York: Harper and Row.

Van Riper, C. (1947). *Speech correction: Principles and methods.* Englewood Cliffs, NJ: Prentice-Hall.

Van Riper, C. (1973). *The treatment of stuttering.* Englewood Cliffs, NJ: Prentice-Hall.

Van Riper, C. (1979). The stutterer's clinician. In J. Eisenson (Ed.), *Stuttering: A second symposium.* New York: Harper and Row.

Wahler, R., Sperling, K., Thomas M., Teeter, N., & Luper, H. (1970). The modification of childhood stuttering: Some response relationships. *Journal of Experimental Child Psychiatry, 3,* 411–428.

Williams, D. (1978). The problem of stuttering. In F. Darley and D. C. Spriestersbach (Eds.), *Diagnostic methods in speech pathology.* New York: Harper and Row.

Wyatt, C. (1969). *Language learning and communication disorders in children.* New York: The Free Press.

Zwitman, D. H. (1978). *The disfluent child: A management program.* Baltimore, MD: University Park Press.

13

The Attitude and Orientation of the Counselor

Carl Rogers

Postscript
Client-Centered Therapy

Julius Seeman

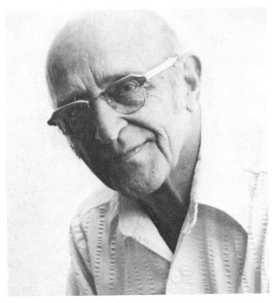

Carl Rogers

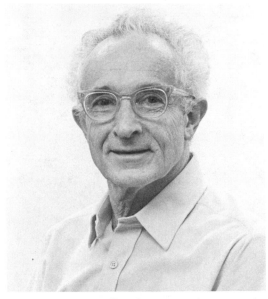

Julius Seeman

Many therapies for stuttering are represented in this book. Perhaps none has had such a pervasive and generic impact on speech pathology in general and on stuttering in particular, than the principles of Client-Centered Therapy, as developed by Carl Rogers. The philosophy and thinking of Rogers surfaces in almost all clinical endeavors dealing with communication disorders, whether we are engaging in case-history taking, parent counseling, or individual client management. His respect for the integrity of the individual, his focus on feelings, and his encouragement of self-responsibility are components of much that we do in the clinical management of stuttering. In his first book, *Counseling and psychotherapy,* Rogers devoted the last chapter entirely to verbatim transcriptions and analyses of clinical interviews with an adult stutterer. His approach to the human condition generally subordinates the symptom (such as stuttering) and instead focuses on helping a person to explore his feelings about himself and to develop an honesty and understanding of how he may experience himself more comfortably and productively. He thinks that each of us has the potential within ourselves to explore ourselves, our feelings, and our behavior; to become responsible for ourselves; and to become comfortable with who we are. His style is warm and supportive, yet honest and tenacious in moving people toward assuming greater responsibil-

ity for examining and managing their lives. Client-centered therapy has been and still is, in and of itself, a therapy for stuttering. However, in addition, its principles have been seen in many other therapies presented in this book. As a philosophy and as a style it has influenced the manner in which other significant therapies are put into effect.

Dr. Rogers agreed to having his earlier published material that describes the principles of his therapy appear in this volume. However, because of other commitments, he recommended a colleague, Dr. Julius Seeman, to write the update. Dr. Seeman in his own right is a well-known client-centered therapist who has considerable experience in applying this therapy to stuttering. Many years ago he published the now famous "Case of Jim," which was a written account of a series of clinical interviews with an adult stutterer, along with an audiotape of those interviews. He is eminently qualified to provide a current view of client-centered therapy as it applies to stuttering. Dr. Seeman not only discusses Dr. Rogers's earlier views, but also traces an evolution of them to their current state. Additionally, Dr. Seeman shares the case of Jim, discusses his therapy in detail from the client-centered perspective, and provides us with specific follow-up information about this stutterer some 30 years after his original therapy.

13

The Attitude and Orientation of the Counselor[1]

In any psychotherapy, the therapist himself is a highly important part of the human equation. What he does, the attitude he holds, his basic concept of his role, all influence therapy to a marked degree. Differing therapeutic orientations hold differing views on these points. At the very outset of our discussion, therefore, it seems appropriate to consider the therapist as he functions in client-centered counseling.

A GENERAL CONSIDERATION

It is common to find client-centered therapy spoken of as simply a method or a technique to be used by the counselor. No doubt this connotation is due in part to the fact that earlier presentations tended to overstress technique. It may more accurately be said that the counselor who is effective in client-centered therapy holds a coherent and developing set of attitudes deeply imbedded in his personal organization, a system of attitudes which is implemented by techniques and methods consistent with it. In our experience, the counselor who tries to use a "method" is doomed to be unsuccessful unless this method is genuinely in line with his own attitudes. On the other hand, the counselor whose attitudes are of the type which facilitate therapy may be only partially suc-

cessful, because his attitudes are inadequately implemented by appropriate methods and techniques.

Let us, then, consider the attitudes which appear to facilitate client-centered therapy. Must the counselor possess them in order to be a counselor? May these attitudes be achieved through training?

THE PHILOSOPHICAL ORIENTATION OF THE COUNSELOR

Some workers are reluctant to consider the relationship of philosophical views to scientific professional work. Yet in therapeutic endeavor this relation appears to be one of the significant and scientifically observable facts that cannot be ignored. Our experience in training counselors would indicate that the basic operational philosophy of the individual (which may or may not resemble his verbalized philosophy) determines, to a considerable extent, the time it will take him to become a skillful counselor.

The primary point of importance here is the attitude held by the counselor toward the worth and the significance of the individual. How do we look upon others? Do we see each person as having worth and dignity in his own right? If we do hold this point of view at the verbal level, to what extent is it operationally evident at the behavioral level? Do we tend to treat individuals as persons of worth, or do we subtly

[1]This chapter is a revision and extension of an article which first appeared in the *Journal of Consulting Psychology* (April, 1949), *13*, 82–94.

devaluate them by our attitudes and behavior? Is our philosophy one in which respect for the individual is uppermost? Do we respect his capacity and his right to self-direction, or do we basically believe that his life would be best guided by us? To what extent do we have a need and a desire to dominate others? Are we willing for the individual to select and choose his own values, or are our actions guided by the conviction (usually unspoken) that he would be happiest if he permitted us to select for him his values and standards and goals?

The answers to questions of this sort appear to be important as basic determiners of the therapist's approach. It has been our experience that individuals who are already striving toward an orientation which stresses the significance and worth of each person can learn rather readily the client-centered techniques which implement this point of view. This is often true of workers in education who have a strongly child-centered philosophy of education. It is not infrequently true of religious workers who have a humanistic approach. Among psychologists and psychiatrists there are those with similar views, but there are also many whose concept of the individual is that of an object to be dissected, diagnosed, manipulated. Such professional workers may find it difficult to learn or to practice a client-centered form of therapy. In any event, the differences in this respect seem to determine the readiness or unreadiness of professional workers to learn and achieve a client-centered approach.

Even this statement of the situation gives a static impression which is inaccurate. One's operational philosophy, one's set of goals, is not a fixed and unchanging thing, but a fluid and developing organization. Perhaps it would be more accurate to say that the person whose philosophical orientation has tended to move in the direction of greater respect for the individual finds in the client-centered approach a challenge to and an implementation of his views. He finds that here is a point of view in human relationships which tends to carry him further philosophically than he has heretofore ventured, and to provide the possibility of an operational technique for putting into effect this respect for persons, to the full degree that it exists in his own attitudes. The therapist who endeavors to utilize this approach soon learns that the development of the way of looking upon people which underlies this therapy is a continuing process, closely related to the therapist's own struggle for personal growth and integration. He can be only

as "nondirective" as he has achieved respect for others in his own personality organization.

Perhaps it would summarize the point being made to say that, by use of client-centered techniques, a person can implement his respect for others only so far as that respect is an integral part of his personality make-up; consequently the person whose operational philosophy has already moved in the direction of *feeling* a deep respect for the significance and worth of each person is more readily able to assimilate client-centered techniques which help him to express this feeling.[2]

THE THERAPIST'S HYPOTHESIS

The question may well arise, in view of the preceding section, as to whether client-centered therapy is then simply a cult, or a speculative philosophy, in which a certain type of faith or belief achieves certain results, and where lack of such faith prevents these results from occurring. Is this, in other words, simply an illusion which produces further illusions?

Such a question deserves careful consideration. That observations to date would seem to point to an answer in the negative is perhaps most strikingly indicated in the experience of various counselors whose initial philosophic orientation has been rather distant from that described as favorable to an optimum use of client-centered techniques. The experience of such individuals in training has seemed to follow something of a pattern. Initially there is relatively little trust in the capacity of the client to achieve insight or constructive self-direction, although the counselor is intrigued intellectually by the possibilities of nondirective therapy and learns something of the techniques. He starts counseling clients with a very limited hypothesis of respect, which might be stated somewhat in these terms: "I will hypothesize that the individual has a limited capacity to understand and reorganize himself to some degree in certain types of situations. In many situa-

---

[2]This whole topic might be helpfully pursued on a deeper level. What permits the therapist to have a deep respect for, and acceptance of, another? In our experience, such a philosophy is most likely to be held by the person who has a basic respect for the worth and significance of himself. One cannot, in all likelihood, accept others unless he has first accepted himself. This could lead us off into various byways, to a consideration of those experiences, including therapy, which assist the therapist to gain an abiding and realistically founded self-respect. We shall leave such a discussion for Chapter 10, limiting ourselves here simply to a description of the philosophical organization which seems to be the most effective foundation for this type of therapy.

tions and with many clients, I, as a more objective outsider, can better know the situation and better guide it." It is on this limited and divided basis that he begins his work. He is often not very successful. But as he observes his counseling results, he finds that clients accept and make constructive use of responsibility when he is genuinely willing for them to do so. He is often surprised at their effectiveness in handling this responsibility. Against the less vital quality of the experience in those situations where he, the counselor, has endeavored to interpret, evaluate, and guide, he cannot help but contrast the quality of the experience in those situations where the client has learned significantly for himself. Thus he finds that the first portion of his hypothesis tends to be proved beyond his expectations, while the second portion proves disappointing. So, little by little, the hypothesis upon which he bases all his therapeutic work shifts to an increasingly client-centered foundation.

This type of process, which we have seen repeated many times, would appear to mean simply this: that the attitudinal orientation, the philosophy of human relationships which seems to be a necessary basis for client-centered counseling, is not something which must be taken "on faith," or achieved all at once. It is a point of view which may be adopted tentatively and partially, and put to the test. It is actually an hypothesis in human relationships, and will always remain so. Even for the experienced counselor, who has observed in many many cases the evidence which supports the hypothesis, it is still true that, for the new client who comes in the door, the possibility of self-understanding and intelligent self-direction is still—for this client—a completely unproved hypothesis.

It would seem justifiable to say that the faith or belief in the capacity of the individual to deal with his psychological situation and with himself is of the same order as any scientific hypothesis. It is a positive basis for action, but it is open to proof or disproof. If, for example, we had faith that every person could determine for himself whether he had incipient cancer, our experience with this hypothesis would soon cause us to revise it sharply. On the other hand, if we have faith that warm maternal affection is likely to produce desirable personal reactions and personality growth in the infant, we are likely to find this hypothesis supported, at least tentatively, by our experience.

Hence, to put in more summarized or definitive form the attitudinal orientation which appears to be optimal for the client-centered counselor, we may say that the counselor chooses to act consistently upon the hypothesis that the individual has a sufficient capacity to deal constructively with all those aspects of his life which can potentially come into conscious awareness. This means the creation of an interpersonal situation in which material may come into the client's awareness, and a meaningful demonstration of the counselor's acceptance of the client as a person who is competent to direct himself. The counselor acts upon this hypothesis in a specific and operational fashion, being always alert to note those experiences (clinical or research) which contradict this hypothesis as well as those which support it.

Though he is alert to all the evidence, this does not mean that he keeps shifting his basic hypothesis in counseling situations. If the counselor feels, in the middle of an interview, that this client may not have the capacity for reorganizing himself, and shifts to the hypothesis that the counselor must bear a considerable responsibility for this reorganization, he confuses the client, and defeats himself. He has shut himself off from proving or disproving either hypothesis. This confused eclecticism, which has been prevalent in psychotherapy, has blocked scientific progress in the field. Actually it is only by acting *consistently* upon a well-selected hypothesis that its elements of truth and untruth can become known.

THE SPECIFIC IMPLEMENTATION OF THE COUNSELOR'S ATTITUDE

Thus far the discussion has been a general one, considering the counselor's basic attitude toward others. How does this become implemented in the therapeutic situation? Is it enough that the counselor hold the basic hypothesis we have described, and that this attitudinal orientation will then inevitably move therapy forward? Most assuredly this is not enough. It is as though a physician of the last century had come to believe that bacteria cause infection. Holding this attitude would probably make it inevitable that he should obtain somewhat better results than his colleagues who looked upon this hypothesis with contempt. But only as he implemented his attitude to the fullest extent with appropriate techniques would he fully experience the significance of his hypothesis. Only as he made sterile the area around the incision, the instruments, the sheets, the bandages, his hands, the hands of his assistants—only then would he experience the full meaning and full effectivness of this tentative hypothesis which he had come to hold in a general way.

So it is with the counselor. As he finds new and more subtle ways of implementing his client-centered hypothesis, new meanings are poured into it by experience, and its depth is seen to be greater than was first supposed. As one counselor-in-training put it, "I hold about the same views I did a year ago, but they have so much more meaning for me."

It is possible that one of the most significant general contributions of the client-centered approach has been its insistence upon investigating the detailed implementation of the counselor's point of view in the interview itself. Many different therapists from a number of differing orientations state their general purposes in somewhat similar terms. Only by a careful study of the recorded interview—preferably with both the sound recording and transcribed typescript available—is it possible to determine what purpose or purposes are actually being implemented in the interview. "Am I actually doing what I think I am doing? Am I operationally carrying out the purposes which I verbalize?" These are questions which every counselor must continually be asking himself. There is ample evidence from our research analyses that a subjective judgment by the counselor himself regarding these questions is not enough. Only an objective analysis of words, voice and inflection can adequately determine the real purpose the therapist is pursuing. As we know from many experiences in therapists' reactions to their recorded material, and from a research analysis by Blocksma (33), the counselor is not frequently astonished to discover the aims he is actually carrying out in the interview.

Note that in discussing this point the term "technique" has been discarded in favor of "implementation." The client is apt to be quick to discern when the counselor is using a "method," an intellectually chosen tool which he has selected for a purpose. On the other hand, the counselor is always implementing, both in conscious and nonconscious ways, the attitudes which he holds toward the client. These attitudes can be inferred and discovered from their operational implementation. Thus a counselor who basically does not hold the hypothesis that the person has significant capacity for integrating himself may think that he has used nondirective "methods" and "techniques," and proved to his own satisfaction that these techniques are unsuccessful. A recording of such material tends to show, however, that in the tone of voice, in the handling of the unexpected, in the peripheral activities of the interview, he implements his own hypothesis, not the client-centered hypothesis as he thinks.

It would seem that there can be no substitute for the continual checking back and forth between purpose or hypothesis and technique or implementation. This analytical self-checking the counselor may verbalize somewhat as follows: As I develop more clearly and more fully the attitude and hypothesis upon which I intend to deal with the client, I must check the implementation of that hypothesis in the interview material. But as I study my specific behaviors in the interview I detect implied purposes of which I had not been aware, I discover areas in which it had not occurred to me to apply the hypothesis, I realize that what was for me an implementation of one attitude is perceived by the client as the implementation of another. Thus the thorough study of my behavior sharpens, alters, and modifies the attitude and hypothesis with which I enter the next interview. A sound approach to the implementation of an hypothesis is a continuing and a reciprocal experience.

SOME FORMULATIONS OF THE COUNSELOR'S ROLE

As we look back upon the development of the client-centered point of view, we find a steady progression of attempts to formulate what is involved in implementing the basic hypothesis in the interview situation. Some of these are formulations by individual counselors, whereas others have been more generally held. Let us take a few of these concepts and examine them, moving through them to the formulation which appears to be most commonly held at the present time by therapists of this orientation.

In the first place, some counselors—usually those with little specific training—have supposed that the counselor's role in carrying on nondirective counseling was merely to be passive and to adopt a laissez faire policy. Such a counselor has some willingness for the client to be self-directing. He is more inclined to listen than to guide. He tries to avoid imposing his own evaluations upon the client. He finds that a number of his clients gain help for themselves. He feels that his faith in the client's capacity is best exhibited by a passivity which involves a minimum of activity and of emotional reaction on his part. He tries "to stay out of the client's way."

This misconception of the approach has led to considerable failure in counseling—and for good reasons. In the first place, the passivity and seeming lack of interest or involvement is experienced by the client as a rejection since indifference is in no real way the same as acceptance. In the second place, a laissez faire attitude does not in any way indicate to the client that he is regarded as a person of worth. Hence the counselor who plays a merely passive role, a listening role, may be of assistance to some clients who are desperately in need of emotional catharsis, but by and large his results will be minimal, and many clients will leave both disappointed in their failure to receive help and disgusted with the counselor for having nothing to offer.

Another formulation of the counselor's role is that it is his task to clarify and objectify the client's feelings. The present author, in a paper given in 1940 stated, "As material is given by the client, it is the therapist's function to help him recognize and clarify the emotions which he feels" (169, p. 162). This has been a useful concept, and it is partially descriptive of what occurs. It is, however, too intellectualistic, and if taken too literally, may focus the process in the counselor. It can mean that only the counselor knows what the feelings are, and if it acquires this meaning it becomes a subtle lack of respect for the client.

Unfortunately, our experience in conveying subtleties of emotionalized attitude is so limited, and the symbols of expression so unsatisfactory, that it is hard accurately to convey to a reader the delicate attitudes involved in the therapist's work. We have learned, to our dismay, that even the transcripts of our recorded cases may give to the reader a totally erroneous notion of the sort of relationship which existed. By persistently reading the counselor responses with the wrong inflection, it is possible to distort the whole picture of the relationship. Such readers when they first hear even a small segment of the recording itself, often say, "Oh, this is entirely different from the way I understood it."

Perhaps the subtle difference between a declarative and an empathic attitude on the part of the counselor may be conveyed by an example. Here is a client statement: "I feel as though my mother is always watching me and criticizing what I do. It gets me all stirred up inside. I try not to let that happen, but you know, there are times when I feel her eagle eye on me that I just boil inwardly."

A response on the counselor's part might be: "You resent her criticism." This response may be given empathically, with the tone of voice such as would be used if it were worded, "If I understand you correctly, you feel pretty resentful toward her criticism. Is that right?" If this is the attitude and tone which is used, it would probably be experienced by the client as aiding him in further expression. Yet we have learned, from the fumblings of counselors-in-training, that "You resent her criticism" may be given with the same attitude and tone with which one might announce "You have the measles," or even with the attitude and tone which would accompany the words "You are sitting on my hat." If the reader will repeat the counselor response in some of these varying inflections, he may realize that when stated empathically and understandingly, the likely attitudinal response on the part of the client is, "Yes, that is the way I feel, and I perceive that a little more clearly now that you have put it in somewhat different terms." But when the counselor statement is declarative, it becomes an evaluation, a judgment made by the counselor, who is now telling the client what his feelings are. The process is centered in the counselor, and the feeling of the client would tend to be, "I am being diagnosed."

In order to avoid this latter type of handling, we have tended to give up the description of the counselor's role as being that of clarifying the client's attitudes.

At the present stage of thinking in client-centered therapy, there is another attempt to describe what occurs in the most satisfactory therapeutic relationships, another attempt to describe the way in which the basic hypothesis is implemented. This formulation would state that it is the counselor's function to assume, in so far as he is able, the internal frame of reference of the client, to perceive the world as the client sees it, to perceive the client himself as he is seen by himself, to lay aside all perceptions from the external frame of reference while doing so, and to communicate something of this empathic understanding to the client.

Raskin, in an unpublished article (159), has given a vivid description of this version of the counselor's function.

> There is [another] level of nondirective counselor response which to the writer represents *the* nondirective attitude. In a sense, it is a goal rather than one which is actually practised by counselors. But, in the experience of some, it is a highly attainable goal, which . . . changes the nature of the counseling process in a radical way. At this level, counselor participation becomes an active experiencing with the client of the feelings to which he

gives expression, the counselor makes a maximum effort to get under the skin of the person with whom he is communicating, he tries to get *within* and to live the attitudes expressed instead of observing them, to catch every nuance of their changing nature; in a word, to absorb himself completely in the attitudes of the other. And in struggling to do this, there is simply no room for any other type of counselor activity or attitude; if he is attempting to live the attitudes of the other, he cannot be diagnosing them, he cannot be thinking of making the process go faster. Because he is another, and not the client, the understanding is not spontaneous but must be acquired, and this through the most intense, continuous and active attention to the feelings of the other, to the exclusion of any other type of attention.

Even this description may be rather easily misunderstood since the experiencing with the client, the living of his attitudes, is not in terms of emotional identification, but rather an empathic identification where the counselor is perceiving the hates and hopes and fears of the client through immersion in an empathic process, but without himself, as counselor, experiencing those hates and hopes and fears.

Another attempt to phrase this point of view has been made by the author. It is as follows:

> As time has gone by we have come to put increasing stress upon the "client-centeredness" of the relationship, because it is more effective the more completely the counselor concentrates upon trying to understand the client *as the client seems to himself.* As I look back upon some of our earlier published cases—the case of Herbert Bryan in my book, or Snyder's case of Mr. M.— I realize that we have gradually dropped the vestiges of subtle directiveness which are all too evident in those cases. We have come to recognize that if we can provide understanding of the way the client seems to himself at this moment, he can do the rest. The therapist must lay aside his preoccupation with diagnosis and his diagnostic shrewdness, must discard his tendency to make professional evaluations, must cease his endeavors to formulate an accurate prognosis, must give up the temptation subtly to guide the individual, and must concentrate on one purpose only; that of providing deep understanding and acceptance of the attitudes consciously held at this moment by the client as he explores step by step into the dangerous areas which he has been denying to consciousness.
>
> I trust it is evident from this description that this type of relationship can exist only if the counselor is deeply and genuinely able to adopt these attitudes. Client-centered counseling, if it is to be effective, cannot be a trick or a tool. It is not a subtle way of guiding the client while pretending to let him guide himself. To be effective, it must be genuine. It is this sensitive and sincere "client-centeredness" in the therapeutic relationship that I regard as the third characteristic of nondirective therapy which sets it distinctively apart from other approaches. (170, pp. 420–421)

RESEARCH EVIDENCE OF A TREND

A research study recently completed would tend to confirm some of the preceding statements (180). Counselor techniques used by nondirective counselors in cases handled in 1947–48 have been analyzed in terms of the categories used by Snyder in analyzing cases handled in 1940–42 (196). This gives an opportunity for direct comparison of counselor methods, and hence the opportunity to note any observable trend. It is found that at the earlier date the counselors used a number of responses involving questioning, interpreting, reassuring, encouraging, suggesting. Such responses, though always forming a small proportion of the total, would seem to indicate on the counselor's part a limited confidence in the capacity of the client to understand and cope with his difficulties. The counselor still felt it necessary at times to take the lead, to explain the client to himself, to be supportive, and to point out what to the counselor were desirable courses of action. As clinical experience in therapy has continued, there has been a sharp decrease in all these forms of response. In the later cases, the proportion of responses of any of these types is negligible. Eighty-five per cent of the counselor responses are attempts to convey an understanding of the client's attitudes and feelings. It appears quite clear that nondirective counselors, on the basis of continuing therapeutic experience, have come to depend more fully upon the basic hypothesis of the approach than was true a half dozen years ago. It seems that more and more the nondirective therapist has judged understanding and acceptance to be effective, and has come to concentrate his whole effort upon achieving a deep understanding of the private world of the client.

Since the completion of the second study mentioned, it seems to be true that there has been more reaching out for a wider variety of therapist techniques. For the most part, however, this has meant a searching for new ways of making it clear that the therapist is thinking and feeling and exploring with the client. It is natural to expect that with increasing security in clinical experience there will be an increasing variety of attempts to communicate the fact that the therapist is endeavoring to achieve the internal frame of reference of the client, and is trying to see with him as deeply as the client sees, or even more deeply than the latter is able at the moment to perceive. In utilizing this increasing variety of responses, it is quite possible that this current formulation of the counselor's role will be discarded, just as previous formulations have been. So far, however, this seems not to be the case.

THE DIFFICULTY OF PERCEIVING THROUGH THE CLIENT'S EYES

This struggle to achieve the client's internal frame of reference, to gain the center of his own perceptual field and see with him as perceiver, is rather closely analogous to some of the Gestalt phenomena. Just as, by active concentration, one can suddenly see the diagram in the psychology text as representing a descending rather than an ascending stairway or can perceive two faces instead of a candlestick, so by active effort the counselor can put himself into the client's frame of reference. But just as in the case of the visual perception, the figure occasionally changes, so the counselor may at times find himself standing outside the client's frame of reference and looking as an external perceiver at the client. This almost invariably happens, for example, during a long pause or silence on the client's part. The counselor may gain a few clues which permit an accurate empathy, but to some extent he is forced to view the client from an observer's point of view, and can only actively assume the client's perceptual field when some type of expression again begins.

The reader can attempt this role in various ways, can give himself practice in assuming the internal frame of reference of another while overhearing a conversation on the streetcar, or while listening to a friend describe an emotional experience. Perhaps something of what is involved can even be conveyed on paper.

To try to give you, the reader, a somewhat more real and vivid experience of what is involved in the attitudinal set which we are discussing, it is suggested that you put yourself in the place of the counselor, and consider the following material, which is taken from complete counselor notes of the beginning of an interview with a man in his thirties. When the material has been completed, sit back and consider the sorts of attitudes and thoughts which were in your mind as you read.

Client: I don't feel very normal, but I want to feel that way. . . . I thought I'd have something to talk about—then it all goes around in circles. I was trying to think what I was going to say. Then coming here it doesn't work out. . . . I tell you, it seemed that it would be much easier before I came. I tell you, I just can't make a decision; I don't know what I want. I've tried to reason this thing out logically—tried to figure out which things are important to me. I thought that there are maybe two things a man might do; he might get married and raise a family. But if he was just a bachelor, just making a living—that isn't very good. I find myself and my thoughts getting back to the days when I was a kid and I cry very easily. The dam would break through. I've been in the Army four and a half years. I had no problems then, no hopes, no wishes. My only thought was to get out when peace would come. My problems, now that I'm out, are as ever. I tell you, they go back to a long time before I was in the Army. . . . I love children. When I was in the Philippines—I tell you, when I was young I swore I'd never forget my unhappy childhood—so when I saw these children in the Philippines, I treated them very nicely. I used to give them ice cream cones and movies. It was just a period—I'd reverted back—and that awakened some emotions in me I thought I had long buried. *(A pause. He seems very near tears.)*

As this material was read, such thoughts as the following would represent an external frame of reference in you, the "counselor."

> I wonder if I should help him get started talking.
> Is this inability to get under way a type of dependence?
> Why this indecisiveness? What could be its cause?
> What is meant by this focus on marriage and family?
> He seems to be a bachelor. I hadn't known that.
> The crying, the "dam," sound as though there must be a great deal of repression.
> He's a veteran. Could he have been a psychiatric case?
> I feel sorry for anybody who spent four and one-half years in the service.
> Some time he will probably need to dig into those early unhappy experiences.
> What is this interest in children? Identification? Vague homosexuality?

Note that these are all attitudes which are basically sympathetic. There is nothing "wrong" with them. They are even attempts to "understand," in the sense of "understanding about," rather than "understanding with." The locus of perceiving is, however, outside of the client.

By way of comparison, the thoughts which might go through your mind if you were quite successful in assuming the client's internal frame of reference would tend to be of this order:

You're wanting to struggle toward normality, aren't you?

It's really hard for you to get started.

Decision-making just seems impossible to you.

You want marriage, but it doesn't seem to you to be much of a possibility.

You feel yourself brimming over with childish feelings.

To you the Army represented stagnation.

Being very nice to children has somehow had meaning for you.

But it was—and is—a disturbing experience for you.

As pointed out before, if these thoughts are couched in a final and declarative form, then they shift over into becoming an evaluation from the counselor's perceptual vantage point. But to the extent that they are attempts to understand, tentative in formulation, they represent the attitude we are trying to describe as "adopting the client's frame of reference."

THE RATIONALE OF THE COUNSELOR'S ROLE

The question may arise in the minds of many, why adopt this peculiar type of relationship? In what way does it implement the hypothesis from which we started? What is the rationale of this approach?

In order to have a clear basis for considering these questions, let us attempt to put first in formal terms and then in paraphrase a statement of the counselor's purpose when he functions in this way. In psychological terms, it is the counselor's aim to perceive as sensitively and accurately as possible all of the perceptual field as it is being experienced by the client, with the same figure and ground relationships, to the full degree that the client is willing to communicate that perceptual field; and having thus perceived this internal frame of reference of the other as completely as possible, to indicate to the client the extent to which he is seeing through the client's eyes.

Suppose that we attempt a description somewhat more in terms of the counselor's attitudes. The counselor says in effect, "To be of assistance to you I will put aside myself—the self of ordinary interaction—and enter into your world of perception as completely as I am able. I will become, in a sense, another self for you—an alter ego of your own attitudes and feelings—a safe opportunity for you to discern your-

self more clearly, to experience yourself more truly and deeply, to choose more significantly."

THE COUNSELOR'S ROLE AS IMPLEMENTATION OF AN HYPOTHESIS

In what ways does this approach implement the central hypothesis of our work? It would be grossly misleading to say that our present method or formulation of the method grew out of the theory. The truth is that, as in most similar problems, one begins to find on the basis of clinical intuition that certain attitudes are effective, others are not. One tries to relate these experiences to basic theory, and thus they become clarified and point in the direction of further extension. It is thus that we have arrived at the present formulation, and this formulation will undoubtedly change as we solve some of the perplexities stated at the end of this chapter.

For the present, it would appear that for me, as counselor, to focus my whole attention and effort upon understanding and perceiving as the client perceives and understands, is a striking operational demonstration of the belief I have in the worth and the significance of this individual client. Clearly the most important value which I hold is, as indicated by my attitudes and my verbal behavior, the client himself. Also the fact that I permit the outcome to rest upon this deep understanding is probably the most vital operational evidence which could be given that I have confidence in the potentiality of the individual for constructive change and development in the direction of a more full and satisfying life. As a seriously disturbed client wrestles with his utter inability to make any choice, or another client struggles with his strong urges to commit suicide, the fact that I enter with deep understanding into the desperate feelings that exist but do not attempt to take over responsibility, is a most meaningful expression of basic confidence in the forward-moving tendencies in the human organism.

We might say then, that for many therapists functioning from a client-centered orientation, the sincere aim of getting "within" the attitudes of the client, of entering the client's internal frame of reference, is the most complete implementation which has thus far been formulated, for the central hypothesis of respect for and reliance upon the capacity of the person.

THE CLIENT'S EXPERIENCE OF THE COUNSELOR

The question would still remain, what psychological purpose is served by attempting to duplicate, as it were, the perceptual field of the client in the mind of the counselor? Here it may assist us to see how the experience seems to the client. From the many statements written or given by clients after therapy one realizes that the counselor's behavior is experienced in a variety of ways, but there appear to be certain threads which are frequently evident.

A first excerpt may be taken from a statement by a professionally sophisticated client who had recently completed a series of five interviews. She had known and worked with the counselor in another professional capacity.

Initially we discussed the possibility of these interviews interfering with our relationship as co-workers. I very definitely feel that the interviews in no way altered this relationship. We were two entirely different people in our two relationships and the one interfered not at all with the other. I believe that this was due in large measure to the fact that we almost unconsciously, because of the nature of therapy, accepted each other and ourselves as being different people in our two relationships with each other. As workers we were two individuals working together on various everyday problems. In counseling we were mostly *me* working together on my situation as I found it. Perhaps the last sentence explains to a considerable extent how I felt in the counseling relationship. I was hardly aware during the interviews of just who it was sitting in the office with me. I was the one that mattered, my thinking was the thing that was important and my counselor was almost a part of me working on my problem as I wanted to work on it.

My most prominent impression of the interviews is difficult to put into words. As I talked I would almost feel that I was "out of this world." Sometimes I would hardly know just what I was saying. This one may easily do if one talks for long periods to oneself—becoming so involved in verbalization that one is not keenly aware of just what one is saying and very definitely not aware of what the words actually mean to one. It was the role of the counselor to bring me to myself, to help me by being with me in everything I said, to realize what I was saying. I was never conscious that he was reflecting or re-stating things I had said but only that he was right along with me in my thinking because he would say to me things which I had stated but he would clear them for me, bring me back to earth, help me to see what I had said and what it meant to me.

Several times, by his use of analogies, he would help me to see the significance of what I had said. Sometimes he would say something like "I wonder if this is what you mean, _____ " or " _____, is that what you mean?" and I was conscious of a desire to get what I had said clarified, not so much to him as a person but through him, clarified to myself.

During the first two interviews he interrupted pauses. I know that this was because I had mentioned before counseling started that pauses made me self-conscious. However, I remember wishing at the time that he had let me think without interruption. The one interview that stands out most clearly in my mind was one in which there were many long pauses during which time I was working very hard. I was beginning to get some insight into my situation and, although nothing was said, I had the feeling by the counselor's attitude, that he was working right along with me. He was not restless, he did not take out a cigarette, he simply sat, I believe looking hard right at me, while I stared at the floor and worked in my mind. It was an attitude of complete cooperation and gave me the feeling that he was with me in what I was thinking. I see now the great value of pauses, if the counselor's attitude is one of cooperation, not one of simply waiting for time to pass.

I have seen nondirective techniques used before—not on myself—where the techniques were the dominating factors, and I have not always been pleased with the results. As a result of my own experience as a client I am convinced that the counselor's complete acceptance, his expression of the attitude of wanting to help the client, and his warmth of spirit as expressed by his wholehearted giving of himself to the client in complete cooperation with everything the client does or says are basic in this type of therapy.

Notice how the significant theme of the relationship is, "we were mostly *me* working together on my situation as I found it." The two selves have somehow become one while remaining two— "we were *me*." This idea is repeated several times; "my counselor was almost a part of me working on my problem as I wanted to work on it"; "it was the role of the counselor to bring me to myself"; "I was conscious of a desire to get what I had said clarified, not so much to him as a person but through him, clarified to myself." The impression is that the client was in one sense "talking to herself," and yet that this was a very different process when she talked to herself through the medium of another person.

Another example may be taken from a report written by a young woman who had been, at the time she came in for counseling, rather deeply disturbed. She had some slight knowledge about client-centered therapy before coming for help. The report from which this material is taken was written spontaneously and voluntarily some six weeks after the conclusion of the counseling interviews.

In the earlier interviews, I kept saying such things as "I am not acting like myself." "I never acted this way before." What I meant was that this withdrawn, untidy, and apathetic person was not myself. I was trying to say that this was a different person from the one who had previously functioned with what seemed to be satisfactory adjustment. It seemed to me that must be true. Then I began to realize that I was the same person, seriously withdrawn, etc., now, as I had been before. That did not happen until after I had talked out my self-rejection, shame, despair, and doubt, in the accepting situation of the interview. The counselor was not startled or shocked. I was telling him all these things about myself which did not fit into my picture of a graduate student, a teacher, a sound person. He responded with complete acceptance and warm interest without heavy emotional overtones. Here was a sane, intelligent person wholeheartedly accepting this behavior that seemed so shameful to me. I can remember an organic feeling of relaxation. I did not have to keep up the struggle to cover up and hide this shameful person.

Retrospectively, it seems to me that what I felt as "warm acceptance with (out) emotional overtones" was what I needed to work through my difficulties. One of the things I was struggling with was the character of my relationships with others. I was enmeshed in dependence, yet fighting against it. My mother, knowing that something was wrong, had come to see me. Her love was so powerful, I could feel it enveloping me. Her suffering was so real that I could touch it. But I could not talk to her. Even when, out of her insight, she said, while she was talking of my relationships with the family, "You can be as dependent or as independent as you like," I still resisted her. The counselor's impersonality with interest allowed me to talk out my feelings. The clarification in the interview situation presented the attitude to me as a *ding an sich* which I could look at, manipulate, and put in place. In organizing my attitudes, I was beginning to organize me.

I can remember sitting in my room and thinking about the components of infantile needs and dependence in maladjustment, and strongly resisting the idea that there was any element of dependence in my behavior. I think I reacted the way I might have if a therapist in an interview situation had interpreted this for me before I was ready for it. I kept thinking about it, though, and began to see that, although I kept insistently telling myself I wanted to be independent, there was plenty of evidence that I was also wanting protection and dependence. This was a shameful situation, I felt. I did not come to accept this indecision in myself until I had guiltily brought it up in the interviews, had it accepted, and then stated it again myself with less anxiety. In this situation, the counselor's reflection of

feeling with complete acceptance let me see the attitude with some objectivity. In this case, the insight was structured rationally before I went to the interview. However, it was not internalized until the attitude had been reflected back to me free of shame and guilt, a thing in itself which I could look at and accept. My restatements and further exposition of feeling after the counselor's reflection were my own acceptance and internalization of the insight.

How shall we understand the counselor's functions as it was experienced by this client? Perhaps it would be accurate to say that the attitudes which she could express but could not accept as a part of herself became acceptable when an alternate self, the counselor, looked upon them with acceptance and without emotion. It was only when another self looked upon her behavior without shame or emotion that she could look upon it in the same way. These attitudes were then objectified for her, and subject to control and organization. The insights which were almost achieved in her room became genuine insights when another had accepted them, and stated them, with the results that she could again state them with less anxiety. Here we have a different, yet basically similar, experiencing of the counselor's role.

It is natural that the more articulate and sophisticated clients would give more complete accounts of the meaning the experience had for them. The same elements appear to be present, however, in the simple and relatively inarticulate accounts of thoroughly naïve clients. A veteran with little education thus writes of his counseling experience.

Much to my surprise, Mr. L. the counselor let me talk myself dry so to speak. I thought he might question me on various points of my problem. He did to a small extent but not as much as I had anticipated. In conferring with Mr. L., I listened to myself while talking. And in doing so I would say that I solved my own problem.

Here again it seems fair to suppose that the counselor's attitude and responses made it easier for the client to "listen to myself."

A THEORY OF THE THERAPIST'S ROLE

With this type of material in mind, a possible psychological explanation of the effectiveness of the counselor's role might be developed in these terms. Psychotherapy deals primarily with the organization and the functioning of the self. There are many elements of experience which the self cannot face, cannot clearly perceive, because to face them or admit them would be inconsistent with and threatening to the current organization of self. In client-centered therapy the client finds in the counselor a genuine alter ego in an operational and technical sense—a self which has temporarily divested itself (so far as possible) of its own selfhood, except for the one quality of endeavoring to understand. In the therapeutic experience, to see one's own attitudes, confusions, ambivalences, feelings, and perceptions accurately expressed by another, but stripped of their complications of emotion, is to see oneself objectively, and paves the way for acceptance into the self of all these elements which are now more clearly perceived. Reorganization of the self and more integrated functioning of the self are thus furthered.

Let us try to restate this idea in another way. In the emotional warmth of the relationship with the therapist, the client begins to experience a feeling of safety as he finds that whatever attitude he expresses is understood in almost the same way that he perceives it, and is accepted. He then is able to explore, for example, a vague feeling of guiltiness which he has experienced. In this safe relationship he can perceive for the first time the hostile meaning and purpose of certain aspects of his behavior, and can understand why he has felt guilty about it, and why it has been necessary to deny to awareness the meaning of this behavior. But this clearer perception is in itself disrupting and anxiety-creating, not therapeutic. It is evidence to the client that there are disturbing inconsistencies in himself, that he is not what he thinks he is. But as he voices his new perceptions and their attendant anxieties, he finds that this acceptant alter ego, the therapist, this other person who is only partly another person, perceives these experiences too, but with a new quality. The therapist perceives the client's self as the client has known it, and accepts it; he perceives the contradictory aspects which have been denied to awareness and accepts those too as being a part of the client; and both of these acceptances have in them the same warmth and respect. Thus it is that the client, experiencing in another an acceptance of both these aspects of himself, can take toward himself the same attitude. He finds that he too can accept himself even with the additions and alterations that are necessitated by these new perceptions of himself as hostile. He can experience himself as a person having hostile as well as other types of feelings, and can experience himself in this way without

guilt. He has been enabled to do this (if our theory is correct) because another person has been able to adopt this frame of reference, to perceive with him, yet to perceive with acceptance and respect.

A By-product

As a somewhat parenthetical comment, it may be mentioned that the concept of the therapist's attitude and function which has been outlined above tends to reduce greatly a problem which has been experienced by other therapeutic orientations. This is the problem of how to prevent the therapist's own maladjustments, emotional biases, and blind spots from interfering with the therapeutic process in the client. There can be no doubt that every therapist, even when he has resolved many of his own difficulties in a therapeutic relationship, still has troubling conflicts, tendencies to project, or unrealistic attitudes on certain matters. How to keep these warped attitudes from blocking therapy or harming the client has been an important topic in therapeutic thinking.

In client-centered therapy this problem has been minimized considerably by the very nature of the therapist's function. Warped or unrealistic attitudes are most likely to be evident wherever evaluations are made. When evaluation of the client or of his expressions is almost nonexistent, counselor bias has little opportunity to become evident, or indeed to exist. In any therapy in which the counselor is asking himself "How do I see this? How do I understand this material?" the door is wide open for the personal needs or conflicts of the therapist to distort these evaluations. But where the counselor's central question is "How does the client see this?" and where he is continually checking his own understanding of the client's perception by putting forth tentative statements of it, distortion based upon the counselor's conflicts is much less apt to enter, and much more apt to be corrected by the client if it does enter.

This principle may be worded in a slightly different fashion. In a therapeutic relationship in which the therapist enters, as a person, making interpretations, evaluating the significance of the material, and the like, his distortions enter with him. In a therapeutic relationship where the therapist endeavors to keep himself out, as a separate person, and where his whole endeavor is to understand the other so completely that he becomes almost an alter ego of the client, personal distortions and maladjustments are much less likely to occur.

Though this point of view has been stated here only in general terms, it has been borne out in the experience of clinical training. Some individuals may be so maladjusted that they cannot perceive experience from the other person's point of view. Clients feel that such counselors-in-training are not understanding and tend to give up the interviews. And such counselors tend to leave the field. With most counselors-in-training, the effectiveness of achieving the internal frame of reference of another is sufficient reward to make this the focus of their effort. Personal problems of their own, which might at first have made it difficult accurately to understand or reflect or accept attitudes, tend consequently to play a smaller and smaller role. The deep emotional entanglement of client and therapist which can occur where the therapist sees his role as an evaluative one is almost absent from our experience.

THE DIFFICULTY OF UNDERSTANDING THE PERCEPTIONS OF ANOTHER

Thus far the explanation of the counselor's function, as it is presently formulated, has been given without particular reference to the special difficulties involved. It has been our experience that there are many clinical situations in which it is genuinely difficult even for the experienced counselor to achieve the internal frame of reference of the client. An excerpt from client material may exemplify some of the problems we have met.

The excerpt is from a third interview with a young man from a psychiatric ward. The material is electrically recorded, and presented as given by the client. If one places himself in the role of the counselor, he may find it something of a problem to perceive with this client.

A good many thoughts, a good many feelings are just right there in my head. I just put them—I just—I don't know—I feel them inside my head, they stop it up. *(Short pause.)* I just get down to the things in my head and thought and mind, but it's just that I—it's just that I—I don't know—what goes on, goes on different, goes on in the inside, that's what stops me up—stops me up quickly. It's just that, I, I'm wondering with real force whether I could go out there back to that ward of mine and really live, really be somebody. I just—it shot right out of my head. I wondered if I could possibly go back there and do that, really be somebody there. *(Short pause.)* I just keep on wondering, keep on thinking about it, and if I ever will be—just come right straight

back to something and do something and be somebody there. *(Short pause.)* It'd probably just help me keep on being different, a different man, a different person back there. Here in this office I generally come out with some commonsense thoughts, and ideas, something with some real feeling in it, a real mind, real thought. Yesterday when I came in here I was just living, and—I will be today. I'm very sure of it. I can just be—I can get away with it just about so much up here, then I—it's just too much.[3]

Here the problem faced by the counselor is the fact that much of the client's expression is confused and expressed in such private symbolism that it is difficult to enter into his perceptual field and see experience in his terms. It would seem that the type of empathic thinking carried on by a counselor who was successfully client-centered in respect to this material would include thoughts of this type:

It seems as though feelings and thoughts block you.
It's the inside thoughts, as I understand it, that stop you up.
It's the question, the puzzle, as to whether you could possibly *be* somebody.
I can understand that that thought leaves you abruptly as well as comes to you.
You wonder and wonder whether you could be a *person,* back on the ward.
You feel that some of your reactions are real, and sensible.
It seems to you that here in the therapy hour you are actually alive.
That thought is just overpowering—more than you can face.

If the counselor maintains this consistently client-centered attitude, and if he occasionally conveys to the client something of his understanding, then he is doing what he can to give the client the experience of being deeply respected. Here the confused, tentative, almost incoherent thinking of an individual who knows he has been evaluated as abnormal is really respected by being deemed well worth understanding.

On the other hand the therapist may find thoughts running through his mind which are of an evaluative nature, judging this material from his own frame of reference, or of a self-concerned nature, in which his attention has shifted from the client to himself. Such thinking might include themes such as the following:

The thinking here is confused and the expressions inarticulate.
There seem to be feelings of unreality.
Is this a schizophrenic?
Am I understanding his meaning correctly?
Should I encourage his desire to be a self?

[3]From a psychoanalytic interview recorded by Earl Zinn, and used by permission.

Here is a striking example of the conscious self struggling to regain a sense of control over the organism.
He reacts with some panic to the thought of living and
being a person.
What will I respond to this?

Such thoughts as these will occur to any counselor at times, no matter how basically client-centered
his views may be. Yet it would appear to be true that
whether the theme is evaluative or self-concerned,
there is slightly less of full respect for the other person than in the thoroughly empathic understanding
previously cited. When the counselor is concerned
with himself and what he should do, there is necessarily a decreased focus upon the respect he feels for
the client. When he is thinking in evaluative terms,
whether the evaluation is objectively accurate or inaccurate, he is to some degree assuming a judgmental
frame of mind, is viewing the person as an object,
rather than as a person, and to that extent respects
him less as a person. On the other hand, to enter
deeply with this man into his confused struggle for
selfhood is perhaps the best implementation we now
know for indicating the meaning of our basic hypothesis that the individual represents a process which is
deeply worthy of respect, both as he is and with regard to his potentialities.

SOME DEEP ISSUES

The assumption of the therapeutic role which has
been described raises some very basic questions indeed. An example from a therapeutic interview may
pose some of these issues for our consideration. Miss
Gil, a young woman who has, in a number of therapeutic interviews, been quite hopeless about herself,
has spent the major part of an hour discussing her
feelings of inadequacy and lack of personal worth.
Part of the time she has been aimlessly using the finger paints. She has just finished expressing her feelings of wanting to get away from everyone—to have
nothing to do with people. After a long pause comes
the following.

S:[4] I've never said this before to anyone—but I've
thought for such a long time—This is a terrible thing
to say, but if I could just—well (*short, bitter laugh;
pause*), if I could just find some glorious cause that I
could give my life for I would be happy. I cannot be
the kind of a person I want to be. I guess maybe I

haven't the guts—or the strength—to kill myself—
and if someone else would relieve me of the responsibility—or I would be in an accident—I—I—just
don't want to live.

C:[5] At the present time things look so black to you
that you can't see much point in living—

S: Yes—I wish I'd never started this therapy. I was
happy when I was living in my dream world. There I
could be the kind of person I wanted to be—But
now—There is such a wide, wide gap—between my
ideal—and what I am. I wish people hated me. I try
to make them hate me. Because then I could turn
away from them and could blame them—but no—It
is all in my hands—Here is my life—and I either accept the fact that I am absolutely worthless—or I
fight whatever it is that holds me in this terrible conflict. And I suppose if I accepted the fact that I am
worthless, then I could go away someplace—and
get a little room someplace—get a mechanical job
someplace—and retreat clear back to the security of
my dream world where I could do things, have
clever friends, be a pretty wonderful sort of person—

C: It's really a tough struggle—digging into this like
you are—and at times the shelter of your dream
world looks more attractive and comfortable.

S: My dream world or suicide.

C: Your dream world or something more permanent than dreams—

S: Yes. (*A long pause. Complete change of voice.*) So
I don't see why I should waste your time—coming
in twice a week—I'm not worth it—What do you
think?

C: It's up to you, Gil—It isn't wasting my time—I'd
be glad to see you—whenever you come—but it's
how you feel about it—if you don't want to come
twice a week—or if you do want to come twice a
week?—once a week?—It's up to you. *Long pause.*

S: You're not going to suggest that I come in often-
er? You're not alarmed and think I ought to come
in—every day—until I get out of this?

C: I believe you are able to make your own decision. I'll see you whenever you want to come.

S: (*Note of awe in her voice.*) I don't believe you are
alarmed about—I see—I may be afraid of myself—
but you aren't afraid for me—(*She stands up—a
strange look on her face.*)

C: You say you may be afraid of yourself—and are
wondering why I don't seem to be afraid for you?

---

[4]Subject, or client.

[5]Counselor.

S: *(Another short laugh.)* You have more confidence in me than I have. *(She cleans up the finger-paint mess and starts out of the room.)* I'll see you next week—*(that short laugh)* maybe. *(Her attitude seemed tense, depressed, bitter, completely beaten. She walked slowly away.)*

This excerpt raises sharply the question as to how far the therapist is going to maintain his central hypothesis. Where life, quite literally, is at stake, what is the best hypothesis upon which to act? Shall his hypothesis still remain a deep respect for the capacity of the person? Or shall he change his hypothesis? If so, what are the alternatives? One would be the hypothesis that "I can be successfully responsible for the life of another." Still another is the hypothesis, "I can be temporarily responsible for the life of another without damaging the capacity for self-determination." Still another is: "The individual cannot be responsible for himself, nor can I be responsible for him, but it is possible to find someone who can be responsible for him."

In the particular excerpt cited, are the counselor responses which indicate an external frame of reference—"I'd be glad to see you," "I believe you are able to make your own decision"—the effective responses, or are the effective responses those which view from within the client? Or is it the deep respect, whether indicated from the external or internal frame of reference, which is the important ingredient?

Does the counselor have the right, professionally or morally, to permit a client seriously to consider psychosis or suicide as a way out, without making a positive effort to prevent these choices? Is it a part of our general social responsibility that we may not tolerate such thinking or such action on the part of another?

These are deep issues, which strike to the very core of therapy. They are not issues which one person can decide for another. Different therapeutic orientations have acted upon different hypotheses. All that one person can do is to describe his own experience and the evidence which grows out of that experience.

THE BASIC STRUGGLE OF THE COUNSELOR

It has been my experience that only when the counselor, through one means or another, has settled within himself the hypothesis upon which he will act, can he be of maximum aid to the individual. It has also been my experience that the more deeply he relies upon the strength and potentiality of the client, the more deeply does he discover that strength.

It has seemed clear, from our clinical experience as well as our research, that when the counselor perceives and accepts the client as he is, when he lays aside all evaluation and enters into the perceptual frame of reference of the client, he frees the client to explore his life and experience anew, frees him to perceive in that experience new meanings and new goals. But is the therapist willing to give the client full freedom as to outcomes? Is he genuinely willing for the client to organize and direct his life? Is he willing for him to choose goals that are social or antisocial, moral or immoral? If not, it seems doubtful that therapy will be a profound experience for the client. Even more difficult, is he willing for the client to choose regression rather than growth or maturity? to choose neuroticism rather than mental health? to choose to reject help rather than accept it? to choose death rather than life? To me it appears that only as the therapist is completely willing that *any* outcome, *any* direction, may be chosen—only then does he realize the vital strength of the capacity and potentiality of the individual for constructive action. It is as he is willing for death to be the choice, that life is chosen; for neuroticism to be the choice, that a healthy normality is chosen. The more completely he acts upon his central hypothesis, the more convincing is the evidence that the hypothesis is correct.[6]

UNSOLVED ISSUES

The preceding paragraphs state the experience of one person, the writer, in a positive (or, as it will seem to some, an extreme) form. Let us drop back to considering a minimal statement regarding the attitude of the counselor, and the effect his attitude has upon the client.

It has been the experience of many, counselors and clients alike, that when the counselor has

---

[6]It will be evident from this discussion that neither in practice nor in theory can we go along with the comment by Green (72) that client-centered counseling is simply a subtle way of getting across to the client the cues which indicate approval of cultural values. His hypothesis could be partially maintained in some of the early client-centered cases, but it does not appear to be supported at all in the present handling by experienced counselors. As client-centered therapy has developed, it becomes more and more clear that it cannot be explained on such a basis.

adopted in a genuine way the function which he understands to be characteristic of a client-centered counselor, the client tends to have a vital and releasing experience which has many similarities from one client to another. A recognizable phenomenon, one that can be described, seems to exist. Whether the present description is an accurate one is another question. Different counselors have used different descriptive terms, and only time and research can indicate which description is the closest semantic approximation to the phenomenon.

Is the crucial element in the counselor's attitude his complete willingness for the client to express any attitude? Is permissiveness thus the most significant factor? In counseling this scarcely seems to be an adequate explanation, yet in play therapy there often appears to be some basis for this formulation. The therapist may at times be quite unsuccessful in achieving the child's internal frame of reference, since the symbolic expression maybe so complex or unique that the therapist is at a loss to understand. Yet therapy moves forward, largely, it would seem, on the basis of permissiveness, since acceptance can hardly be complete unless the counselor is first able to understand.[7]

Another type of formulation would stress the fact that the essential characteristic of the relationship is the new type of need-satisfaction achieved by the client in an atmosphere of acceptance. Thus Meister and Miller describe the experience as "an attempt on the part of the counselor to offer the client a new type of experience wherein his cycle of unusual responses may be disrupted since the counselor does not supply the reinforcement by rejection which other social contacts have provided. The client's report of his behavior, his actual behavior, and his need to behave as he does—all are 'accepted.' Thus in the counseling relationship itself the client adopts a new mode of response, a different mode of need-satisfaction." (131, pp. 61–62)

Still another formulation places the emphasis upon the counselor's level of confidence or level of

expectancy in regard to the individual. This view raises the question: Is it not the counselor's full confidence in the ability of the person to be self-directing to which the client responds? Thus in the case of Miss Gil, cited earlier, the counselor statement, "I believe you are able to make your own decision," would be regarded as a chance verbalization of the effective counselor attitude which was crucial for the whole relationship. From this point of view it is the expectancy of the counselor that "you can be self-directing" which is the social stimulus to which the client responds.

Still another type of formulation might be that offered by Shaffer, in which psychotherapy is seen as "a learning process through which a person acquires an ability to speak to himself in appropriate ways so as to control his own conduct." (181) From this point of view the counselor attitude might be seen simply as providing an optimal atmosphere for the client to learn to "speak to himself in appropriate ways."

Yet another description is that the relationship is one which provides the client with the opportunity of making responsible choices, in an atmosphere in which it is assumed that he is capable of making decisions for himself. Thus in any series of counseling interviews the client makes hundreds of choices—of what to say, what to believe, what to withhold, what to do, what to think, what values to place upon his experiences. The relationship becomes an area for continuing practice in the making of increasingly mature and responsible choices.

As will be observed, these differing formulations are not in sharp contrast. They differ in emphasis, but probably all of them (including the formulation given in this chapter) are imperfect attempts to describe an experience about which we still have too little research knowledge.

AN OBJECTIVE DEFINITION OF THE THERAPEUTIC RELATIONSHIP

It will have been painfully evident that the material of this chapter has been based upon clinical experience and judgment rather than upon any scientific or objective basis. Almost no research has been done upon the complex problems of the subtle client-therapist relationship. A beginning was made by Miller (132) in a small study based upon eight interviews—two psycho-analytic, one "non-nondirective," and five nondirective. Using transcribed typescripts as a basis

---

[7]Since the writing of the above, a different explanation has been pointed out to the author. It is quite possible that the child assumes that the therapist perceives the situation as he does. The child, much more than the adult, assumes that everyone shares with him the same perceptual reality. Therefore when there is permissiveness and acceptance, this is experienced by the child as understanding and acceptance, since he takes it for granted that the therapist perceives as he does.

If this description is accurate, then the situation in play therapy differs in no essential way from the description of the relationship which has been given throughout the chapter.

for analysis, judges endeavored to make objective discriminations as to how the counselor responses were experienced by the client (as separate from the counselor's intent). The judges were to decide whether the counselor's statement was experienced as (1) "accepting," defined as respecting or admitting the validity of the client's position, (2) supporting, (3) denying, or (4) neutral. By analysis of variance technique it was shown that the differences between judgments were not great, particularly in relation to the nondirective interviews. In fact, the categories seemed more suitable for these interviews than for the others. The basic finding was that the nondirective interviews were largely characterized by a client experience of acceptance, rather than of neutrality or support. It was also found that in an interview regarded by the counselor as unsuccessful, there were as many responses experienced as denying or rejecting as there were in the interviews from other orientations. The fact that responses may be cast in a nondirective form does not, in other words, prevent them from being, or being experienced as, denial or rejection. This study is the first to make the attempt to measure the relationship from the client's point of view.

Another study has just been completed which is not only important in itself, but holds much promise for continuing objective analysis of many of the subtle aspects of the relationship between the therapist and the client. It is a coordinated pair of researches by Fiedler (57, 58), which may be described briefly in the following paragraphs.

Fiedler started from the assumption, held by almost all therapists, that the relationship is an important element in facilitating therapy. Consequently, all therapists are endeavoring to create what they regard as the ideal relationship. If there are in fact, several different types of therapeutic relationship, each distinctive of a different school of therapy, then the ideals toward which experienced therapists of these different schools are working will show relatively little similarity. If, however, there is but one type of relationship which is actually therapeutic, then there should be a concordance in the concept of an ideal relationship as held by experienced therapists. One would in this case expect more agreement between experienced therapists, regardless of their theoretical orientation, than between the experienced therapist and the novice within the same school of thought, since greater experience should give keener

insight into the elements of the relationship.

To test this somewhat complex series of hypotheses, Fiedler first made a pilot study using eight therapists, and then a more carefully defined study in which ten persons were involved. In this main study there were three therapists who were analytically oriented, three from a client-centered orientation, one Adlerian, and three laymen. The task of these individuals was to describe the ideal therapeutic relationship. This they did through the use of the "Q" technique devised by Stephenson (201, 202).[8] Seventy-five statements were drawn from the literature and from therapists, each statement descriptive of a possible aspect of the relationship. (To illustrate, three of the statements were "Therapist is sympathetic with patient," "Therapist tries to sell himself," "Therapist treats the patient with much deference.") Each of the ten raters sorted these seventy-five descriptive statements into seven categories, from those most characteristic of an ideal relationship to those least characteristic. Since this meant that each rater had assigned a value of from one to seven to each item, the sorting made by any rater could now be correlated with that of any other rater.

The results hold much of interest. All correlations were strongly positive, ranging from .43 to .84, indicating that all the therapists and even the nontherapists tended to describe the ideal relationship in similar terms. When the correlations were factor analyzed, only one factor was found, indicating that there is basically but one relationship toward which all therapists strive. There was a higher correlation between experts who were regarded as good therapists, regardless of orientation, than between experts and nonexperts within the same orientation. The fact that even laymen can describe the ideal therapeutic relationship in terms which correlate highly with those of the experts suggests that the best therapeutic relationship may be related to good interpersonal relationships in general.

What are the characteristics of this ideal relationship? When all the ratings are pooled, here are the items placed in the top two categories.

Most characteristic
   The therapist is able to participate completely
   in the patient's communication

[8]See not only the references indicated, but page 140 of Chapter 4, in which another study using this technique is described.

Very characteristic

> The therapist's comments are always right in line with what the patient is trying to convey.
>
> The therapist sees the patient as a co-worker on a common problem.
>
> The therapist treats the patient as an equal.
>
> The therapist is well able to understand the patient's feelings.
>
> The therapist really tries to understand the patient's feelings.
>
> The therapist always follows the patient's line of thought.
>
> The therapist's tone of voice conveys the complete ability to share the patient's feelings.

Here, from the point of view of this chapter, is outstanding corroboration of the importance of empathy and complete understanding on the part of the therapist. Some of the items also indicate the respect which the therapist has for the client. There is unfortunately little opportunity to judge the extent to which reliance is placed upon the basic capacity of the client, since very few items regarding this were included. From the rating of these few characteristics it may be said that such reliance is only moderately characteristic of this heterogeneous group of therapists.

At the negative end of the scale are placed those items which describe the therapist as hostile to or disgusted by the patient, or acting in a superior fashion. At the extreme negative pole is the statement, "Therapist shows no comprehension of the feelings the patient is trying to communicate."

In a second major aspect of this research Fiedler has endeavored to measure the type of relationship which actually is achieved by different therapists, and the degree to which the actual is similar to the ideal. In this study four judges listened to ten electrically recorded interviews, and for each interview sorted the seventy-five descriptive items to indicate the extent to which they were characteristic of that particular interview. Of the ten interviews, four were conducted by psychoanalytically oriented therapists, four by client-centered therapists, two by Adlerians. In each group, half of the interviews were conducted by experienced therapists, half by nonexperts.

The findings, based on the various correlations, were as follows:

1. Experts created relationships significantly closer to the "ideal" than nonexperts.

2. Similarity between experts of different orientations was as great as, or greater than, the similarity between experts and nonexperts of the same orientation.

3. The most important factors differentiating experts from nonexperts are related to the therapist's ability to understand, to communicate with, and to maintain rapport with the client. There is some indication that the expert is better able to maintain an appropriate emotional distance, seemingly best described as interested but emotionally uninvolved.

4. The most clearly apparent differences between schools related to the status which the therapist assumes toward the client. The Adlerians and some of the analytic therapists place themselves in a more tutorial, authoritarian role; client-centered therapists show up on the opposite extreme of this factor.

The primary significance of these two studies is not the findings alone, since the studies are based upon small numbers, but the fact that a start has been made in this subtle and complex area. As the methodology becomes more refined, it appears entirely possible that objective answers may be found to some of the perplexing questions which are raised about the therapeutic relationship.

It would also appear, from the point of view of this chapter, that the findings of these studies confirm in a general way some of the elements stressed in the preceding sections. The importance of complete and sensitive understanding of the client's attitudes and feelings, as they seem to him, is supported by Fiedler's work. As to the importance of reliance upon the client's capacity the study is silent, but it is obvious that there is now no barrier to the exhaustive study of such an issue. This increase in methodological skill and sophistication makes possible research which has hitherto seemed impossible. It is this promise for the future which makes Fiedler's study basically important. It appears clear that in time this chapter on the attitude of the therapist, and his relationship with the client, can be rewritten in objective, verified terms, based upon clinical hypotheses scientifically tested.

Corroborative Evidence for the Basic Hypothesis

In concluding this chapter, it may be well to return to its fundamental premise, and to examine it, not as related to therapy alone, but as related to our general experience. A basic hypothesis has been stated concerning the capacity of the individual for self-initiated, constructive handling of the issues involved in life situations. This hypothesis is not yet definitively proved or disproved by research evidence from the field of therapy. So far as clinical experience is concerned, some clinicians state that their clinical experience supports this hypothesis, but others look upon it with considerable skepticism and indicate that in the light of their experience any such reliance upon the capacity of the individual is of very doubtful validity.

In this situation, unsatisfactory from a scientific point of view, it may be worth our while to examine the scattered evidence, from fields outside of psychotherapy, which has relevance to the hypothesis. There is a certain amount of objective evidence, and some experiential evidence, from other fields.

In the well-known study of autocratic, democratic, and laissez faire groups conducted by Lippitt and others (118), it was found that in the democratic group where the leader's role was one of interest and permissiveness, the group took responsibility upon itself, and in quantity and quality of production, in morale, and in absence of hostility, it exceeded the records of the other groups. In the laissez faire group, where there was no consistent structure, and no leader interest, and in the autocratic group where behavior was controlled by the leader's wishes, the outcomes were not so favorable. While this study is based on small numbers, and is perhaps lessened in value by the fact that the leaders were genuine in their democratic functions and role-playing in other groups, it is nevertheless worthy of consideration.

In a study made many years ago by Herbert Williams (223), a classroom group of the worst-offending juvenile delinquents in a large school system was brought together. As might be expected, these boys were retarded in intelligence (average I.Q. 82) and in school achievement. There was no special equipment save for a large table on which a variety of readers and textbooks for various ages were placed. There were but two rules: a boy must keep busy doing something, and no boy was permitted to annoy or bother others. Here is a situation of genuine permissiveness within broad and realistic limits, with responsibility clearly placed upon the individual. Encouragement and suggestions were given only after an activity had been self-initiated. Thus if a boy had worked along artistic lines, he might be given assistance in getting into a special art class; or if activities in mathematics or mechanics had engaged his interest, arrangements might be made for him to attend courses in these subjects. The group remained together for months, though some were not in the group for the whole period. During the four months the measured educational achievement increased 11.2 months in reading age, 14.5 months in arithmetic age, and similarly in other subjects. The total increase in educational ages was 12.2 months, and if three members are omitted whose attendance was short, the average increase is 15.2 months—more than four times the normal expectation for a group with this degree of retardation. This was in a group in which reading and other educational disabilities abounded.

In a very different area, a study of food habits was made during the war, under the supervision of Kurt Lewin (112). It was found that when groups were urged by a lecturer to make use of little-used meats—hearts, kidneys, brains—few (10 per cent) actually carried out the suggestion in practice. In other groups the problem of war scarcities was discussed with the group members and simple information about the meats given to them, following which the group members were asked to make their own decisions about serving the meats in question. These decisions, it was found through a follow-up study, tended to be kept, and 52 per cent actually served one or more of these meats. Self-initiated and responsible action proved far more effective than guided action.

A study by Coch and French (41) comes to the same conclusion regarding industrial workers. With conditions of pay held constant, some groups of workers were shifted to a new task and carefully instructed in the way to handle it and in ways of increasing efficiency on the new task. Other groups were shifted to the new task, and permitted to discuss, plan, and carry out their own way of handling the new problem. In the latter groups productivity increased more rapidly, increased to a higher level, held a higher level, and morale was definitely higher than in the groups which had been instructed.

A study of supervision in an insurance company was made by the Survey Research Center (206).

When units in which productivity and morale were high were compared with those in which they were low, significant differences were discovered in the methods and personalities of the supervisors. In the units with high productivity, supervisors and group leaders tended to be interested primarily in the workers as people, and interest in production was secondary. Supervisors encouraged group participation and discussion and group decisions in matters affecting their work. Finally, supervisors in these "high" units gave little close supervision to the work being done, but tended to place the responsibility upon the worker.

Other industrial studies (62, 116, 126, 207), though less objective in nature, bear out the two that have been cited. Various industries, in this country and in Great Britain, have found that in quite divergent industrial situations there is improvement in effectiveness and in morale when workers are trusted as being capable of responsible handling of their own situation. This has meant a permissiveness toward their active participation in thinking about the issues, and a willingness for them to make, or participate in making, the responsible choices and decisions.

In addition to such industrial evidence there is significant social experience which bears upon the topic. The way in which the self-directing capacities of small communities were utilized in the development of the TVA project is well described by David Lilienthal (115). In a very different problem-situation, that of training a striking force of Marines, General Carlson relied very heavily upon the self-directing capacities of the individual, in developing the famous Carlson's Raiders.

In dealing with juvenile delinquency there is similar experience. The Area Projects, developed by Clifford Shaw in delinquency areas, were found to be successful when they built upon the strength of the group. If the leader was a catalyst, a person genuinely able to accept the neighborhood as it existed and to release the group to work toward its real purposes and goals, the result was in the direction of socialization. The gangster, the petty politician, the tavern keeper, when given the opportunity to express real attitudes, and the full freedom to select goals, tended to choose goals which moved the group toward more social objectives. On the other hand,

> attempts to produce these changes *for* the community by means of ready made institutions and programs planned, developed, financed, and managed by persons outside the community are not likely to meet with any

more success in the future than they have in the past. This procedure is psychologically unsound because it places the residents of the community in an inferior position and implies serious reservations with regard to their capacities and their interest in their own welfare. What is equally important is that it neglects the greatest of all assets in any community, namely the talents, energies, and other human resources of the people themselves. . . . What is necessary, we believe, is the organization and encouragement of social self-help on a cooperative basis. (183)

In quite another area—that of dealing with health problems—we find further relevant social experience. The famous Peckham Experiment in London provides an opportunity to study the basic hypothesis from a fresh vantage point. The Peckham Centre is a center organized for family health and recreation by a group of biologists. In attempting to promote health and richness of living for individuals and families, the sponsoring group has learned many lessons which are deeply relevant to our understanding of psychotherapy. Let us first listen to the manner in which the handling of the facts of the medical examination has developed.

> Another outstanding characteristic of the biological overhaul [health examination] must be emphasized. The facts elicited and their significance are as far as possible presented to the family in their entirety, in lay terms. *No advice is volunteered.* To the layman this may appear but natural, since no advice is sought; but to anyone trained in the medical profession—that is specifically to give advice—it is a most difficult attitude to achieve. Indeed "to give advice" seems to be a wellnigh irresistible impulse to most human beings in a situation of authority. We try then not to give advice and to refrain from assuming the authority of special knowledge. As one of the members put it, "The doctor simply tells you how you stand." It is thereafter left to their own degree of intelligence to act. It is an intensely interesting study to watch and note the various actions undertaken (often at considerable sacrifice in some other direction) as the family intelligence is brought to bear on the facts stated to them after examination. It is seldom the individual but nearly always the family as a whole that responds. A technique leading to this result seems to be fundamental, because it gives to the family an opportunity of exercising the responsibility that it so deeply feels. It is difficult to understand, indeed, why a laissez-faire attitude to a mouthful of decaying teeth should change as the result of the new circumstances, but it does; or why a complacency to a useless overweight in either a man or a woman should change—but it does; with results in either instance of marked benefits both to the individual and to the family. It was found in practice that when the examinations were conducted in a spirit which led up to conclusions which were bits of advice, often no action was taken; whereas by leaving it to spontaneity in the individual

and to his own sense of responsibility, action is taken in the overwhelming majority of cases. This very action represents the exercise of a faculty that has been largely in abeyance. With exercise of a faculty, health develops. The faculty for responsibility is no exception to this rule. (145, pp. 49–50)

With this type of handling, with a deep respect for the right and capacity of the individual to be responsible for himself, 90 per cent of the individuals in whom some disorder is discovered go for treatment.

Not only in regard to health activities is this hypothesis found to be effective. It is also the purpose of the Centre to give families an opportunity for recreational enrichment of living. The description of the experience in moving realistically toward this goal provides an interesting parallel to the progression of thinking in the formulation of client-centered therapy.

Our problem is the "man in the street." He is the man without egotistic drive; he is the diffident and the meek. Because he seems to lack initiative he is left to his own resources—of which he seems to have none. To attract him to any organization is difficult enough; to keep him in it is still another problem. But because he forms the bulk of the public he is most worth study, for on him the success of any social organization depends.

The first tentative approach to encouraging the members to do things was based on the common assumption that ordinary people like to emulate their betters; that an exhibition of a high degree of skill, of relative perfection, would stimulate the imitative faculty and lead to like action. That method of approach we have found useless; the assumption is not bourne out by the experiment.

Primarily, individuals are conscious only of their own capacity and act accordingly. They may admire, they may even be envious of outside standards, but they do not use them even as stimulants to try out their own capacity. Skill beyond their own capacity tends to frighten, to inhibit rather than to attempt them to emulation. The status "teacher" tends inevitably to undermind self-confidence. Our failures during our first eighteen months' work have taught us something very significant. Individuals, from infants to old people, resent or fail to show any interest in anything initially presented to them through discipline, regulation or instruction which is another aspect of authority. (Even the very "Centre idea" has a certain taint of authority and this is contributing to our slow recruitment.)

We now proceed by merely providing an environment rich in instruments for action—that is, giving a chance to do things. Slowly but surely these chances are seized upon and used as opportunity for development of inherent capacity. The instruments of action have one common characteristic—*they must speak for themselves*. The voice of the salesman or the teacher frightens the potential users.

How does this fact reflect on organization and the opportunity for experimental observation on this material?

Having provided the members with a chance to do things, we find that we have to leave them to make their own use of them. We have had to learn to sit back and wait for these activities to emerge. Any impatience on our part, translated into help, has strangled their efforts—we have had to cultivate more and more patience in ourselves. The alternative to this cultivation of patience is, of course, obvious—the application of compulsion in one or other of its many forms, perhaps the most tempting of which is persuasion. But having a fundamental interest in the source and origin of spontaneous action—as all biologists must—we have had to discard even that instrument for initiating activities. Even temptation, the gentlest form of compulsion, does not work because human beings, even children, recognize carrots for what they ultimately mean; we have at least progressed beyond the donkey!

We do not suggest that communication, teaming, regulation, system, discipline, authority and instruction are not desirable things but neither can we agree that there is anything wrong with those who spurn these things; we are not missionaries seeking to convert people to desirable things, but scientists seeking the truth in the facts.

Civilization hitherto has looked for the orientation of society through an imposed "system" derived from some extrinsic authority, such as religion, "cultural" education, or political suasion. The biologist conceives an order emanating from the organism living in poise in its environment. Our necessity, therefore, is to secure the free flow of forces in the environment so that the order inherent in the material we are studying may emerge. Our interest is in that balance of forces which sustains naturally and spontaneously the forms of life we are studying.

The Centre is the first experimental station in human biology. It asks the question—"What circumstances will sustain human beings in their capacity for full function (i.e. in health); and what orientation will such fully functioning entities give to human living (i.e. to society)?" (145, pp. 38–40)

Here is obviously a basic willingness on the part of the sponsors of this Centre for people to be themselves—even when that involves differing from the values held by the sponsors. To leave the person free to choose or reject what we regard as "desirable things" requires an inner questioning of basic attitudes which is no easier for the biologist than for the psychotherapist, as the following statements indicate.

The training of the staff is difficult. It is in fact no easy thing for the individual as a scientist to place himself as an instrument of knowledge completely at the disposal of any and every member, and at the same time, without exercising authority, to assume his right and proper position in the community as a social entity. But he is also there to make observations. This the members have readily come to accept, jokingly describing themselves as the biologist's "rats."

They soon come to appreciate that the scientist's primary concern is *to be used by the members as a means of reaching and sustaining their own maximum capacity for health.* Moreover, they come to sense that in carrying on their own activities and inaugurating new ones through the method of self-service, many of them are in fact step by step themselves growing into important members of the staff. (144, p. 78)

The active-passiveness of the observer is not easy to attain without the essential extension of the laboratory scientist's discipline which allows facts to speak for themselves. In human biology the facts are actions which seriously complicate the problem but do not put it beyond the possibility of solution.

The biological necessities of the situation then compel us to leave the members to themselves, to initiate their own activities, their own order of things. We have no rules, regulations nor any other restriction of action, except a very fluid time-table. Within eighteen months the seeming chaos and disorder is rapidly developing into something very different. This is apparent even to our visitors, one of whom on leaving described the life in the Centre as being like a stream allowed to form its bed and its banks according to the natural configuration of the land. (145, p. 41)

Here in this community effort is seen the emergence of the same type of hypothesis upon which the client-centered therapist bases his work. Not only is the hypothesis the same as regards the person, the client, but the conclusion in regard to the role of the "leader" also has many striking similarities.

Is there any unity in these bits of evidence gathered from such diverse sources? Is there anything relevant to our concern with psychotherapy in studies which cover such remote issues as whether people eat kidneys, or decide how an industrial shop unit shall be run? I feel that there is. If we consider the central thread which runs through these highly varied studies and experiences, it would seem that it may be summarized in an "if-then" type of statement.

If the individual or group is faced by a problem;

If a catalyst-leader provides a permissive atmosphere;

If responsibility is genuinely placed with the individual or group;

If there is basic respect for the capacity of the individual or group;

Then, responsible and adequate analysis of the problem is made;
responsible self-direction occurs;
the creativity, productivity, quality of product exhibited are superior to results of other comparable methods;
individual and group morale and confidence develop.

It would appear that the hypothesis which is central to this chapter, and basic to the function of the client-centered therapist, is an hypothesis which has been and is being investigated in other types of human relationships as well, and that the evidence in regard to it has a significant and positive similarity no matter what the field of endeavor.

SUGGESTED READINGS

The reader who wishes to consider in more detail his own attitudes as they actually operate in his reactions with others, and the means of implementing his basic attitudes in therapy, will find rich food for thought and a wealth of practical help in Porter's book, *An Introduction to Therapeutic Counseling* (148). An earlier consideration of implementation is contained in chapter six of *Counseling and Psychotherapy* (166).

A thorough discussion of the psychology of the therapeutic relationship, covering both its description and its dynamics, is contained in the article by Estes (54). For other accounts of the attitude and orientation of the therapist, three references might be particularly pertinent. The first two are psychoanalytic, the third the viewpoint of a religious counselor. They are: the chapter on "What Does the Analyst Do?" by Horney (89, pp. 187–209); Reik, *Listening with the Third Ear* (161); Hiltner, *Pastoral Counseling* (83, Chapter 7).

For a knowledge of the research regarding the counselor's function, one might read Porter's study (149, 150) or Snyder (197) as early examples. Seeman (180) and Fiedler (58, 57) represent recent work in this area, Fiedler's studies being particularly significant for their new methodology.

For an example of the evidence from other sources regarding the basic hypothesis of client-centered therapy, the little study by Coch and French (41) would be a start.

Client-Centered Therapy

Julius Seeman

At the time of this writing, the person-centered approach is nearing the half-century point in its formal existence. Its public beginnings came in 1942, with the publication of Rogers's *Counseling and psychotherapy.* This chapter will describe the essential elements of this approach as it applies to psychotherapy, provide some sense of historical perspective to aid in understanding the approach more fully, and illustrate aspects of the approach as it has been used with persons who were experiencing speech difficulties.

Client-centered therapy characteristically has not been construed as a problem-specific approach. The therapy is envisioned rather as a growth-enhancing experience in any personal domain that the client chooses to explore. In this context it is altogether relevant for a client-centered therapist to work with persons who have concern about their speech. Its relevance will become clear as this chapter unfolds.

Part of the history of this approach is reflected in its terminology, which involves three phases of evolution. The terms corresponding to these phases are *nondirective therapy, client-centered therapy,* and the *person-centered approach.* In the earliest phase, Rogers's experience and writing may best be understood in dialectic terms. He was increasingly dissatisfied with the concept of therapist as expert and as interpreter of another's experience. He was impelled to explore alternative ways of relating to clients in which he would rely less upon himself as arbiter of experience and more upon the client's own potential for growth.

Thus, the earliest formulations were couched in terms of contrast, and the name given to this approach was *nondirective.* The name made sense at the beginning because it was seen as an antithesis to "directive" therapy. It was a natural, perhaps inevitable, way for the dialectic process to begin and for the new therapy to unfold.

This early development on Rogers's part was very much an empirical, rather than a theory-based, process. On the basis of his clinical experience, he had come to see that clients had surprising possibilities for exploring and comprehending their own areas of pain, but there was no body of knowledge and certainly no research that supported such a premise. These elements were to come later but the early development came from Rogers's direct clinical experience.

From today's standpoint, there was much that was primitive in these early therapeutic efforts. Because a theoretical grounding had not yet evolved, the vocabulary and concepts that guided the therapy were still quite simple. This lack of theory, along with the presence of the new verbatim recording technology, fostered an emphasis on verbal techniques as a core element in the therapy. Moreover, the concept "nondirective" placed a strong value-laden emphasis on the verbal technology.

But the dialectic process has a way of evolving and creating new syntheses. And so it was with this therapy. As new levels of understanding took place, the earlier polarities and contrast themes were no longer needed, and the term "nondirective" was less functional. In its place came a name that described in more precise and affirmative terms the essence of this therapy. The term "client-centered" came to be the term of choice. It described with simple accuracy exactly what the core of the therapy was meant to be; namely, an approach in which the therapist *centered attention upon the world of the client's immediate experiencing.* In this sense, the therapy came to be understood as an altogether phenomenological therapy, a process in which the therapists's total attention was focused upon the internal frame of reference of the client. There was a parallel development of personality theory that sought to explain the conceptual underpinning of the therapeutic process. A detailed analysis of the relationship between theory and therapy will illuminate the importance and the role of personality theory in providing a structure for the therapeutic task. This material will be presented in a later section of this chapter.

SOME THEORETICAL VARIANTS OF CLIENT-CENTERED THERAPY

In any living system, it is natural that new experimentation and new emphases should develop over time. This phenomenon has been true for client-centered therapy. Variations have in fact evolved along two dimensions. One dimension concerns the relative emphasis on preconceptual experiencing on the one hand and cognitive processes on the other. The second dimension concerns the extent to which the therapist introduces structure into the therapeutic task.

With respect to the relative roles of preconceptual experiencing and cognitive processes, distinctive emphases on the former are evident in the work of Gendlin (1962, 1978) and on the latter by Wexler (1974) and by Rice (1974, 1984). Gendlin has made basic contributions to our understanding of the phenomenon of experiencing. He has argued that experiencing is the fundamental process necessary to personality change. He has explicated the theoretical basis of his argument and has evolved a technology designed to facilitate the experiencing process.

Postscript 13

In the description of Gendlin's work it becomes clear that he sees the roots of experiencing as a preconceptual organismic phenomenon, an internal movement or "felt sense." The therapist's task is to help the client focus on this internal process. Implicit in the therapist task is the premise that the client has access to knowledge and understanding that is not merely a cognitive function but a total organismic function. This view is akin to the Reichian and Gestalt concepts that persons have experience and information stored throughout their bodies and not just in their heads. The therapist helps the client gain access to these data in the focusing process.

The writings of Wexler and of Rice place stronger emphasis on the cognitive end of the precognitive–cognitive continuum. Both of these contributors characterize therapy as an information processing experience. Wexler begins by offering a critique of the traditional client-centered view of experiencing and self-actualization, arguing that these concepts are ill-defined and nonoperational. He advances a view that places cognitive processes at the core of the therapeutic task, suggesting that "Experience . . . is created by the functioning of cognitive processes" (1974, p. 59). He further argues that cognitive processes are the active agents that transform information and make it usable. Implicit in this view is that people get into psychological trouble when they have inadequate or ineffective ways of organizing and integrating information. In this sense, a major task of the therapist is to help the client make information more usable. More specifically, the therapist's goal is to help the client do a more effective job of differentiating and integrating the meaning inherent in thought processes.

Rice sets the parameters of therapy in her assertion that the therapeutic task involves cognitive-affective reprocessing. Her use of the term *cognitive-affective* indicates that both cognition and precognitive feeling and experiencing are elements of the therapeutic process. She pictures therapy as a process of exploration that leads not only to the discovery of hitherto unexpressed feelings, but also to a new understanding of self. The latter goal in particular comes about through reprocessing and reconstructing data.

The second major dimension on which variations in client-centered theory and technology have occurred is in the domain of therapist structure. In Rogers's formulation of client-centered therapy, therapist structure is minimal. The therapist's task is to attend to whatever material the client offers, to enter into the client's world as he or she explores this material, and to go wherever the client leads. One can think of this process as naturalistic. Modifications of this naturalistic process take the form of therapist structures designed to facilitate the therapy. There are two such structural variants in the published literature, those by Gendlin (1978) and by Rice (1974). In each case, the structure follows the theoretical frames that I have just described.

Gendlin argues that, since experiencing is an essential component of therapy, it is wasteful to leave the process to chance, and more efficient to set the process in motion intentionally. Consequently, Gendlin becomes in effect a teacher of the process—that is, he offers instruction in effective client experiencing. He does this by teaching the client the techniques of *focusing.* I will not try to go into detail here on how this technique is taught, but indicate simply that there are a series of specific steps that direct the client's attention and awareness inward toward his or her bodily representations of experiential data.

Rice similarly follows her theory of reprocessing by offering structure. She argues that there are problematic areas in a client's life that represent difficulties for the client, that the client calls the therapist's attention to these areas, and that these problematic areas are best dealt with by having the therapist and client stay with these areas in order to work on the task of reprocessing. In this sense the therapist directs attention to such areas even when the client may be moving away from them or treating them unsystematically. The specific focal behavior of the therapist remains in the client-centered mode in that it is the phenomenology of the client that largely governs the moment-to-moment process.

In my own work as a therapist, my experience has been that Rogerian self-theory serves as a highly useful framework to guide my behavior. Repeatedly I have seen that experiencing becomes the avenue to new discoveries about the self, with consequent reorganization of the self-structure. The significance and power of this reorganization is validated in research findings about the self. For example, in major studies of adult maturity conducted by Heath (1965, 1977), he reported that "the four most powerful predictors of the maturity of men in three different cultures were measures of the self-concept."

With respect to variations in classical client-centered procedures, the single most significant modification for me has been in the use of procedures that focus and intensify the immediate experiencing process. In this connection I have found two procedures useful: the Gendlin focusing procedure already mentioned, and the Gestalt dramatization procedure described by Perls, et al. (1951). I find these procedures altogether compatible with a phenomenological approach. The cues for the use of these procedures come from the clients as I see them struggle to reach and comprehend their own immediate experience. My role at that point is to offer ways that may assist them in enhancing the experiencing process. Both Gendlin and Perls work at precisely this level.

THE PERSON-CENTERED APPROACH

In the third level of development of the client-centered approach there was a recognition that the therapeutic relationship described by Rogers need not be limited to therapy but in fact had generic qualities. The elements of that relationship were seen to be constructive and enhancing not only in therapy but in many other kinds of interpersonal settings. This recognition had been voiced early in the development of the client-centered approach (e.g., Rogers, 1951) but it was strongly expanded in the 1960s when Rogers left the academic setting and moved into a community setting—specifically, when he joined the Western Behavioral Sciences Institute.

Postscript 13

This move opened more direct opportunities for him to work with individuals who in no way defined themselves as "clients" or as persons in need of help. For many of these persons, a group experience was seen as a challenging and enriching personal growth experience. In this context, the term *client-centered* simply did not fit. Yet it was the case that the principles and concepts originally developed in the context of therapy were regarded as relevant to many kinds of interpersonal encounters. The term *person-centered* constituted an appropriate bridge from therapy relationships to other kinds of relationships.

The idea that self-theory and basic client-centered theory was applicable beyond the context of therapy has had wide acceptance among professionals with a client-centered orientation. Concepts and applications have extended to work with parents, to theories of education, to industry, and to government. Rogers's own interests have recently centered on the possibilities of the person-centered approach as a resource for conflict resolution in international relations. It is thus clear that the boundaries of relevance for the person-centered approach are broad, and that the limits are as yet unknown.

A CASE ANALYSIS

This section consists of a basic theoretical formulation and a series of verbatim passages from a therapy experience of a young man.

The Theory

Rogers (1951, 1961) has in a number of publications emphasized that a central construct in the personality theory associated with client-centered therapy is the construct *the self.* Studies of psychotherapy records have permitted us to observe persons in varying stages of disturbance, change, and integration. From the resulting evidence we can observe that a core determinant of personal development concerns the relationship between a person's experiences and his or her concept of self. In this connection we may conceptualize the self in terms of two components: the *experiential self* and the *conceptual self.* The experiential self may be defined as the sum total of the individual's personally relevant experiences. The conceptual self represents the emergent view of self, the self-definition that evolves from these experiences. There is a selective process involved, for the person is not always able to use all experiences as a basis for defining the self. Some experiences may be too dangerous, too painful, or too threatening, to accept, and so the person may deny or distort these experiences to make them tolerable. Yet there is a risk in this selectivity. Though such a process may make the self more acceptable and life more tolerable, the process also deprives the person of the reality data that helps the person make accurate observations, accurate judgments, and realistic decisions. Thus a person may pay a high price for self-consistency, in the form of blind spots and distortions in his or her view of self and the world. But that is not all. These needs to fend off reality sometimes exact another toll, in the form of anxiety and stress, for it takes work and energy to maintain the self in the face of recurrent threats, challenges, and contradictory experiences. When this stress becomes too painful, the person may seek help in the form of psychotherapy.

What, then, can the therapist do? The terms of the theory provide not only the explanation of what has gone wrong, but also the structure of the helping process. Let us review the core of the theory and note the way in which the theory provides a structure for the behavior of the therapist. Concretely, let us sketch the self-structure of Person A, a male in his mid-twenties. In Figure 13–1, Circle I represents the experiential self, the sum total of the person's significant experiences; Circle II represents the person's conceptual self.

Segment *b* is the component of self in which Person A has been able to integrate his experiences into his concept of self. But it is also evident that a significant proportion of his experiences, as represented by segment *a*, has not entered into his self-definition—that is, segment *a* comprises those experiences that are too dangerous, too unacceptable, or too vaguely understood, to be integrated and utilized as an acceptable aspect of self. Segment *c* has a significance of its own. It represents that aspect of the self-concept that is not validated by experience. It is a segment that is an amalgam of an idealized image and introjected views of self, views that have been instilled by significant others and adopted by the person, yet without a basic foundation within Person A himself.

One way to think about the self-structure depicted in Figure 13–1 is to think about Person A as a scientist. Circle I represents the observational and experiential data from which he forms the theory or concept represented by Circle II. If he utilizes all of the data, an accurate theory is likely to result. But if he is selective and omits data, his theory will not represent all of reality and hence will be less comprehensive and indeed perhaps defective.

If we now construe this formulation in terms of the therapist's task, we see that the task of the therapist is to help Person A get in touch with the unknown or unacceptable aspects of his experience—that is, segment *a*—and integrate these experiences into his conceptual self. If such a process is successful, by the end of therapy Person A will be able to utilize most of his experiences as a basis for self-definition, as in Figure 13–2.

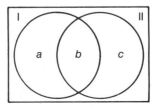

Figure 13-1. Self-structure pre-therapy.

Postscript   13

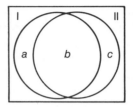

Figure 13-2.   Self-structure post-therapy.

We can see in this post-therapy diagram that Person A has integrated a much larger portion of his experiential self into his conceptual self. In the process several other important processes have taken place:

He has learned that his experiences are less dangerous and unacceptable than he earlier thought.

He has learned to trust the *process of experiencing*—that is, he has learned to pay attention to his own signals.

He has learned that he can be the source of his own valuing process.

He has come to like himself more and to accept himself more fully.

He finds other people less threatening and can thus relate to others more freely and fully.

It will be useful now to take a closer look at the way in which the self theory set forth here helps to provide a framework for defining the therapist's task. Rogers (1958) has described this task in terms of three components provided by the therapist: unconditional positive regard, empathy, and congruence. With respect to the first component, unconditional positive regard, several considerations prompt this criterion. First and foremost, the acceptance of other persons as they are is in its simplest essence a matter of human dignity. Such acceptance in no way implies endorsement of or agreement with their views, but simply a matter of relating to the person in nonjudgmental terms. A by-product of this attitude leads to an important precondition of change in therapy; namely, the creation of a climate of safety and trust in which the client can dare to venture into exploration that may be threatening.

But safety is often not enough. The therapist can also serve as a resource for helping the client not only explore and experience new feelings but also enhance the understanding of those experiences. A powerful technology for doing this is available to the therapist in the form of empathic understanding. The therapist can enter into the internal frame of reference of the client, attempt to perceive the world of experience just as the client is experiencing that world, and in that process illuminate what the client is trying to feel and comprehend.

The third and final component of the therapist's behavior is congruence—that is to say, the therapist's inner feelings and outer behavior in harmony with each other. The therapist helps to foster a real relationship rather than a role relationship, and can do so best when he or she is at one with self.

AN ILLUSTRATION OF THE THERAPEUTIC PROCESS

The illustration that follows presents passages from the counseling experience of a 25-year-old man whom I shall call Jim. When Jim first came for counseling, he had a pronounced pattern of stuttering, a pattern that affected deeply his view of himself and his relationships with others. The increasing distress that he was feeling led him to seek psychotherapy. Jim was in therapy for two years. In order to capture the scope of the process, I shall present four passages spaced along this two-year span. I have added footnote comments that are designed to emphasize the way in which the theory that I have sketched earlier helps us to comprehend the therapeutic process. It will be possible, I think, to note the close fit between theory and therapy.

Passages from Interview One*

C1: Well, I'm I'm having q-q-quite a bit of trouble in class talking and it s-seems like I—well, I want to talk in class but I'm unable to. I, oh I just get sc-scared and tied up and oh, everything else.[1]

T1: Is it that you want to so much and yet the very thought of it is frightening? Is that the way it works?[1]

C2: Yes, I, I, oh I just get scared and I begin to sweat and I I have—and my stomach bothers me and everything else and w-well when I t-try to get the word out somethin' gets st-stuck in my mm-mouth or something. I, I just, I just feel like quitting school.[2]

T2: It's a terribly discouraging thing to you when it happens this way?

C3: Yeah, I t-try so hard and—well, it seems like the harder I try the more trouble I have.

T3: It must seem unfair to you that, here you try, you do the best you can, and still you can't get anywhere—I mean there's something pretty awful about that thought.[3]

C4: And, oh, when I have trouble I feel like I'm sorta dumb, sorta worthless, and I think everybody else thinks I'm stupid or something. (Pause). It's talking, and I guess it's just about, I guess it's about in everything I do, I just feel like I'm no good, I just sorta crack up when I try hard. I don't know, I guess there isn't any use in trying hard anymore.

---

*The passages of this counseling experience are quoted from *The Case of Jim,* a booklet written by the author of this paper. Publisher: Counselor Recordings and Tests of Nashville, Tennessee, 1957.

[1]When we consider all of the different responses that the counselor might have made to Jim's opening statement, one may well wonder why the counselor made this particular response. The point of the response is that the counselor intends from the very start to enter the client's world of experience—i.e., to comprehend the client's internal frame of reference. The response also portrays a nonjudgmental empathic response.

[2]Notice that the counselor's response is followed by further exploration.

[3]When the counselor says "There's something pretty awful about that thought" he is not expressing his own personal view but trying rather to capture the sense of Jim's feeling of defeat expressed in C3.

Postscript 13

T4: You get to feeling worthless yourself, and you're sure that everybody else just thinks the same way about you, is that the way you feel?[4]

C5: Everybody else thinks that I'm, "Oh well, he's crazy, or there's something wrong with him, he can't talk right, he can't do anything right. So, well, we'll just simply let him go. Oh, well, I guess we'll be nice to him but he's no good, he's just sorta worthless." That's the way I feel other people think about me; they think I'm crazy or something; I don't know, I guess I am.

T5: Is it that you come to feel those things yourself, about yourself, too?[4]

C6: Well, whenever I'm alone I feel so depressed, oh, it seems like nobody loves me, nobody cares for me anymore. Well, when I'm out with, when I'm out in a crowd I feel so lo-lo-lonely, and all by myself, and oh, it seems like I want to talk, and I don't want to make a fool of myself either.

T6: No matter what you do, you feel very deeply alone when you're with people.[4]

C7: I don't know, I get tight and I sweat, I'm sweating now; and my voice is jerky and shaky, and I feel all tight and stuff and everything and my heart seems to be beating faster and everything else.

T7: It seems like everything comes together at that very point where you have to speak, where it seems like a big crisis for you, doesn't it?

C8: Yeah. It seems like every time I talk it seems to be quite an ordeal, I guess. It seems like s-something, something very important in my life. Might as well get a job in some factory or something. Just quit the whole thing.

T8: I'm sure there are times when you just feel like giving up the whole business of trying to get anywhere.

C9: Yeah, OK, I think—

T9: OK, yeah, I think it's about time—   *(End of Session)*

Passages from Interview 18

C10: Well ah, I've been th-thinking about my ag-aggression.—It's—I'm beginning to s-s-s-well, I'm— not beginning to see more, I'm beginning to feel more that I might be showing a lot of aggression in my st-stuttering toward other people because I know now ah, the other person suffers even more than I do sometime. And it's, I don't know, I guess I am doing it to make the other person suffer. I mean this is something I could never—I could never admit before. I mean, I mean it would—if I just said it, it would just be a lie, but I'm beginning to see now maybe it isn't a lie, maybe I do have a lot of aggression in myself. That's the way I'm showing it toward other people. I know I used to feel quite bad about my speech. But ah, it's it's something s-so new that I'm probably showing aggression in my speech. I need to say it over and over again. It's, I'm just trying to work it through. I-It surprises me so much.[5]

[4]The counselor's general intention becomes more clear as one studies these responses. His continuing purpose is to understand Jim's inner feelings, and to make it safe for Jim to continue more deeply into an exploration of these feelings. One may have expected the counselor to offer more sympathy, or to suggest specific remedial steps to Jim. The counselor, however, is not inclined to look upon feelings of distress and inadequacy as negative feelings to be soothed or avoided, but rather as feelings to be explored, experienced, and understood. Hence his continuing purpose is to turn further "inward" with Jim as he deals with these feelings.

[5]We see here a fascinating illustration of a way in which personality change begins to take place in counseling. Jim is examining his own conception of himself and beginning to realize that there are elements in his make-up which had never been acceptable to him before. We shall see that in this entire interview Jim is trying to test and integrate these new ways of looking at himself.

In terms of the earlier diagram, Jim is evidently exploring segment *a* of his experiential self, and discovering new elements.

T10: It's an idea you have to keep close to you. . . .[6]

C11: I do.

T11: . . . and play around with because it's new, and it seems like it hits you rather strong too.[6]

C12: Yes, it has. I didn't know, well, I mean, oh, I've read about it before. But I always want to hurry and get over to the next sentence, you know.

T12: That was for somebody else.

C13: Yes. That was for the other guy, that wasn't for me. But I'm beginning to see it, I guess it is for me. I rather enjoy—I didn't want to be a person, I didn't want to be a self. But I am now and the t-times that I feel bad now are when I do not become an individual. (Pause) Do you know, I just can't realize, I just can't realize that I had a lot of aggression in me. Gee, I mean it's so new yet. (sounds surprised) I mean I have to go back and talk about it again and again. It's just, boy! I'm aggressive. Even now, no, I'm not aggressive. Yes I am. I mean I just said I was, but I just don't want to quite accept it yet. I am aggressive—or am I? I'm beginning to doubt. M-hm. That's also—gee, I thought I'd be going out of here admitting that I was ag-ag-aggressive. But now I don't know whether I'll be able to or not. You know—well, I mean—I could admit to you I was aggressive, OK, you moved up one, made some progress. But I'm not interested in making progress. Hm, I'm not interested in making progress. That's something new. Before, I thought gee, I wanted to make some progress in here, going to improve. That was *important,* I mean that was important for me to make progress in here, in therapy. But now it isn't. It isn't important. Hmm. That is also something new now that I'm feeling. That was something that sort of threatened me before, too. It sure was, whether I was going to make progress or not. Yeah, that was *really* something. Because if—I knew if I would not make any—well, gee, that was—I wouldn't want to like that. I wouldn't be able to accept that at all.

T16: It was one of your biggest fears. . . .

C17: Yeah, you know that (slightly laughing) was. I thought gee, I'm going to take therapy and I—boy, you'd better make progress, if you don't why you're screwy or something, you're nuts. Mhmm. Things are sure changing around, boy! Boy, I can't even predict my own behavior around here anymore (laughing)—something I was able to do before. Now boy, I don't know what I'll say next. Man, it's a real—you know, that's quite a feeling. Not to be able to predict your own behavior; that is quite a feeling. Something I haven't been able to do before. I mean well, I'll just say, well, what I want to say. I, I thought I was doing that all along here. But I guess I wasn't. Hmm. Just let come what may. Really, let come what may. Are you really—Now I'm beginning to doubt that. I'm beginning to wonder whether—[7]

T17: Can you be that free?

C18: Yes. Can I really be that free or am I sort of just kidding myself again that I am that free? I'm back again to where I'm beginning to wonder about this whole thing. By jove! Really something (softly) I'm beginning to enjoy this now, I'm getting a big kick out of it. Before I used to get—it was work. Now, I'm beginning to enjoy this, now. It's adventure,

---

[6]The counselor is responding to what he considers important in counseling; namely, the awareness of an immediately experienced feeling. Note that the counselor hardly refers to the context of Jim's comments, but focuses on the *experiencing process.* The therapist's attention is centered on the immediately given "livingness" of the client—i.e., the point at which the client's energy is being utilized.

[7]I found this passage to represent a fascinating moment in therapy. When Jim says, in an elated tone, "Things are sure changing around, boy! Boy, I can't even predict my own behavior around here anymore . . ." he is letting us know that he has become more open to new experiences and new discoveries about himself. The old fears, the old vigilance, the old tightness of self-definition, are giving way. Importantly, he is learning how to experience in the present.

Postscript   13

happiness. Well, I'm joyful about it, let's say I'm joyful. Even about all these old negative things, I don't want to make progress, that I'm aggressive, I'm, I'm, I'm, joyful with my aggression. Sad and mo-mo-mournful, mournful, mournful about it (keeps repeating the word voluntarily). There the third time, why I'll do it, you just give me plenty of time (laughs). That's something I wasn't able to do before; I would have just said mo-mournful once and hurried to something else. But—[8]

T18: Now, you're saying to me, "OK, so I'll let you know I have trouble with my speech and I'm going to keep on working, right in front of your face."[9]

C19: Right! That's right! I don't care what you think about it. Maybe I'm showing ag-ag-ag-aggression like that. Maybe I am. Maybe I'm, I'm just gonna make you hurt. (leans very close to therapist, voice raising) I'm just gonna hurt you all I can with this stuttering. That's some—hmm, I'm surprised I said that. I'm just going to hurt you all I can with my speech. I'm just gonna st-st-st-stutter all I c-c-c-can. (voluntarily imitates stutter) That wasn't an actual block, I imitated those, but I'm able to do it and I'm able to s-s-show ag-ag-aggression (real stutter) towards you like that. Gee! I showed quite a bit of aggression even toward my therapist, toward my therapist. Boy this is surprising.[10]

T19: You never knew you felt that?

C20: I never knew I could do something like that. I'm surprised you're not klopping me on the head or something. "Mustn't do that man, mustn't do that." I'm surprised you're not rejecting me, you're not punishing me, I'm surprised.

T20: Surprised that I'm not giving. . . .

C21: (Talking at the same time) I am, I'm terribly surprised (slightly laughing).

T21: Surprised that I'm not coming back at you.

C22: Yeah, that you're not. I can't believe it. (softly) I can't (slightly laughing) I can't, I can't believe it. (laughing to relieve tension) You're not jumping all over me. You're not angry at me. You're not. (laughing) For once somebody's not angry at me. I don't have to worry whether you feel angry at me or not. This is the first time I ever felt this. That you're not angry at me. It surprises me. (Pause) All this aggression I've shown towards you. Yet I'm, showing it in my speech. That is the thing that is more surprising than ever. That's the thing that surprises me that I sh-showed aggression by my stuttering. By my stuttering I've showed aggression. Something I've tried to get rid of all the time. Something I didn't want to do all the time. I mean before this was—I never thought of this. It was just something, well, it just did-didn't exist.

T22: Of all the things you're doing with your speech is showing aggression.

C23: By—that is right! M-hm. That is really a revelation. That really surprises me. My goodness! Sure does, sure does.

T23: This is what speech meant to you. It really must surprise you.

[8]Jim's zestful attitude about his negative feelings is interesting. He is telling us that once he is really able to experience them they give him a sense of freedom and release.

[9]This response illustrates one of the elements of client-centered technology. The stereotype of client-centered technology as a repetition or echo of the client's statement is in no way descriptive of the therapist's real task. I have always defined my task as listening for the emergent but unformed feelings that the client is struggling to experience and comprehend. T18 is an example. What I sensed in Jim's earlier statement (C18) was a note of assertiveness, even defiance. Note that my comment on T18 captured that note of defiance, and released Jim to move more deeply into expression of hostile feelings.

[10]Jim senses a rise in his hostility and tries out directly the experience of being openly attacking and aggressive toward the therapist. Jim's use of the relationship to try out the experience of hostility represents one of the unique aspects of counseling. It is through the avenue of such direct experiences in the relationship that much new learning by the client takes place in counseling.

C24: That is what speech means, to be aggressive. And I was proudly trying to hold it in. Sp-speech is aggression. Speech is aggression. When I'm—When I talk I'm being ag-ag-aggressive. Something I never wanted to be. Maybe that's the reason I didn't want to talk. Yeah, but yet when I was quiet, I didn't want to be that way either. (pause)

T24: Jim, let's stop for today.

All right, let's do.   *(End of Session)*

Passages from Interview 63

C25: I guess—I guess that was what I was sort of worried about. . . . sort of had the feeling that I might lose her. But you know, I don't feel like—I don't feel like crying. I just get mad now. Gee whiz I feel sort of guilty about that. You know I sort of feel guilty about that, ashamed of myself about what I said, by golly, I do. By golly I'm not going to be pushed around by anyone. In other words, I don't—you know—this is it, you know, I always used to beg. I'd always—be nice and proper and I'd be a gentleman and you know everything the way you're supposed to do.

T25: Please like me.

C26: Yea, yea that's it, that's right, that's it by golly that's it; by golly, please like me, please like me, I'll be a good boy, I'll be a good boy if you'll like me; if you like me I'll be good, I'll be good. . . . you know that's awfully new. Please like me, as if I was sort of playing up—they were something—something I had to look up to; y-yea before when I would lose a girl I would, gee I would just, you know, I would f-feel like I was deserted or rejected again as if, as if my mother rejected me again. There's, gee there's a lot of similarity to that feeling there. Oh here's, here's something. My masculinity used to depend on whether I had a girl or how successful I was with the opposite sex. If I was su-successful with the girls, if they liked me well then I would assume that I'd be masculine. Hell, if they wouldn't like be that would be a threat to my masculinity. So, in other words my masculinity is not determined by my relationships with the girls. It's something within me. It's the way I look at everything—at the women, at men, kids and everything else. It's the way I look at myself, it's the way I act. It isn't dependent on heterosexual relations anymore; I mean it isn't dependent on whether the girl likes me, therefore, I feel like I'm masculine. If she doesn't like me therefore I feel, what's the matter. Yea, if they don't like me, it would be, it would be a threat to my masculinity. That's it. . . .[11]

T26: It would be like telling you, you're not really a man.

C27: That's it, by golly that's it (claps) by golly that's it. By golly that's it, that's right (laughs).

T27: No wonder you never knew.

C28: (laughs) I never knew whether I was a man or a woman. . . . That's awful true by golly. In other words, I-I like that by golly. Boy, I'm proud of that.

T28: You're saying by golly you're the one who decides it.

C29: Yeaaa. That's it. Boy, that's it. That's it, by golly nobody's going to question it. I don't care. By golly I'll go out and slug somebody. (Pause) You know man I'm getting awfully defensive about this now ain't I? Sort of funny, as if I've got to prove it yet, yeah, as if I have to go around proving it. Boy, that's sure a change-about.

---

[11]Jim is saying that his view of himself was once determined largely by the values of others, but that he can now depend upon his own direct experience to guide him.

Postscript 13

T29: You feel suddenly like you're insisting on it an awful lot.

C30: Yea, that's it. Gee, that's sure awful funny.

T30: You've still got to insist on it or it's in danger?

C31: Yea, that's it. That's right. But that hurts a little. That's right, I have to insist on it. But, you know here's the thing, here's the thing by golly. I'll go out and fight for it; before I always, it always had to sort of come from without but by golly I'll go out and fight for it. You know I been sort of wondering you know, I been—you know—within the last several days I felt I could be a bachelor the rest of my life and wouldn't question my masculinity whereas before I had to hurry up and get married so I would appear masculine. That's right, but no more. In other words I don't have to have a crutch. I'd sure like one but somehow I can (pause) sort of think about not becoming married without becoming too overwhelmed by my own loneliness. Your know I have been able to talk about these things, I mean I've been able to put these things all into words. Man, I've been able, gee, I've been able to feel a lot of things here today. Gee, I don't know whether it's all clear or not, but I've been able to feel a lot of things. In other words, before I wasn't able, I wasn't even able to admit this to you. Because gee that was something to hide, behind here again but I mean I've been able to paint it on the walls so that you could also take a look at it. I happen to be doing, oh a horrible job of painting but somehow you've been able to see this thing, too. Th-that's what I did here today I think. *(End of Session)*

Passages from Interview 120 (The Final Interview)

C32: This is the last one. I feel a little depressed about it. It just began to hit me now.

T32: Just as you came in?

C33: Yes, just as I came in. I happened to think, I sure been in here a lot and a lot of times.

T33: It is sure hard to think of cutting it off and leaving, isn't it?

C34: Oh, it is. Gee, I mean I didn't think much about it until now. You know there's a lot of things been happening to me in the last few days. You know I'm not afraid of losing control any more. In other words, I'm not afraid of my feelings anymore. And uh, I just, man I just feel like I-I well, like I'm worth somebody. . . . Well, maybe somebody really, really likes me. I mean not as a little boy but as a man. I hate to say that in a way because it's so darn true. Yea, yea, in a way it hurts to say that but—

T34: Why, it hurts—

C35: It hurts that, man, I had to wait so long before I finally grew up.

T35: I see. It took such a long time for you to be able to say that.

C36: Yea, I mean everything I've been missing.

T36: Uh-huh.

C37: That's the reason that—for some of this, some of these things, by golly if I couldn't have them in the right ways that I was going to have it in the wrong way. In other words, as I mentioned before, there wasn't any reward in being good.

T37: By golly, you were going to do it anyhow.

C38: That's right.

T38: I think that was accompanied by a lot of anger on your part, wasn't it?

C39: Yea, boy there was; I mean I, boy I thought of that again and again. In other words, I did that because I was so mad and I was going to prove that I was going to be a man and also there was some element of punishment towards myself in that, or of self hate. But there was also this aggression and also this self hate; it was also going to be, well by golly, I'm going to prove that I'm not a little boy. (Pause) Then you know the wonderful thing is I—I don't have any fear of losing control any more. And the funny thing was—I was, let's see—last few days I didn't have to hold myself. In other words, I mean I could set and let my feelings go free and I wasn't afraid of myself. That was so wonderful. The feelings were not intense or anything like that.[12]

T39: Is it you feel like you can have those feelings and that's all right?

C40: Uh-hum.

T40: And that's why you don't feel like you're going to lose control, is that it, because the feelings are okay to have?

C41: Uh-hum, also they weren't as powerful as I imagined them to be. . . .Really, I mean, well, that's it and it's over. In other words there isn't anything that builds up. That's it, nothing builds up. I mean when it's over, that's all.[12]

T41: Uh-hum.

C42: In other words I can—well, it isn't a take it or leave it, but I can have the feelings and they're over. I mean they're not very intense or anything but before they used to be intense and I would try to fight it. But I mean I'm not fighting them now and they ain't intense. (Pause) I happened to think about the last two years. Boy, what a struggle that's been. I think I remember the first session here. Gee, I was afraid. I was afraid I might—I was afraid I might let something get out that I didn't want to. And sure a lot of things got out that I didn't want to. Boy, but I feel so different now, so different. I—gee, I—yet in some ways I feel different and in some ways I feel the same. But yet I don't feel the same. (Pause) Probably one reason was—was I never tried something because well because I was afraid of it. But I, well, I just feel pretty good now. You know, I feel like I'm really broken somehow, really, really broken yet I feel pretty good about it.[13]

T42: In what way do you mean that, broken? I'm not sure I understand.

C43: By that I mean I don't have anything to hide any more. I don't feel like I'm always walking on edge, and anytime ready to go over. You know, in other words, I mean everything sort of widened out. In other words I'm not afraid of myself, anymore.

T43: That everything widened out makes me feel like this walking on a straight thing, that you felt like you were in danger.

C44: Boy, that is right, yeah.

T44: And now with everything widened, it is just much safer to just do more things.

C45: That's right. It sure is, much safer. Boy you've really treated me good, you know that. Boy we've really had some hard battles in here haven't we? Really, really had some hard battles. Boy, I used to get really mad at you. You, boy oh boy, you really used to threaten me. I don't mind leaving either, don't mind leaving. But you know, the wonderful feeling is that I can always come back again. You know, that is something.

T45: Something reassuring about that?

C46: It really is. I'll probably be back here next summer.[14]

---

[12]We see here one kind of learning which takes place in counseling. Jim is saying that he has learned to deal with feelings which have made him anxious in the past and to make a more complete response to these feelings even in the face of anxiety.

[13]Here we get some further understanding of Jim's anxiety. He tells us that he had feelings of which he was afraid or ashamed.

[14]Jim's wish to maintain some contact with the counselor is not at all unusual. Clients often need to try themselves out after counseling. It is not at all unusual, either, for clients to re-open counseling after a time out of therapy. As a matter of fact Jim returned a year later for a brief series of interviews.

Postscript   13

T46: I'm glad I could work with you and any time you want to write or if you drop in here. . . .

C47: Well, you know what I'm going to do? Sometime I'll write you a letter but I don't want you to answer it. I mean, if you want to answer it that's okay but that's not the purpose of my writing. Ok, well, good-bye, and thank you.[14]   *(End of Session)*

A LOOK AT THE PROCESS

There are strong sequential elements in the therapeutic process, and those elements are illustrated in Jim's counseling experience. I shall now highlight the sequential flow of the integrative process as I see it in the transcript.

1. The Capacity to Explore One's Feelings in the Face of Anxiety

Self-reorganization involves the exploration of feelings that are often unknown to the person and often by their nature threatening. The individual's tendency is to avoid pain, and thus to avoid looking at threatening feelings. Individuals in counseling learn to explore feelings in the face of anxiety because they also learn that self-discovery is freeing and rewarding.

Jim describes such a process within himself in C39, when he tells us that he can let his feelings go free without fighting them. It is interesting to note, parenthetically, that Jim found these feelings less intense than he imagined them to be. This experience is not uncommon with clients. Jim himself described some of the dynamics of this phenomenon when he explained that he no longer allowed the feelings to build up within him.

2. The Capacity to Experience Fully the Range of Attitudes Within the Person

This facet of integration is linked closely to the previous one, and may be considered a further development of the earlier point. We are referring here to the capacity of individuals to let themselves experience fully the feelings that relate to them as persons. It has already been pointed out that the reverse tendency, that of denial, is associated with tension and disturbance.

We may now bring together the first two hypotheses, those of exploration and experiencing, by recalling the second passage in the record. In C10, Jim is exploring his feelings of aggression in a tentative way. We can see the struggle he has in dealing with this concept. In C16, Jim comes back to the idea of his aggression and continues to explore its relation to him. You may recall that he is "trying it on for size" when he says, "I am aggressive—or am I?" In the last phase of the interview we come to Jim's full experiencing of his aggression, when, in C19, he attacks the therapist verbally. This sequence illustrates vividly what we mean by exploring and experiencing.

3. The Capacity to Symbolize Accurately One's Immediate Experience

This hypothesis refers to the individual's ability to give meaning to experience through words or behavior. It is a kind of "labeling" process; as such it may be less important than the experience itself. This hypothesis seems more abstract than the others, and so an example may be especially useful here.

Perhaps you will recall C15, where Jim is feeling the pain involved in his conflict with his speech. He feels the need to identify what he is feeling, and gropes for the word. Finally, he comes through with the word *stress.* One can hear in the record the sense of release which Jim felt when he found the word that symbolized accurately his inner emotional state. Clients have often expressed this sense of release when they have been able to identify exactly what they are feeling. It is questionable whether the intellectual activity of labeling or naming feelings is alone integrative. The important factor, rather, is the appropriate blend of affect and intellect, of feeling and knowing. One of the important factors here too is congruence. It is the congruence between experience and symbol that constitutes the sense of discovery. This experience has been referred to aptly as an "aha" experience.

4. The Capacity to Assimilate New Experiences into the Concept of Self

Here we have a continuation of the processes described in the hypotheses above. Individuals who are able to experience and symbolize attitudes rather than inhibit them are also in a position to evaluate their meaning. They can ask, just as Jim did, "Is this part of me? Am I this way?" Thus the person has an opportunity to deal with contradictory experiences and assimilate them. He or she can, in other words, evaluate and revise a self-concept on the basis of new experiences. This implies that some degree of fluidity or flexibility in one's self-organization is part of being an integrated person.

5. The Capacity to Develop an Integral Locus of Evaluation

This hypothesis is closely related to the previous one. We are referring here to the ability of individuals to use their own experiences as a basis for evaluating self and developing self-conceptions. This ability is what we mean by internal locus or source of evaluation. This point may seem self-evident until we examine more closely the ways in which a person develops self-conceptions. It has been suggested earlier than an alternative source of self-evaluation arises from appraisals of others. Individuals who function through internal threat and denial tend to distrust their own experiences as a source of evaluation and use appraisals of others.

It should be made clear that this process is not an either/or process—that is, we do not mean to imply that a person develops a self-concept either through

Postscript   13

self-appraisal or appraisals of others. People are very much social beings, and appraisals by others are part of the way people learn about themselves. The point is, however, that the maladjusted person tends to give up personal experiences as a source of self-learning. The integrated person, on the other hand, can use all of the evidence, from self and others, and in the long run reach a conclusion based on an internal synthesis of the evidence.

Jim illustrates the concept of internal locus of evaluation very clearly in the third excerpt. In an eloquent passage (C26), Jim says, "My masculinity used to depend on whether I had a girl or how successful I was with the opposite sex. If I was su-successsful with the girls, if they like me well then I would assume that I'd be masculine. Hell, if they wouldn't like me that would be a threat to my masculinity. So, in other words my masculinity is not determined by my relationships with the girls. It's something within me. It's the way I look at everything—at the women, at men, kids and everything else. It's the way I look at myself, it's the way I act."

Let us return now to the relation between experiencing and evaluation. Persons who can experience their feelings fully are also the persons who are learning most about self. They have a maximum basis for self-evaluation. On the other hand, persons who do not dare to base a self-concept on internal evaluation are precisely the persons who tend to deny threatening experiences, and thus the persons who have the least basis in direct experience for such evaluation.

We shall see in the next hypothesis that there is another way in which experiencing and self-evaluation are linked.

6. The Capacity to Accept One's Self and Others

Individuals who have the ability to experience feelings and use them to develop self-conceptions are also secure and self-trusting persons. It follows almost as a matter of definition that they are self-accepting persons. This does not mean at all that the integrated person is complacent or self-satisfied. It does not mean, either, that the integrated person does not have strong feelings or conflicts. What it does mean is that the self-accepting person need not deny such feelings, but can see them all as part of self.

One interesting corollary of self-acceptance is acceptance of others. The individual who is internally secure also finds it easier to accept other people. This, too, does not mean that the person exudes sweetness and light, is never hostile, or never disagrees with others. But it does mean that such persons are less threatened by others, and can perceive differences in others without feeling that such differences restrict them in some way.

7. The Understanding of One's Own Self-Boundaries

Therapy is not only a process of self-discovery, but also one of self-definition. People not only learn what they are like, but also learn to identify more clearly their own self-boundaries, to differentiate more clearly between self and nonself. This capacity to understand the boundaries of the self, which characterizes integrated persons, has profound implications for interpersonal relationships. No doubt all of us can recall examples of the reverse phenomenon. We have seen it in parents who have not differentiated clearly between themselves and their children and who consequently find it difficult to allow autonomous development. We have seen it in people whose security depends upon their control of others, or in people who are threatened by the actions of others and withdraw. The person who understands the sense of personal separateness as an individual is not likely to be involved in such relationships. This separateness does not in any degree imply a sense of distance or aloofness. Quite the contrary; it is only out of the understanding of one's self-ness that one person can be freely close to another without threat, obligation, need, or fear. Putting the matter this way makes clearer the close connection between this concept of self-boundaries and acceptance of others.

A Thirty-Year Follow-Up

When Jim completed two years of therapy, he left to take a professional position that was interpersonal in nature. I have kept in touch with him through occasional letters. In preparation for writing this chapter, I invited him to take a retrospective look at what the counseling experience meant to him. His own first-person account follows.

> My therapy with Dr. Seeman had a profound effect on me in terms of my developing my identity or self-concept. However, I also have suffered from depression for the rest of my life. This was not constant by any means, but would loom up during periods of stress. Because of this I have had counseling intermittently since then.
>
> The one factor in all of the above counseling experiences is that they were short-term, provided support, allowed me to share my feelings, and feel more competent and whole. I was able to move into a therapeutic relationship very quickly, work through a problem quickly, and be on my way. This suggests that the long-term process of counseling of 30 years ago enabled me to move very quickly in one or two sessions and get instant results. Also the various counselors found me an easy client to work with.
>
> My counseling on a long-term basis 30 years ago enables me to use very short-term counseling, as if I were getting a "booster shot" for some disease. Another aspect of my long-term counseling experience of 30 years ago is that I have become an effective helping person, a skill that has not left me.
>
> In regard to my stuttering, it is no longer the central part of my life nor do I see my speech defect or stuttering as the most important part of my personality or self-concept. Counseling certainly was important in making this change. However, as I developed into a more successful adult, other people looked beyond my speech handicap and thought "if he made it this far, he cannot be a total failure." The results of long-term competence in a profession adds to one's self-esteem and self-concept.

Postscript 13

> I now have a very close, affectionate, friendly, and good-time relationship with my father, something I did not have 30 years ago. He has and shows much love for me.

CONCLUSION

An examination of the therapeutic process that occurred with Jim suggests that his experiences in therapy, and the outcomes of therapy for him, are congruent with the theoretical expectations set forth here. Changes that occur in central aspects of a person's self-definition affect other aspects of the person's life. That is what appears to have happened for Jim.

The foregoing outcome is also compatible with human-system theory, which postulates that central elements of the person's behavioral systems are integrally linked. Consequently, it should be possible to intervene at different points in the human system and affect other behavioral systems within the person. In this sense, experiential processes in psychotherapy had a positive effect for the degree of impediment in Jim's speech. What I noticed particularly was a reversal that Jim effected at the immediate point of speech blockage. Whereas at the start of therapy, Jim exerted more effort and strain at the point of blockage, late in therapy he had spontaneously taken to reducing effort and to relax at the instant of blockage. His pauses became almost imperceptible. It appears to me that, as smooth speech became less urgently necessary as a test of personhood for Jim, he was able to put his speech issues into more useful perspective.

REFERENCES

Gendlin, E. T. (1962). *Experiencing and the creation of meaning.* New York: The Free Press of Glencoe.

Gendlin, E. T. (1978). *Focusing.* New York: Everest House Publishers.

Rice, L. N. (1974). The evocative function of the therapist. In D. A. Wexler and L. N. Rice (Eds.), *Innovations in client-centered therapy.* New York: Wiley and Sons.

Rice, L. N. (1984). The tasks of the therapist. In R. Levant and J. M. Shlien (Eds.), *Client-centered therapy and the person-centered approach.* New York: Praeger.

Rogers, C. R. (1942). *Counseling and psychotherapy.* New York: Houghton-Mifflin.

Wexler, D. A. (1974). A cognitive theory of experiencing, self-actualization, and the therapeutic process. In D. A. Wexler and L. N. Rice (Eds.), *Innovations in client-centered therapy.* New York: John Wiley and Sons.

Wexler, D. A., & Rice, L. N. (1974). *Innovations in client-centered therapy.* New York: John Wiley and Sons.

Rogers, C. R. (1951). *Client-centered therapy.* New York: Houghton-Mifflin.

Systematic Desensitization Based on Relaxation

Behavior Therapy of Stuttering: Deconditioning the Emotional Factor

Postscript
Systematic Desensitization

Joseph Wolpe

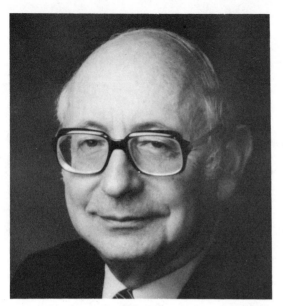

Joseph Wolpe

In the late 1950s and 1960s, Systematic Desensitization as a therapy for stuttering enjoyed a sharp surge of interest in the British Commonwealth, including Australia, Great Britain, and South Africa, as well as in various parts of Europe, Scandinavia and the United States. Under the leadership of its founder, Joseph Wolpe, and with the work of Lazarus, Yates, Lazovik, Lanyon and Lang, Brutten and his students, and Salter, this therapy became firmly established both in psychotherapy (especially for phobias) and in work with stutterers. In a sense, Wolpe's work was a major pioneering effort to break away from psychodynamic perspectives in clinical psychology to focus on neurosis and its therapy as processes of behavior. Wolpe was espousing the cause of changing behavior and eliminating symptoms rather than developing insights into etiology and the more traditional psychotherapeutic tactics. Stuttering was viewed as a symptom of anxiety about talking, and the therapy focused on reducing that anxiety by developing and using behavior that competed with it, while gradually and progressively experiencing visual representation of anxiety-provoking stimuli.

Wolpe as its developer was the obvious and natural selection to discuss systematic desensitization therapy and to provide an update on his current thoughts about its application to stuttering. In this chapter by Dr. Wolpe, there is a presentation of his original conceptualizations and discussions about this therapy for stuttering. He follows this with his views and assessments of its current applications, more than a quarter of a century later.

14

Systematic Desensitization Based on Relaxation

Joseph Wolpe

Of the methods of therapy considered in this book the present parallels most closely the experimental procedure of feeding cats in the presence of increasing "doses" of anxiety-evoking stimuli (described in Chapter 4).

An anxiety hierarchy is a list of stimulus situations to which a patient reacts with graded amounts of anxiety. The most disturbing item is placed at the top of the list, the least disturbing at the bottom. These hierarchies provide a convenient framework for systematic desensitization, through relaxation, to increasing amounts of anxiety-evoking stimuli.*

The theory may be summarized like this: If a stimulus constellation made up of five equipotent elements $A_1A_2A_3A_4A_5$ evokes 50 units of anxiety response in an organism, proportionately less anxiety will be evoked by constellations made up of fewer elements. Relaxation that is insufficient to counter the 50 units of anxiety that $A_1A_2A_3A_4A_5$ evokes may be well able to inhibit the 10 units evoked by A_1 alone. Then if the anxiety evoked by A_1 is repeatedly inhibited through being opposed by relaxation, its magnitude will drop, eventually to zero. In consequence,

a presentation of A_1A_2 will now evoke only 10 units of anxiety, instead of 20, and this will similarly undergo conditioned inhibition when opposed by relaxation. Through further steps along these lines the whole combination $A_1A_2A_3A_4A_5$ will lose its power to arouse any anxiety.

The raw data for a hierachy are obtained in several ways. The patient's history frequently reveals a variety of situations to which he reacts with undue disturbance. Further areas of disturbance may be revealed by perusal of his answers to the Willoughby questionnaire. Then he is given the "homework" task of making up a list of everything he can think of that is capable of frightening, disturbing, distressing, or embarrassing him in any way, excepting, of course, situations that would frighten anybody, such as meeting a hungry lion. Some patients bring back extensive inventories, others very scanty ones; and with the latter a good deal of time may have to be spent during interviews eliciting further items.

Confronted at last with anything between about 10 and 100 heterogeneous items, the therapist peruses them to see whether they belong to one or more thematic categories. If there is more than one theme, the items of each are grouped together. For example, one patient had a subdivision into enclosement, death, and bodily-lesion themes; another into social disapproval, disease, and aloneness; a third

*A basic assumption underlying this procedure is that the response to the imagined situation resembles that to the real situation. Experience bears this out. People are anxious when they imagine stimuli that are fearful in reality. This is in keeping with Stone's observations (1955) in another context.

Note: Reprinted from PSYCHOTHERAPY BY RECIPROCAL INHIBITION by Joseph Wolpe, M.D. with the permission of the publishers, Stanford University Press. Copyright © 1958 by the Board of Trustees of the Leland Stanford Junior University.

into trauma, death, and being in the limelight; a fourth into rejection and scenes of violence.

The subdivided list is now handed to the patient, who is asked to rank the items of each sublist in descending order according to the measure of disturbance he would have upon exposure to each. The rearranged list constitutes the hierarchical series that will be used in treatment. Modifications or additions may of course be made later.

At the first desensitization session the patient, already trained in relaxation, is hypnotized and in the trance is made to relax as deeply as possible. He is then told that he will be required to imagine a number of scenes which will appear to him very vividly. If he feels disturbed by any scene, he is to raise his hand as a signal. The weakest scenes from the hierarchical series are now presented in turn, usually for between two and three seconds each in the beginning. The raising of the left hand or any manifestation of increased bodily tension leads to the immediate curtailment of the ongoing scene. When it is judged that enough scenes have been given, the patient is roused from the trance and asked how clear the scenes were and whether any of them were disturbing. Even if he has not raised his hand during the trance, he may report having been very slightly to very considerably disturbed by one or more of the scenes. (Patients almost never raise their hands to a disturbance that is only slight.)

At the second desensitization session, a day or more later, the procedure is largely determined by what happened at the first. A scene that produced no disturbance at all is omitted and the next higher item in the hierarchy presented in its place. A scene that was slightly disturbing is presented again, unchanged. If there was considerable disturbance to the weakest scene from any hierarchy, a still weaker stimulus must now be substituted. Suppose, for example, that the disturbing item was seeing a funeral procession. Typical weaker substitutions would be the word "funeral," seeing the procession from a distance of 2300 yards, seeing an isolated and presumably empty hearse, or a *very brief* presentation of the original scene. The verbal substitution would usually be the weakest of these and would therefore be preferred. No harm is ever done by presenting a stimulus that is too weak. A stimulus that is too strong may actually increase sensitivity, and, especially during early experiments with the method, I have occasionally produced major setbacks in patients by prema-

ture presentation to them of stimuli with a high anxiety-evoking potential.*

In most patients, when the same scene is presented several times during a session there is a weaker reaction to each successive presentation. When this occurs, it accelerates therapy.† In other patients there is perseveration of anxiety responses, so that the anxiety produced by a second presentation summates with that from the first, the repetition tending thus to have a sensitizing effect rather than a therapeutic one.

With suitably cautious handling some headway will be made in the hierarchies at each session, and *pari passu* with this the patient will report a progressive decrease of sensitivity to the relevant kinds of stimulus situations encountered in the normal course of his life. The total number of sessions required varies greatly but is usually between 10 and 25.

The introspections of a clinical psychologist who was treated by this method are of interest:

> Most typically the emotion associated with a situation tended to diminish or disappear between one session and another. On three or four occasions, however, the desensitization seemed to occur quite suddenly in the course of a session. On these occasions the change was subjectively a dramatic one: I would feel, all at once, a sense of separation, or apartness, or independence of the situation; a feeling that "I am *here*, it is *there*." To say simply that I attained greater objectivity, or more simply that the emotional component of the image disappeared, would be accurate but not quite as descriptive of my subjective experience as the preceding sentence.
>
> The change, even when sudden, never seemed to constitute an "insight." My insight into my difficulties was perhaps fairly good initially, and was not altered one way or the other by the desensitization process *per se*. It might be said, however, that my "perception" of situations changed.

Patients who cannot relax will not make progress with this method. Those who cannot or will not be

---

*When sensitivity is increased as a result of an error of this kind, no scenes must be presented at the next session or two, and during these the hypnotic trance should be utilized merely to relax the patient as deeply as possible. At subsequent sessions scenes are introduced very cautiously from far down in the hierarchy whose subject matter produced the setback.

†I frequently inquire whether the reaction is weakening or not by saying after, say, the third presentation of a scene, "If your reaction has been decreasing, do nothing; if not, raise your hand." If it has been decreasing, I present the same scene two or three times more.

hypnotized but who can relax will make progress, although apparently more slowly than when hypnosis is used. The method necessarily fails with a small minority who are unable to imagine the suggested scenes. A few, perhaps about 5 per cent, do not make progress because although they can visualize clearly, they do not have the disturbed reaction to the imagined scene that they would have to the reality. Experience has shown that most of these can arouse the relevant emotions by *verbalizing* the scenes, and they then progress in the same way as other patients.

Occasionally, one comes across a patient who, having been desensitized to a hierarchy list, reveals a range of further, previously unrecognized sensitivities on a related but distinct theme. After desensitization to the latter, a third theme may become evident, and so on. It is surmised that this profusion of variations is due to unusually numerous and severe past stresses having brought about a conditioning of anxiety responses to an extaordinarily large number of aspects of certain situations. In these cases, abreaction is sometimes a valuable adjuvant because it involves the whole of the original conditioning situation (see pp. 195-98).

THE CONDUCT OF DESENSITIZATION SESSIONS

An account will be given of the exact details of procedure at one patient's desensitization sessions—her first session and two successive sessions when therapy was well under way. This patient had the following anxiety hierarchies (the most disturbing items being on top, as always):

Hierarchies

A. Fear of hostility

1. Devaluating remarks by husband
2. Devaluating remarks by friends
3. Sarcasm from husband or friends
4. Nagging
5. Addressing a group
6. Being at social gathering of more than four people (the more the worse)
7. Applying for a job
8. Being excluded from a group activity
9. Anybody with a patronizing attitude

B. Fear of death and its accoutrements

1. First husband in his coffin
2. At a burial
3. Seeing a burial assemblage from afar
4. Obituary notice of young person dying of heart attack
5. Driving past a cemetery
6. Seeing a funeral (the nearer the worse)
7. Passing a funeral home
8. Obituary notice of old person (worse if died of heart disease)
9. Inside a hospital
10. Seeing a hospital
11. Seeing an ambulance

C. Fear of symptoms (despite *knowing* them to be nonsignificant)

1. Extrasystoles
2. Shooting pains in chest and abdomen
3. Pains in left shoulder and back
4. Pain on top of head
5. Buzzing in ears
6. Tremor of hands
7. Numbness or pain in fingertips
8. Dyspnea after exertion
9. Pain in left hand (old injury)

First Desensitization Session (12th Interview)*

Before this interview the patient had learned to relax most of the muscles in her body. At our last meeting hypnosis had been discussed, and as she was afraid of it, I had tried to reassure her.

After some discussion about other matters, I told her that we would now try to have a hypnotic session. As she was comfortably seated, I said, "Rest a hand on each thigh. In response to suggestions that I shall give you, you will notice various things happen to your hands. However, if at any time you feel anxious at what is happening, you will be able to interrupt the proceedings immediately. You will at no stage lose consciousness."

*The hypnotic induction procedure follows Wolberg (1948).

Her hands having settled comfortably on her lap, I went on, "Look at your hands and keep on looking at them. At the same time I want you to give your fullest attention to the sensations in your hands, whatever they may be. At this moment you may be aware of the texture of your skirt, of the warmth between your fingers and in your thighs, of tingling sensations, perhaps an awareness of your pulse, or the movement of air over your fingers. There may even be other sensations. Concentrate on your sensations, give them your complete attention, no matter what they are, and continue to do so. As you go on watching you will notice small movements appearing in your fingers. It will be interesting to see which finger moves first—maybe the thumb or little finger or index finger or the middle finger or even the fourth finger. *(Right index finger moves.)* There, your right index finger moved, and now, as you go on watching, you will notice other fingers move, and the general effect of these movements will be to spread the fingers farther and farther apart. *(Movements appear in other fingers of the right hand.)* Now you begin to notice that as the fingers spread apart, a feeling of lightness appears among the other sensations in your hand and soon you will observe that your right hand begins to rise. Your right hand will become lighter and lighter and it will begin to lift. There, we can already see some slight arching of the right hand. Your hand goes up higher and higher. *(Hand rises.)* As it rises you will notice that the palm begins to turn slowly inward, because it is going to rise to your face. When your hand touches your face, you will be aware of a profoundly pleasant, heavy feeling throughout your body. Then, or even before then, your eyes will close. *(Her hand slowly rises to her face and her eyes close.)* Now you feel so pleasantly heavy and drowsy, you become heavier and heavier.

"Now let all the muscles of your body relax. Let relaxation grow deeper and deeper. We shall concentrate on the various zones of your body in turn. Relax the muscles of your forehead and those of the rest of your face. *(Pause.)* Relax all the muscles of your jaws and of your tongue. *(Pause.)* Relax the muscles of your eyeballs. *(Pause.)* Now relax your neck. *(Pause.)* Let the muscles of your shoulders and your arms relax. *(Pause.)* Relax the muscles of your back and your abdomen. *(Pause.)* Relax the muscles of your thighs and your legs. *(Pause.)* Let go more and still more. You become so calm, you feel so comfortable, nothing matters except to enjoy this pleasant, calm, relaxed state. *(Pause.)*

"Now I am going to give you some scenes to imagine and you will imagine them very clearly and calmly. If, however, by any chance anything that you imagine disturbs you, you will at once indicate this to me by raising your left hand two or three inches. First I am going to give you a very commonplace scene. Imagine that you are sitting alone in an armchair in the living room of your house. It is a very pleasant sunny day and you are sitting in this chair perfectly at ease. *(Pause of about 5 seconds.)* Next I want you to imagine the printed word 'Dentist.' *(Pause of about 3 seconds.)* Stop imagining this word and concentrate on relaxing your muscles. *(Pause.)* Now imagine that you are reading the newspaper and that your eye falls upon the headline 'Prominent citizen dies at 86.' *(Pause of about 3 seconds.)* Stop imagining those words, and again concentrate on your muscles. Let them go completely. Enjoy this calm state."

After a minute or two, I said to the patient, "In a few moments, I'll count five and then you will wake up feeling very calm and refreshed. *(Pause.)* One, two, three, four, five."

She now opened her eyes and to my "How are you?" said that she felt quite calm. Replying to further questions, she said that all three of the scenes had been clear and the only one that had disturbed her was the third one and the disturbance had even in this case been very slight. It may be noted that the first scene had nothing to do with the items on the hierarchy list. It was inserted as a kind of control, and a street scene or a flower or almost anything else which has no obvious relevance to the hierarchy items could equally well have been used. The word "dentist" was used as a kind of sensitivity test because of its vague associations with hospitals and illness.

17th Desensitization Session (32d Interview)

Since desensitization to the fear of hostility (sublist A) had progressed much more rapidly than the others, at the last few sessions this sublist had been set aside and our attention concentrated on the death fear and fear of symptoms. Six sessions before, we had begun to deal with funerals (B-6) on the hierarchy list. On the first occasion, the word "funeral" had alone been presented, and thereafter actual funerals had been presented, starting from two blocks away and then at decreasing distances as her reaction declined. At the previous session she had been made to imagine a funeral passing in the street in front of her and this had caused slight disturbance. Imagining a pain in her left shoulder had been just perceptibly disturbing. A scene of a woman in a film weeping had also been introduced because of its association with the idea of death and she had reacted very slightly to it.

At this session she was hypnotized in the same way as in the first session, but, as would be expected, the procedure took much less time. When she was deeply relaxed, I spoke as follows: "I am going to present a number of scenes to your imagination which you will imagine very clearly. It goes without saying that, if by any chance any scene should disturb you, you will indicate it by raising your left hand. First, I want you to imagine that you are standing at a street corner and a funeral procession passes you. You may have some feeling of sadness, but apart from this you are absolutely calm. *(Brief pause.)* Stop the scene. *(Pause of about 4 seconds.)* Now I want you to imagine the same scene of the funeral passing in the street before you. *(Pause of 6 or 7 seconds.)* Now just relax. Think of nothing but your muscles. *(Pause of about 15 seconds.)* Now I want you to imagine the same scene of the funeral again. *(Pause of about 8 seconds.)* Stop imagining that scene and just relax. If the last presentation of that scene disturbed you even to the slightest degree I want you now to raise your left hand. *(Hand does not rise.)* Good. Now let yourself go still further. *(Pause of about 15 seconds.)* Now I want you to imagine last time's scene of the woman in the film weeping bitterly. *(Pause of about 4 seconds.)* Now stop imagining this scene and just relax. *(Pause of about 15 seconds.)* Now I want you again to imagine the scene of the weeping woman. *(Pause of about 8 seconds.)* Stop that scene and again think of nothing but relaxing. If the last presentation of that scene disturbed you in the slightest, please raise your left hand. *(Hand does not rise.)* Good. Relax. *(Pause of about 15 seconds.)* Now I want you to imagine that you have a pain in your left shoulder. *(Pause of about 10 seconds.)* Now stop that pain and think only of relaxing. *(Pause of about 15 seconds.)* Now again imagine you have a pain in your left shoulder. *(Pause of about 10 seconds.)* Stop that pain and think of your muscles only. Soon I'll count five and you will wake. *(Pause.)* One, two, three, four, five."

The patient was not asked during the trance to indicate if she had been disturbed by the shoulder pain, because I assumed—wrongly, as it turned out—that

there would be no disturbance. (As stated earlier, patients usually do not spontaneously signal *mild* disturbances.) On waking, she stated that there had been a very slight disturbance to the first presentation of the funeral scene, less to the second, and none to the third. The weeping woman had not disturbed her at all, but each presentation of the pain in the shoulder had been very slightly disturbing.

18th Desensitization Session (33d Interview)

The hypnotic session was, as usual, preceded by a discussion of the patient's experiences of the past few days.

At this session the funeral scene and the one of the woman weeping were abandoned because it had been possible to present them without any disturbance whatever at the previous session. They were replaced by two new scenes, slightly higher on the hierarchy. The pain in the left shoulder was again presented because its presentation had not been completely free from disturbance last time. Having hypnotized the patient and made her relax, I spoke as follows:

"First we are going to have something already well familiar to you at these sessions—a pain in your left shoulder. You will imagine this pain very clearly and you will be not at all disturbed. *(Pause of about 4 seconds.)* Stop imagining this pain and again concentrate on your relaxing. *(Pause of about 15 seconds.)* Now again imagine that you have this pain in your left shoulder. *(Pause of about 10 seconds.)* Stop imagining the pain and again relax. *(Pause of about 15 seconds.)* Now I'd like you to imagine the pain in your left shoulder a third time, very clearly and calmly. *(Pause of about 10 seconds.)* Now stop this pain and focus your attention on your body, on the pleasant relaxed feeling that you have. If you felt in the least disturbed by the third presentation of this scene, I want you now to indicate it by raising your left hand. *(The hand does not rise.)* Go on relaxing. *(Pause of about 15 seconds.)* Next I want you to visualize the following. You are in your car being driven by your husband along a pleasant road in hilly country. On a distant hillside you can clearly see the gray stones of a cemetery. *(Pause of 2 or 3 seconds.)* Now stop imagining this scene and think only of relaxing. Let yourself go completely. *(Pause of about 15 seconds.)* I want you again to imagine the same scene of the distant hillside cemetery. *(Pause of 4 or 5 seconds.)* Now stop imagining the scene and again think of your muscles and of letting them go still more. *(Pause of about 15 seconds.)* I want you to imagine that while you are standing in a queue at a drugstore you begin talking to the woman next to you and she tells you that her husband has been very short of breath since he had his heart attack. *(Pause of 2 or 3 seconds.)* Now cut that scene short and relax. *(Pause of about 15 seconds.)* Now I want you to imagine the same scene again very clearly and calmly. *(Pause of about 4 seconds.)* Stop imagining this scene and relax."

On waking, the patient reported that the first presentation of the pain in her left shoulder had been very slightly disturbing but by the third presentation it had not disturbed her at all. The first presentation of a distant cemetery had been fairly disturbing but the second much less so. The woman in the drugstore whose husband had had a heart attack had disturbed her considerably the first time and somewhat less the second time.

Two remarks must be made here. First, it was not imperative to present the two new scenes only twice each, but experience with this patient had shown that new scenes did not entirely lose their power to disturb at the first session at which they were given, so that to force the pace would have taken up time and gained nothing.

Second, it will have been noticed that although the scenes presented follow the general idea of the hierarchy list, they do not conform to it absolutely and the therapist may introduce variations according to his discretion and his knowledge of the case.

14

Behavior Therapy of Stuttering: Deconditioning the Emotional Factor

Joseph Wolpe

Temple University School of Medicine, Philadelphia, Pennsylvania

I am particularly happy at the convocation of this seminar because it represents a significant stage in the *social* advancement of behavior therapy. In saying this, I do not underrate the *scientific* importance of the seminar, but in a therapeutic field scientific findings are valuable only insofar as they can be applied. To make behavior therapy available to all who may benefit from it many therapists will have to be trained in its methods. Widespread training can only be instituted with federal support; and support depends on recognition by governmental agencies of the social potential of behavior therapy. The sponsorship of this seminar by the Vocational Rehabilitation Administration is the first concrete manifestation of federal recognition. This is something to be very pleased about. Nevertheless, my pleasure falls short of jubilation, for there is a long way to go, many more steps to take, and many obstacles to surmount before we find ourselves in a position to offer training in behavior therapy to all who would and should have it. At Temple Medical School we are in the process of trying to establish a behavior therapy center where first and foremost teachers may be trained, and I am hopeful that the present seminar foreshadows the provision of federal support for this.

To give perspective to the topic of my paper, which is based on the proposition that neurotic anxiety is a determinant of most stuttering, I should like to give a brief, broad picture of behavior therapy against its experimental background. I think this is particularly desirable for the sake of those here who are new to this approach or who have viewed its applications to stuttering too narrowly. Let me start with a definition. "Behavior therapy" is a collective term for psychotherapeutic methods that have been derived from experimentally established principles of learning. These methods are generally applied to psychiatric conditions that are essentially a matter of maladaptive habits acquired by learning. The commonest subgroup of such maladaptive habits is the *neuroses,* and it is to their treatment that behavior therapy has most often been applied.

A neurosis is a very special kind of habit. Excepting a few unusual cases of hysteria, its outstanding feature is that it is primarily an *emotional* habit. This means that it involves primarily the autonomic nervous system, most characteristically in the form of anxiety (fear). The fear is usually unmistakable, but the emotion may take strange forms—variations of anxiety that the patient may describe as depression; or the feelings may be unfamiliar ones for which there are no words; and their strangeness may lead to further anxiety. "Normal" anxiety is distinguished from neurotic anxiety in that while the stimuli to the former indicate real danger, those to the latter do not. It is normal to be afraid when one's boat is sinking or

Note: From *Stuttering and the conditioning therapies,* pp. 15–27, B. B. Gray and G. England (Eds.). Monterey, CA: Monterey Institute for Speech and Hearing. Reprinted with permission.

if one is threatened with a major material loss; but neurotic to be afraid of being alone at home or entering a crowded living-room. Fear in such objectively nondangerous situations leads to avoidance of the situations as well as to other secondary effects that I shall refer to shortly.

To assert that a neurosis is a matter of "mere" habit, is of course heresy to psychoanalytic ears. Psychoanalysis teaches that the core of a neurosis is a complex of ideas whose painful content has caused them to be "repressed" into the "unconscious mind," and that neurotic manifestations are due partly to devious channeling of the emotional energy assumed to be attached to the repressed complex and partly to the effects of forces of "resistance" that keep the complex submerged. If this account were true, behavior therapy could not possibly be fundamentally effective, and any improvements if achieved would sooner or later be followed by relapse or symptom substitution, as indeed the psychoanalysts frequently proclaim. But the proof of a pudding is in the eating of it. What is the long-term prognosis when a neurosis is treated as a matter of habit? Experience has not upheld the psychoanalytic expectation. I can today point to a dozen cases of my own that, followed up for 12–18 years after behavior therapy, have displayed neither relapse nor symptom substitution. When, in other occasional cases, symptoms have recurred, they have always been traceable to new learning experiences; and have never been seen to arise insidiously from depths of the alleged "unconscious".

That neurotic behavior is based on emotional habits first became clearly evident from observations on experimental neuroses in animals. Anxiety manifested by motor agitation and such autonomic reactions as mydriasis, pilo-erection, and urination, can be elicited in an animal by giving it a painful (but not damaging) shock in a small cage. As the shock is repeated, anxiety at increasing levels is observed in the cage *in the absence of the shock.* Conditioning of anxiety to stimuli from the cage is thus clearly going on. After several shocks the anxiety is so intense that the animal will not touch food in the experimental cage even after a day or two of starvation. In its living cage or in an open courtyard it is entirely at ease and eats readily. In the laboratory in which the experimental cage stands, anxiety is also observed, but less than in the cage. There is also anxiety in other rooms according to their degree of physical resemblance to the laboratory. These conditioned anxiety reactions persist indefinitely—i.e., they do not extinguish even after prolonged evocations during repeated visits to the experimental cage.

Human neuroses display the same basic features as those of the animal. Anxiety is most frequently their dominant manifestation. It also usually turns out to be the basis of syndromes in which it is not always immediately obvious—such as stuttering, impotence, psychosomatic disorders, and the so-called character neuroses. It is a further point of resemblance to the animal neuroses of the laboratory that the origin of human neuroses can usually be traced to specific conditioning experiences. Whatever aspects of the conditioning situation make a strong imprint on the person become triggers to anxiety responses and maintain this function indefinitely. For example, a student had an attack of paroxysmal tachycardia that he interpreted as a heart attack. When a doctor he consulted failed to reassure him, he panicked, and an anxiety habit was conditioned. Fifty years later, at the age of 70, he still had severe anxiety whenever, for any reason, his heart beat rapidly.

The neurotic habits of experimental animals can consistently be overcome by feeding them under conditions of weak anxiety. In the experiments described above, among the various rooms which resembled the experimental laboratory, it proved always possible to find one where anxiety was weak enough not to inhibit eating. The eating of repeated portions of food there was correlated with a gradual diminution and eventually complete elimination of anxiety. The animal would then accept food in a room more like the experimental room and the same treatment would be applied. After further intervening stages, eating became possible in the experimental cage, enabling the anxiety responses to be overcome there too.

METHODS OF DECONDITIONING NEUROTIC EMOTIONAL HABITS

Techniques based on the principle of inhibiting anxiety by a response that (like eating) can "compete" with it, were subsequently found to be widely applicable to human neuroses. In man, a considerable number of responses are capable of inhibiting anxiety. Those that have found most extensive use are assertive responses and deep muscle relaxation. Since at this seminar much will be said by others about techniques that utilize these particular responses, I shall give only a very brief account of them; and then make mention of some other techniques. Full descriptions have been provided by Wolpe (1969).

The term "assertive" is applied to any behavior which gives overt expression to spontaneous and appropriate feelings *other than anxiety.* Expression of these feelings is instigated by the therapist when he perceives that undue anxiety is evoked in the patient by interchanges with other people. Each time the patient manages to express these feelings he inhibits his anxiety to some extent, and in consequence somewhat weakens the anxiety-response habit. The feelings most commonly involved are anger and resentment, but anything from affection to revulsion may be relevant.

Relaxation responses are often valuable when used directly in the life situation, but have their most effective application in a technique that closely parallels the treatment of experimental neuroses to which I referred. This is called *systematic desensitization.* It is a method of bringing about the specific deconditioning of anxiety elicited by defined stimulus situations and most often to situations of a kind to which no direct action on the part of the patient is relevant. If a man is anxious in crowds, there is no kind of *assertive* action that he can be advised to take to inhibit his anxiety. The patient is taught to relax by an abbreviated version of Edmund Jacobson's technique (1939, 1964) during 15-minute periods in the course of 5 or 6 interviews. Most of the remainder of these interviews is devoted to defining the stimulus areas (or "themes") of inappropriate anxiety arousal, assembling varied situations on each "theme," and then arranging the situations in a rank order determined by the amount of anxiety each elicits.

When relaxation has become adequate and when the hierarchies are ready, one begins the central procedure, which is to present the weakest scene from a hierarchy to the *imagination* of the deeply relaxed patient for a few seconds, repeating presentations until the imagined item no longer evokes any anxiety at all. At each presentation the weak anxiety evoked by the scene is to some extent inhibited by the relaxation so that at the next presentation its evocation is weaker still, until it is eventually at zero. The therapist then proceeds to the next scene, and so on, until the whole hierarchy has been dealt with. There is almost always complete transfer of the deconditioning

of the anxiety from the imaginary situation to the corresponding situation in reality.

At least a score of different behavior therapy techniques exist. Several of them are variants of systematic desensitization, which are usually introduced only when relaxation has proved to be ineffective. One technique involves the use of non-aversive electrical stimulation, and evidently depends upon external inhibition in the Pavlovian sense. The patient is asked to imagine items in hierarchical order, and when he signals that he has a clear image of a prescribed item, one or two mild galvanic shocks are passed into his forearm. The sequence is repeated until it is found that the item no longer evokes any anxiety. Another related technique involving the use of pleasant emotions in the place of relaxation as the counterconditioning agent was introduced by Lazarus and Abramovitz (1962) under the label *emotive imagery.* These techniques and many others are described in a recent text by Wolpe (1969).

In neuroses in general the clinical effects of these techniques have seemed to be impressively superior to those of psychoanalysis and other traditional methods. In a personal total of over 200 cases of neurosis (Wolpe, 1958), I have reported a rate of recovery or marked improvement that approaches 90% with a mean number of interviews in the region of 30. While there is no certainty that these cases are comparable with those reported in psychoanalytic series in which about 60% recover in 600 or so sessions, it is encouraging to note that recent comparative control studies involving specified phobic conditions have also yielded significantly superior results for behavior therapy techniques (e.g., Lang, Lazovik and Reynolds, 1965; Paul, 1966).

BEHAVIOR THERAPY IN STUTTERING

Let us now consider behavior therapy in relation to the special matter of stuttering. Even though anxiety is the core of most neuroses, it is by no means always foremost among the complaints that bring the patient to the therapist; for it may have repercussions on particular organs or particular functions that are more distressing than its directly felt effects. We know from psychophysiological studies that normal people show great variation in the extent to which different bodily systems participate in anxiety responses. Special complications are apt to occur when the anxiety response is channeled to an unusual degree along particular pathways. Whether the neural dispositions that underlie such channeling are established by maturation or by learning or by both is not known. But there are undoubtedly stomach reactors, nose reactors, pulse reactors, blood pressure reactors, and so on (Wolff, 1950). In other individuals anxiety interferes with specific motor functions: and interference with the speech mechanism produces stuttering.

That anxiety has a key role in *most* stuttering is shown by the fact that *most* stutterers speak perfectly fluently when they are alone, and many do also in the presence of congenial categories of people that can be specified; but the presence of human beings of other categories evokes anxiety, as a little investigation soon shows, and it is this that appears to impair the functioning of the speech mechanism. Speaking to people without stuttering is made possible for these subjects by eliminating their neurotic anxiety habit of response to people.

However, it is not always exclusively by an attack upon the anxiety habit that stuttering can be reduced. It seems clear that the possibility of operant control also frequently exists. There are at least two mechanisms through which anxiety may be conceived to impair speech. These are explicated by Figures 14–1 to 14–3. Figure 14–1 shows the normal speech response situation—where smooth speech follows a stimulus to it (S_s). Figure 14–2 illustrates how tension in the vocal apparatus may *per se* produce stuttering by direct physical interference with speech movements. In Figure 14–3 we see how stuttering may be the response to a stimulus compound made up of a stimulus to speech (S_s) and the internal (proprioceptive) stimuli (S_P) produced by an anxiety response (R_A) evoked by its conditioned stimulus (S_A).

To the extent that stuttering is a function of physical interference with the vocal apparatus, it can only be corrected by removing that interference. To the extent that the stutter is a response to an $S_s \cdot S_a$ compound, it is subject to operant control. It would appear, on the basis of the experiments of Goldiamond (1965) and Migler (1966), that compound stimulus operant conditioning is at work in some cases at least. But it is not impossible that both mechanisms are relevant, and that both may sometimes operate in the same case.

In stutterers, as with all other cases he treats, the first task of the behavior therapist is to determine what stimuli control the maladaptive behavior. Usually, it is early obvious that the stutter occurs only in definable social contexts, and a little probing reveals that these are contexts in which anxiety is aroused. There are, of course, a minority of patients who in all circumstances stutter to much the same degree; and it is likely that in them anxiety reactions have no relevance to the stutter. These are perhaps pure cases of operant stuttering. But in those cases in which anxiety does play a part, the exact stimuli that are its antecedents need to be identified. In some cases, like the first that I shall shortly describe, the dominating anxiety sources are in interpersonal contexts that call for assertive training. In other cases the sources are phobic-like; and then some kind of systematic desensitization is indicated. These stimuli are not always obvious, and a great deal of careful exploration may be needed. For example, in a case I am currently treating, although it was soon clear that some social situations produced the stammer and others did not, the patient denied experiencing anxiety in the former. But when details were defined, it became evident that he was anxious at being scrutinized; and the greater the number of people of certain categories who observed him, the greater was the anxiety and the more pronounced the stutter. As a rule, when primary anxiety has been deconditioned, anxiety secondary to the stutter ceases to be a problem.

I shall now give you my examples of cases of stuttering markedly and lastingly benefitted by deconditioning of anxiety habits. In the first case assertive

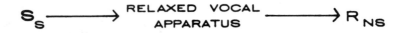

Figure 14-1. The S-R chain in normal speech.

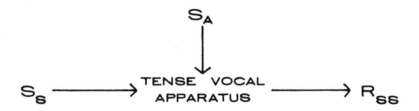

Figure 14-2.   Stuttering as a product of nonspecific tenseness.

training was the main instrument; in the second; systematic desensitization.

In May, 1952, Mr. A., a 31-year-old clerk was referred for treatment of a severe stutter which had begun at the age of five.* Almost every sentence was repeatedly interrupted by the stutter, and each interruption marked by violent facial contortions. He was worse during any "unhappiness, worry, uncertainty, or work under pressure". The first three interviews were devoted to history-taking and data-gathering. A great many inter-personal situations could arouse anxiety in him and it was hypothesized that to the extent that the anxiety could be detached from these, the stutter would improve.

At the fourth interview I described to Mr. A. how neurotic reactions are conditioned and explained the reciprocal inhibition principle of therapy. It was evident that the anxiety associated with direct dealings with people needed our first attention. Because of it he frequently endured aggression from others for long periods without protest until sometimes, his bottled-up emotions exploded in ill-directed rage. I told him that he had rights as well as duties. I drew attention to the failing helplessness embodied in his delayed rage reactions, and emphasized the need for reactions of protest to be expressed as soon as possible if real mastery of situations was to be gained.

Three days later he reported that he had been less permissive to his assistants at work and had insisted on their getting things done. However, he had found it difficult to be firm consistently. I assured him that practice would produce consistency. He had also for the first time asked his wife to help him with work he had brought home from the office.

Four days later he gave the following example of counter-anxiety expressive behavior. While playing a card game with some friends, he had made an error, for which his companions had laughed at him, upsetting him so badly that he was left trembling. After a while he realized that he ought to be expressing his annoyance, and answered back sharply, soon to find that his trembling had disappeared completely. In the past he would have felt hurt and downtrodden and have remained completely passive in such a situation. In correlation with increasingly consistent exteriorising of feelings in relevant contexts he developed an increasing feeling of inner freedom and his speech lost its stutter except occasionally with his boss, and in conditions of unusual stress. The facial contortions ceased entirely.

He was seen two years later and spoke without any suggestion of stutter.

The second case I shall give you also received some assertive training, but only showed *major* improvement when specific anxiety sources were treated by systematic desensitization. I had also at an early stage applied to him the method of rhythmic speaking described by Andrews and Harris (1965).

*This case is reported at greater length in *Psychotherapy by Reciprocal Inhibition* (1958), pp. 128–130.

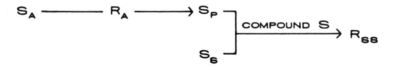

Figure 14-3.   Stuttering as a conditioned response to a compound stimulus.

In typical fashion, this method very soon produced noticeable control of the stutter, which in two or three weeks decreased by about 50%, whereafter the most assiduous practice failed to improve it further.

The patient, Mr. B., was a man of 25 who, like the foregoing case, had stuttered quite severely, since he was 5 years old. He said that he had always been worse with strangers. It is interesting to note that his score on the Willoughby Neuroticism Schedule was 13, which is within normal limits, indicating that he was free from neurotic anxiety in many interpersonal situations. Correspondingly, he had no difficulty asserting himself in these situations. When a person has some assertive skills, it is relatively easy, as a rule, to extend the assertion to other situations in which he has habitually been inhibited; and this proved to be the case with Mr. B.

Investigation revealed that most of his neurotic interpersonal anxiety was related to humiliation or the threat of it, in the general context of appearing clumsy or foolish—for example, knocking something over or making an error in adding. The degree of anxiety evoked by a given "blunder" was greatly influenced by the identity of his "audience". He was relatively comfortable with certain friends, less with others, and much less with strangers; but the most distressing witness was his father.

Mr. B. was taught relaxation, and hierarchies dealing with the subject of humiliation were drawn up. After desensitization to situations involving less threatening individuals had been accomplished, scenes that featured his father began to be introduced. One of the weaker scenes was sitting with his father in a restaurant and knocking over the salt. More disturbing scenes were knocking the salt off the table; knocking over the water; making an erroneous statement. After 9 desensitization sessions in the course of four months his fear of these "humiliation" situations steadily declined and his speech was judged to have improved 90–95%. He then terminated therapy for financial reasons. About a year later his improvement was found to have been maintained, both as judged by me and as reported by his wife.

Psychophysiological studies are, of course, needed to determine whether the changes obtained in the speech of these patients are really due to emotional deconditioning. At present I can only say that in the dozen or so cases I have treated over the years, there has apparently been a constant relationship between anxiety reduction and speech improvement; and this fits in with the observed relationship between anxiety-evoking social situations and stuttering.

Accepting the relevance of anxiety, we have to consider how it is possible to reshape speech in the persistence of anxiety. To the extent that, as illustrated in Figure 14–3, stuttering is a motor habit of response to stimulus compounds made up of stimuli instigating speech and the proprioceptive stimuli due to the anxiety that certain social situations elicit, stuttering could be overcome *either* by subtracting the anxiety *or* by changing the stuttering habit of response to the compound. We know, of course, from the work of Goldiamond (1965) that the stuttering habit can be modified by operant control. Experiments recently conducted by Migler (1966) at Haverford State Hospital, near Philadelphia, indicate that the control can to a significant extent be transferred to the life situation. On the theory that stuttering is reinforced whenever the stutter is followed by an emergence of the word, Migler adopted the procedure of having the patient speak in the consulting room and then shocking him on each occasion on which the word was *successfully* produced after a stutter. He found that there was marked improvement in the consulting room with partial, but quite considerable transfer to the life situation. He subsequently found that by having the patient make tapes of his speaking at home, and then punishing him according to the number of times that the stutter was reinforced, he achieved much greater change in the life situation. The cases are still being treated and continue to improve, and at least one of them is more than 90% improved in the life situation.

It may well be that speech habit factors and direct physiological interference factors contribute in varying proportions to the malfunction in those persons in whom anxiety is the basis of stuttering. If this is so, attempts to decondition the stuttering reaction to the stimulus compound that elicits it would rarely eliminate the malfunction entirely, would usually ameliorate it considerably, and would sometimes be without effect.

The question of the specificity of deconditioning methods applies in the same way to stuttering as to all other cases in which anxiety habits are the focus of treatment. Therefore, studies which do not involve stuttering have relevance to stuttering. A recent study by Dr. Gordon Paul (1966) seems to rule out the possibility of attributing the changes of behavior therapy to "transference" or other nonspecific or inadvertent interpersonal processes. In a large class of students who applied for training in public speaking he found a considerable number who were highly anxious in situations of public scrutiny. Many of these agreed to take part in a therapeutic experiment. Paul obtained the services of five experienced and well reputed psychotherapists whose orientation ranged from Freud to Sullivan. They each treated nine of the students in groups of three, using three different techniques—1) the therapist's own variety of insight therapy, 2) support and suggestion ("attention-placebo"), and 3) systematic desensitization, in which they had to be trained *ab initio*. Each patient received five therapeutic sessions. When, at the end of treatment, the patients were evaluated, 20% of the insight group were much improved, none of the support and suggestion group, and 86% of the desensitization group. Thus, despite their inevitably negative bias towards desensitization, the "dynamic" therapists did significantly better with it than even the method in which they had been trained.

Much remains to be learned. We have reached a stage in the evolution of methods of behavior change that is both rewarding now and exciting in promise. There is a rapidly growing volume of research reflected by the success of the journal *Behavior Research and Therapy* established by Hans J. Eysenck in 1963. It is safe to predict that in a decade from now behavior therapy practices both in relation to stuttering and in general will be greatly refined and extended by this research.[1]

REFERENCES

Andrews, G. & Harris, M. (1965). The syndrome of stuttering. London.

Goldiamond, I. (1965). Stuttering and fluency as manipulatable operant response variables. In L. Krasner and L. P. Ullman (Eds.). Research in behavior modification. New York: Holt, Rinehart, and Winston.

Jacobson, E. (1938). Progressive relaxation. Chicago: University of Chicago Press.

Jacobson, E. (1964). Anxiety and tension control. Philadelphia: Lippincott.

Lang, P. J., Lazovik, A. D. & Reynolds, D. J. (1965). Desensitization, suggestibility and pseudotherapy. *Journal of Abnormal Psychology, 70*, 395.

Lazarus, A. A. & Abramovitz, A. (1962). The use of 'emotive imagery' in the treatment of children's phobias. *Journal of Mental Science, 108*, 191.

Migler, B. (1966). Personal communication.

Paul, G. L. (1966). Insight vs. desensitization in psychotherapy: An experiment in anxiety reduction. Stanford: Stanford University Press.

Wolff, H. G. (1950). Life stress and cardiovascular disorders. Circulation, *1*, 187.

Wolpe, J. (1958). Psychotherapy by reciprocal inhibition. Stanford, CA: Stanford University Press.

Wolpe, J. (1969). The practice of behavior therapy. New York: Pergamon Press.

[1]A second journal, *The Journal of Applied Behavior Analysis* has recently appeared, and a third *The Journal of Behavior Therapy and Experimental Psychiatry,* is scheduled for August, 1969.

Postscript   14

Systematic Desensitization

Joseph Wolpe

In the sixteen years since the seminar on which Gray and England's 1969 book was based, the value of behavior therapy has been increasingly recognized in syndromes in whose origin, learning has a role—in stuttering not least. At the seminar it was seen to be crucial to have a functional conception of speech that, taking account of the varied bases of stuttering, would provide a framework for appropriately varied therapeutic strategies. The trend of most recent work has, by contrast, been empirical: treatments are proposed and carried out with little or no interest in the mechanisms of speech. This regressive approach, which Gray and England foretold (p. 5), is now quite widespread. The strategic advantage that exists in using knowledge of physiological processes and of experimentally established principles of learning has been largely disregarded.

In this chapter, I will return to the orientation of the Monterey seminar and examine how recent methods of treatment can be integrated with a revised functional conception.

REVISED SCHEMAS FOR THE MECHANISMS OF STUTTERING

The schemas shown in Figures 14–4 to 14–8 are a revision and extension of those put forward in 1969 (see pp. 346–347). What determines the presence or absence of stuttering is in every case the functional state of the vocal apparatus. In the diagrams, the stuttering is characterized as being determined by *tension* in the vocal apparatus, a feature partially inferred from the very commonly observed correlation between stuttering and emotional tension. (Key to symbols: S_{SD} = speech demand stimulus, S_{AN} = nonspecific anxiety stimulus, S_{AAP} = anxiety-arousing person.)

Not everybody develops disfluency in relation to social anxiety. Therefore, a predisposition must exist. The evidence for predisposing factors has been well presented by Brutten and Shoemaker (1967.)

Figure 14–4 portrays, by way of background, the "normal" situation in which a relaxed vocal apparatus mediates normal speech, so that disfluency is minimal.

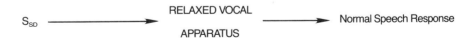

Figure 14-4.   The S-R chain in normal speech.

Figure 14–5 illustrates the well-known fact that many people who are ordinarily without speech impediment stutter to a varying extent in circumstances of emotional stress. The presumption is that in these people emotional stress tenses the vocal apparatus to a degree sufficient to result in stuttering. Such anxiety has an unlimited number of possible antecedents.

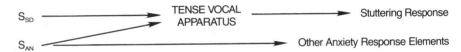

Figure 14-5.   Stuttering due to severe anxiety affecting the speech of a nunstutterer.

Figure 14–6 shows the commonest mode of clinical stuttering, seen as caused by tension in the vocal apparatus due to speech-related anxiety. The discriminating anxiety stimulus is usually a person, but it may also involve other elements such as telephones, variously compounded with proprioceptive and other bodily stimuli; and frequently the act of speaking is by itself in different measures a stimulus to anxiety. The anxiety consists of a widespread constellation of bodily responses, but it implicates significantly, and perhaps especially, the vocal musculature.

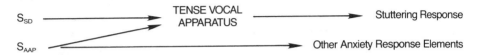

Figure 14-6.   Habitual stuttering caused by anxiety response to particular persons. The anxiety need not be severe, but affects especially the vocal apparatus.

In Figure 14–7 we see how tension of the vocal apparatus may occur as a conditioned response to the compound stimulus of speech demand and a particular person or class of persons who do not evoke generalized anxiety, though they

Postscript 14

may at one time have done so. Clearly, in such cases the vocal tension is an operant and its habit strength is unlikely to be affected by treatments designed to decondition anxiety.

Compound

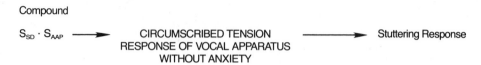

Figure 14-7. Stuttering as a conditioned operant in response to a compound stimulus. The anxiety-arousing person no longer evokes general anxiety.

Figure 14–8 illustrates a special case of the foregoing. Here speech demand *alone* elicits vocal tension and therefore stuttering occurs *whenever* the subject speaks, even when alone. Again, since generalized anxiety is not present, anxiety deconditioning will not be a relevant treatment.

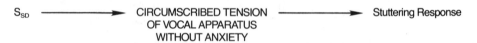

Figure 14-8. This is a special case of the situation illustrated in Figure 14-7. Speech demand alone elicits vocal tension; the person stutters even when alone.

THE PREDOMINANCE OF THE EMOTIONAL FACTOR AND THE NEED FOR INDIVIDUAL DIAGNOSIS

Practically without exception, the contributors to the Monterey seminar perceived an emotional factor behind the majority of cases of stuttering. However, there has to this day been no evaluation of the incidence of the emotional factor, although a project to do this was adumbrated by Brutten and Shoemaker (1966) and Brutten (1969).

Numerous treatments have been directed at changing speech itself. Examples are the shadowing method of Cherry and Sayers (1956), the feedback "punishment" of Goldiamond (1965), the massed trials procedure of Shoemaker and Brutten (1969, p. 74), and the more recent metronome-controlled and breathing-regulated methods to be described in this chapter.

It is natural for a therapist to attribute favorable results to the methods that he uses; but in those cases of stuttering that anxiety underlies, beneficial change must be more closely related to the emotional impact on the patient of the therapeutic situation than to the speech-directed measures as such.

The frequent beneficial effect that follows such measures (directed at changing speech itself) seems at first glance to rule out a very high incidence of emotionally based cases of stuttering. But it is important to realize that all of these treatments have emotional accompaniments that might beneficially change those cases of stuttering that are emotionally based. In addition to the direct emotional impact of the therapist, the performance of stuttering-free speech itself has emotional consequences. The very achievement of nonstuttering speech, no matter how, has powerful anxiety-countering effects. The speech therapist can be as easily misled about the way in which his methods take effect as psychotherapists have been misled in their treatment of neuroses (Eysenck, 1952). The crucial fact here is that with treatment other than behavior therapy about 50% of cases are markedly improved despite wide differences of method. The therapists can scarcely be right in attributing their similar results to their methods, which are far more likely to be due to emotional effects on the patient that occur during all the methods. This supposition is supported by the fact that with the addition of the deliberate emotion-directed methods of behavior therapy, the recovery rate for psychotherapy of the neuroses rises to 80% or more (Wolpe, 1982, p. 328).

Of course, in accordance with the observation of Shoemaker and Brutten (1967), and as indicated in Figures 14–7 and 14–8, those cases that do have an operant basis would be most appropriately treated by the use of operant techniques, or perhaps by one of the speech-control methods described later in this chapter. But if a therapist treats *all* cases by the same formula or the same operant method, he or she does not know which successes are attributable to that method and which to the simultaneous emotional events. It would be advantageous, both from the scientific point of view and in the interest of economy of effort, for therapists to know in advance to which of the two diagnostic subclasses each case belongs. A certain number of cases have both bases. This means that sometimes emotional deconditioning will leave a residue of operant stuttering; it will then need to be treated accordingly.[1]

A SURVEY OF RECENT TECHNIQUES

Recent years have witnessed the emergence of innovative programs that lend themselves to wide and economical application. One of these is a systematic use of rhythm; and two others employ breathing control in different ways.

An effective and flexible therapeutic method based on the elicitation of rhythmic speech was developed by Brady (1968, 1969, 1971). [See also Burns and Brady (1978).] He built upon Barber's (1940) experience of the diminution of disfluencies when speech becomes rhythmic. This observation had been made a century earlier and had even then led to the therapeutic use of metronomes (Colombat de l'Isere, 1831), but methods of transfer to daily life were nonexistent until the work of Meyer and Mair (1963) and Andrews et al. (1964). Meyer and Mair introduced a miniature metronome attached to the ear, which permitted the

---

[1] Operant conditioning methods are distinguished from the conventional psychotherapies in having a clear target of change in specified behavior. Emotional change may nonetheless follow; there is an interesting similarity to the diminution of anxiety often noted with other motor-focused training methods, such as those of the Alexander technique.

Postscript 14

transfer of fluency to the life situation that in some cases continued without the use of the device. Andrews and Harris instituted a verse-like scanning of speech with similar success. Encouraged by these favorable results, Brady evolved a logically constructed program whose central feature was a miniature electronic metronome resembling a hearing aid that patients could wear behind the ear and that could be used under all ordinary life circumstances. Although the immediate focus of action was modifying the character of speech, Brady was constantly aware of the implication of his procedures for deconditioning anxiety.

The first step of Brady's routine is to find conditions under which the patient can speak fluently with the aid of a desk metronome. In the case of a severe stutter, fluency may not be achieved until, with the patient alone with the therapist, each syllable is paced to the beat of a loud metronome, set, perhaps, as slow as 40 beats per minute. It is almost always possible to find conditions in which the patient can speak easily and fluently. Once fluent verbalization has been attained at a slow rate, the next task is to move towards the rate and cadence of normal speech. Using fluency as the guide, the metronome is speeded up in steps until a rate of 80 to 100 beats per minute is reached.

Achieving fluency at a rapid rate with the desk metronome usually results in a substantially enhanced mood and a sense of hope, especially in severely afflicted stutterers who may not have experienced fluent speech for many years. The patient is warned that a great deal of work lies ahead before the improvement can be transposed to the normal environment. He is instructed to practice speaking with a desk metronome at home for at least 45 minutes daily. At any time when he feels hard-pressed because of the speed of the metronome, he may consider some beats as signalling voluntary pauses, giving himself a chance to relax.

When considerable proficiency has been obtained, the miniature metronome is attached to the ear, initially to replace the table metronome at home and in the office; and afterwards to extend the patient's fluency in an increasing range of life situations. Extending the range is guided by knowledge of the amount of anxiety that various situations elicit. This knowledge is obtained by careful questioning. The situations are listed in increasing order of anticipated speaking difficulty, an order that depends in part on the relative strength of anxiety that the patient experiences in the situations and in part on the relative severity of stuttering. For example, the mildest situation on a particular patient's list was speaking to a friend, and the most severe making a peroration at a business meeting.

While making efforts to achieve fluency through direct exposure to graduated situations, it is quite common for the patient to have unexpected difficulty from time to time. The cause can usually be traced to anxiety related to previously unidentified conditionings (which are practically always present, and certainly to be expected, given the complexity of human life). When setbacks of this kind occur, it is extremely important to enable the patient to regain fluency as soon as possible. One may set about this either by going back to a slower rate of speech, or by retreating to more rigid pacing (one syllable or one word per beat). Sometimes it is necessary to backtrack to the situation on the hierarchy that was the last to have been "conquered." The resumption of control must be insisted upon even though it may impose on the therapist a great deal of effort in guidance and coaching. What may also be necessary is behavior rehearsal in the therapist's office, simulating outside speaking situations in which the therapist takes the role of one or more other persons in the life of the patient. This procedure not infrequently facilitates progress even without the occurrence of setbacks.

In patients whom the miniature metronome has enabled to speak fluently, an attempt is made to discontinue progressively the use of the instrument, starting with those speaking situations in which the patient has the least difficulty. Many find it helpful during this phase to pace their speech to an imaginary metronome. If there is appreciable difficulty at any point, the patient must at once return to stricter pacing of his speech, at first without the metronome. If this does not alleviate the difficulty, he may have to resume using the device.

It is reasonable to expect that the metronome procedure will have its greatest relevance to stuttering elicited by anxiety that is produced either by speech itself or, much more often, by social situations that impose speech demand, and this applies to most cases. However, in certain patients in whom there is difficulty in extending metronome-aided fluency into a particular situation or class of situations, it has been found helpful to employ systematic desensitization (p. 337) adjunctively. In other cases, assertiveness training (p. 344), often with behavior rehearsal, is a major adjuvant.

The efficacy of Brady's program was studied in 26 severe chronic stutterers ranging in age from 12 to 53 years (Brady, 1971). All of them had been stuttering from early childhood, and all had had various forms of therapy in the past, which in no case had improved the patient's speech. In 21 of these cases, treatment had diminished disfluency by an average of 67%. Of the failures, three terminated therapy after a few sessions without giving reasons; and two terminated because they were moving some distance from Philadelphia. Almost all of the successful patients continued to improve after the conclusion of active therapy. The follow-up psychiatric interview, which took place between 6 and 44 months after the end of treatment (with a mean of 13.8 months), revealed that all patients regarded themselves as speaking much more fluently and were pleased with their change. All were more self-confident and better able to deal with the challenges of daily life. However, three of these patients were still using the miniature metronome "most of the time," and eight "some of the time."

REGULATED BREATHING METHODS

The proponents of these methods, Azrin and Nunn (1974) and Schwartz (1976), have claimed an extraordinarily high degree of success, although their programs differ markedly in detail.

Azrin and Nunn conceptualize their treatment as based on the same general principle they have applied to a variety of other undesirable habits—countering

Postscript 14

the problem behavior by an incompatible activity. In the case of stuttering, however, the behavior employed in the treatment does not appear to be incompatible in the same direct manner as that utilized for such other conditions as fingernail biting or hair pulling. Inhibition of speaking, by pausing, for example, would have been directly incompatible, but Azrin and Nunn found, in their preliminary efforts, that simple pausing was not sufficient to affect the stuttering; and therefore added other activities, particularly changing the breathing pattern, self-induced relaxation, and the formulation of one's thoughts.

The following is an outline of the procedure Azrin and Nunn adopted. The only direct personal contact with the patient occurs during a single session about 2 hours in duration. The first step is to make a detailed review of the inconveniences and annoyances that the stuttering has caused in order to heighten the patient's motivation "to engage in the necessary training effort." As part of this effort, the patient is asked to stutter deliberately, and then to describe in detail the kinds of words on which he has stuttered and the accompanying unpleasantness, including associated body movements such as blinking; and dwelling on the situations and persons that for him are most closely associated with stuttering. This is meant to maximize attention to relevant circumstances and factors. The patient is also taught to alert himself to the likelihood of stuttering and to indicate to the counselor when he feels that a stutter is imminent.

Next he is shown a number of ways in which to relax when tension rises—by slouching slightly; by learning to breathe deeply, slowly, and regularly; and by telling himself to relax by letting abdominal and throat muscles go as limp as possible while continuing to carry out the breathing instructions.

Against this background a speaking routine is instituted. The patient is instructed to formulate in advance the words he is going to use. Then, after exhaling, he slowly takes a deep breath, inhaling while constantly relaxing the chest and throat muscles, and is told to start speaking as soon as the inhalation is complete. In speaking, he must emphasize the initial part of the statement and must at first settle for short durations, gradually to be increased as he becomes more fluent. If at any moment he starts stuttering, he must recommence the routine. He is also asked to carry out the routine while *imagining* himself in stuttering-prone situations.

Several types of structured practice are given. The patient first practices the relaxation exercises without speaking. Then he uses the breathing drill as a means to increase progressively the number of words he can speak fluently, while reading out of a book or speaking to the counselor. At first he breathes after each word and later after an increasing number, until he can read long passages before pausing for breath. He is instructed to telephone friends each day for the first few weeks for further practice of breathing and speaking. The counselor telephones the patient about three times during the first week to give encouragement and to answer questions, and intermittently thereafter. These conversations at the same time enable the counselor to evaluate the quality of speech.

The results that Axrin and Nunn obtained are impressive. On the first day after treatment, stuttering was reduced by an average of 85% in the 14 subjects. The improvement reached 97% after one month, remaining at this level after four months in the 8 subjects who were followed up for that length of time. They reported that it had taken a great deal of effort to adhere to the program during the first few weeks, but that afterwards the new manner of speaking became automatic.

A very different manner of using breathing to control speech has been proposed and popularized by Schwarz (1976). The subject is trained to initiate speech only towards the *end* of an easy expiration of a sighing character; stretching the first syllable to make the sound a smooth-flowing movement that blends imperceptibly with the exhalation. He is also taught to speak more slowly. The results that Schwarz claims are ostensibly comparable to those of Azrin and Nunn, between 83% and 92%.

The striking results reported for these breathing methods merit their receiving the most serious attention. Unfortunately, in the several years since their description, no independent replications seem to have appeared, to say nothing of controlled studies.[2] It is conceivable that these methods may be effective *both* for stuttering that is emotionally based and stuttering dependent on operant mechanisms; but we do not know.

THERAPEUTIC MECHANISMS OF THE NEW METHODS

We must consider the question of how the breathing routines and Brady's rhythm method accomplish their effects. At their initiation, they are clearly nothing but coping techniques, altering the technique of speaking in an essentially mechanical way. In the case of the rhythm method, it seems clear from Brady's careful and long-continued observations that what is predominantly achieved in successful cases is a deconditioning of speech-related anxiety. In terms of the schemata presented previously, it must be postulated that when recovery is incomplete, it is because some anxiety conditioning remains, or there is an undealt-with operant factor, or both.

In respect to the breath-control techniques, the basis of change is much less clear. It may be that to a great extent these continue to be coping techniques, requiring the subject to go on employing them indefinitely, even though with practice the activity becomes increasingly automatic and decreasingly strenuous. At the same time, one may reasonably expect that in consequence of the mastery of speech that results from this "coping," there is a progressive deconditioning of anxiety. It seems likely that research will reveal that after such treatment some

---

[2]The exception is a six-subject report by Andrews and Tanner (1982) on the Azrin and Nunn method, with significant but disappointing results including two failures.

Postscript 14

subjects need additional emotional reconditioning through assertiveness training or systematic desensitization, and others need the application of formal operant methods (*see* Boudreau & Jeffrey, 1973).

Actually, the Azrin and Nunn procedure is not confined to the control of speaking through breathing, but explicitly incorporates relaxation and other techniques that are routinely used to counteract anxiety in behavior therapy. The effect of these would be to add to the anxiety-diminishing effect of the mechanical control of speech. Here again future research may reveal the need for further emotional reconditioning in some cases and for operant methods in others.

REFERENCES

Andrews, G., & Harris, M. (1964). *The syndrome of stuttering. Clinics in Developmental Medicine, No. 17.* London: Heinemann.

Andrews, G., & Tanner, S. (1982). Stuttering treatment: An attempt to replicate the regulated breathing method. *Journal of Speech and Hearing Disorders, 47*, 138–140.

Azrin, N. H., & Nunn, R. G. (1974). A rapid method of eliminating stuttering by a regulated breathing approach. *Behavioral Research and Therapy, 12*, 279–286.

Boudreau, L. A. & Jeffrey, C. J. (1973). Stuttering treated by desensitization. *Journal of Behavior Therapy and Experimental Psychiatry, 4*, 209–212.

Barber, V. B. (1940). Studies in the psychology of stuttering–XVI: Rhythm as a distraction in stuttering. *Journal of Speech Disorders, 5*, 29–42.

Brady, J. P. (1968). A behavioral approach to the treatment of stuttering. *American Journal of Psychiatry, 125*, 843–848.

Brady, J. P. (1969). Studies on the metronome effect on stuttering. *Behavior Research and Therapy, 7*, 197–204.

Brady, J. P. (1971). Metronome-conditioned speech retraining for stuttering. *Behavior Therapy, 2*, 129–150.

Brutten, G. J. (1969). *Stuttering: Reflections on a two-factor approach to behavior modification.* In B. B. Gray and G. England (Eds.), *Stuttering and the conditioning therapies.* Monterey, CA: Monterey Institute for Speech and Hearing.

Brutten, E. J., & Shoemaker, D. J. (1967). *The modification of stuttering.* Englewood Cliffs, NJ: Prentice-Hall.

Burns, D., & Brady, J. P. (1978). Stuttering and speech disorders. Symposium on behavior therapy in psychiatry. *Psychiatric Clinics of North America, 1:2.*

Cherry, C., & Sayers, B. (1956). Experiments upon the total inhibition of stammering by external control, and some clinical results. *Psychosomatic Research 1*, 233–246.

Colombat de l'Isere, M. (1831). *Du begaiement et de tous les autres vices de la parole traites par de nouvelles methodes.* (2nd ed.) Paris: Mansut.

Eysenck, H. J. (1952). The effects of psychotherapy: An evaluation. *Journal of Consulting Psychology, 16*, 319.

Goldiamond, I. (1965). Stuttering and fluency as manipulatable operant response classes. In L. Krasner and L. P. Ullman (Eds.), *Research in behavior modification* (pp. 106–156). New York: Holt.

Gray, B. B., & England, G. (1969). *Stuttering and the conditioning therapies.* Monterey, CA: The Monterey Institute for Speech and Hearing.

Meyer, V., & Mair, J. M. M. (1963). A new technique to control stammering: A preliminary report. *Behavior Research and Therapy, 1*, 251–254.

Schwarz, M. (1976). *Stuttering solved.* New York: McGraw-Hill.

Shoemaker, D. J., & Brutten, E. J. (1969). *A two-factor approach to the modification of stuttering and related behaviors.* In B. B. Gray and G. England (Eds.), *Stuttering and the conditioning therapies.* Monterey, CA: The Monterey Institute for Speech and Hearing.

Wolpe, J. (1982). *The practice of behavior therapy* (3rd ed.). New York: Pergamon Press.

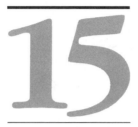

Modification of Behavior

Charles Van Riper

Postscript
Modifying Stuttering Behavior

Harold L. Luper

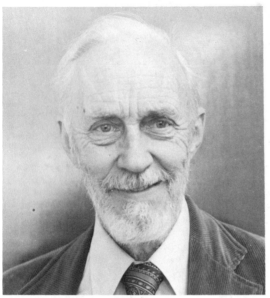

Charles Van Riper

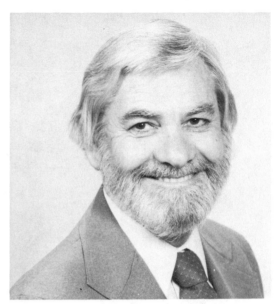

Harold L. Luper

The work of Charles Van Riper on stuttering has been at the inner core of this problem for over 50 years. As teacher, as researcher, as theorist, as therapeutic innovator, and as a clinician, this man has provided a standard and a model that has had an influence and generated a loyalty among clients, students, and clinicians alike throughout the world. From all of his many significant contributions, we as editors felt that his therapeutic philosophy, tactics, and innovations stood out for presentation in this volume. One reason for this inclusion is that in many ways it contrasts sharply with other therapies presented in this book. But in other ways, Van Riper's work could be viewed as the forerunner, the pacer, in anticipation of many current views and perspectives about therapy for stuttering. Where most of us may address only a few issues, Van Riper has covered the waterfront of critical issues about this problem. Whether it is therapy for children, therapy for adults, therapy for parents of stutterers, environmental manipulation, motor-mechanics, learning, counseling, relapse—he has been there, both with his clients and in his writings. When a reader moves through Van Riper's writings over the years one can identify certain persistent themes that keep coming through. These themes are most evident in the prepublished material that appears in this next chapter. His is a toughening, accepting, no-nonsense, anti-avoidance, honest, and tenacious approach to therapy for advanced stages of stuttering.

He attacks self-deception and avoidance, he empathizes with feelings of guilt and embarrassment, he encourages self-confrontation and self-acceptance as a stutterer. Although he warns against seeking fluency, he therapeutically attacks those variables that reinforce stuttering and avoidance. One can't help but wonder if Van Riper had one agenda for the toughening therapeutic experiences for the stutterer, but another more theoretical (and clinical) agenda that would eventually lead to fluency, as a consequence of not seeking it.

When Van Riper was contacted about participating in this book, he was excited about its possibilities and significance for the literature on stuttering. Although he gave the editors permission to republish some of his earlier work, he had already reached emeritus status as a professor and admitted himself to an emeritus status on the topic of stuttering. He was busy writing on other topics, far from the vineyard where he had planted so many seeds.

As a result he recommended that Dr. Harold Luper, a researcher, author, and authority on stuttering in his own right, as the person to write and interpret and update the Van Riper perspective. Fortunately for all of us, this was both a compliment and a challenge that Dr. Luper graciously accepted. Therefore, in this chapter, we have a blending of the thoughts of two men who at one point shared similar points of view.

15

Modification of Behavior, Part One

Charles Van Riper

EXPLORING THE PROBLEM

So far we've been trying to help you understand the problems you'll encounter when you begin to help the stutterer overcome his communication difficulties. Now we come to the nitty-gritty of actual therapy. We'll try to tell you what to do, how to do it, when to do it, and why it should be done. Now this is, of course, an impossible set of goals. The uniqueness of each individual clinician and each stutterer prevents any specific recommendations from being universally applicable. Nevertheless, we can certainly give you enough basic guidelines and practical illustrations of therapy procedures to let you devise a therapy program for your client that's tailored to his special needs. We hope the activities we suggest will stimulate you to invent better ones, more appropriate ones. That being said, let's get started.

How Should You Begin

Stuttering often presents such a complicated picture that many clinicians aren't sure where or how to begin. We think we can help. In another book published by the Speech Foundation of America called *To the Stutterer* twenty-four speech pathologists, psychologists, and psychiatrists who themselves had been severe stutterers were asked to answer this question: "What advice would you give to a stutterer who, for one reason or another, can't get professional speech

therapy?" Surprisingly, there were several things most of them agreed on, and one of these was that the stutterer should study his own stuttering. They expressed this in different ways but the emphasis was clear. If the confirmed stutterer remains unclear and confused about his behaviors and the feelings associated with them, his prognosis will be poor. This makes sense. The clinician's job is to facilitate learning and unlearning. If the client is to change his abnormal reactions to the anticipation or presence of fluency breaks, he has to learn what those reactions are. Also, when the client starts to explore his problem he looks closely at it, touches it, examines it, and often confronts it directly for the first time. He reverses the tendency to hide from it and to hide it from others. These confrontations are the beginning of desensitization. Therapy with the older stutterer should therefore begin with this confrontation and analysis. There are some real advantages in beginning this way and we'll describe them later. But first, here are some examples of activities you might use.

Some of these suggestions will be inappropriate for certain clients. Some of them will be appropriate at one point in therapy but not at another. Too many clinicians feel uncertain about what they can do at this stage of therapy. That's because there's no way to get around the fact that each client has different needs, and his needs change throughout therapy. You'll have to use your clinical judgment about what procedures to use then, but here are some things you can do.

Note: From *Therapy for stutterers,* C. Starkweather, ed. Memphis, TN: Speech Foundation of America.

Some Procedures

1. During the diagnostic examination, provide a running commentary on what you observe the stutterer doing. 2. Demonstrate some of the anticipatory and release reactions that you've seen in other stutterers and then ask your client to identify those that he too has experienced. 3. Play some audio or video recordings of other stutterers and have your client join you in their analysis. 4. Your client's own recordings can then be scrutinized in the same way. 5. Read and discuss descriptions from the literature on stuttering of the common feelings stutterer's have. 6. Before entering a feared situation, such as making a phone call or asking a stranger for directions, the client can write out or verbalize his expectations and feelings. 7. After he's entered feared situations try to express how you think your client felt and then ask him to correct any false impressions or, if you're lucky, you may be able to get him to describe what happened. 8. Tell your client you need to put his stuttering behaviors into your own mouth so you can understand them, and ask him to teach you how he stutters until your reproductions are fairly close. 9. Get him to collect samples of easy, unforced stutterings or to identify them in your own speech. 10. Have him say a stuttered word repeatedly to show him how his stuttering changes with adaptation. 11. From one of his recordings, have him count his stuttered and nonstuttered words so that he sees how much of his speech is fluent. 12. Use a stop watch to show him how long his stutterings really are. 13. Have him underline feared words before he reads a passage out loud, and then underline actual stutterings while listening to a recording of it; he may come to recognize the invalidity of some of his word fears. 14. Jointly make a catalog of the *variety* of his stuttering behaviors and then ask him about the purposes they may serve. (Why did he say "ah, ah, ah, ah," before that long prolongation on the /m/?) 15. Look with him for the presence of improper coarticulation in his repeated syllables; see if he used a schwa vowel rather than the vowel that should have been there. 16. Explore with him on videotape, or in front of a mirror, the abnormal mouth, jaw, or tongue postures he uses just before his speech attempt, comparing them with what he does when the word is spoken normally. 17. Explore his tremors, areas of tension, his avoidances, postponement, starter, and release behaviors. 18. Investigate with him his feelings of frustration, fear, shame, or hostility. 19. Determine the situational or phonemic or positional cues that trigger his fears of stuttering. 20. If possible, determine the vague outlines of his self-concept.

Selecting Procedures

We've given a few of the many activities that can be used in this exploration phase. We're certain you can invent ones that are more appropriate for the specific stutterer you're working with. Also, we've listed these suggestions in random order. You'll have to arrange these confrontation experiences so your client won't be overwhelmed. Generally, you should begin with experiences that are least likely to produce resistance, anxiety, or other forms of emotional distress. Then you should sequence other exploratory activities according to his ability to tolerate or profit from them. Have him help you make these decisions. Have him rank a set of activities in the order of their threat, stress, or difficulty. Usually the client knows better than you what to confront first and what to postpone for later sessions. He may also be able to devise better experiences than you can. The important thing is to involve him immediately in the therapy process. He's not passive clay in your hands to be moulded to your liking. From the first, you should define his role as a co-therapist. He'll need some training first in how to be his own clinician, but both of you know you can't be with him all the time and that most of the work of therapy will have to be performed and designed by him. Sooner or later he'll have to become fully his own clinician, so it's best to get started and introduce this role as soon as possible. You're a guide, not the Magical Monarch of Moo.

Why Begin This Way?

Some clinicians jump into the thicket of stuttering by asking too much of their clients too soon. They forget how emotional the adult stutterer is about his stuttering. They forget the blind hate he has for it. They forget how often he's tried to ignore it, disguise it, or pretend it doesn't exist. When climbing a long ladder it's better to put a foot on the bottom rung than to try to leap to the top. It's wise, then, to begin by stimulating the client's curiosity about what goes on when he stutters or expects to. If you can get him really interested in exploring his problem, you'll find some real pay-offs. First, he'll reduce the amount of running away, and hiding, and disguising he does because he's reluctant to expose his stuttering. If he's going to explore his stuttering, he'll have to seek it out. To examine it, he must be temporarily willing to experience it. Second, by exploring his stuttering in the presence of a warmly interested clinician who is permissive and not threatening, his fears, frustration, and shame will begin to decrease. Third, the disorder itself will lose some of the mystery that surrounds it. Finally, because of these things, some stutterers will show an immediate reduction in the amount of stuttering they exhibit while others may stutter more frequently but less severely. But even if no immediate change occurs in the severity or frequency of the stuttering, some basic changes in your client's attitudes toward his disorder are probably taking place. He's always been mystified and terrified by his stuttering. Now, in the relative safety of the therapy room, with you as a companion, guide, and co-explorer, one who is objective and analytical, interested rather than rejecting, he can touch the untouchable and scrutinize the inscrutable. Rapport, that indispensible ingredient of all therapy, is achieved more easily in such an atmosphere.

Ways of Confronting Stuttering

Your client may prefer to talk in generalities about his stuttering than to exhibit it. All right, let's do that talking after he's given you some specific samples that can be discussed. Here are some things you can do to get those samples. With most stutterers, we recommend beginning with the oral reading of a passage about some aspect of the disorder, and as soon as a moment of stuttering has occurred, you should first duplicate it and then ask the client to do so too, before either of you talk about it. Ask him to describe the feelings he had before, during, and after the speech attempt. Reflect these feelings and try to clarify them. Ask him why he did what he did. What purpose, if any, is served by a head jerk or a sudden exhalation of air. Give him some possible explanations and have him choose from them or ask him to volunteer some explanations of his own. State your ideas as hypotheses not as certainties, as inferences that must be checked out and tested. Have him compare the abnormal mouth posture he started to say the word with to the posture he used when saying the word normally. What was he really afraid of, if he was afraid? Were there old memories of past difficulty on that particular word or sound? What are some possible explanations for his eye closing or looking away? Where did the tension begin and how did it

spread? What happened just before the final utterance of the word? Though we phrase these in terms of questions, they're for your use, not his. In discussing behaviors with your client, try not to cross-examine him. Try instead to get him to volunteer this information and to be interested in it. Try also to get him to use descriptive rather than evaluative language in his analysis. These are just suggestions. You may find better ways of helping him to know what he's doing or feeling.

Although we've found it wise to begin with oral reading, we soon shift to the narrative monologue as the material from which samples of overt and covert stuttering behaviors can be procured. Have him talk about himself, the people who play important roles in his life, and about his stuttering experiences. We often tape record these sessions and then play them back to the client so that bits of behavior or expressions of feeling can be identified and discussed. Don't succumb to the temptation to lecture your client. Try to get him to say what he thinks before you offer your own commentary, then play the sample again for checking or for revising. Then use a mirror (preferably a full length one) or a videotape recorder to aid in the objective scrutiny.

Next, we recommend that you use conversational dialogue as the vehicle for exploring, analyzing, and cataloging. The topics of the conversation should again be stuttering as a disorder, his own particular stuttering behaviors and the feelings associated with them, or the goals and processes of therapy. Often at this time you'll find him talking about his feelings about you. He may even do some testing to see if you're really competent or really committed to his welfare. Without being defensive, reflect these feelings as being entirely natural and show that you are interested and accepting. Though the ostensible purpose of all this exploration is to compile a catalog of the stutterer's common responses to the anticipation or occurrence of stuttering, you're also trying to build a good working therapeutic relationship, and you're beginning to desensitize him at the same time. Additionally, you should use phone calls to provide samples for exploration. Or you can invite some friend or stranger to join you. The stress you produce this way may bring on stuttering responses you haven't seen before. Also, these situations may provide a useful transition to speaking situations in the outside world.

Since the world outside that therapy room is where the stutterer must do most of his living, we insist that, as soon as it seems appropriate, you and he get outside that room. If you don't make an effort to do so, you may never know how that stutterer really stutters, nor will he. As you know, stuttering can vary widely in its severity from one speaking situation to another. Ordering a cup of coffee in a restaurant, asking a bus driver a question, or asking for information at the airport, will bring on behaviors and feelings you could never have obtained through interviews in your office. You won't have to do much of this, but you certainly should do enough to get an impression of how valid his reports are. What's even more important, you'll be able to assess his strength so you won't overload him.

Perhaps most important, your willingness to share his outside problems, will help convince him that you're committed and dedicated to his welfare. Stutterers often doubt and mistrust their clinicians. If you're willing to go with him into feared situations, he won't feel so alone. Then too, after these outside experiences have been shared and discussed objectively in terms of the new information they provide, you'll have created a model of the sort of self-scrutiny you want him to do. If, in addition, you're also willing to enter another situation and duplicate the kind of stuttering your client has and then follow up with an objective analysis of what took place, he'll be tremendously impressed. Much of his resistance will disappear. Even one or two of these joint experiences can make a remarkable difference. From this time on, he'll not only be much more willing to explore on his own but you can also feel more confidence in what he reports as having occurred.

When to End Exploration

We can't tell you when to end the exploratory phase. Only you can make that judgment, but here are some guidelines or goals. Can the client duplicate his stutterings with reasonable fidelity? Can he talk about their major features and dynamics? Can he discuss his feelings of anxiety, frustration, hostility, or shame? Has he brought, for your examination, trophy-samples of behaviors that have occurred outside the therapy room? Has he attained reasonable success in analyzing his behaviors during monologue, conversation, or on the telephone when you're with him? Has he become curious about and interested in what he does or feels when he expects or experiences stuttering? Has some of his testing and resistance declined? Does he value your companionship as a co-explorer? Is he becoming impatient to get on with the modification of the stuttering?

We know that these questions may be hard to answer but they are the guidelines most clinicians use in deciding when to move to the next phase of therapy, the desensitization phase. In making this decision, you shouldn't expect your stutterer to have accomplished anything. Though we begin with exploration, analysis, and identification, we keep using them throughout the rest of therapy as well. Over and over again the client will have to confront himself objectively. By beginning this way we make it easier

15

Modification of Behavior, Part Two

Charles Van Riper

CALMING AND TOUGHENING THE STUTTERER

Your next goal is to devise a program that will desensitize the stutterer to his stuttering. Some of this desensitization has already occurred during exploration and identification, but most stutterers also need intensive therapy focussed directly on cutting down their reactions to the expectations or actuality of stuttering. Great gains in fluency usually appear as they learn to calm themselves, but the big payoff comes later in the facilitation of new learning and unlearning they must do when they start to modify their stuttering behaviors. No stutterer can learn new ways of stuttering or better ways of living if he keeps getting bowled over by emotional reactions when he tries to talk. If you can toughen him to his stuttering; if you can help him learn that he doesn't have to panic when stuttering is threatened or experienced, progress will come more swiftly.

How the Stutterer Feels

These emotions are mainly fear, shame, and frustration. As you know, stutterers fear certain speaking situations more than others, and they also fear certain words or sounds. These fears can be very strong, sometimes to the point of complete panic, and we must provide experiences that reduce their intensity and frequency. The stutterer's shame often shows up in his hesitancy to exhibit his disorder and in the many avoidance and disguise behaviors he uses to keep other people from recognizing him as a stut-

terer. Most stutterers find it hard to disclose these feelings of stigma except to someone they can really trust. Finally, you'll have to deal with your client's continual experiences of frustration. You musn't ignore these feelings of frustration, for they may be even more important than the more evident feelings of fear and shame. Being unable to say what you want to, finding your breathing blocked, finding that you can't untangle your tongue, finding yourself mute, or realizing that you're hanging onto the same sound or syllable interminably when you want desperately to get on with your message is a devastating experience. When it happens hundreds of times a day, the cumulative frustration builds up until you can hardly keep from exploding. As a speech clinician, you've got to understand this frustration if you're going to help the stutterer.

So your job, in this phase of therapy, is to help the client learn how to increase his tolerance of communicative frustration, to reduce his feelings of shame and embarassment, and to weaken his fears. How can you do it? There are several approaches and you'll have to decide, based on what you know of your client, which one or ones is best for his needs and capacities.

Calming Him Down

Oddly enough, until a clinician helps them learn how, few stutterers ever try to calm themselves when confronted by the threat of stuttering. Yet, if a series of speaking situations is arranged in a hierarchy or ascending order of difficulty, and your client is asked to try to remain as calm as possible *while he's stuttering;* as he climbs each step of this therapeutic ladder, he'll discover to his surprise that he can control his emotions to a remarkable degree. The important ingredient in this kind of desensitization therapy is that your client must stay on each successive step of the hierarchy, trying repeatedly to remain calm, until he's finally successful. Then he goes on to the next step and does his speaking *and his stuttering* in this situation until again he finds success. The emphasis is not on being fluent in these graded speaking situations but in remaining fairly calm whether he stutters or not. Indeed, you should give strong approvals when your client does stutter yet shows no signs of emotional reaction and says that he felt pretty calm. There will be occasions when he won't seem to be able to stay calm. Don't accuse him of not trying hard enough. You've been pushing him too fast. You may need to revise the hierarchy by inserting some new substeps or rungs in the ladder of difficulty. There will also be times when your client will have to stay on one rung of that ladder for some time or even go back to an earlier step before he can progress. But sooner or later, if you're warm and approving when he makes some headway and reassuringly patient when he doesn't, he'll learn that it's possible to expect or experience stuttering without getting upset.

How long should your stutterer stay on one step before tackling the next most difficult speaking situation? We think he should keep on entering and re-entering the situation until he says and his behavior indicates that he has remained relatively calm during his stuttering moments. We can't describe exactly what the signs of calmness are, for they vary with each stutterer, but in general you'll find that the amount of forcing and struggling is lessened, the panicky avoidance and postponement and recoil behaviors are decreased, and he stutters more easily. His breathing is less disturbed. He says he's more calm. When these and other signs begin to appear with consistency, he's ready to tackle the next most difficult speaking situation in the hierarchy.

One of the best ways to help your client realize that it's possible to climb this ladder is to climb it yourself. You should do some pseudostuttering, especially on the early steps of the hierarchy, and show him that you can do so fairly calmly. Make sure you do this without offending the client, but do it. It's easier to touch a hot stove if someone else shows you he can touch it without getting burned. You'll be modeling a calm and objective attitude for your client. If you find it hard to provide this model, well, you'd better learn to desensitize yourself if you want to help stutterers.

Testing Reality

Another important way to help the stutterer lose his speech anxiety and shame is to use the principle of deconfirmation. Most stutterers rarely examine those times when they expect a lot of difficulty but have little or none. All they remember are the times when their morbid expectations were confirmed. They'll tell you that they always have trouble, for example, on words beginning with the /p/ sound, or that they always stutter when talking on the telephone and so on. This isn't true, of course, but the stutterer believes it. Your job is to help him test reality. Help him get experiences in which he'll first predict the amount of difficulty he'll have in a speaking situation and then check, via tape recording or some other means, how often and how severely he actually stuttered. Or if he tells you that other people laugh at him when he stutters or that they show signs of impatience, or revulsion, again have him predict and then check. Over and over again, your stutterer will discover to his surprise that he rarely stutters as often or as severely as he expects to and that very few of his listeners really show the reactions he attributes to them.

Eye Contact

Most stutterers base their expectations on just a few of their worst experiences (and there always are some, of course) but his usual expectations of evil are often exaggerated and even morbid. It's a good idea to give your client a chance to look closely and objectively at what happens when he stutters. This is why many speech clinicians work hard to get their clients to look at their listeners instead of lowering their gaze when they stutter or expect to. This habitual averting of the eyes during stuttering can be very powerful and compulsive, and it's hard to change. The stutterer dreads the pity, rejection, impatience, or other reactions of his listeners, so he looks away. Unfortunately, if he keeps doing so, his listeners will conclude that he's ashamed of his difficulties, and this makes things worse. By learning to look at his listeners while he's stuttering, your client can not only test the validity of his fears but also put his listeners at ease. Moreover, by maintaining eye contact the stutterer demonstrates that he's accepting, not rejecting, his stuttering as a problem to be solved. When he looks away he's denying the problem. It must be faced in the mirror of the listener's eyes.

Self-Disclosure

The amount of energy most confirmed stutterers spend hiding their disorder is tremendous. They devise intricate strategies of avoidance and disguise. They assume masquerades of all sorts in the hope, usually a vain hope, that their listener won't recognize that they're stutterers. This burden is a heavy one and it only makes communication more difficult. You have to help your client stop pretending that he's a normal speaker and stop hiding the fact that occasionally he has some real difficulty talking. Help him experience the great relief that comes when he accepts his stuttering not as a miserable curse but as a problem that he's trying to solve. Now this doesn't mean that he should be willing to stutter but that he should be willing to show that he's working on his stuttering.

Pseudostuttering or Faking

Another way of helping the client face up to his problem is by pseudostuttering, or, as it is sometimes called, faking. You can't just ask your stutterer to start doing it in all speaking situations. You have to first help him understand why it's useful and what the ultimate pay-off will be. You should plan for him to use it gradually and in a series of graded situations. You should be able to use some pseudostuttering yourself in speaking with him and in outside situations where he can watch you calmly exhibit stuttering as severe as his own. He'll see that most of your listeners don't penalize you. We suggest that at first you ask him to use pseudostuttering only on nonfeared words and that simple syllabic repetitions or fairly short prolongations should be the first kind to use. Again he should try to remain as calm as possible while exhibiting these voluntary disfluencies. Occasionally he should deliberately say the stuttered word again as though correcting himself, thus showing his listener that he's accepting his problem and working on it.

Later on, when he shows real progress in desensitization, the client should duplicate some of the features of his own habitual stuttering reactions. At this point, he may tell you that some of his faked stuttering turn into "real, uncontrollable stuttering blocks." This is an opportunity for you to tell him to try to keep the pseudostuttering entirely voluntary, even during the emotional reaction, and if he can he'll make great gains. He may have to pseudostutter more slowly, more deliberately, more strongly, more consciously, but he can learn that it's possible to maintain control. Once again, you should patiently clarify the reasons and goals for using pseudostuttering, and provide necessary approvals for progress. No desensitization procedure takes effect immediately; there are delays, slippage, and other fluctuations in progress. Through all this your client will need your support if he's going to learn that he can touch his stuttering, that he can deliberately put it into his mouth and exhibit it before strangers without having the skies fall down on his head. No one dies of a moment of stuttering, certainly not of a moment of pseudostuttering, but your clients have to learn to touch the untouchable and toughen themselves. By gradually learning to stutter on purpose and without pain, your client will lose a lot of the negative emotions that color his disorder; when this occurs, he'll find great relief.

Tolerating Frustration

Much of the gross abnormality your stutterer shows is a reaction to his feeling that his utterance is being blockaded or that his syllables are recycling themselves out of his control. These abnormal reactions to communicative frustration have been learned, and they can be unlearned. No one has to stutter grotesquely, but your client probably won't have discovered this when he comes to you. His head jerks, gasps, and contorted features are usually reactions to frustration. It's immensely frustrating for him to open his mouth and find that he's mute. He'll tell you that it's a miserable experience to find his lips jammed together when he wants to open them, or to hear himself prolonging a yard of an /s/ sound when he knows that only a fraction of an inch of it is appropriate. By the time he comes to you, he may be automatically and involuntarily responding to these unpleasant frustrations with recoils, forcings, head jerks, or any number of other reactions that contribute to his audible or visible abnormality. Later on, you'll try to help him modify these behaviors, but at this phase of therapy your main job is to desensitize him to the frustration. If you can help him build up his tolerance to feeling blocked, he'll be able to bear his fixations or oscillations without instantly reacting in his old abnormal ways, and this is a great gain.

Freezing

How can this tolerance to communicative frustration be learned? There are many ways of doing it, and you'll have to decide which ones are appropriate for the stutterer you're working with. One technique we've found useful is called freezing. Find a signal you can use the instant your client starts to prolong or repeat a sound or its posture. When he sees the signal he should freeze or immobilize his articulators (or continue to repeat the syllable if that's what he's doing), as long as your signal is being given. Make sure you have him hold the abnormality long enough to watch it in a hand mirror, or have it replayed on a delayed feedback apparatus or recorder, or while you duplicate it, or comment about it. Since the idea is to build up the stutterer's tolerance to the frustration and to prevent its triggering the recoil, forcing, or the other abnormal responses, you should gradually increase his freezing or holding so that he can tolerate more and more of it. Sometimes it's wise to have your client first give you the signal as you duplicate some of his characteristic behaviors, and when the signal is turned off, you should move forward into the rest of the word easily rather than using his characteristic responses. Make sure that he understands why he's doing what he's doing, that he must toughen himself to these frustrating stimuli that trigger so much of his abnormality. Stutterers tend to go haywire when they feel blocked or reverberating and they do all sorts of maladaptive things that only make their problem more severe. If they can learn to touch the snake of stuttering without flinching, if they can make gains in tolerating communicative frustration, all sorts of good things happen.

The Stuttering Bath

Another approach uses the principle of flooding. With a few especially courageous stutterers, a "bath of stuttering" can produce desensitization. The client is asked to collect a large number of moments of stuttering in a given time period or a large number of situations in which he stutters before he can go to bed or eat a meal. You can decide whether to accept pseudostutterings as fulfilling the quota at first, but it's best to insist on "real stutterings" as soon as possible.

What usually happens is that the stutterer, for perhaps the first time in his life, wants to stutter, for each new instance of stuttering brings him closer to fulfilling his quota and getting reward or relief. This approach isn't for all stutterers. Many would refuse or sabotage the assignment simply because they couldn't bear the experience. Nevertheless, if your stutterer can accept the challenge and does it to desensitize himself, the experience can produce some dramatic and favorable changes in his attitude toward his disorder and its treatment.

For most stutterers, the adaptation principle can be used. Have them repeat the stuttered word over and over again while trying to remain calm. There will be times when, after the word has been said fluently two or three times, the fear will build up again and more stuttering will result. You should try to arrange it so that he ends on a successful utterance and has signalled his feeling of calmness not only during the utterances of the word but in the stuttering period just prior to the attempt. Have him make a collection of some of the words he has stuttered on during the previous day and use these for adaptation practice.

There are other ways of decreasing the stutterer's fears, frustration, and shame. Some clinicians try to teach the stutterer to assume a state of deep relaxation while he imagines himself in a hierarchy of feared speaking situations or as he attempts to speak. Some use strongly assertive and even aggressive behaviors to countercondition these negative emotions. Some use humor to counteract the fear or embarrassment. Some prefer to seek out and provide ventilation or resolution for the other anxieties or conflicts that augment the stutterer's communicative distress. Some feel that the stutterer will be less emotional if he examines his speech output realistically to determine the amount of fluent speech he already possesses. Most stutterers pay little attention to this fluent fraction of their speech output and tend to notice only the moments of abnormality. They often exaggerate and pump up their fears. By helping them look at their speech objectively, these clinicians hope that the stutterer will become less hypersensitive and morbid. All of us do all we can to build up our client's self-esteem and to reduce whatever seems to be lowering it, for we know that when his morale is high he's less vulnerable to stress and negative emotions. If we can help him solve some of his other problems, his problem of stuttering becomes more soluble.

Finally, we want to re-emphasize your role in this desensitization therapy. If you can accept his stuttering as a problem and if he finds in you a warm, trustworthy companion and guide, he too will come to acquire this attitude. As he exhibits his stuttering before you and finds that you don't penalize or reject him for it, his stuttering loses much of its evil emotional coloring. For once in his life he's found another person who understands how he feels and who's dedicated to his welfare. He's no longer alone. There's no better healing medicine than this.

15

Modification of Behavior, Part Three

Charles Van Riper

MODIFYING THE STUTTERING

If your stutterer has made some real gains in identifying what he does when he expects to stutter or when he finds himself stuttering, and if he's found ways to stay calm during these episodes, he's ready to tackle a new set of goals. These concern the modification of his overt stuttering behaviors. Since the bulk of his abnormality usually consists of habitual responses to the expectation and experience of fluency breaks, your client will inevitably become more fluent if he unlearns them.

The First Goal

We have found it wise to begin by aiming our therapy at the reduction or elimination of the stutterer's avoidance and postponement responses to feared words and situations because these seem to be more under his control. Often they're used deliberately as well as automatically. Nevertheless, you should expect some resistance when these responses are attacked, and if you know why he resists giving up his avoiding and postponing, you won't be upset. For many years your client has been able to minimize his suffering by refusing to enter feared situations, by substituting easy words for hard ones, or by revising his sentences. By vigilantly scanning approaching speaking situations or prospective utterances, he has sometimes managed to escape the frustration or social penalities that otherwise might have occurred. Indeed, this avoidance has often been the only way he's found to reduce his distress. Avoidance re-

sponses can be very strong. You don't just tell him to stop avoiding. Even though he might like to or try to—and many stutterers hate themselves for always having to run away—at that last crucial moment of speech attempt, his old avoidance responses will dominate. And then he'll think of himself as a coward as well as a stutterer. He needs your help to eliminate them and he needs a systematic program to unlearn them.

What we've said about avoidance also holds true for postponement. The repeated use of an "ah" or an "um" or a "well, well, well-uh" just before attempting speech may be a large part of his abnormality, and it's clear that if these could be eliminated, much of his deviance would disappear. When he approaches a feared word, backs up, pauses, says previous words or phrases several times, it's obvious that these behaviors are impairing his over-all fluency and that he'd be better off if he didn't use them. Or perhaps he postpones saying the feared word by coming to a dead halt, a pause that not only breaks the flow of utterance but also produces frustration in the listener and the stutterer himself. Surely, you think, if he could eliminate these gaps in his speech, the stutterer would be more fluent. But these postponement behaviors have been very useful to him. Often they've helped him hide the fact that he stutters. Often, if he's been able to stall long enough before attempting a feared word or situation, he's discovered that indeed he didn't stutter. He'll ask you why this happens and you'd better have an answer. One explanation is simply this—fears, like other emotions, tend to fluctuate. They vary in intensity as time passes. At one moment the situation or word fear may be very intense; a moment later it may weaken. It flares and subsides like the flames in the fireplace. It rarely maintains itself at a peak level very long. The stutterer has simply discovered that, by postponing, he can sometimes manage to make the speech attempt at emotional ebb tide, at that fleeting instant when his word fear has declined almost to zero, and that when he can do so, little stuttering occurs. Yes, postponing occasionally keeps him from stuttering but the precision of timing is hard to achieve. More often than not, the very act of finally attempting the word causes the word fear to flare up again, and then he'll only have added the abnormality of his stalling to the stuttering it did not prevent. It's your job to help him realize vividly how rarely his avoidance, postponement, and disguise behaviors yield any real relief, and how often they contribute to the listener's impression of abnormality, how much they fracture his fluency, and how they actually reinforce his fears. Ducking and dodging and stalling and pretending are the things to be avoided—not the stuttering. If your stutterer is going to learn how to modify his stuttering, he simply has to come to grips with it.

Stopping Avoidance

By now, you should have achieved a good therapeutic relationship and we hope your client prizes your approvals and is not indifferent to your disapprovals, for these are your major tools. They're the basic tools of every competent clinician. If you're operant-minded, you may want to devise an appropriate program that will decrease these behaviors. If so, you'll have to outline it carefully, defining the behavior you want to decrease, deciding on scheduling, criteria, sequential steps, etc., and be prepared to do the necessary counting and plotting of responses. If operant conditioning isn't your bag, you still have to administer your approvals and disapprovals carefully, using them to facilitate your client's acceptance of the necessity to give up avoiding, postponing, and pretending he doesn't stutter. You'll use your approvals and disapprovals to help him become his own clinician with all the responsibility for planning and performance that this role requires. Help him devise and revise subgoals and strategies. Share your expectations and ease his hurt when he fails to corroborate them. We've had stutterers stop avoiding as soon as they realized that they were losing more than they gained from its use, but this insight rarely comes immediately or easily. Much of our effort is expended in creating conditions so that this insight can occur.

We now provide a list of some suggested experiences that have proved useful for most of the confirmed stutterers we've worked with. 1. During oral reading, ask your stutterer to try to use synonyms as substitutes for all words beginning with /p/ so that the garbling of his speech is made vivid to him. 2. Make a telephone call in his presence and, as you speak, duplicate the kinds of avoidances, postponements, and disguise tricks he uses. Discuss. 3. Engage him in conversation, and when he shows any of these behaviors, have him say the sentence they occurred in twice over, duplicating the behaviors the first time, and then without them, before he can continue talking. 4. Using oral reading, have him rewrite the passage so that it includes all his characteristic avoidance, postponement, and disguise devices. You can use the format of the drama script with stage directions *(Look away and pretend to think here. Put hand over mouth)* to indicate the disguise responses. Have him help you design the passage. 5. Use a similar preparation for what he says when he makes a phone call. 6. Fill your own speech full of his characteristic avoidance, postponement, and disguise behaviors as you make a long phone call while he watches. 7. Using some recordings of his speech, have him identify and count how frequently these reactions were used and perhaps how long they lasted. 8. Analyze with him some appropriate recordings made by other stutterers so he can see how much of their speech abnormality was produced by the postponement and avoidances they used. Then scrutinize one of his own recordings from the same point of view. 9. Using a reading passage or prewritten sentences for paraphrasing or phone calls, have him load these excessively with the behaviors, then speak them over and over again *ad nauseum* until he's thoroughly sick of using them. 10. Devise a signal upon which he is to continue performing these behaviors until you signal again. Have your client use it on you first as you insert some postponement device of his into your own speech; then you apply it to him. Progressively increase the demand for continuation of the undesired behavior until it becomes distasteful.

Reinforcement and Punishment

The activities described above are devoted primarily to building a vivid awareness of the behavior the stutterer should try to reduce, and to help him see that he should not be using it. We now suggest some other activities that use positive and negative reinforcement or mild punishment to decrease these responses. 1. Use the time-out procedure by insisting that your stutterer come to a dead halt and pause for five or ten seconds whenever one of these behaviors appears. 2. Turn your head away, shut your eyes, or cover your ears the moment you detect one of them in his speech. 3. Whenever he demonstrates one of them, duplicate it in your own speech or behavior simultaneously and continue it for a minute or so even as he continues talking. 4. Say "no, no" or give some other kind of disapproval whenever such a behavior occurs, then have him say it too when it appears. 5. Devise experiences in which your administered penalty or his own self-administered penalty is contingent on a certain quota of these reactions in a certain situation involving stress or during a certain period of talking time. Example: Have the client make ten phone calls before breakfast and postpone eating it (for a specified time) if he uses more than a certain number of word substitutions, etc. Have him select the time of the delay and set the number of word substitutions that would demand the penalty. 6. Have him signal each time he anticipates a feared word. Show him your approval when he says it without the old reactions. 7. After setting up a substantial quota of assigned oral reading time, paraphrasing, or phone calls, one that will ensure a considerable amount of labor and perhaps distress, reward him for each instance of direct attack on a signaled feared word by deducting a portion of that quota. For example, every time he refuses to substitute or postpone, the oral reading time is reduced by five minutes. 8. Have him stand on one leg until he has been able to read aloud for a set number of minutes without postponing. 9. With his help, devise a substantial reward for entering a certain number of feared situations that normally he would have avoided. 10. For every speaking situation he confesses avoiding, have him devise an appropriate penance such as a certain amount of paraphrasing, oral reading, or phone calls.

Let's reiterate that these are just suggestions and that they may not be at all appropriate to the needs of the particular stutterer you're working with. They simply illustrate the kinds of things that could be done. As we've indicated, it's wise to have him help you plan the activities and set the performance quotas for the application of reinforcement or punishment. We structure the relationship as a co-therapist

one. We work out these tasks and goals together, often setting maximum and minimum subgoals. We work hard to get the stutterer to administer his own approvals and disapprovals. When emotional reactions arise, we're there to help him weather them. A concerted attack on his avoidance, postponement, and disguise behaviors can't help but reduce them markedly, often to zero. Again, let's stress the need to achieve this reduction not only in the oral reading monologue and conversation that occur in the therapy room and in your presence but also in his everyday life.

Fluent Stuttering

Your efforts to strip away the stutterer's defensive strategies for coping with his fears won't be effective unless you can offer something better to take their place. If he isn't going to avoid or postpone, *what is* he going to do? Your answer to this question should be very simple but direct: "Start saying the word you fear. Start saying its first sound. Start saying its first syllable. Sound out that word. Work through its motor sequence in a forward direction without interruption or recoil and do this slowly, deliberately, and strongly. Enter the speaking situations you formerly avoided, start talking and talk as much as you can and as often as you can. Instead of hiding and disguising the fact of your stuttering, display it openly but with this important difference—display it as a problem that you're obviously trying to solve." This is what the stutterer has to learn. These are the positive behaviors that you, as his clinician, must clarify and reinforce.

When should these goals be introduced? It's difficult to generalize, but usually we incorporate them after the stutterer has shown a fairly substantial reduction in the avoidance, postponement, and disguise behaviors. However, don't wait until they've entirely disappeared. Indeed they may not disappear until the stutterer has made some progress in learning to approach his feared words and situations more directly and openly. You'll have to be the judge of this, of course, but you should know that it's possible to strengthen the new replacement behaviors at the same time that the old ones are being extinguished. You can, for example, give your approval whenever the stutterer begins a feared word by attempting its first sound even though he prolongs it and show your disapproval when he prefaces the attempt by "ah . . . ah . . . ah . . ."

Where should this work be done? Again, it's wise to begin in the comparative safety of the therapy room and in your presence. The stutterer will need you there to help him know why he should do what you're asking. There will be failures that you may need to interpret or assuage. You'll have to provide models of the behaviors desired. The stutterer will need your support and your information and your feedback. We suggest, as before, that the speaking of individually feared words, oral readings, monologue, conversation, and phone calls should be used as the vehicles of this new learning. We recommend that you accompany your client out into the real world a few times, enough times, to show him that he can function differently there too.

How can you help him learn these new behaviors? If your basic orientation lies in operant conditioning, you can find examples of procedures and programs by Bruce Ryan and George Shames in another Speech Foundation of America publication, *Conditioning in Stuttering Therapy,* and we don't have to expand upon their contributions here. Instead, we'll present the rationale for the experiences we hope you can provide your client and then describe some of them.

There are a great many different kinds of stuttering behaviors. One stutterer shows one set of them; other stutterers show different sets. Even the stutterer you're now working with or planning to work with may stutter differently from time to time and it's almost certain that the variety of stuttering behaviors he shows now are unlike those he demonstrated when he was a child. Sometimes his struggling is very severe, but there are other instances when he seems to stutter easily. These easy effortless stutterings can be found occasionally in his speech and they're the goal models you should now try to set up for him. If he can always stutter in this easy way, the interruption to his speech flow will be minimal. These easy stutterings won't frustrate him and they won't frustrate his listener. He won't be penalized for them since they have little abnormality and so he'll feel no shame. And he won't fear having to exhibit this kind of stuttering. If he can learn to stutter in this way, the vicious spiral can be unwound. If he can lose his fears, shame, and frustration, you can be sure that he won't stutter so often. By shaping the kind of stuttering he does so that it comes closer and closer to this model and finally reaches it, he can become a fluent speaker even though some residue of stuttering remains. At worst, he'll view his stuttering as a minor nuisance that he and others can easily tolerate; at best, he may attain the self-concept of being a mildly disfluent normal speaker and stop thinking of himself as a stutterer, for even normal speakers have their disfluencies too. You may ask, and the stutterer may ask you, if it's possible to learn to stutter in this new way. All we can say is that we've helped many to do so.

Clarifying the Model

Your first task is to make it clear to the stutterer what it is he's supposed to learn. We've described the characteristics of this easy stuttering before but let's be more specific. The stutterer in attempting a feared word must try to begin it with the articulatory posture and movement that fits the first sound and syllable of that word when it's spoken normally. He shouldn't cock his mouth into an abnormal posture that might trigger a tremor. He shouldn't start it suddenly but as slowly as he can. Some stutterers who have learned it call this new kind of stuttering "slow-motion stuttering." He doesn't necessarily have to *talk* slowly but he should stutter slowly. The client should also learn how to make *strong* movements, not weak ones, but this doesn't mean that he should abnormally tense his lips, tongue, etc. One stutterer said that he had discovered he could "stutter loose as a goose," whatever that means, probably that he no longer squeezed his lips or pressed his tongue or shut his ventricular folds tightly and then tried to blow the barriers open with a blast of air from a suddenly compressed chest. In this easy stuttering, most of the contacts are light, not squeezed firmly shut. Always, the movement is forward, the stutterer "sounding out" the successive phonemes sequentially. Once he begins the feared word, he doesn't stop; he keeps going—going forward in slow motion. The shifts from posture to posture are gradual, not sudden. No sound is elongated more than the others; all are slowed down proportionally. All this description is unduly detailed and you certainly don't need to explain it to the client. We might as well describe how he should learn to skate. We provide it for your guidance, not his. Your job is to show him how to shape his stuttering so that it comes to resemble the new form.

As we've said, there are times when he already stutters this way and it really isn't a new way. If you have him say the same word over and over again, he will often be using the model a time or two before he becomes fluent. You can show him how to stutter this easy way by simply doing it and without any explanation at all. We've often taught young stutterers to do it by putting enough samples into our own mouth and then asking them to imitate us. Some stutterers have called it "the slide"or "the glide" or "sounding out." Most just call it "slow-motion stuttering" or "easy stuttering." What they are really doing, of course, is trying to say the word without avoidance or struggle. It really isn't necessary to stutter hard or abnormally.

Activities for Easy Stuttering

Now let's sketch a few of the many possible activities you might use to help him learn this easier way. 1. In your own speech, fake a few samples of your client's characteristic behaviors, then say the word again with the slow-motion, easy stuttering, then say it normally before proceeding. Have him "shadow" you, doing what you're doing as you say the word several times. 2. When he's talking and stuttering in his old way, repeatedly provide the model of the new form simultaneously with his stuttering. 3. Insert some duplications of his stuttering into your own speech and have him show you over and over again how you could use the new form as you continue your duplication. 4. Demonstrate one of his old abnormal trigger postures (lip protruding, etc.) and show him how to shift from this into a more normal beginning posture. 5. Have him assume one of these abnormal postures and change it several times back and forth into normal and abnormal positions before beginning the word. 6. Have him follow your model of shifting from tight lip or tongue contacts to light ones in the utterance of isolated feared words beginning with lip or lingual sounds in isolated words and then in sentences. Usually, when he adopts the tight contacts they will turn into tremors and he'll then feel that he's stuttering but this won't happen if the looser contacts are being produced. 7. On a feared word and especially one that begins with a vowel, you may notice that he shows a complete stoppage of airflow or phonation. This usually means that his ventricular folds (false vocal cords) are occluded. Most stutterers either recoil from this "blockage" experience and start over again or use an "ah" or inhalatory gasp or other means of opening the airway. There are better ways than these for opening that sphincter and one of them is to start with vocal fry and blend it into true

phonation. Teach him to *search* for the adjustments he needs to make rather than to struggle blindly. 8. Provide your simultaneous modeling of a shift from high tensed oral musculatures into relaxed ones when he shows such marked tensions. 9. Reinforce with your approval all stutterings that are continuous rather than interrupted, all those that move forward even though at first certain sounds are abnormally prolonged but, as soon as you can, give him the idea that he should be making movements, strong ones but slow ones, as he works his way through the utterance of that word. Often the prolongation of the first sound of a stuttered word is only a disguised postponement behavior, the stutterer hanging onto it until the fear ebbs enough to decrease the probability of further stuttering. 10. Teach him to time the moment of speech attempt with a slow, strong jaw movement and help him know something about the appropriate co-articulation of the attempted syllable. Often the stutterer, consumed with fear of the initial sound, will be trying to say a syllable containing the schwa vowel rather than the vowel that's required. He tries to say the word "paper, for example, by producing the /p/ that belongs to the syllable "puh" rather than the right one. Sometimes you can help him get the proper co-articulation by having him pre-form the correct vowel in pantomime as he makes the speech attempt on the word.

We could provide many other suggested activities like this to help you solve some of the problems you may encounter but surely these will at least illustrate the general procedures. Your job is to start with the behaviors your client demonstrates and then modify and shape them until finally they approximate the goal behaviors. Often, to keep the model of easy stuttering before him, it's wise to ask the stutterer to fake frequently both the old and new forms on nonfeared words, thus providing the needed contrast. Sometimes it's wise to have him fill his speech with these easy slow-motion stutterings, saying all his words in this way for short periods to vivify the goal.

In this phase of therapy, then, the emphasis is on problem solving, on finding better ways of approaching and uttering the words he expects to stutter on. Your stutterer needs your observations and commentary if he's to make the necessary changes or even to discriminate what they should be. He'll also need your faith and support when temporary or partial failures occur. Some stutterers learn this better way of "stuttering" very easily; others need a lot of help and a lot of appropriate reinforcement. One way or another your job is to teach him that he can attempt his feared words without using the old avoidance and struggle reactions that constituted so much of his abnormality and disrupted fluency.

Beginning Response Alteration

After your client has the model of new easy stuttering clearly in mind, and after he's had some vivid experiences in putting it into his mouth as well, we recommend that he use it in the process we've called cancellation. We refer to the practice of following each word on which the old forms of stuttering occur with an obvious pause and then repeating that word using the new form of easy stuttering on it before continuing. The sequence is 1. old form of stuttering; 2. definite pausing; 3. new form of stuttering. The cancellation is only a strategy you can use to help your client extinguish his old form of stuttering and strengthen the new. The pause functions as a mild punishment (time-out) but it also provides the time needed by the stutterer to help him identify what he did wrong and the time to make plans for demonstrating the contrasting new kind of stuttering when he says the word again. The latter, the new easy stuttering, must be done before the stutterer can continue speaking, so it's this that gets rewarded most strongly. Moreover, by using the cancelling process, the stutterer shows to himself and to the world that he's willing to work openly to change his abnormal way of speaking. And there are many other good reasons for using this strategy. You should at least explore its utility as a means of habituating the new easy way of stuttering. Even though the stutterer has shown you that he now has the capacity to stutter in this new way, this doesn't necessarily mean that he'll immediately be able to use it consistently wherever and whenever he wants to. Some of the old stuttering behaviors are bound to occur for some time. Cancellation can take care of them. Train your client to use it consistently in monologue, conversation, phone calls, and in outside speaking situations, both in your presence and when he's on his own.

Better Reactions

Once your stutterer is willing and able to cancel his old abnormal responses and can do so with some consistency, it's wise to move toward their modification while they're still occurring. Show him how to release himself from his sticky, prolonged mouth postures or compulsive repetitions of a syllable in a less abnormal way. Perform his stuttering behaviors and then demonstrate better ways of releasing, of moving forward slowly and easily. Throw yourself into his characteristic fixations or tremors, then without stopping and trying again, loosen the tight contacts that he so often uses, get the air and sound flowing, and progress gradually from the sound to the correct syllable and through the utterance of the word. Do what he does when he stutters severely, then show him how to search for the correct articulatory posture, for the easing of hypertensed muscles, for the proper co-articulation of the syllable.

Often we've stuttered right along with our stutterers as they begin a moment of stuttering but then we release ourselves in better, less abnormal ways than those he's using. This stuttering in unison except for the better release you're demonstrating will soon teach your client to follow your example. Or you can assume his characteristic form of "blocking" and continue doing it until *he* shows *you* the kind of release you've been trying to teach him. Don't let him try and stop and then try again. Teach him to stay with his abnormality and work out of it in a more appropriate way. Help him modify his old stuttering patterns *while they're occurring* and reward all progressive approximations toward the easy, slow-motion, forward flowing response he's learned in the cancellation phase of therapy.

You needn't be alarmed if your client finds some initial difficulty in working out of his "blocks" in this new way. Reward the partial successes; clarify the goals; give him feedback so he can recognize not only what he's done wrong but also what he's done well. He's bound to get some partial successes if he keeps trying to change the way he usually responds to the experience of finding himself stuttering. For years he's just surrendered helplessly at these moments; now he's "wrestling with his demon" instead. Win or lose, it's a better feeling and a healthier one. When, for example, you find him beginning to say a /p/ word by protruding and squeezing his lips and then shifting to the new response of voluntarily retracting and loosening them before working through the rest of the word, you'll know that he's on his way. And so will he. Only a few experiences of this sort can make a tremendous difference. Though at first it may take a tremendous voluntary effort to resist the old manner of responding and to substitute the new, we've often been surprised to find how soon the latter becomes easy and automatic. Indeed there are some stutterers who learn it by themselves as soon as they've learned to cancel. It isn't necessary to struggle blindly when you feel yourself stuttering. It's possible to stutter easily and with very little abnormality. There are thousands of ways of stuttering. Help your client find a better one. Many stutterers don't even call this way of talking "stuttering."

Getting Set

There's no need for your client to cancel or wrestle with his stuttering for the rest of his life. If this were all we had to offer, the prospect would be a life sentence to hard labor and we wouldn't offer it. Fortunately it's possible to get set to say the feared word in the new way and then to say it in that new way. Many stutterers discover this by themselves; some need teaching. You may have to help him do some motor planning or rehearsing of the new easy stuttering before the speech attempt. Certainly you can clarify the model and provide the necessary challenge. Again, he'll occasionally get a few successes along with some failures and the former can be strongly reinforced. But what if he fails and finds himself in one of his old "blocks"? Well, then he can wrestle with it and modify it. And what if he doesn't do that either? Have him cancel it. And what if he doesn't even do that?

Write down the word for him and have him use it again in another sentence some other time. Bind up his wounds and stay with him. The Rome of an easier way of stuttering isn't built in one therapy session. All therapy has its temporary failures. Progress never moves in a straight line. Though it oscillates back and forth it may still move forward. You'll find that as your client discovers the real fluency that comes when he can stutter easily rather than grotesquely any momentary set back won't matter much. Soon he'll be using the easier form of stuttering automatically and habitually and then he'll find it so much fun to talk you'll have to hide from him.

We've sketched the outline of one way you might help your stutterer to decrease his abnormality and increase his fluency. It's not the only way. It may not even be the right way for we can't know your client's personal characteristics, or his present stuttering behaviors, or his other personal problems. But far too many clinicians approach the responsibility for doing stuttering therapy with reluctance because they lack a comprehensive plan or because they have no rationale for what they do. If you're going to guide your stutterer out of the morass of his difficulties, you need to have some kind of a map. We've provided one for you. It's roughly drawn and not very detailed but it shows some of the routes both you and your stutterer might follow. Many have found fluency at the end of this trail.

Modifying Stuttering Behavior

Harold L. Luper

I'm not certain why Dr. Van Riper chose not to write the postscript to his earlier work or why he suggested me as the person to do it. Even though Dr. Van Riper is officially retired from Western Michigan, he continues to write and turn out new material. Perhaps, as I have heard him admit about some of his other writings, he finds it difficult to go back and re-read material that he wrote earlier. Most likely it was because he's now concentrating on writing short stories about his youth in northern Michigan.[1] Perhaps he suggested my name since I was associated with the Speech Foundation of America project in which the material reproduced here was included. Or maybe I was chosen because I am a long-time advocate of his form of therapy, even though I have never used it in exactly the same manner as he did. Whatever the reasons, I am honored to be asked to write this postscript and I'll try to do it justice.

Before looking at the three sections he wrote under the general topic of "Modification of Behavior," it may be helpful to put Van Riper's contributions in perspective. Dr. Van Riper's professional writings in speech pathology have been voluminous, especially on the topic of stuttering. In addition to his descriptions of therapy in the six editions of his widely used textbook, *Speech correction principles and methods* (1939 through 1978), Van Riper has written many articles, chapters, and three lengthy volumes on stuttering (*The nature of stuttering*, 1971 and 1982, and *The treatment of stuttering*, 1973). Because his textbooks have been so widely adopted in college courses, his opinions on stuttering therapy have had wide acceptance, especially during the period from the early 1940s through the middle 1970s. No other single individual has appeared to have the influence he has had on stuttering therapy unless it would be Wendell Johnson, a fellow student and professional colleague of Van Riper. Van Riper and Johnson were part of what Bloodstein (1981) has called "The Iowa Development" in ref-

---

[1]See *The Northwoods Reader* (1977) and *Tales of the Old U.P.* (1981) by Cully Gage (pseudonym for C. Van Riper). Published by Avery Color Studios, AuTrain, Michigan.

erence to the contributions of these (and other) individuals in the early days of the speech pathology program at the University of Iowa. Bloodstein describes the importance and uniqueness of "The Iowa Development" as follows:

> In brief, the new therapeutic approach for which Bryngelson, Johnson, and Van Riper opened the way was one that aimed at a reduction in the fear and avoidance of stuttering while at the same time attempting to reduce the stuttering itself directly through gradual modification based on study and understanding of the behavior of which stuttering consisted. This approach represented a sharp departure from the philosophy on which the traditional methods were based. Bryngelson, Johnson, and Van Riper were severely critical of these methods. They argued that they merely gave the stutterer a temporary crutch on which to lean and that quick recovery almost inevitably portended sudden relapse. Above all, such methods served in the long run to intensify rather than decrease fear because in effect they said to the stutterer, "Don't stutter". "Swing your arms or talk in some odd and unnatural way, but whatever you do don't stutter." And the implication was that hardly anything was more unusual or grotesque or more to be feared and avoided than stuttering. By contrast, the new approach was to say to the stutterer "Go ahead and stutter. But learn to do so without fear and embarrassment and with a minimum of abnormality." (Bloodstein, 1981, p. 344.)

Although Van Riper, Johnson, and Bryngelson are lumped together in this description of stuttering therapies, Bloodstein is careful to identify some of the individual contributions from each of the three men. Bryngelson was known more for his introduction of voluntary stuttering and the "objective attitude," Johnson for his emphasis on perceptual and evaluative reorientation, and Van Riper for his attempts to find better ways of modifying the stuttering behavior itself. The three men were friendly protagonists professionally, each arguing his own beliefs with vigor but respecting and frequently using ideas from the others.

The 1974 description of modification of stuttering behavior needs to be put into still another perspective: that of the purpose for which it was written. The material was prepared for a publication of the Speech Foundation of America entitled *Therapy for stutterers.* The Speech Foundation has long attempted to provide helpful suggestions on therapy to clinicians in practice. Largely at the insistence of the Director of the Foundation, Mr. Malcolm Fraser, the Foundation has sought to present material to clinicians in a more simplified and practical manner than is often found in college textbooks. The sections that have been reproduced here are essentially a simplified, easier-to-read version of the therapy program he presented in much more detailed fashion in Chapters 8 through 13 of *The treatment of stuttering* (1973). Readers who find some of the 1974 material too simplified may wish to read the lengthier chapters in *The treatment of stuttering* text.

My intent in this postscript is to look at the three sections reproduced at the start of this chapter, pointing out statements that appear to need clarification in terms of today's ways of looking at stuttering therapy and emphasizing aspects that most characterize Van Riper's approach. I will then briefly indicate what

Postscript   15

changes, if any, I would suggest. Finally, I'll take a stab at guessing at what changes Van Riper would make were he updating this material at this time.

COMMENTS ON MODIFICATION OF BEHAVIOR
Part One—Exploring the Problem

In other writings Van Riper has called this stage of therapy *Identification* (Van Riper, 1973; 1978). "Exploring the problem" perhaps expresses better the type of attitude Van Riper hopes to instill in the client as he looks at his own stuttering. Van Riper thinks that most stutterers really do not know what they are doing when they stutter. They may be aware of the fact that they are "stuck" or they may feel they "can't get the word out" but they remain largely unaware of the specific things they are doing when they stutter or when they expect to stutter. One of the reasons for beginning with identification, according to Van Riper, is that the stutterer needs to learn what his abnormal reactions are if he is going to change them.

But identification as an aid in learning what to change is not the only reason Van Riper begins this way. Note his emphasis on the value of having the stutterer confront his stuttering. There are probably many reasons a stutterer is often unaware of all of his stuttering behaviors. Few of us are completely aware of all of our mannerisms, especially in highly habitualized behaviors. Stutterers may have even a greater reason for being unaware since frequently they are so panicked during the moment of stuttering that they can think only of the embarrassment and fear they are feeling. Van Riper believes that one of the major reasons for this lack of awareness on the part of the stutterer is denial of the symptom. He thinks that most stutterers have endured countless frustrations, embarrassments, and feelings of shame and guilt because of their stuttering. The shame and guilt are unpleasant feelings, and thus the act of stuttering is highly unpleasant to the stutterer. The pattern of avoidance and concealment that so often characterizes the stutterer leads naturally to a tendency to deny the problem. If one can't escape this unpleasant event, one can at least act as if it doesn't exist. And if one does this frequently, the pattern of denial may soon grow to the point where the speaker does not recognize even those behaviors that should be quite obvious.

I have seen hundreds of examples of such unawareness. One that stands out in my memory was a college student with a very loud vocalized inhalation as part of his stuttering repertoire. I thought it would be best for him to identify this bizarre behavior rather than my pointing it out to him. But it took many sessions of our studying his behaviors together before he came to recognize the breathing abnormality. All he was aware of was the fact that he was "having trouble getting the word out."

Van Riper feels that the emotions attached to the stuttering—the fears, shames, hostile feelings, and embarrassments—that have led to the denial of the stuttering must be confronted directly before the stutterer can eliminate them.

In his words, the stutterer must "touch the untouchable and scrutinize the inscrutable" (Van Riper, 1974, p. 49). There is an advantage in doing this. Confrontation, in Van Riper's view, leads to some degree of desensitization.

Note that his exploratory or identification phase is not directed only at the speech behaviors. Van Riper wants the stutterer to identify his feared words, feared situations and even his feelings of anxiety, frustrations, shame or fear.

Many clinicians have complained that it is difficult to begin therapy in this manner. They feel clients have an aversion to studying their stuttering in such detail. Many clinicians think it is too much to ask of a client and may even be unnecessary. Most who use fluency-shaping procedures place little emphasis on self-study of stuttering behaviors other than making certain that the stutterer can identify when he stutters so that he can monitor his own speech and self-reinforce or self-consequate at appropriate times. Webster has this to say about the self-study of stuttering:

> It has been common practice in "stutter fluently" therapies to emphasize the client's study of his disfluent speech as a condition of therapy. . . We have found that time allocated to the examination of disfluent speech is time removed from our therapeutic process. Although knowledge of targets may be facilitated by familiarizing clients with properties of their disfluent speech, we have not witnessed evidence that supports this notion. (Webster, 1979, 218).

Learning what one does when one stutters perhaps is more important for those therapies like Van Riper's that seek to teach the stutterer ways to modify his stuttering than for programs that seek to "replace" stuttered speech with another set of speaking behaviors.

Perhaps the clinician's own aversions to having a stutterer observe and talk about things he hates in himself explain why many prefer some of the more recent behaviorial approaches. It also seems possible that not all stutterers have feelings of fear and shame to the degree that they could not benefit from therapy without such confrontation. Guitar and Peters speak to this issue in their book *Stuttering: An integration of contemporary therapies* (1980). They suggest that stutterers whose stuttering is not maintained by strong emotions may not need to confront their fears in this manner.

Certainly, if one feels, as Van Riper does, that stuttering is maintained primarily because of the intense fears, shames, and embarrassments associated with it, then some means of reducing those feelings seem in order. Studying and confronting them seem appropriate ways, though not the only ways, to begin reducing those feelings.

Part Two—Calming and Toughening the Stutterer

Van Riper has long been known for his colorful writing and for his descriptions of the inner feelings of the stutterer. Nowhere is this demonstrated any better than in the second of his three sections on "Modification of Stuttering." After briefly

Postscript   15

explaining that the primary reason for this phase of therapy is to reduce the stutterer's emotional reactions to the point where the learning of new behaviors is facilitated, Van Riper describes in detail how he thinks the stutterer feels. The importance he places on attempting to describe these feelings is a clear indication of his belief that successful therapy depends in large part on reducing or eradicating the stutterer's feelings of fear, shame, and frustration. Van Riper feels that the average clinician does not understand these feelings, and that this lack of understanding is a major cause of ineffective therapy. So, in Part Two, we see Van Riper both describing what he sees as the stutterer's feelings and presenting in simplified fashion some techniques for modifying the feelings and associated reactions.

"Calming and toughening" are goal-centered substitute terms for what Van Riper has previously described as *Desensitization* (Van Riper, 1978; 1973). Remaining calm to the threat or experience of stuttering is a new response to be learned in place of the former patterns of panicky avoidance, postponement, forcing, struggling or recoiling. How is the new calm reaction learned? There are a number of ways including: (a) deconfirmation experiences (finding out that one doesn't always stutter as much or as often as he expected to), (b) maintaining eye contact with the listener even when stuttering (to test the validity of his fears and to put his listeners at ease), (c) openly admitting to others that he is working on his stuttering, (d) pseudostuttering first in less feared situations and later in situations where more difficulty is expected, (e) "freezing" or deliberately immobilizing the articulators upon signal during moments of stuttering, (f) attempting to stutter in a large number of situations or on a large number of words within a short period of time (the "stuttering bath"), or (g) by remaining calm during repeated utterances of stuttered words (adaptation).

Note that these types of desensitization experiences are similar to but still somewhat different from those typically used in "systematic desensitization" (Wolpe, 1958). Elsewhere Van Riper (1973) has described his desensitization activities as "in vivo desensitization" to emphasize the fact that the stutterer learns to change his reactions while actually entering feared situations rather than by imagining himself in stress situations, as advocated by Wolpe. The general principles of arranging the experiences in a hierarchy from least feared to most feared and not proceeding to the next higher level until successful on the present one are still followed. Van Riper places the emphasis not upon being fluent as the stutterer goes through these speaking situations but on remaining calm whether or not he stutters. As in systematic desensitization, if the stutterer is unsuccessful in remaining calm in a particular situation on the hierarchy, the clinician is to move the stutterer back to a less feared situation for awhile. Observable signs that the stutterer is remaining calm are given to help the clinician make this judgment. These include a reduction in the amount of struggling or forcing and in the amount of postponement and recoil behaviors. Breathing should also be less disturbed.

The emphasis on desensitization activities advocated here characterized Van Riper's therapy long before Wolpe (1958) described the techniques he called "Systematic Desensitization." For example, in the 1946 version of *Speech correction principles and methods,* Van Riper describes his emphasis on decreasing the emotional reactions associated with stuttering as follows:

> One of the most important phases of the treatment of the secondary stutterer is that which attempts to change the shame and embarrassment which are associated with the act of stuttering. . . . It is usually wise to ask the stutterer to recall the most unpleasant experiences and to recount them to a group of fellow stutterers. When these formerly traumatic situations are re-experienced on an adult and objective level, much of the attendant emotionality tends to disappear. . . . (Van Riper, 1946 p. 362)

> The attitude taught to the stutterer as a substitute for the old reactions to his blocks is that of unemotional admission of his speech difference as a problem to be solved. . . .In summary, we may say that the stutterer must (1) learn to adopt an objective attitude toward his disorder, and (2) gradually diminish the shameful and embarrassed reactions which accompany it. (Van Riper, 1946, p. 363)

It is also interesting that this 1946 description of his therapy includes many, if not most, of the activities advocated in 1974 for desensitizing the stutterer. Specific mention is made in the 1946 chapter of deconfirmation experiences, the value of maintaining good eye contact with the listener, pseudostuttering, the "bath" of stuttering experiences, and open admission of the disorder. In summary, about the only change seen in terms of desensitization is in the way it is labeled. The term "eradicating the mal-attitudes of shame and embarrassment" (Van Riper, 1946, p. 362) has given way to "calming and toughening" in the 1974 version, but the methods advocated for achieving these changes appear to be about the same.

Part Three—Modifying the Stuttering

It may be confusing to some readers for Van Riper to label the third phase of his therapy program "Modifying the Stuttering" when his overall program is labeled in this publication as "Modification of Stuttering." The redundancy between the use of "modifying" as a title for this section and "modification" as the name for the entire therapy approach was probably done intentionally to emphasize his belief that real changes in habitual ways of approaching feared words or stuttered words cannot be achieved until the stutterer is successful in confronting his problem and analyzing it, and can remain relatively calm during its occurrence. Everything in the stuttering therapy program is aimed at teaching the stutterer how to modify and cope with his fears and tensions, but the real changes in the speech behaviors themselves must await prior changes in how one looks at and reacts to his problem.

Typically, Van Riper attempts to simplify the process for the neophyte clinician by suggesting a sequence for what and how the stuttering behaviors should

Postscript 15

be modified. He suggests beginning with reducing or eliminating the stutterer's avoidance and postponement responses. His rationale is that these are more under the stutterer's voluntary control and therefore more amenable to change. He discusses the fact that the stutterer may resist giving up these ways of coping with stuttering because they have been somewhat successful in evading the full force of the stuttering or in delaying the embarrassment and frustration accompanying the stuttering. Most of his suggestions for stopping avoidances involve ways to make the behaviors unpleasant and the use of positive reinforcement for any attempts the client makes to utter his feared words without avoidances or postponements.

As Van Riper acknowledges, new responses are seldom made habitual simply by inhibiting certain behaviors. Rather, some behaviors that the stutterer actively attempts need to be learned to replace the old habitual responses. Saying this differently, a successful speech response is not just "not struggling and not avoiding." Instead, the stutterer needs to approach speaking with several active steps in mind. The type of response that Van Riper seeks to instill contains several features including: beginning the feared word with the appropriate articulatory posture and movement, starting the movement slowly, making strong articulatory movements through the word, and using loose articulatory movements and shifting gradually from one sound position to the next. As one looks at the features of the desirable speech response, it is easy to see similarities in the speech modification techniques Van Riper advocates and those used in so called "fluency-shaping" programs. The slow motion movements advocated by Van Riper seem similar in function to many of the methods used to slow overall speaking rate. In both instances there appears to be a desire to reduce the negative effects of time pressure on the stutterer and to get him to use a type of speech production that gives him more time to make the necessary coordinations among respiratory, phonatory, and articulatory processes. Likewise, the use of "loose articulatory movements" (often called "loose contacts" by Van Riper therapists) appear to be similar to Cooper's "smooth-speech" fluency-initiating gesture (Cooper, 1979) or Webster's "reduced-pressure" target (Webster, 1975). In fact, it is my opinion that few, if any, of the specific speech modification goals of the currently popular fluency-shaping approaches are new or unique to the treatment of stuttering. The distinction, then, is not so much on what the stutterer is taught to do, but on when and how the stutterer is encouraged to modify his speech attempts. Because of the importance Van Riper places on fear and avoidance behaviors as key elements in the maintenance of stuttering, he does not advocate teaching the stutterer a new way to approach speaking attempts until the stutterer has demonstrated that he can face his problem openly and with little emotion. Most of the fluency shaping approaches seem to feel that permanent changes can be made in the stutterer's speech by beginning with speech modification changes. And although some fluency shaping approaches initially placed little emphasis on attitudinal changes for maintaining fluency, there now appears to be a strong movement to include steps to alter attitudes on the part of several current fluency shaping approaches (e.g., Shames & Florance, 1980).

Note that Van Riper calls the desirable, new speech response "easy stuttering" probably because he does not want the stutterer to continue seeking a way of not stuttering. Van Riper's belief is that the stutterer's tendency to avoid stuttering will be reinforced less if he thinks he is working for easy stuttering than if he is working for nonstuttered or fluent speech. In the section entitled "Activities for easy stuttering," Van Riper gives a number of suggestions for techniques that lead to voluntary control of the speech mechanism during stuttering. As presented in this section, the stutterer is encouraged to search for ways to *vary* his speech behaviors until they approximate the fluent forms of stuttering that Van Riper considers as the ultimate target. The emphasis on *variation* in attempting to develop more habitual ways of approaching feared words reminds one of the acronym he used so long for his therapy steps, "MIDVAS," which stood for motivation, identification, desensitization, variation, approximation, and stabilization (Van Riper, 1963, 1972, 1978).

The material beginning with the subheading "Better Response Alteration" and continuing to the end of the chapter is a brief description of what I consider the heart of Van Riper's modification approach. Suggestions are first given for teaching the stutterer to modify his speech during a cancellation. In this technique the stutterer is asked to begin by first using his old form of stuttering. After completing the stuttered word, he is to have a definite pause in which he tries to calm himself and figure out what he needs to modify to produce the word fluently. He is then to try the new form of the fluent stuttering. Once the stutterer is using cancellations consistently, he should be taught how to modify his stuttering while it is occurring. The material presented under the subheading of "Better Reactions" is what Van Riper long ago labeled as "pulling out" of the stuttering. After the stutterer has learned to modify his stuttering successfully during the stuttering act, he can learn to prepare before he attempts the feared word to use the modifications he has learned under the previous steps of cancellations and pullouts. He now attempts, as described under the heading, "Getting Set," to plan ahead with new motor sets so that the word is uttered in a slow-motion, fluent manner without any of the old abnormality. I'm not sure that Van Riper would agree with me, but I have always thought of the three steps of cancellations, pullouts, and preparatory sets as *steps in learning how to control stuttering,* while the various suggestions given for how to change the speech mechanism so that speech will be uttered smoothly rather than being blocked up (such as using loose, articulatory movements or planning ahead for the position of the sounds that follow a stuttered sound) are *techniques for controlling stuttering.*

In the last half of the first paragraph under "Getting Set," Van Riper stresses his belief that the stutterer should feel there is always something that he can and should do about his stuttering. Unsuccessful attempts to get set for a stuttered word should not be left to reinforce feelings of failure; rather, these should be-

Postscript   15

come signals to the stutterer that he needs to wrestle with and try to "pull out" of his block. Or if his attempt to pull out of the block fails, he should be prepared to try to cancel the attempt by trying it again with conscious effort to modify what he is doing. This attempt to instill in every stutterer the attitude that he can and should work on all his stuttered words is probably the major factor underlying Van Riper's maintenance program.[2]

A BRIEF PEEK AT THE CRYSTAL BALL

If Doc Van, as Van Riper is affectionately known, were writing this today, what would he say differently from what he wrote in 1974? It's always risky to pretend to know what someone else is thinking—especially someone as creative and productive as Van Riper. But sometimes a future position can be predicted by tracking the path a person has trod in earlier stages. This method is frequently used in economic projections. Experiences of the past are graphically plotted to develop a curve that is extended to project a future point. Fortunately Van Riper has written so much that we have access to his thinking at many different points in his career. Let's look at a few of these points for a clue on where he would be today and where he and others in his camp of stuttering therapy will be in the future.

Several years ago, Van Riper (1958) summarized his therapy program during his first 20 years at Western Michigan in a chapter entitled "Experiments in Stuttering Therapy." In this remarkable chapter, Van Riper described his therapy program as it evolved year by year from 1936 through 1956. Not only had he made extensive notes on what he did each year in therapy, Van Riper had also included judgments on the progress made by his clients at the time and for several years later. This classic chapter should be considered "must" reading for all serious students of stuttering therapy.

We'll begin the base of our projection curve with 1936, his first year at Western Michigan. Here's how he describes the rationale for his treatment program at that time:

> In 1936 we believed that the essence of stuttering lay in a neuromuscular blocking or inability to move the paired speech musculatures at a specific moment in time. These blockings, however, were seen as being of extremely short duration, lasting but a fraction of a second, and precipitated by a latent dysphemia activated by situation and word fears. The *greater* part of the stuttering abnormality was viewed as consisting of *learned* reactions to the threat or experience of these blockings, as avoidance or frustration responses. These, it was felt, could be unlearned through proper training methods, thereby decreasing the severity of the disorder. With the severity decreased it was hoped that the frequency would subsequently be reduced, with less unpleasantness in speaking since less fear and frustration would occur. In short, our aim was to "whittle down" the stuttering to its neuromuscular blockings, thereby achieving a fluency adequate for everyday communication.

[2]Although Van Riper usually included a "stabilization" phase as an important component of his therapy program, it was omitted in the 1974 booklet in favor of a chapter on "Transfer and Maintenance" written by Harold L. Luper.

Influenced by our psychoanalytic experiences and by the concept of a *margin* of cerebral dominance which could operate the speech mechanism fluently so long as it was not reduced by ego-destructive stresses, we felt that any therapeutic program should include activities which would enhance that margin and increase the individual's ego strength. We also felt that the stutterer could be trained and toughened to resist the specific disturbing influences which impaired that margin of cerebral dominance or which reduced that ego strength. Any experience which would do either should decrease the frequency of the stuttering blocks.

It should be noted that the basic assumptions upon which this rationale rested were these: (1) Stuttering consists largely of learned behavior and can be modified and reduced through training procedures. (2) Stuttering consists largely of avoidance and frustration responses, both of which reinforce the stuttering. (3) The stutterer's self-concept can be altered so that less stuttering will occur. Both the stuttering and the stutterer were viewed as being modifiable. (Van Riper, 1958, pp. 277–278)

So how was this view of stuttering translated into therapeutic methods? Stutterers were urged to reduce bimanual activities and were taught new unilateral skills to build up a greater margin of cerebral dominance. Each client performed daily exercises of simultaneous talking-and-writing, in which he wrote the first letter of a word suddenly and in time with the utterance of that word. (I well remember the hours spent in talking-and-writing required in 1946 when I entered Van Riper's therapy program.) Stutterers were also taught to use voluntary stuttering (a deliberate repetition of the first sound or syllable of a feared word) in order to begin learning how to change involuntary stuttering into voluntary control of the stuttering. And, as Van Riper describes it, "some fairly superficial psychotherapy was also given" (Van Riper, 1958, p. 281).

Van Riper continued evaluating his success in therapy and making experimental variations in his approach. He added the technique of having the stutterer prewrite any utterances in which stuttering was expected. He modified the use of psuedostuttering, having the stutterers use it on nonfeared rather than feared words as a way of aiding desensitization and for finding an easier form of stuttering. Emphasis was continued on discouraging the use of any avoidance behaviors and on encouraging the stutterer to go directly into his feared words and find easier ways to work his way through them. Many activities designed to help the stutterer resist any disturbing influences that increased his anxiety about talking were conducted. And gradually, over a period of years, the procedures of cancellations, "pull-outs," and preparatory sets were introduced as ways of helping the stutterer learn to modify his stuttering. The basic steps in therapy, as explained to the stutterer, looked like this in 1949:

> We will now outline the therapy. Our basic aim is to teach you *how to stutter, and without obvious abnormality, in a way which does not interrupt the flow of your speech.* If you can do this, it should solve your speech difficulty. It should eliminate most of your fears, both of speaking situations and of difficult words. Free speech then is the by-product rather than the goal of our therapy. We want to teach you how to stutter so quickly, effortlessly, and unnoticeably that your stuttering will be

Postscript   15

no impediment whatsoever. You probably have observed before this that no two stutterers stutter in exactly the same way. Is there then still another way which has less abnormality in it? We hope to show you.

It would be pleasant for all of us if this goal could be achieved instantly, but our experience shows us that it cannot. You have been stuttering in your present fashion too long. You have strong fears and habits and attitudes which cannot be erased so easily. First of all we must weaken the old reactions, the long-practiced form of stuttering which you now possess. Right now you stutter automatically, almost involuntarily. You have little control either of your speech or of your emotions. Therefore, we must proceed up a long ladder of sub-goals each of which takes you closer to the conquest of your speech defect.

Here is the ladder, beginning with the bottom rung:

1. You must understand the over-all plan of treatment.
2. You must, for the time being, be willing to stutter openly and without embarrassment.
3. You must acquire the ability to keep good eye contact with your listener throughout your moment of stuttering.
4. You must stop avoiding feared words and speech situations.
5. You must stop postponing, half-hearted speech attempts, and retrials.
6. You must be able to analyze your own stuttering in terms of its varying symptoms.
7. You must learn how to cancel. This refers to a technique wherein you go right through your old stuttering block, then pause during which you study the block you have just had, then try the word again in a different way.
8. You must master the principle of negative practice. By this we mean that you must be able to duplicate or initiate at will each typical sample of your own stuttering.
9. You must uncondition or weaken your habitual reactions of approach or release.
10. You must learn how to pull out of your old blocks voluntarily, to get them under voluntary control before uttering the word.
11. You must learn how to prepare for the speech attempt of feared words, so that they can be spoken without interruption or abnormality.
12. You must learn how to build barriers against disturbing influences.
13. You must learn to fill much of your speech with voluntary loose movements of your tongue, lips and jaws.
14. You must learn how to reinforce your new fluency each day. (Van Riper, 1949)

Looking next at the fourth, fifth and sixth editions of *Speech correction principles and methods* (Van Riper, 1963; 1972; 1978), we see that Van Riper used the acronym, MIDVAS, to explain the basic stages in therapy in which M stands for motivation, I for identification, D for desensitization, V for variation, A for approximation and S for stabilization. These stages are essentially the same as those in the 1974 version "Modification of Behavior" except that the motivation and stabilization sections were by other writers and thus were not included in the material reprinted here. Although some new techniques such as use of biofeedback are incorporated, most of the activities recommended by Van Riper appear to be basically organized around the same purposes from approximately 1949 to 1978. The asymptote of our projection line appears to have been reached sometime around 1949. This is not to suggest that Van Riper did not make changes in his therapy after that time; but it does appear that the basic form of his therapy was established by about 1949, and that the changes that came after that time were less drastic. Gone was the emphasis on unilateral activities and talking-and-writing that were advocated in 1936. The systematic procedures for learning to modify stuttering that are described in 1949, however, are still present in the 1974 and 1978 versions of his therapy. The emphases on confronting the problem and decreasing sensitivity about stuttering, however, seem to have been present from even the earliest days of Van Riper's therapy. The record speaks for itself. Van Riper remained true to his 1936 assumptions that the stutterer and his speech were both modifiable, although he changed considerably some of the aspects he thought should be modified, and he altered in many ways the activities used to change the stutterer's speech and feelings.

During the mid-1970s and the early 1980s, stuttering specialists frequently divided stuttering therapists into two major camps. One camp, championed by individuals such as Shames (1969), Perkins (1973), Ryan (1974), and Webster (1974), utilized principles of operant conditioning to establish, transfer, and maintain stutter-free speech. Most of the members of this camp tended to deny the necessity of working directly on attitudes and feelings, hoping instead to obtain any necessary changes as a by-product of increased fluency. Fluency was normally measured in units such as the absence of repetitions and prolongations over time. A speech pattern that would result in few repetitions and prolongations was sought, frequently through very abnormal ways of talking such as the use of very slow speech rates. Once nonstuttered speech was obtained, efforts were made to transfer it to other stimulus situations and to maintain the fluency over long periods of time without resorting to continued therapy. The opposing school of thought, led by Van Riper, but including many stuttering therapists such as Sheehan (1970), Gregory (1973), and Luper and Mulder (1964) was more inclined to emphasize anti-avoidance techniques, control of stuttering behaviors through direct confrontation and conscious manipulation, and reduction of fears and other negative emotions about speaking. This group of therapists tended to distrust most of the techniques used to establish fluency, such as slow rate, rhythmical talking, and use of delayed auditory feedback procedures, because it was felt these fluency-producing devices would probably not lead to permanent reductions in stuttering, and because they were not preceded by activities to alter the stutterer's fears and tendencies to avoid stuttering. As Van Riper stated it in one publication:

> Does [the stutterer] need to learn how to talk normally or does he need to learn to stutter? In our view the basic problem involves learning better ways of coping with the stuttering when it is threatened or occurs. This is what the stutterer must learn. Merely giving him a period of fluency will not help him know what to do

Postscript 15

when he expects or experiences stoppages in the flow of his speech. Indeed such a period of fluency may make him even more helpless when the stuttering does return, as alas it usually does." (Van Riper, 1973, pp. 206–207)

As in most controversies, intermediate points of view began to emerge. Some clinicians who had begun from a nonavoidance, stuttering-modification school of thought became impressed with data published by the fluency-shaping clinicians that showed long-term gains in fluency and changes in attitudes about communication among stutterers who had received fluency-shaping therapies. On the other hand, after the initial glamour of a supposedly new approach had worn off, some of the fluency shapers were forced to admit that not all of their clients had significant, long-term improvements with the operant approaches and, furthermore, that changes in communication attitudes seemed to be related to long-term improvements in fluency (Guitar & Bass, 1978). So, efforts to integrate concepts from both types of programs began to appear. Notable among these were publications by Guitar and Peters (1980), Starkweather (1980), and Shames and Florance (1980). Guitar and Peters pointed out advantages and disadvantages of either approach, suggested criteria for selecting which approach to emphasize, and recommended a "combined approach" for most stutterers. Starkweather pointed out that stuttering has two major components: feelings that accompany the stuttering and speaking behaviors that result in stuttering. As Starkweather states:

> Both the feelings and the overt behavior have to be treated. If only the feelings are treated the client is likely to relapse because many of his original overt behaviors remain intact, even though they may be reduced in severity. When they occur, the stutterer is likely to react to them all over again and become resensitized. Desensitization alone is not enough. Conversely, if only the overt behaviors are treated, there is another danger of relapse. If the fear of being disfluent is still present, normal disfluencies can provoke the old reactions of struggle and avoidance and the relearning of the old overt behaviors." (Starkweather, 1980, p. 327.)

Starkweather goes on to advocate a multiprocess behaviorial approach to stuttering therapy in which recognition is made of several ways in which stuttering can be learned and in which both nonavoidance and fluency-shaping techniques are utilized.

The Shames and Florance (1980) therapy approach developed over a period of years in primarily a behavioral framework. However, as Shames and his coworkers sought to find better ways of helping the stutterer maintain his gains in therapy, increasing attention was placed not only on helping the stutterer develop stutter-free speech, but also on helping him change those attitudes that were thought to maintain stuttering.

To return to our crystal ball–gazing, what can be our best guess as to what positions on these questions members of the nonavoidance, stuttering modification camp will take as we approach the last decade of the 1900s? I think the Guitar and Peters (1980) and Starkweather (1980) publications are a good indication. I believe the descendents of Van Riper's philosophy will still place a great deal of importance on helping the stutterer feel differently about how he talks. I think they will continue to recognize the value of the stutterer not avoiding his feared words and feared situations, but they will probably accept the notion that attitudinal changes can occur as a by-product of increased fluency and do not necessarily have to precede real changes in speech behavior.

The nonavoidance, stuttering modification group will not be satisfied with a form of speaking that is fluent only by adoption of an unusual method of speaking, such as an extremely slow rate. But, in this regard, neither do most fluency shapers see this as a final goal. Most of the people who follow the Van Riper way of thinking about therapy will not be content to measure improvement solely by a decrease in number of stuttered words. They will look for other positive signs such as greater spontaneity in verbal expression, reduction of avoidance and struggle behaviors, and freedom from undue concern over fluency as marks of the rehabilitated stutterer.

Van Riper's influence on stuttering therapy will long be felt. But a healthy, vigorous, scientifically-oriented discipline is not content to rest on the laurels of the past. Improvements, modifications, and varying emphases will continue so long as we have persons who stutter and clinicians who seriously seek answers to the stuttering problem. Van Riper improved his therapy techniques by observing their effects on the stutterers with whom he worked. He expects other clinicians to do the same.

REFERENCES

Bloodstein, O. (1981). *A handbook on stuttering* (3rd ed.). Chicago: National Easter Seal Society.

Cooper, E. B. (1979). Intervention procedures for the young stutterer. In H. Gregory (Ed.). *Controversies about stuttering therapy.* Baltimore, MD: University Park Press.

Gregory, H. (1973). *Stuttering: Differential evaluation and therapy.* Indianapolis: Bobbs-Merrill.

Guitar, B. & Bass, C. (1978). Stuttering therapy: The relation between attitude change and long-term outcome. *Journal of Speech and Hearing Disorders, 43,* 392–400.

Guitar, B. & Peters, T. J. (1980). *Stuttering: An integration of contemporary therapies.* Memphis, TN: Speech Foundation of America.

Luper, H. L. & Mulder, R. L. (1964). *Stuttering: Therapy for children.* Englewood Cliffs, NJ: Prentice-Hall.

Perkins, W. H. (1973). Replacement of stuttering with normal speech, II. Clinical procedures. *Journal of Speech and Hearing Disorders, 38,* 283–294.

Ryan, B. P. (1974). *Programmed therapy for stuttering in children and adults.* Springfield, IL: Charles C. Thomas.

Shames, G. H., Egolf, D. B., & Rhodes, R. C. (1969). Experimental programs in stuttering therapy. *Journal of Speech and Hearing Disorders, 34,* 38–47.

Postscript   15

Shames, G. H. & Florance, C. L. (1980). *Stutter-free speech: A goal for therapy.* Columbus, OH: Charles E. Merrill.

Sheehan, J. G. (Ed.). (1970). *Stuttering: Research and therapy.* New York: Harper and Row.

Starkweather, C. W. (Ed.) (1974). *Therapy for stutterers.* Memphis, TN: Speech Foundation of America.

Starkweather, C. W. (1980). A multiprocess behaviorial approach to stuttering therapy. In W. Perkins (Ed.), Strategies in stuttering therapy. *Seminars in Speech, Language and Hearing, 1,* 327–338.

Van Riper, C. (1939). *Speech correction principles and methods* (1st ed.). Englewood Cliffs, NJ: Prentice-Hall.

Van Riper, C. (1946). *Speech correction principles and methods* (1st ed., 6th printing). Englewood Cliffs, NJ: Prentice-Hall.

Van Riper, C. (1949). To the stutterer as he begins his speech therapy. *Journal of Speech and Hearing Disorders, 14,* 303–306.

Van Riper, C. (1958). Experiments in stuttering therapy. In J. Eisenson (Ed.), *Stuttering: A symposium.* New York: Harper and Row.

Van Riper, C. (1963). *Speech correction principles and methods* (4th ed.). Englewood Cliffs, NJ: Prentice-Hall.

Van Riper, C. (1971). *The nature of stuttering* (1st ed.). Englewood Cliffs, NJ: Prentice-Hall.

Van Riper, C. (1972). *Speech correction principles and methods* (5th ed.). Englewood Cliffs, NJ: Prentice-Hall.

Van Riper, C. (1973). *The treatment of stuttering.* Englewood Cliffs, NJ: Prentice-Hall.

Van Riper, C. (1974). Modification of behavior. In C. Starkweather (Ed.), *Therapy for stutterers.* Memphis, TN: Speech Foundation of America.

Van Riper, C. (1978). *Speech correction principles and methods* (6th ed.). Englewood Cliffs, NJ: Prentice-Hall.

Van Riper, C. (1982). *The nature of stuttering* (2nd ed.). Englewood Cliffs, NJ: Prentice-Hall.

Webster, R. L. (1974). A behavioral analysis of stuttering: Treatment and theory. In K. Calhoun, et al. (Eds.), *Innovative treatment methods in psychopathology.* New York: John Wiley & Sons.

Webster, R. L. (1975). *Clinician's program guide: The precision fluency shaping program.* Roanoke, VA: Communications Development Corporation.

Webster, R. L. (1979). Empirical considerations regarding stuttering therapy. In H. Gregory (Ed.), *Controversies about stuttering therapy.* Baltimore MD: University Park Press.

Wolpe, J. (1958). *Psychotherapy by reciprocal inhibition.* Stanford, CA: Stanford University Press.

16

Evolution of a Target-Based Behavioral Therapy for Stuttering

Postscript
Stuttering Therapy from a Technological Point of View

Ronald L. Webster

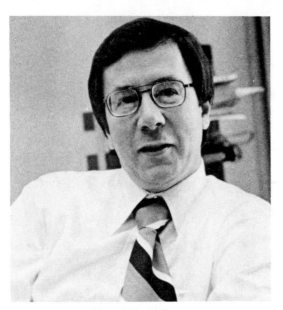

Ronald L. Webster

In a relatively short period of time Webster has had a profound impact on a large number of clients, mostly adult stutterers, who have enrolled in his treatment programs at Hollins College. He has built a careful procedure from simple sound-making behaviors through gradually more complex combinations and rates to ultimately more natural and spontaneous conversational speech. In the process, Webster takes advantage of the relatively unthreatening oral tasks of meaningless sound production and of a rate of utterance that is so slow as to be boring, thereby facilitating fluency from the outset of the program. Webster also relies on the social reinforcements and practice opportunities available to groups of stutterers who participate in a residential treatment program intensively for a period of weeks.

He views therapy as a technology of self-management and feedback to the stutterer about his own speaking behavior. He minimizes human judgment and error relative to meeting criteria for gentle onset of speech utterances by use of computer technology. The full responsibility is on the stutterer for responding to his own self-generated information about his speech. Initial overlearning is the key to ultimate, automatic fluency.

Webster has painstakingly gathered and analyzed data leading to progressive change and refinement of his program. For Webster, as well as for other behaviorally oriented contributors to this volume, the ultimate criterion for evaluating the success of therapy is the overt performance of the client and the eventual emergence of fluency. He is sensitive and responsive to the data emerging from his program as evidenced in his concerns with simplifying the tasks for the stutterer by reducing the number of behaviors that the client tracks at any one time. Webster has not allowed himself to be swayed by bias or sentimentality. Instead he has judiciously invoked the principles of the scientific method in his search for continuously improved clinical technology.

16

Evolution of a Target-Based Behavioral Therapy for Stuttering*

Ronald L. Webster

Hollins Communications Research Institute, Hollins College, Roanoke, Virginia

INTRODUCTION

The purpose of this chapter is to relate certain aspects of the work which led to the development of a behaviorally based speech reconstruction program for the treatment of stuttering. Note at the outset that the thrust in program evolution has been toward a physically oriented therapy technology that is applicable on a standardized basis to stutterers in general. The treatment at focus in this report has been designated as the "Precision Fluency Shaping Program: Speech Reconstruction for Stutterers" (Webster, 1974a). In the course of this therapy's development, specific behavioral and electronic technologies were derived that treat stuttering in an objective and effective manner.

As a result of our work on the development of our therapy, it now appears clear that no special theoretical foundations are required in order to establish a practical treatment for stuttering. At its simplest level, the theoretical basis for stuttering therapy seems to require only one readily testable assumption—that the speech response complex of stuttering can be altered through the application of learning principles in an effort to generate normal sounding, fluent speech. The term "fluent speech" as used in

this chapter refers to normally fluent speech (3% or less disfluency rate) and not to a technically perfect absolute fluency. Other higher level suppositions regarding possible determining variables of stuttering have not been shown to aid in therapy development (Van Riper, 1973). It seems particularly important to assess the extent to which the systematic empirical reconstruction of speech response details in stutterers can contribute to the creation of effective therapeutic processes. This report deals with a series of empirical analyses of the behaviors and training methods which were eventually found to be clinically useful in enhancing the long-term retention of normal fluent speech in large numbers of stutterers.

Our present stuttering therapy was derived through a sequence of five prior programs. Each successive version increased the specificity of what was taught in therapy, improved the application of learning principles to the behavior-change task, and made the acquisition and long-term retention of fluent speech more reliable and easier for the client to attain. A concomitant finding was that the reliability of clinician performance across successive clients also improved. As the program became established in terms of identifiable technologies, relevant dimensions of clinician behavior also became more discernable and more clearly specified in the context of therapy. Progress in the effectiveness of the therapy

*Presented at the First Annual Multidisciplinary Approach to Stuttering, Stuttering Center, Department of Neurology, Baylor College of Medicine, May, 1979.

program across successive versions was clearly demonstrated to be a function of the extent to which a careful, empirical orientation was maintained. There were countless occasions when we ventured into the cul-de-sac of theory and concept. As we learned and then relearned again and yet again, advances in the adequacy of therapy were linked to our ability to observe, measure, and manipulate relatively tiny behavioral details.

PROGRAM I

We began our project on stuttering therapy during the early months in 1966. Thanks to discussions with my colleague, Bobby Boyd Lubker, I became interested in the problem of stuttering. Our initial purpose was to replicate the operant conditioning study reported by Goldiamond (1965). In our replication, two severe stutterers participated over a period of approximately four to six months. Baseline data on oral reading tasks were collected. Word-per-minute rates and percent of words containing disfluencies were determined. Baseline data were used for making subsequent comparisons of the effects induced via treatment variables. Treatment was initiated by establishing a slow speech rate using a paced, oral reading task. Words were extended in duration until an overall speech rate of approximately 30 words per minute was attained. It was observed that fluent speech was attained during the periods when the prolonged speech was in use. When disfluencies occurred occasionally during oral readings, delayed auditory feedback (DAF) was switched on temporarily and the speech rate was slowed. After a short period of time, DAF was faded out and oral reading continued. The oral reading pace was gradually accelerated until rates of approximately 120–160 words per minute were reached. After attaining the 120-word rate, participants were asked to transfer their improved speech fluency to conversational settings in the laboratory and in outside settings as well. The results were mixed. The positive result was that excellent fluency (disfluency rates for 20-min speech samples were under 1%) was demonstrated in the reading tasks. Improved fluency was observed in conversations held in the laboratory, but the disfluency rates were generally not below 3%. Transfer of speech to contexts outside the laboratory was very poor. In addition, home practice sessions were used in order to enhance transfer, but when these activities involved

the use of a tape recorder, the disfluency rates were indicative of poor retention of what had been taught in therapy.

PROGRAM II

The version of the therapy program introduced a number of changes. The basic fluency generating mechanism was still prolonged speech. Again, an oral reading task was used in therapy beginning with the slow reading rate of 30 words per minute. DAF was still used, but now in a different manner. This condition was used continuously during the first therapy session after the collection of baseline data and was gradually faded out during the first hour. The simple expediency of turning down the volume control constituted the fading technique. Reading rate was also controlled now through instructions and the pacing procedure was dropped because it proved to be rather cumbersome in use. The step in this program, which now in retrospect appears to have been most important in terms of its future consequences, involved "smoothing out" the slow speech that had been established in the first hours of therapy. The basic approach involved instructing the participant to reduce the speed and the amplitude employed in making consonant sounds while at the same time sustaining vowel durations. This smoothing procedure seemed to facilitate the client's acquisition of fluency. During practice sessions in the clinic, the participant worked diligently to smooth out his sounds within words, phrases, and sentences. The smooth-flowing quality of speech was enhanced by this procedure. In the event any stuttering was observed to occur, an instruction was given to smooth speech. In the event the instruction was not immediately effective, the speech rate was slowed until it was smooth and fluent and was then gradually speeded up again. After the speech rate was increased to approximately 110 words per minute, a rate discrimination training procedure was introduced. The participant read for a period of 2 min at a rate of approximately 110 words per min, and then switched to a slower rate (approximately 75 words a minute) for 2 min. Once performance had stabilized (disfluency rates below 1%) conversational training was initiated. The procedure used to simulate conversation involved having the subject describe pictures. This technique was highly productive of conversation. First, single sentences were used and then gradually two- and three-sentence conversations were developed. The next step involved having the participants converse with the experimenter in the laboratory. After approximately 5–8 hr of conversation in the laboratory context, an attempt was made to initiate fluent conversations in outside settings. An all-or-none transfer procedure was employed in which the person was instructed to use the new fluent speech pattern in conversations at home. If he was successful, he was to continue what he was doing. On the other hand, if he was initially unsuccessful, he was instructed to move completely to the pattern he had used most recently in the laboratory or was instructed to forget about the laboratory-taught behaviors altogether and rely on his prior nonfluent form of speech. In general, once fluent speech was initiated in the home, the transfer of these skills to other settings was attempted relatively quickly. Subjects monitored their own speech; when they reported that they had fewer than five major disfluencies a day in daily conversation, therapy was terminated. A total of 16 subjects went through Program II. Therapy time ranged from a low of 10 hours to a high of 40 hours.

Seven of the first eight clients who entered this program attained disfluency scores less than 1%; one had a 2% score (Webster, 1970). The dependent variable was the percent of words in which at least one disfluency was observed. Although these results were encouraging, a more careful analysis revealed mixed results. Good fluency had been observed in laboratory reading and conversation. Moderate success was seen in transfer to outside situations. The most important finding was that retention of fluent speech was difficult to maintain. The participants reported that they had substantial problems in concentrating on the production of fluent speech. In addition, we had observed that there was a noticeable reluctance on the part of more than half of the participants to actively seek out new transfer situations. We concluded that Program II was more effective than Program I but it was obvious that the generality of our procedures was inadequate and that the tasks required of the participants were not totally suitable for therapy.

VARIATIONS ON PROGRAM II

We made several attempts to enhance the efficacy of Program II. These variations were extremely important in the eventual development of the program. The

positive value of these efforts resulted from our exhaustion of attempts to enhance the essential characteristics of Program II. First, in an attempt to improve transfer to outside settings, we attempted to create finer task gradations while making the transition from oral reading to conversation. Great care was used to select a sequence of pictures which led logically into a conversational theme. In addition, efforts were made to simulate conversation by using popular plays. This manipulation showed some slight improvements in transfer with some of the treated cases but it also showed that we had clearly not provided a general enhancement of the therapy program. Our next venture involved providing extrinsic reinforcement for the use of fluency acquired in the treatment program. The procedure involved taking people through Program II; at those times in transfer activities when fluent speech was used, nickels were dispensed from the experimenter's coin dispenser. Although this was effective in encouraging participants to enter the transfer context, there was not a reliable performance increase in transfer. Retention of fluency was not generally improved. The apparent amount of concentration required to sustain fluent speech had not diminished.

Our next variation attempted to focus the participants' attention on fluency during transfer by providing mild punishment when fluent speech was not used. A remote control shocker provided a mild but uncomfortable shock to the forearm of the participant when the experimenter pressed a button. In transfer, the procedure was to provide a brief shock for each instance where disfluencies occurred. The most striking outcome of this procedure was that it suppressed conversational efforts. While there were powerful theoretical and practical reasons not to attempt to use punishment in the long-term control of behavior, we had considered the possibility that the brief use of punishment in transfer might focus the person's attention on the specific tasks involved in the production of fluent speech. Again, we had made a wrong choice. There were no noticeable improvements in transfer and the already somewhat negative aspects of transfer were further enhanced by the use of a punishment procedure. Therefore, we once again altered our thinking and sought another reasonable therapeutic variation.

Our next choice was based on the premise that anxiety has a major role in the genesis of stuttering behavior (Williams, 1968). Although we had no evidence from our data that anxiety was interfering with transfer activities, we considered the possibility of anxiety was a far more subtle and pervasive factor than we had previously assumed. We established a hierarchy of outside activities that involved speech. We taught muscle relaxation and presented the hierarchies during the periods of relaxation. Our relaxation technique was effective; we were frequently able to induce sleep in the participants. However, relatively little progress in transfer was accomplished with five different stutterers who used this variation. Several mild stutterers had an increased ease of transfer but the overall results of this approach were disappointing.

Another variation on Program II merits comment. Perhaps this variation was more indicative of our fatigue than our creativity. We decided that a cognitive approach might be beneficial and proceeded to employ "the power of positive thinking." The participants were taught to envision themselves standing in each transfer context, producing the very specific behaviors that they had learned in the laboratory. Instructions were given to see oneself as being successful, powerful, competent, and confident. Several participants were aided slightly by our exhortations, but no substantial measurable improvements in transfer were observed.

The main results of the Program II variants were negative. Essentially, we noted that a variety of careful manipulations was sometimes effective with some stutterers. Given the lawfulness observed in the establishment of fluency with the operant shaping procedures in the laboratory, it had appeared that the essential problem involved transfer. As a result, we had focused on transfer, per se, and had failed to consider the nature of the tasks used in therapy. We made progress when we examined the behaviors involved in the early stages of the therapy process.

PROGRAM III

This version of our evolving therapy tested the idea that perhaps difficulties previously observed in transfer and retention of fluency with our earlier programs were related to the inadequate specification of the responses that were to be learned in therapy. We had begun to suspect that fluent speech represented a set of behaviors that was too complex to learn well in therapy, particularly when working with long chains of behavior such as those involved in the production of phrases and sentences. We reasoned that the complexity inherent in speech was responsible for a type of learning that was relatively fragile and susceptible to interference when the participant was asked to use these behaviors under normal life conditions. We went on to attempt simplification of the behaviors taught in the program.

Once again, baseline data were collected during oral reading tasks and disfluency counts and reading rates were obtained. Therapy was initiated by having a participant stretch the duration of a spoken word. This time, however, single words were presented instead of a continuous oral reading task. Each word was stretched for 3–4 sec by prolonging vowels. After stabilizing performance on individual words, the gentle initiation of speech sounds was taught. This particular behavior was derived from earlier efforts to smooth speech. We found that gentle initiation of speech sounds was a powerful fluency-generating response in this version of our program. We also learned that the exaggeration of the responses taught in therapy permitted both the experimenter and the participant to note the details of vowel prolongation and the gentle initiation of consonants. In addition, the experimenter's evaluation of each individual response could be immediately presented to the participant. This is an important point. The feedback of information to the learner immediately after a single-word utterance was more accurate and more timely than when we attempted to call attention to some event embedded within a phrase or sentence. As a next step, a long progression of single words (300–500 words) was presented. Word durations were gradually shortened until a slow normal speech rate (about 120 words per minute) was obtained. Transfer of fluent speech into conversation occurred by having the participant first create short phrases from single-word cues. A gradual change was made to the production of longer sentences and then into spontaneous conversation. Fluent conversation was then transferred into a variety of settings in our laboratory. Finally, transfer of fluent speech to the home environment was scheduled and practiced at certain times and at certain places. A fairly rapid extension into the use of fluent speech throughout the day occurred.

The results of this program were better than our previous ones—this was obtained in oral reading in the laboratory settings. The transfer process was less noxious and participants were more willing to attempt a variety of transfer activities than with our prior therapies. The main advantage of this therapy version was that the participants reported a more developed sense of what they did to sustain fluent speech. The results of this program encouraged us to extend the specification of behaviors that should be at focus in therapy.

PROGRAM IV

A number of changes were introduced in this program. The first alteration involved standardizing the size of the response unit used in therapy. The previous program had used single words comprised of various numbers of syllables. We decided to test the utility of the syllable as the basic element to be manipulated in therapy. Thus, after establishing baseline measures, we started participants in therapy by stretching one-syllable words and then moved on progressively to two-syllable words, three-syllable words, short self-generated sentences, longer sentences, and then finally conversation in the laboratory and the subsequent transfer of fluent speech to outside settings.

A change in the instructional procedure was also introduced. We had previously observed that the experimenter often served as a strong cue for the participant's use of fluent speech. In some ways, it appeared as if the experimenter actually inhibited the transfer of fluent speech to everyday life settings. We considered the possibility that the nature of the interaction between the experimenter and the participant was at fault. We introduced a procedure for returning information to the participant that used a system of signal lights instead of the usual conversational exchange. The experimenter sat in the room with the participant, and after each speech response the participant pressed a button which was held in his hand. If the response was judged to be correct by the experimenter, he closed a switch and a green light came on when the participant pressed his button. If the response was judged to be incorrect, nothing happened when the participant pressed his button. It was necessary after a missed response for the participant to self-correct. That is, instead of having the experimenter step in and explain what had gone wrong, the participant had to determine the specific behaviors that were to be corrected and then he had to repeat the response. These changes in the specification of the behavior and the instructional

procedures were found to enhance the power of the program. The acquisition, transfer, and retention of fluency occurred with substantially greater ease for the participant. The experimenter's task was also made easier. The enhanced specificity of the behaviors to be learned in therapy resulted in a more explicit form of training and a more highly developed form of control on the part of the speech of the participants.

PROGRAM V

The behavioral analyses conducted through four versions of the therapy had indicated to us the importance of enhancing the definition of basic fluency-generating skills that were used in therapy. We continued to extend these efforts in the development of Program V by carefully examining the speech sound characteristics of approximately 60 stutterers. A series of manipulations of articulatory and phonatory characteristics were conducted. Particular attention was paid to those behavior changes that resulted in the reliably fluent production of various sounds. From these tests we were able to determine tentative definitions of "target" behaviors which appeared to be precursors to fluent speech. These fluency targets were incorporated in our fifth program.

With this version of the program, our essential concept in therapy began to move away from fluent speech as the therapy goal and toward the attainment of rather specific phonatory and articulatory behaviors which appeared to be antecedent to the production of fluent speech. We were beginning to appreciate the extent to which fluency represents a term that is applied to the appearance of certain forms of speech responses. We were at last beginning to define the substrate of those behaviors that were in fact responsible for fluency. Note that while fluency was the consequence of attaining target behaviors, the target behaviors themselves were now moved to the heart of therapy.

The fifth version of the program was assembled during the Summer and Fall of 1969. The basic structure of the program involved establishing a very slow speech flow in which syllables were prolonged for two seconds. This exaggerated form of slow-motion speech was used only in the laboratory. The next step involved teaching the client a series of skills that were associated with various sound classes. Vowel sounds were dealt with first. Each vowel sound was presented in isolation. The client's task was to learn to attain the correct amplitude versus time contour for these sounds. The skill to be acquired involved the gentle initiation of voicing. The second class of sounds involved syllables with consonants in the initial position. All consonants in this sound class were voiced continuants and involved the target behaviors of increased consonant duration, increased vowel duration, and the gentle onset of voicing. The third sound class dealt with the production of syllables initiated with voiceless fricatives. Reduced intraoral air pressures were taught followed by gentle onset of the succeeding sound. The last sound class, plosive consonants, involved reduced intraoral pressures, soft lip and tongue contact, and the gentle onset of voicing.

After the basic phonatory and articulatory skills were established, one-syllable words were introduced and all targets previously taught were practiced in a series of randomly presented sequences. The slowed speech flow was also transferred into laboratory settings. Subsequently, two-syllable words, three-syllable words, short self-generated sentences, and spontaneous speech were undertaken. During this portion of therapy, syllable durations were systematically reduced. By the time spontaneous conversation was reached, a slow-normal speech rate (about 120 words per minute) had been attained.

The transfer portion of therapy was somewhat different for each client. Each person was first given the opportunity to use the telephone for the purpose of calling local businesses with messages that had been determined by the therapist. When this phase of the transfer activities was judged to be successful, the subject went out into the community and talked with merchants in a variety of settings. Tape recordings were made during these transfer settings and were checked by both the therapist and the client. If any difficulties were experienced by the client, the therapist identified the specific target behaviors that had been deficient in their production and additional practice was provided in the laboratory prior to returning to transfer activities. In the course of working out the transfer activities, it was found that the careful transfer of the fluency-generating targets into the laboratory context seemed to be important. Therefore, steps were inserted to provide parallel transfer training of laboratory skills into conversation in the laboratory. This single step seemed to enhance the ease with which transfer could be undertaken at the end of the program.

The daily laboratory routine consisted of from 10 to 18 20-min periods during which the client worked in the program under the guidance of a therapist. Progress from one stage of the program to the next was made after the client had attained an accuracy of better than 84% on the skill being practiced for two successive 20-min periods. A running record of correct versus incorrect responses was kept during each work period. The results of this therapy program have been reported elsewhere (Webster, 1974b). A total of 56 stutterers (47 males and 9 females) participated in the early stages of work on Program V. Their ages ranged from 8 to 59 yr. The mean pretreatment disfluent word rate for all participants was 15.8%. The mean posttreatment disfluent word rate was 0.9%. The total time in therapy for these participants averaged 50 hr. A follow-up study conducted two years posttherapy on 20 randomly selected cases out of the 56 treated yielded a mean disfluency score of 2.4%.

With the improved definition of fluency-generating skills attained in Program V, it seemed reasonable to attempt the quantification of what we judged to be the most important of those skills. The role of the gentle voice onset became increasingly important as we continued our work on stuttering. With Program V, we learned a great deal about specific movement patterns involved in fluent production of the sounds and syllables of American English. In particular, we began to establish reliable subjective standards for accepting or rejecting attempts to produce gentle voice onsets. It occurred to us that we could ease the task of the therapist, improve the accuracy with which judgments were made about the correctness of the subject's voice onsets, and increase the efficiency of the client's performance in the program if we could establish a computer system that could make judgments about speech sounds. Thanks to my colleague, Professor Keith Hege (Department of Physics, Hollins College), and Reggie Schoonover, one of our graduate students, we were able to establish a computer-based evaluation system for voice onsets. An analog speech signal was run through a series of circuits which amplified and then digitized the incoming speech signal and fed it to the computer. The properties of the incoming signal were read by the computer and stored in memory. Next, the computer searched its memory to find the appropriate reference values for the specific sound that the stutterer was making. Finally, in just a brief part of a second, the computer compared the incoming signal with the standard and made a decision about its adequacy. If the incoming signal met certain criteria, the computer indicated to the user that the speech sound had been made properly.

In January, 1971, we began to use the computer as a regular adjunct in the fluency shaping program. The stutterers were very positive in their evaluations of their interactions with the computer. They believed that the computer was consistent and fair in its judgments about the adequacy of their speech responses. Previously, we had been asking our therapists to make decisions about rather minute characteristics of behavior; it was no surprise to find that the computer was a more reliable judge of minute behavior characteristics than were the human therapists. One of the important results of using the computer was particularly that the stutterers learned more quickly the specific movement patterns involved in producing speech sounds. The transfer of these skills to laboratory and outside settings was also enhanced with the introduction of the computer.

PROGRAM VI

A number of developments occurred within Program V that eventually led to the definition our sixth therapy program during the Fall of 1974. By this time it had become clear to us that the objective, physical definition of target behaviors improved the reliability of therapy and the consequent retention of fluency. Target definitions were tightened, self-measurement of syllable durations with stopwatches was introduced, and the general-purpose laboratory computer was replaced with a specially constructed voice onset computer designated as the Voice Monitor. The therapy sequence assumed a well-standardized format and programmed texts were published. Nonpublished versions of texts had been introduced in Programs IV and V. An overview of Program VI is shown in Table 16–1.

A series of studies yielded two important refinements for Program VI. Advancement criteria were determined for each target in therapy. The attainment of the quantitatively specified criteria permitted the client to progress from one step to the next. Performance norms were also established. The number of 20-min therapy sessions spent by 100 stutterers on each program segment was compiled to provide normative data regarding the acquisition time for each of the therapy segments. Means and standard deviations were computed in order to facilitate the assessment of progress by a client in therapy with the normative data.

Other refinements were also introduced. In previous therapy versions we had attempted to change respiratory behaviors in selected clients by teaching diaphragmatic control of breathing. However, as we continued to attempt to identify those clients who would benefit from this training, we found increasingly that our "pick-and-choose" approach was less reliable than the simple expediency of teaching all the stutterers respiratory control. This became an important general principle in the program. Because of the reliance on the human clinician as the diagnostic entity, and because of the difficulty in relating specific forms of disfluencies to the amount of practice that might be required to establish a given target behavior, the attempts to individualize therapy by selecting targets that might be needed for some stutterers and not others was replaced by a different procedure. With Program VI, all target behaviors were taught to all stutterers. The transfer activities were also standardized. We had learned that with the careful parallel transfer of fluency targets into the laboratory environment, transfer no longer required a menu of activities that served as a basis for selecting a particular one that might or might not work for a given stutterer. The standardized transfer process in the last segment of the therapy program begins with single-message telephone calls spoken at a slow-normal speech rate. Short single-message calls are used and followed by trips to shopping centers where, again, single-message interactions are involved. The transfer process then becomes more complex as double-message telephone and double-message personal contacts occur. The transition to multiple messages on the telephone and in outside settings proceeds very rapidly and routinely for most participants.

Another important form of learning took place when we began identifying the central values for targets and the permissible range of variation. Special attention was directed to controlling the variability of behavior as the clients begin to learn specific targets. As a general finding, we observed that the restriction of variability to specified limits during therapy, when compared with procedures which did not control variability, facilitated both the acquisition of target behaviors and their transfer to other settings. Several of the events that facilitated control of variability involved training clinicians more carefully in target values and their tolerances, introducing standardized

Table 16-1. Overview of the precision fluency shaping program: Speech reconstruction for stutterers.

Part I

Assessment of speech characteristics and self-report data
    500 words oral reading
    300–500 words conversation
    Perceptions of Stuttering Inventory and other tests

Establishment of slow-motion speech flow

Training in diaphragmatic control of respiration
    Coordination of diaphragmatic breathing with slow-motion flow (Transfer)
    Coordination of gentle voice onset with production of voiced continuants (Transfer)
    Coordination of gentle voice onset with production of voiceless fricatives (Transfer)
    Coordination of gentle voice onset with production of plosives (Transfer)

Part II

Integration and consolidation of targets—one-syllable words (Transfer)

Integration and consolidation of targets—two- and three-syllable words/
Reduction in exaggeration of target values (Transfer)

Short self-generated speech chains (Transfer)

Part III

Intensive outside transfer I
    Single message—Telephone
                —Personal contact

Intensive outside transfer II
    Double message—Telephone
                   —Personal contact

Intensive outside transfer III
    Multiple messages—all contacts

Posttreatment assessment
    500 words oral reading
    300–500 words conversation
    Perceptions of Stuttering Inventory and other tests

At-home practice program—1 wk

instruction sets for use in therapy, and employing Voice Monitors and stopwatches as instruments to aid in the measurement of the behaviors being learned.

It became evident during the course of Program V that perhaps we had been expecting clients to complete therapy in less time than was actually needed to acquire effective control of fluency generating skills. Therefore, the total amount of time involved to complete therapy for Program VI was increased to approximately 100 hrs.

We conduct this therapy program over a 3-wk period. Approximately 1,000 stutterers have partici-

pated in Programs V and VI. A comprehensive report on the detailed structure of the program and long-term results is in preparation.

A summary of results obtained with 200 randomly selected cases as shown in Table 16–2. The response measure is a count of spoken words which contained at least one disfluent event. The speech samples used for obtaining these scores included standardized 500-word reading passages (different passages were used for the pretreatment, posttreatment and follow-up) and from 300 to 500 words of spontaneous conversation. The follow-up data were obtained through the use of surprise telephone calls to clients who had previously completed the therapy program. The time between entry and posttreatment samples was 19 consecutive days. The average time between the posttreatment sample and follow-up sample was ten months. However, the range in time out of therapy was 41 months. In addition, self-report data have been derived with a variety of tests and inventories. One of the more important self-report inventories used was the Perceptions of Stuttering Inventory (PSI). The PSI is a 60-item checklist developed by Woolf (1967). The pretreatment mean PSI score for those 200 cases already mentioned was 30.4. The posttreatment means PSI score was 5.7 and the follow-up PSI score was 9.2. PSI scores of ten or under are regarded as being in the normal range. The speech performance data and self-report data are in agreement regarding the nature of the behavior changes induced by stutterers' participation in therapy.

CONCLUSION

In this presentation, I have reviewed the evolutionary steps that led to the emergence of our Precision Fluency Shaping Program. The development of a specialized technology for treating stuttering requires the concomitant development of dissemination mechanisms that carry the relevant information to the clinical community. We have found that written reports and oral presentations are inadequate for providing clinicians with the skills required for effective implementation of therapy. The learning of target values, permissible variations in targets, and the discrimination of targets at various levels of exaggeration are skills that can be established only through specialized training of the would-be program user. The lack of these skills has been firmly linked to incorrect and inadequate program administration. The

measured presence of these skills at high levels is associated with effective program implementation.

Thus, we now have some appreciation for the technical skills that are required for effective clinician performance in the administration of this program. The identification of a set of specific clinical skills and the measurement of these skills appears to provide a way of assessing the clinician's contribution to the reliability and validity of the therapeutic process. Also, the separation of the clinician from the technology enhances our understanding of the respective contribution of each.

The reliable implementation of fluent speech with target behaviors seems to imply that the central events in stuttering must be the distorted gestures of articulation, phonation, and possibly respiration. While there is little doubt that accessory speech responses, accessory nonspeech responses, and personal reactions to others or self are important in the eventual understanding of the stuttering complex, our experience suggests the primacy of distorted articulatory and phonatory gestures in the definition of stuttering. While it has been a theme in the literature on stuttering that the current approaches to manipulating speech-response details are nothing but a dusting off of older procedures, I must take exception with that point of view. The precision with which responses are manipulated in the therapy outlined here, the physical specifiability of the responses that are precursors to fluency, and the high reliability of the manipulative procedures themselves suggest that the efficacy of therapy is likely to be enhanced when we focus with even more precision on the measurement of behavior and the change procedures used with these behaviors. I have provided a preliminary organization of the stuttering complex elsewhere (Webster, 1978). In this definition, the central features of stuttering are represented directly and only in motor events which occur at the level of the larnyx and the vocal tract. A

Table 16-2. Pretreatment, posttreatment and follow-up disfluency scores for combined oral reading and conversational samples in 200 randomly selected cases.

	Pretreatment	Posttreatment	Follow-up
Mean percent disfluent words	15.2	1.3	3.2
Percent of cases with disfluency scores at or below 3%	3.0	92.0	80.0

rationale for suggesting this specific organization for the stuttering phenomenon has been derived from the repeated observation that targets propagate fluent responses in stutterers. In addition, the improvements in therapy that have been consistently associated with refinements in the definition and manipulation of phonation and articulation also suggest their importance in the identification of central features in stuttering.

I believe that the primary goal in stuttering therapy is essentially the same as that in basic research on stuttering—to increase our understanding of the phenomena involved in the problem. Through the search for understanding we can expect to find increased knowledge of lawfulness in stuttering and eventually an enhanced ability to treat the disorder.

REFERENCES

Goldiamond, I. Stuttering and fluency as manipulatable operant response classes. In Krasner, L. and Ullmann, L. P. (Eds.), *Research in Behavior Modification: New Developments and Implications.* New York: Holt, Rinehart and Winston, 1965.

Van Riper, C. *The Treatment of Stuttering.* Englewood Cliffs, New Jersey: Prentice-Hall, 1973.

Webster, R. L. Stuttering: A way to eliminate it and a way to explain it. In Ulrich, R., Stachnik, T. and Mabry, J. (Eds.), *Control of Human Behavior: Volume II.* Glenview, Illinois: Scott, Foresman, 1970.

Webster, R. L. *The Precision Fluency Shaping Program: Speech Reconstruction for Stutterers.* Roanoke, Virginia: Communications Development Corporation, Ltd., 1974a.

Webster, R. L. A behavioral analysis of stuttering: Treatment and theory. In Calhoun, K. S., Adams, H. L. and Mitchell, K. M. (Eds.), *Innovative Treatment Methods in Psychopathology.* New York: Wiley, 1974b.

Webster, R. L. Empirical considerations regarding controversies in stuttering therapy. In Gregory, H. (Ed.), *Controversies about Stuttering Therapy.* Baltimore, Maryland: University Park Press, 1978.

Williams, D. E. Stuttering therapy: An overview. In Gregory, H. (Ed.), *Learning Theory and Stuttering Therapy.* Evanston, Illinois: Northwestern University Press, 1968.

Woolf, G. The assessment of stuttering as struggle, avoidance, and expectancy. *The British Journal of Disorders of Communication, 1967, 2,* 158–171.

Stuttering Therapy From a Technological Point of View

Ronald L. Webster

TECHNOLOGY AND STUTTERING THERAPY

A technology is represented by a specific set of procedures applied to a given problem in order to solve it. Technologies are typically drawn out of empirical analyses of problems. They focus on practical, replicable aspects of problem-solving rather than on creating or maintaining theoretical formulations. The comments in this brief presentation have been strongly conditioned by the recognition that stuttering therapies are technologies. Considering therapies to be technologies seems to have considerable relevance for the future treatment of those who stutter.

There are at least two long-standing and widely held assumptions about stuttering that are encountered as barriers when one assumes a technological orientation toward stuttering therapy. In my view, these related and interacting assumptions, as noble, as desirable, and as eloquently argued as they may be, constitute serious impediments to developments in both stuttering therapy and basic research on stuttering. The functional consequences of these assumptions are unrealistic burdens on clinicians and the direction of attention away from issues that lie at the heart of stuttering therapy.

One assumption that is so strongly held that to question it is to invite attack is what might be called the "clinical imperative." It states that the individual clinician will do all within his or her power to meet the needs of the client. While I presume that few of us would argue the merits of the statement, the practical problems associated with its fulfillment are enormous. There is virtually no uniform system for identifying the individual needs of stutterers (Van Riper, 1971, 1973; Bloodstein, 1975; Wingate, 1976). From a practical point of view there is essentially no agreement on how specific needs of stutterers are to be met (Gregory, 1979). All this is complicated further by the relative paucity of useful clinical experience that student trainees have with stutterers. Clinician training in many respects emphasizes a general clinical method based on the intuitive selection of one "therapeutic approach" or another. Clinicians are reminded to be sensitive to the merits of new "approaches" and to select from any such approaches

---

Postscript 16

---

those aspects of treatment that can be melded with others used by the clinician. It seems to me that the clinical imperative provides a basis for much of the frustration voiced by those who work professionally with stutterers. Well-meaning, well-motivated individuals are simply not equipped with the tools to define and meet the individual needs of their clients who stutter.

A second major assumption is that each stutterer presents a unique problem. Clinicians are urged to be alert to differences between and among their clients and to accommodate therapies to these differences. This assumption about the presumed individuality of stutterers flies in the face of a significant tenet of the scientific method—which simply stated says that we search for common elements in seemingly disparate events. In addition, the practical consequences of this assumption place staggering burdens upon the clinician. If there are only eight different kinds of stutterers and only ten different intervention procedures to draw from, then the odds are approximately one in forty that a correct match would be made. These numbers seem to place an awesome responsibility on the shoulders of the clinician. One can reasonably assert that the clinician is faced with a virtually impossible task if there is to be reliable matching of therapy approaches to stutterers.

The merits of a technological analysis of stuttering therapy seem substantial. Perhaps the single most important strength inherent in the idea is the sustained practical, empirical emphasis on what is actually done by the clinician and what is actually learned by the client. I believe that the arena of stuttering therapy has been excessively concerned with theory, assumption, and speculation (Webster, 1977). Little will be lost and much might be gained if a thorough-going technological analysis is directed toward various forms of stuttering therapy.

GENERAL PROPERTIES OF TECHNOLOGY

A simplified general outline of the major stages in technology development is presented here as a preface to discussing specific aspects of the behavioral and electronic technologies represented in the Precision Fluency Shaping Program. Note that behavioral technology is judged to be properly included within the broader discussion of technology. Stuttering therapies are behavioral technologies.

Developing a technology begins with an empirical definition of a problem requiring resolution. The key word here is empirical—the definition focuses exclusively on events lying within the direct sensory experience of the observer. To the extent possible, quantification of the problem and its associated dimensions is desirable. In general, the more adequate the level of quantification achieved, the greater is the likelihood that results of technological development can be assessed. A next step, or in fact what is likely to become a long series of steps, involves generating and testing a set of alternative tentative solutions to the problem. A number of consequences may be associated with the tests. Those tentative solutions that fail to advance the actual solution to the problem are discarded. Those that are somewhat successful are revised for further testing. Those that are successful are kept for later use and integration in more completely formulated solutions. It is also not unusual to find that the definition of the problem undergoes refinement as tentative solutions are tried out and better approximations are found. The practical side of the developing technology is emphasized with continuing attention to results. The quality and reliability of the results is the overriding concern that guides further developments. Development of a complex technology is often a long and expensive process.

Technology Development in the Precision Fluency Shaping Program

Early work on our therapy program was concerned with the practical goal of establishing fluent speech in stutterers. The major procedure initially tested in Program I used the shaping of prolonged speech during oral reading into fluent speech at normal rates of speaking. Insufficient progress was observed in client transfer of fluent speech into conversations both in the laboratory and nonlaboratory settings. A series of modifications in procedure were tried in Program II and its variants. Once more, even though some progress was noted, the replicability of results with large numbers of stutterers was not adequate. Programs III and IV led to a gradual redefinition of the procedures used. Smaller response units were identified, and instructional methods were improved. Noticeable improvements in the reliability of fluency acquisition, transfer, and maintenance were observed. Program V was based on a shift in the definition of the problem at focus in therapy. The goal shifted from establishing fluent speech, per se, to establishing specific response elements identified at the level of speech and respiratory gestures. Fluent speech was now seen to be the direct result of attaining certain physical values in the force, acceleration, and position of specific gestures. The emphasis in treatment became training clients to produce these specific gestures. The physical specification of targets was attained at a level of objectivity that permitted increased reliability of clinician instruction, increased observability of responses by the clients, and the use of a computer to measure aspects of voice onsets during therapy. As I noted in the preceding article, "advances in the adequacy of therapy were linked to our ability to observe, measure and manipulate relatively tiny behavioral details." I wish to underscore the importance of that observation here. It was clear that by the time we had reached Program V an objectively based stuttering therapy technology was attainable. It was also clear that we were nowhere near being finished with developing the therapy.

A more complete therapy technology was attained with Program VI. In addition to identifying specific fluency-generating targets for respiration, phonation, and articulatory gestures, and their sequences of use in therapy, we tentatively defined permissible ranges of variation in targets during their acquisition by clients. It was recognized that clients learned errors in target attainment in much the same way that correct responses were acquired. Clients who demonstrated excessive variability during the initial stages of target learning were observed to have difficulty in adding subsequent targets to the sequence used in

Postscript 16

therapy. Transfer of target-based fluent speech to outside the clinic and long-term retention of fluent speech were less adequate in those clients who acquired targets with excessive variation than in those who demonstrated reduced variation.

Instruction sets were refined, standardized, and then empirically validated. Each program step had its own written instruction set developed and tested for client comprehension. Instruction sets that were difficult for more than about 15% or more of the clients were revised until they were comprehended by approximately 85% or more of the clients. Standard instruction sets reduced clinician variability in guiding client's target acquisition and increased the efficiency of the therapy process.

The reader may not clearly understand the concept of standardization in clinical instruction. The point here is not that standard instruction sets are complete and are never to be varied. However, the need for specific variations can be defined through program use, and the necessary variants can be prepared and made available within the original instruction set. Variations in instruction can be introduced on a controlled, empirical basis and their consequences related to those of the standard instructions. Variation in clinical instruction was needed less often than any of us had anticipated. This observation may stem from the relatively complete specification of respiration, phonatory, and articulatory targets on which the therapy is based.

Each of 49 separate program segments were examined in order to define advancement criteria and performance norms that would have practical clinical relevance. Advancement criteria for each segment were established on the basis of clinical observations regarding client stability in target usage and included the number of practice trials in each segment and the number of correct responses required in order to move to the next segment. These criteria are minimum trials required for client mastery of the target presented in each segment. Continued experience with the program has indicated that advancement criteria will be revised further in the near future. General performance norms were provided so clinicians could readily evaluate client learning at each program segment. These norms were created by measuring the amount of time required for 100 clients to complete each program segment. Means and standard deviations were calculated to provide a basis for comparing the behavior of a client in therapy with the norms. In this manner, the clinician has information that permits continuing evaluation of a client's progress in each segment of the therapy program against known standards. Deviations in client performance can be readily detected and appropriate adjustments made in instruction or practice procedures. Performance norms also provide a standard basis for evaluating how well clinicians who are attempting replications of therapy are proceeding with their efforts. Finally, performance norms yield a standard background against which clinical judgments can be made.

Phenomena in nature have their own dimensions. An understanding of natural phenomena is necessarily predicated upon learning enough about relevant dimensions to create a sense of how different variables fit together. The development of a technology also functions the same way. Relevant dimensions of the problem at focus must be discerned and their interrelationships probed. We are beginning to have a sense of the many empirical dimensions that yield a relatively reliable and efficient stuttering therapy. One such dimension involves time—the amount and distribution of time spent involved directly with the therapy process. Early on in our work, with Programs III through V, we made an observation that has been quite important in our subsequent structuring of therapy. It appears, given the characteristics of the PFSP, that clients who spend less then ten hours per week practicing the behaviors taught in therapy progress relatively slowly. The clearest example of this point lies in an examination of therapy dropout rates. With the intensive three-week therapy program now used at our institution, the dropout rate is less than 1%. However, with the versions of the program involving less than ten hours of practice per week, therapy dropout rates rose to between 25% and 50%.

Another aspect of practice time is important. It seems desirable to have a stuttering therapy program that constitutes a single, intensive experience for the client. One apparent requirement for such a therapy is that clients have sufficient time to learn, overlearn, and integrate the particular skills taught in therapy. The information that we have acquired to date regarding the amount of time required for successfully completing therapy indicates that probably between 100 and 120 carefully supervised hours are needed for most clients. Less time in therapy seems to be associated with less stable transfer and retention of fluency skills.

Combining Behavioral and Electronic Technologies

Objectivity in behavior specification carries with it the possibility that physical measurement of the behavior can be achieved and used for practical purposes. A central target behavior in the PFSP involves the controlled onset of voicing. Specific amplitude versus time values were established as criteria for each of the three major program segments. The Voice Monitor, a special-purpose computer designed to measure these criteria in either single utterances or connected speech, was created in order to increase the objectivity and efficiency of therapy. We found that client reliability in gentle voice-onset target acquisition was markedly enhanced when the Voice Monitor became a standard component in therapy. Stable criterion values were used with the client from trial to trial. This procedure improved client awareness and control of the gestures responsible for vocal production. The integration of the gentle voice-onset target with other target behaviors was facilitated since the Voice Monitor could be used in all the major therapy segments. It seemed quite clear that the immediacy, reliability, and accuracy of feedback to clients learning the gentle voice-onset target provided an "electronic boost" to the fundamental learning principles on which the therapy was based. We were pleased to find that clients quickly accepted the addition of an electronic technology to the behavioral technology represented in therapy.

Postscript 16

Additional forms of feedback were used during the clients' learning of other target behaviors. For example, stopwatches were introduced as a means of measuring syllable durations, thereby adding to the control of variability in syllable production. Clients used the watch at various stages of therapy to monitor specific syllable durations that were to be achieved at each stage. A respiration trainer has also been developed for the purpose of facilitating client acquisition of diaphragmatic breathing and its coordination with other targets.

Multiple technologies can be readily combined as long as care is taken to join them in a manner that attains the overall goals set for the project. In fact, synergism often results.

TECHNOLOGY AND BASIC SCIENTIFIC PRINCIPLES

Technologies frequently employ principles derived from basic scientific research. Developments in modern drug technologies flow largely from an extensive knowledge of basic chemistry. The production of microchips containing tens of thousands of switching circuits is based on the knowledge of principles involving complex gas laws; conditions that govern state changes in various molecules used in depositing layers of conducting, semiconducting or nonconducting materials on the chips; and laws that govern electron flow at junctions in the circuits. In a similar manner, basic principles of learning have been used to establish and transfer fluency skills involved in the PFSP.

Response shaping is used extensively in the therapy. Responses are taught as small units, usually specified at the level of individual gestures or small groups of gestures. There is an orderly concatenation of small response units into complex behavior sequences. All behaviors are established initially with exaggeration sufficient to permit client monitoring and control of tiny movement details. Each response unit is overlearned and then integrated with other units that are in turn overlearned in combination with each other. Immediate information feedback is provided by instruments and the trained clinician during the acquisition and integration of fluency generating targets. Response generalization is controlled, and parallel transfer procedures have been developed to maximize stimulus generalization of fluency skills from clinic to nonclinic settings. Gradual changes in response requirements and stimulus conditions that exert stimulus control over behavior are faded in or out as required by the structure of therapy.

CONDITIONS NECESSARY FOR TECHNOLOGY
DEVELOPMENT

Special conditions are often required to develop complex technologies. For example, the technology for growing large quantities of living mammalian cells that can be used to synthesize medically significant proteins such as interferon and monoclonal antibodies has special requirements. Specialists in biochemistry, biophysics, and physics were among the professionals that worked to develop the technology. Particular laboratory conditions had to be maintained and special apparatus had to be developed. In addition, a substantial long-term commitment of financial resources was made. Few of us would expect such a sophisticated technology to be developed by an individual medical practitioner. However, in the area of stuttering, it appears to be a common expectation that the individual clinician can indeed synthesize a reliable and valid therapy that will meet the needs of the client.

Our experiences suggest that an effective stuttering therapy technology is likely to be complex. It has become increasingly evident that special circumstances are required if reliable and valid stuttering therapies are to be developed. Some of the relevant conditions are discussed briefly as follows.

Personnel are central to the development of any technology. At various times our work has involved contributions by psychologists, speech pathologists, otolaryngologists, physicists, electrical engineers, and computer scientists. Particular biases were shared by these persons. All were empirically oriented, most were seriously interested in data collection and the techniques of data analysis, and most were intrigued with the idea that a standard therapy could be attained for stuttering. Participation by these individuals was usually on a full-time, professional basis.

Another important requirement for the development of a stuttering therapy technology involves the availability of stutterers in numbers sufficient to provide adequate tests of specific procedures and instruments. More than 1,600 stutterers have participated in various facets of our work. Without the cooperation of large numbers of stutterers, there is no truly effective way to evaluate the reliability, validity, or generality of therapy programs.

Still another critical condition conducive to the development of a stuttering therapy technology was a long-term commitment of institutional resources to the problem of stuttering. The Hollins Communications Research Institute at Hollins College, Roanoke, VA, was established as a center dedicated to the development of research and treatment programs on stuttering. Financial resources have been developed specifically for a substantial effort in this area, and work has been sustained now for approximately 10 years.

LIMITATIONS IN A TECHNOLOGICAL APPROACH TO STUTTERING THERAPY

It is clear that the technology of stuttering therapy is not without problems. We have found, for example, that the therapy is rather difficult to disseminate. The therapy is based heavily upon specific clinician skills that depend on accurate, rapid multiple discriminations of targets at rapid speech rates. We have found that clinicians vary rather widely in their abilities to discriminate target values, and therefore, a specialized form of training appears to be necessary for potential clinician users of the program.

We have also found that clinicians using the program require a certain amount of sustained practice with the therapy if appropriate skill levels are to be

Postscript   16

developed and maintained. A learning curve has been observed with effective clinician users of therapy. This learning curve seems to be closely related to the quality of their initial training and the support provided as clinicians initiate use of the program in their own working environments.

We have found in our own work that there are additional problems that can occur with the clinical staff. One serious problem is that the sustained iteration of a standard therapy program becomes rather stale after an intensive involvement with that therapy for a period of 3–5 years. Therefore, special schedule requirements and variations in clinical routines are necessary if clinicians are to be protected against this burnout phenomenon.

We also feel that the targets employed in the therapy program need further objectification and quantification. We are directing research efforts at this problem at the present time, and hope to see some improvements in the near future. At the present time it is quite clear that the subjective evaluation of target values by the clinician contributes a certain amount of variability to the feedback clients receive. Better observation and measurement of target values will improve our knowledge of exactly what is being learned by clients in therapy and the quality with which skills are being learned.

We are not satisfied with the current level of development manifested in our therapy technology. There are stutterers who, for reasons that are not clear, acquire the therapy skills and then seem to lose the discrimination of the relevant behavior dimensions. There are some stutterers who appear to have extensive difficulty in integrating a number of target behaviors within the speech flow at normal rates. There are also stutterers who have fundamental difficulties in acquiring certain of the target behaviors. Finally, there are some stutterers, a few in number, who indicate that they are motivated to acquire fluent speech, but their behavior in fact belies their claims. On the whole, the fact that approximately 90–95% of the stutterers who enter therapy are capable of acquiring the fluency skills at reasonable levels strongly encourages the approach that we have taken. Rather than cast about for new "approaches" to stuttering therapy, we are finding that our most productive path lies in elaborating and refining our knowledge of the behavior dimensions that seem to be fundamental to the propogation of fluent speech in those who stutter.

REFERENCES

Bloodstein, O. (1975). *A handbook on stuttering*. Chicago: National Easter Seal Society for Crippled Children and Adults.

Gregory, H. (1979). *Controversies about stuttering therapy*. Baltimore, MD: University Park Press.

Van Riper, C. (1971). *The nature of stuttering*. Englewood Cliffs, NJ: Prentice-Hall.

Van Riper, C. (1973). *The treatment of stuttering*. Englewood Cliffs, NJ: Prentice-Hall.

Webster, R. L. (1977). Concept and theory in stuttering: An insufficiency of empiricism. In R. Rieber (Ed.), *The problem of stuttering: Theory and therapy*. New York: Elsevier.

17

Operant Procedures Applied to Stuttering Therapy for Children

Postscript
Operant Therapy for Children

Bruce P. Ryan

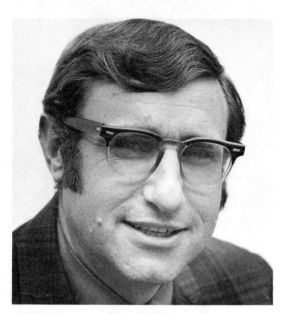

Bruce P. Ryan

Over a period of 15 years Ryan has been conducting clinical research in operant therapy for stuttering children, gradually refining his management programs in accordance with his findings. He is a careful and thorough worker who in the opinion of his colleagues has become one of the foremost authorities in operant programming for this population. At the same time that he has been varying the conventional parameters of behavior modification programs: step size, reinforcement schedules, criteria for advancement, branching, etc., Ryan has also begun to explore covert variables such as attitude and motivation. In addition, he is working on the important therapeutic phases of maintenance and transfer, where operant programs have received criticism.

Ryan is an articulate expositor of his approach whose personal style has won over his audiences for years, and his writing is also convincing. He has explored a number of tactics for obtaining the initial change in the stutterer's speech. These may all be characterized as fluency-shaping procedures. From his research the GILCU program has emerged as a viable, easy-to-administer, and popular procedure. Moving from simple or molecular responses to more natural, complex, and spontaneous ones has long been a component of many programs in speech pathology, but it remained for Ryan to formalize the procedure in his Gradual Increase in Length and Complexity of Utterance Program.

Ryan's operant perspective has not been limited to the problem of stuttering, as evidenced by his authorships of the Monterey Programs for language and articulation problems in children. The same strategies for instatement, transfer, and maintenance of target behaviors appear to have generic application across disorders. With Van Kirk he has applied these programs to the public school context, gathering considerable data to support, popularize, and justify his enthusiasm about the outcome of his therapy programs.

17

Operant Procedures Applied to Stuttering Therapy for Children

Bruce P. Ryan

University of Oregon, Eugene, Oregon

This report concerns operant stuttering therapy programs for five children ranging in age from six to nine years. The programs included programmed desensitization, delayed auditory feedback, and gradual increase in the length and complexity of the speech utterance. Reinforcing events ranged from social reward to points which could be exchanged for toys. The programs varied in length from 15 to 73.3 hours. They were all successful in helping the children to establish fluent speech. Special transfer and maintenance programs were necessary for some of the children. Follow-up measures indicated that the children had maintained their fluency. The value of viewing stuttering as operant behavior was demonstrated.

A number of studies have reported that operant conditioning speech therapy has been effective in establishing fluent speech in adults who stutter (Goldiamond, 1965; Martin, 1968; Haroldson, Martin, and Starr, 1968; Curlee and Perkins, 1969; Perkins and Curlee, 1969; Shames, 1969; and Shames, Egolf and Rhodes, 1969). Several different programs were described in these reports.

Rickard and Mundy (1965) and Leach (1969) reported on operant procedures with children who stuttered. Basically, their procedure was to gradually increase their subjects' fluency by reinforcing them with points or money for fluent utterances. Both of these studies reported relapse after therapy was discontinued.

Thus far, studies of operant conditioning therapy for children and adult stutterers have shown that it is possible to effectively, consistently establish fluent speech, but that this fluent speech is difficult to maintain. As an answer to the problem, Ryan (1968) suggested three phases of stuttering therapy: establishment, transfer, and maintenance.

The goal of the establishment phase is fluent conversation in the presence of the clinician. Establishment programs may take from five to 50 hours. The establishment phase is that period of time in therapy during which the clinician working individually with the child helps him to converse fluently in the clinician's presence for a specified period of time.

The transfer phase has as its goal fluent speech in a wide variety of situations in the stutterer's natural environment and may take 10–20 hours over several weeks. The transfer phase is that period of time in therapy during which the clinician helps the child to speak fluently in a wide variety of situations. With children, this transfer of fluency often occurs spontaneously.

The maintenance phase is to provide for permanent fluency. This phase may encompass 15–20 hours over several months and possibly years. It is that period of time in therapy during which the clinician helps the child to continue to speak fluently in a wide variety of situations. The clinician gradually discontinues therapy contacts and encourages the child and the important people in his environment to continue to provide for fluent speaking.

This paper reports on operant therapy with five children who stuttered. The operant principles of stimulus control and contingency management were

---

Note: From *Journal of Speech and Hearing Disorders, 36,* pp. 264–280. Reprinted with permission.

combined with successive approximation procedures. Prescribed schedules of reinforcement were employed. The results of this combination of principles were several different programs. Some of the steps in the programs used such traditional procedures as prolongation, desensitization, rate control, and increase of the complexity of tasks. The therapy was designed to establish, transfer, and maintain fluent speech. Several different programs for establishing fluent speech were used. Transfer and maintenance programs were quite similar, generally, but differed in specific details.

All five children were seen for a standard interview composed of 29 tasks including imitation, reading, talking while gesturing, and conversation. Three observers, including the person who administered the interview, counted and classified stuttered words. The percentage of agreement among the observers averaged about 80% on counts of stuttered words. The interview was used to decide whether a child was a candidate for therapy, and as a pretherapy measure of stuttering severity; occasionally, it was repeated as a posttherapy measure of stuttering severity.

The clinician working with the child was "calibrated" for correct counting of stuttered words. This was done by the author, who counted the child's stuttered words, listening either to tape recordings or "live" with the clinician. Such "calibration" continued until the individual clinicians and the author reached 90% agreement or better on three consecutive one-minute samples of reading and/or monologue and/or conversation.

Baseline procedures were conducted prior to the child's starting a therapy program. These procedures entailed having the children read and/or monologue and/or converse for 5 to 20 minutes for sessions with no specific contingencies. The programs themselves consisted of a series of steps or tasks which the children engaged in with reinforcement until they demonstrated a stuttering rate of 0.5 stuttered words per minute (one stuttered word every two minutes) or less in each step. Then they moved on to the next step. Some steps consisted of single words, while others required several minutes of conversation. The results of the programs were graphed in the manner described by Mowrer (1969).

The establishment phase (fluent conversational speech with the clinician) was carried out in a university speech clinic setting with student speech clinicians. The transfer and maintenance phases consisted of clinic contacts (gradually reduced in number) and activities outside the clinic.

CASE 1

The first case, RA, was an eight-year-old male. During the initial standard interview RA demonstrated a stuttering word rate of a mean 13.3 SW/M (stuttered words per minute), with a range of 0 to 24 SW/M. In conversation the rate was 16.2 SW/M. His stuttering consisted of part-word repetition, whole word repetition, prolongations, and audible exhalation of air preceding an utterance. Beginning the spring quarter, 1968, RA was asked to read, engage in monologue, and converse with the clinician. These three modes were used in tandem, for 10 minutes each, each session. The clinic sessions averaged 40 minutes in length. The program consisted of identification of stuttered words, instructions to prolong each word and speak fluently, and the delayed auditory feedback technique described by Goldiamond (1965) and Curlee and Perkins (1969). RA read, engaged in monologue, and conversed wearing earphones and hearing his voice delayed. In five steps the delayed auditory feedback was gradually reduced from 250 to 0 msec until he was able to read, engage in monologue, and converse fluently without the equipment. This program is shown in Table 17–1. The reinforcers were social—"Good," "That's right" —and points which could be exchanged for released time from the therapy. The reinforcement schedule was 100%. This was especially rewarding to this boy because he could return to baseball practice as soon as he had completed his speech therapy session.

The results of this program are shown in Figure 17–1, which shows that during the base operant level sessions, RA's stuttering averaged 10 SW/M. The rate was similar in all three modes of reading, monologue, and conversation. Introduction of the program in Session 4 brought a reduction in stuttering rate to 0.7 in all three modes. By Session 6, his stuttering rate was 0.5 or less in all three modes. RA's rate of talking became normal and fluent. This low rate continued until Session 17. The establishment phase was concluded at this point. RA's mother, teacher, and school speech clinician all reported spontaneous transfer of fluent speech to his home and school. No formal transfer was deemed necessary.

It was not possible to see RA during the summer quarter, 1968. In the fall of 1968 RA was seen again

Table 17-1.   Program using delayed auditory feedback (DAF) for RA.

Step	Stimulus (Clinician)	Response (Child)
1	Instructions to count each stuttered word	Count stuttered words at 75% accuracy or better for 5 minutes
2	Instructions to continue counting and to speak* slowly and fluently. DAF setting at 250	Read (or speak slowly and fluently for 10 minutes
3	Same, but DAF setting at 200	Same
4	Same, but DAF setting at 150	Same
5	Same, but DAF setting at 100	Same
6	Same, but DAF setting at 50	Same
7	Same, but DAF setting at 0	Same
8	Same, no DAF equipment	Same

*Instructions were "Read" during the reading time, and "Speak" during monologue and conversation time.

for a standard interview, during which he demonstrated a stuttering rate of 2.8 overall and 11.5 in conversation. He was seen for four sessions during the fall quarter, 1968, when, with only instructions to speak slowly and fluently, he reduced his rate in all three modes to 0.2 SW/M or less. His teacher reported that his stuttering was still noticeable at school, especially on Monday mornings and after vacation periods. It had not been possible to secure full

cooperation of his parents; therefore, it was decided to institute a school maintenance program. RA had already demonstrated transfer of fluent speech, but he could not maintain it. In the winter of 1969 a university speech clinician visited RA's fourth-grade classroom and taught the class and teacher to count stuttered words and to graph. They were also taught to instruct RA to speak fluently in a prolonged manner if he stuttered. The clinician conducted a six-

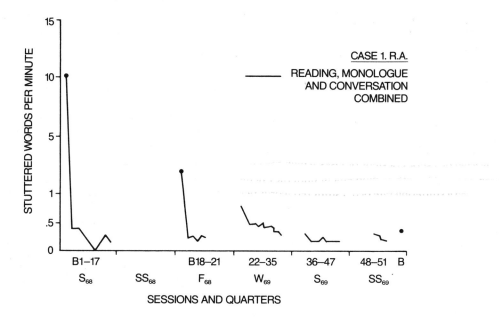

Figure 17-1.   Mean number of stuttered words per minute for Case 1, RA during a 51-session fluency training program over a 15-month period.

minute training period with RA in front of the class one day a week, and the teacher carried out another one each week. Reinforcement was social. There were 14 sessions conducted in the classroom. The results shown in Figure 17-1 indicate that RA's stuttering rate averaged less than 0.5 SW/M in all three modes. Reading was eventually excluded because RA was so fluent. This program was continued during spring, 1969, and the 12 sessions recorded show an average rate of 0.2 SW/M or less. RA and his classmates also reported that the latter were helping him with his speech intermittently during the day. The last measure, made in summer 1969, 15 months after the first session, indicated that RA could and would read, engage in monologue, and converse at 0.4 SW/M or less if given appropriate instructions. It still was not possible to gain the cooperation of the parents to continue this program in the home. There was a total of 51 sessions—25 in clinic and 26 in classroom. It was possible to establish fluent reading, monologue, and conversation in a relatively short time (less than 12 hours). Transfer occurred spontaneously, but it was necessary to continue a maintenance program over a relatively long period (one year). Such a program may need to continue for some additional time if RA is to maintain his present fluency. Teaching him some self-control procedures might also be helpful.

CASE 2

The second case, MH, was a six-year-old male who had been seen in the clinic for two previous quarters (50 sessions) for speech and language therapy. The standard interview revealed an overall rate of 8.6 SW/M with a high of 14 SW/M in conversation. His stuttering consisted of part-word repetition, whole-word repetition, vowel prolongation, and struggle behavior. The two programs devised for this child were modeled somewhat after the Rickard and Mundy (1965) procedure, but added more steps. Both programs will be shown in order to demonstrate similarities and differences. The first program had 19 steps which proceeded from MH's echoing of partial carrier phrases to 45 seconds of fluent utterance with the clinician. Reinforcement consisted of social reinforcers and points which could be turned in for game-playing time. The reinforcement schedule was 100%. The sessions were 50 minutes in length.

The first program is shown in Table 17–2. MH had to emit 10 consecutive correct responses before moving to the next step. The results for MH are shown in Figure 17–2. It can be seen that the program was effective in reducing stuttering behavior and increasing fluent speech throughout the 19 steps of the program. This program required 37 sessions, and the mean stuttering rate during the program was 1.6 SW/M. However, steps 13 (questions by the child) and 17 (two sentences in response to two spoken words) were extremely difficult. In addition, the standard interview administered after the program revealed an overall rate of 3.9 with a high of 8.0 SW/M in conversation.

This program was continued in the summer of 1968 for 12 sessions. MH did not attend more sessions, because he was struck by a car in the middle of the summer and suffered a brain concussion and transient aphasia. He averaged 1.3 SW/M during the summer program. In the fall of 1968, MH seemed to have completely recovered from his accident and again returned for therapy. Because of the difficult steps and failure to reach the establishment phase goal of fluent conversation, Program One was revised to Program Two. Program Two is shown in Table 17–3.

Program Two utilized only 13 steps (many of them were review for MH) and left out the troublesome question step. Question behavior occurred in the conversational activities. Program Two was completed within 22 sessions and transfer to conversation with the mother began in Session 62. MH's rate was 0.2 SW/M throughout this program. This continued throughout the end of the quarter. In winter quarter 1969, MH worked on conversational speech with his mother and the clinician for 17 additional sessions. During this phase his stuttering rate averaged 0.6 SW/M. Besides intermittent positive verbal statements by the clinician contingent on fluent utterances (words, phrases, and sentences, at various steps in the program), MH was also asked to repeat any stuttered words (cancellation). His mother was trained in this process and carried it out daily at home. In spring term 1969, MH was seen weekly by his school clinician, who carried out the same program. These two procedures constituted the transfer program for MH. He was observed at school and demonstrated no stuttering behavior. His teacher also reported that she did not observe any stuttering behavior. Transfer had occurred simply by training

Table 17-2. Program One for developing fluent speech for MH.

Step	Stimulus (Clinician)	Response (Child)
1	Picture and carrier phrase "This is a (name of picture)."	Different picture and same carrier phrase "This is a (name of picture)."
2	Picture and carrier phrase "This is a (name of picture)."	Different picture and different carrier phrase "Here is a (name of picture)."
3	Object and carrier phrase	Different object and different carrier phrase
4	Action and carrier phrase with action being done while phrase is stated	Different action and carrier phrase with action being done while phrase is being said
5	Pictures and carrier phrase with fill-in phrase "I have a big, red car."	Pictures and carrier phrase with fill-in phrase "This is a long, white string."
6	Picture and nursery rhyme	Nursery rhyme said in unison
7	Picture and original sentence	Different familiar picture and original sentence from steps 1, 2, and 5
8	Picture and original sentence	Different unfamiliar picture and original sentence
9	Picture and spoken word	Sentence using the word
10	Spoken word (same set as in step 9)	Sentence using the word
11	Word (different set of words)	Sentence using the word
12	Name of TV show	Sentence about the show
13	Object	Questions about the object
14	Four action pictures in sequence	Four sentence sequence
15	Pictures (same as in steps 1, 7, 8, 9)	Two sentences
16	Unfamiliar pictures	Two sentences
17	Two spoken words about home, e.g. *dinner time*	Two sentences
18	One spoken word (same as in steps 1, 7, 8, 9)	30-sec utterance about the word
19	One spoken word (words from his environment such as *school, lunch, brother*)	45-sec utterance about the word

MH, his mother, and his school speech clinician. An evaluation of his speech at the end of the summer 1969 revealed 0.3 SW/M during a 10-minute sample of monologue and conversation. His mother had not worked with him very much but reported that he was speaking fluently at home. Another evaluation made in April 1970 revealed that his fluent speech has continued for another eight months with no additional special maintenance program.

This program demonstrated the necessity for small, sequential steps. A breakdown in fluency means that branching or new steps must be devised.

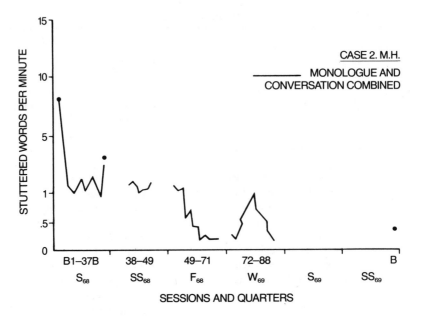

Figure 17-2. Mean number of stuttered words per minute for Case 2, MH, during an 88-session fluency training program over a 15-month period.

Again, it was noted that the maintenance of fluent speech is a critical element. Some level of therapeutic contact and/or school and/or home program must be continued to insure the permanency of the fluency gained in establishment programs. MH was seen for 88 50-minute sessions to complete the two programs. This process brought him to fluent conversational speech, in a wide variety of settings, which was maintained after 14 months without therapy. These programs were similar to Van Riper's "desensitization therapy" (1954) procedures for children who stutter. The programs were also similar to those described by Rickard and Mundy (1965) except that there were many more steps and transfer and maintenance phases.

CASE 3

The third case, CE, was an eight-year-old girl. During the standard interview, she demonstrated a rate of 2.5 SW/M. This low overall rate reflected her extremely fluent reading behavior. Her conversational rate was higher (7.3 SW/M). Her stuttering behavior was composed of part-word repetitions and prolongations with a rising pitch. She was seen for the initial interview one month before therapy began. As "first-aid"

treatment before therapy started, it was recommended to her mother that she speak in a slow, prolonged manner in CE's presence. This was done because, traditionally, parents of stuttering children have been counseled to speak more slowly and easily in front of the children (Van Riper, 1954) and because recent research has suggested that slower speech enhances fluency (Goldiamond, 1965; Curlee and Perkins, 1969). When CE began therapy one month later, a high rate of slow, prolonged speech was observed, particularly in monologue. She went through nine base-rate sessions of monologue and conversation to determine the possible positive effects of the slow, prolonged speech. It was hoped she might become more fluent if she continued the prolongations. Reading was not employed because CE read so fluently. Although there was variation throughout the base-rate sessions, it appeared that she would not become fluent simply by emitting prolongations. The two clinicians working with her also reported extreme difficulty in getting her to talk. It was decided to develop a program for CE which would both increase the amount of her talking and decrease the rate of stuttering. A summary of this program is shown in Table 17–4. Social reinforcement, for example, "Good," "Good talking," was given, contingent upon fluent utterances (utterances

Table 17-3. Program two for developing fluent speech for MH.

Step	Stimulus (Clinician)	Response (Child)
1	Nursery rhymes said one sentence at a time	Nursery rhymes said one sentence at a time in unison with the clinician
2	Pictures	Carrier phrase and name of picture "This is a _____."
3	Pictures and objects	Varying carrier phrases and name of picture or object
4	Pictures	Shorter, medial carrier phrase plus two fill-ins "_____ are for _____."
5	Pictures	One phrase
6	Pictures	One sentence
7	Action picture	One sentence
8	Spoken word	One sentence
9	Picture sequence	Short monologue (15 sec)
10	Spoken word	Short monologue (30 sec)
11	Short phrase infrequently	Conversation
12	Longer phrases more frequently	Conversation
13	Conversation (50%) of talking time)	Conversation (50% of talking time)

which contained no stuttered words). The schedule of reinforcement was 100%. The sessions with CE were 50 minutes in length. This program, too, resembled the desensitization technique described by Van Riper (1954). The results are shown in Figure 17–3.

CE demonstrated 0.1 SW/M throughout the 43-step program. A postprogram standard interview in Session 28 revealed an overall rate of 0.2 SW/M with a conversational rate of 0.8 SW/M.

After a spring-quarter break, the program was resumed. The initial sessions were used for review. From then on, they were all in the conversational mode. In Session 36, two clinicians attended, to provide a larger audience. In the 38th and following sessions, the mother attended. Observations at both home and school revealed 1.5 SW/M (these were

short part-word repetitions and prolongations with little or no struggle) and 0.0 SW/M, respectively, in those settings. Both the parent and the classroom teacher said that CE was no longer stuttering. No formal transfer program was deemed necessary. The summer maintenance program consisted of three rechecks (Sessions 56–58). CE continued to maintain fluent speech for three months after the conclusion of the formal program (Session 56).

In 58 50-minute sessions of therapy with CE it was possible to establish fluent speech which transferred spontaneously to the natural environment and was maintained with minimal contact over a three-month period. A brief recheck of CE later (April 1970) revealed that she was still fluent, eight months after therapy had been terminated.

Table 17-4.   Summary of program for increasing verbalization and fluency for CE.

Step	Stimulus (Clinician)	Response (Child)
Series A 1–7	Picture, nursery rhyme (7 steps)	Speak in unison, after the clinician, and in response to questions
Series B 8–14	Picture, statements and questions about pictures (7 steps)	Statements, answers to questions, 1-min monologue
Series C 15–23	Addition problems, flash cards, for speed, inattention and competition (9 steps)	Answers to flash card problems under varying conditions of speech, clinician inattention and competition
Series D 24–31	Blackboard, chalk, pictures drawn by clinician and case (8 steps)	Draws, labels pictures, describes pictures, monologue and conversation
Series E 32–36	Stories, tell a story, starts a story, finishes a story (5 steps)	Repeats a story, finishes a story, starts a story
Series F 37–43	Conversation, one sentence, one question, normal conversation (7 steps)	One question, one sentence, normal conversation
Total	(43 steps)	

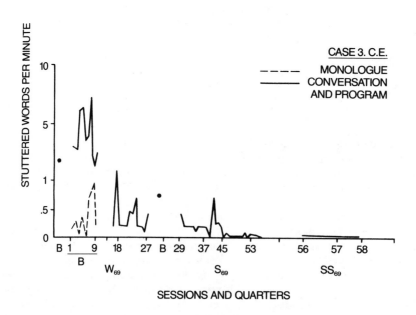

Figure 17-3.   Mean number of stuttered words per minute for Case 3, CE, during a 58-session fluency training program over a 9-month period.

CASE 4

The fourth case, RM, was a nine-year-old male who had been seen for diagnostic evaluations and parent counselling. No formal, direct speech therapy had been attempted because the home situation was very unstable and the boy was not doing well in school. The clinicians initially yielded to the psychological implications of the problem and followed through on a joint program with the school counselors and remedial reading teachers. After two years the stuttering behavior of RM persisted at about the same level. A standard interview demonstrated an overall rate of 2.8 SW/M with a high of 9 SW/M in conversation. Baseline data collected during the first seven sessions reflected the initial interview: his stuttering rate was 0.9 SW/M in reading, 10.3 SW/M in monologue, and 11 SW/M in conversation. The rate was low in reading because RM was an extremely poor and slow reader.

The program for RM is shown in Table 17–5. The sessions were 30 minutes in length. Part I was carried out in Sessions 7–21, Part II in Sessions 22–48, and Part III in Sessions 46–61. The criterion for advancement was 0 SW/M. RM was required to say one fluent sentence 10 times (10 fluent sentences), then two

fluent sentences 10 times, and so on (different sentences each time). Reinforcement was social, for example, "Good job," "That's fine." The reinforcement schedule was 100%. The results of the program are shown in Figure 17–4. Stuttering immediately decreased. In Session 48 in Part II, the clinician put the small handcounter which she was using to count stuttered words in front of RM during their conversation. He was told its purpose. This overt counting of his stuttered words appeared to depress the stuttering rate slightly and the procedure was continued until the end of the program. His mother came into the program in Session 50 and carried out a similar conversation-counting program for five minutes a day at home until the end of the spring term (Session 61). This was the only transfer program for RM. His mother reported that he did extremely well at home. His teacher reported that she still observed stuttering from time to time. A recheck in the summer quarter, three months after the last clinic session, revealed a monologue and conversation rate of 0 SW/M in the clinic setting. His mother reported that he had been speaking very well the past three months, although she only occasionally practiced with him. The program required 61 sessions, or 30.5 hours, to

Table 17-5. Program of gradual increase in length of utterance for RM.

Step	Stimulus (Clinician)	Response (Child)
	Part I	
1	Instructions to speak slowly and fluently about a picture	1* fluent sentence
2–6	Instructions to speak slowly and fluently about a picture	2–6* fluent sentences
7–8	Instructions to speak slowly and fluently about a picture after the picture is removed	7–8* fluent sentences
	Part II	
9	Instructions to speak slowly about anything, occasionally using pictures to stimulate monologue	15 sec of fluent monologue
10	Instructions, etc.	30 sec of fluent monologue
11	Instructions, etc.	45 sec of fluent monologue
12–22	Instructions, etc.	1–20 min of fluent monologue
	Part III	
23–33	Instructions, conversation	15 sec to 10 min of fluent conversation

*Different sentence each time.

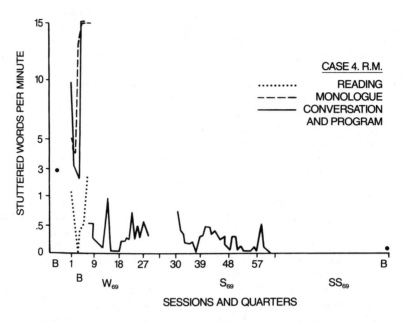

Figure 17-4. Mean number of stuttered words per minute for Case 4, RM, during a 61-session fluency training program over a 9-month period.

complete. Eight months later (April 1970) the mother reported by telephone that RM was continuing to speak fluently. There had been no special maintenance program, but his mother occasionally practiced with RM.

CASE 5

The fifth case, BH. was a nine-year-old male who had been seen for several diagnostic evaluations for 18 months previously. His parents were counseled to speak slowly around him, decrease conflicts in the home, and so on. He received nine months of daily speech therapy in a small group in his school. None of these activities eliminated the stuttering behavior, although there was a reduction from a rate of 16.6 in the standard interview to 9.6 SW/M, with the conversational rate of 13.0 SW/M. His base rate before the program was 4.0 SW/M in reading, 9.5 SW/M in monologue, and 15.0 SW/M in conversation. His stuttering consisted mostly of part-word repetitions and prolongations. Because the family was moving from the state in a few months, it was decided to engage in a crash program to eliminate his stuttering. The parents brought him to the university clinic on Saturday mornings for three-hour sessions and engaged in a

daily home program for five minutes a day which paralleled the clinic program. His school clinician also carried out a similar program in his school daily. Points were used as reinforcers for fluent utterances. These could be exchanged for toys. For each stuttered word, points were subtracted and BH was required to repeat each stuttered word fluently. His program is outlined in Table 17–6. The schedule of reinforcement was gradually changed as BH went through the program. Initially he received a point for 30 seconds of fluency which was given with social reinforces, such as "Good," "That's right," "Fine." The schedule was gradually changed until a point was given only for each five minutes of fluent utterance. The branch steps were devised when BH demonstrated that he could not think of anything to talk about and became upset in the clinic session. These branch steps consisted of 16 steps which started with one fluent word and progressed to 150 seconds of fluent talking, at which point BH was put back in the regular sequence. He was reinforced for each correct step in the branch sequence with a point.

The home and school programs carried out each week were important parts of the transfer program. In addition, another part of the transfer program which involved the entire family was initiated after BH had completed the conversation mode (Step 18).

This program is shown in outline form in Table 17–7.

To provide for maintenance of fluency, the parents were instructed to continue giving BH points for fluent utterances until he earned enough for a bicycle he wanted. These points were so arranged that he could earn only a maximum number per day, which would permit a gradual accumulation of points to coincide with his birthday some four months after the last session. BH also sent in weekly postcards from his new home reporting on his fluency and listing the points he had earned for the week.

The results of the program are shown in Figure 17–5. The immediate reduction in stuttering behavior can be seen in Session 1, which worked through reading and started monologue. It was possible to review reading, finish monologue and start conversation in Session 2. In Session 3, reading and monologue were reviewed and conversation was completed. In Session 4, all three modes were reviewed and the transfer program was begun. In Session 5, the transfer program was completed. BH came in one final Saturday two weeks after Session 5. His parents were checked on the maintenance program and the standard interview was readministered to BH. He demonstrated 0.0 SW/M. The amazing, rapid reduction in stuttering both in and out of the clinic during this 15-hour program was undoubtedly due in part to excellent cooperation and concurrent home and school speech therapy programs.

Observation in BH's classroom revealed a similar decrease in stuttering. Postcards sent by BH and his parents for three months after the clinic program was completed reported a continued low rate. A letter from the parents received six months after the conclusion of the clinic program stated that BH was doing well although he had slipped a little since receiving the bicycle. A tape recording received 12 months later indicated that he was speaking with less than 0.5 SW/M.

DISCUSSION

A summary of all five programs with the five children is shown in Table 17–8. All of the programs were effective in establishing fluent conversational speech. The length of time taken to establish fluent conversation varied greatly from program to program due to initial steps in some of the programs and to lack of expertise in early programs. Spontaneous transfer of fluent speech was demonstrated by at least four of the five children. Williams[1] in his research has made the same observation of spontaneous transfer by children who stutter. Maintenance of fluent speaking is an important phase in therapy, as demonstrated by all cases, but especially RA, MH, and BH. The children's

[1]D. E. Williams, personal communication (November 1969).

Table 17-6. Program of gradual increase in length of utterance with positive reinforcement and punishment for BH.

Step	Stimulus (Clinician)	Response (Child)
1	Instruct to read fluently book to read	Read fluently 3 min
2	Instruction and book	Read fluently 4 min
3	Instruction and book	Read fluently 5 min
4	Instruction and book and parent	Read fluently 5 min
5	Parent gives instructions, book	Read fluently 5 min
6	Parent gives instructions, book (clinician out of room)	Read fluently 5 min
A	Branch program consisting of 16 steps which led from 1-word utterance to 150 sec of utterance	
7	Instructions to speak fluently	Speak fluently 3 min
8–12	Repeat steps 2–6 in monologue	Speak fluently 3–5 min
B	Branch program consisting of 16 steps which led from 1-word utterance to 150 sec of utterance	
13	Instructions to converse fluently	Converse fluently for 3 min
14–18	Repeat steps 2–6 in conversation	Converse fluently 3–5 min

Table 17-7.   Transfer program for BH.

Step	Stimulus	Response
1	Parent 1, clinician, conversation different physical settings outside therapy room	10 min fluent conversation in the different settings
2	Parent 2,* clinician, conversation in therapy room	10 min fluent conversation
3	Parent 2, clinician, conversation different physical settings outside therapy room	10 min fluent conversation
4	Parent 2, clinician, 1 male peer and 1 female peer in conversation (substeps in which various combinations of these people were present) in therapy room	10 min fluent conversation (2 min at each sub step)
5	Parent 2, clinician, 1 male peer, 1 female peer in conversation in different physical settings outside the therapy room	10 min fluent conversation
6	Parents 1 and 2, siblings, clinician (substeps in which various combinations of these people were present) conversation in the therapy room	10 min fluent conversation
7	Parents 1 and 2, siblings, clinician conversation in different physical settings outside the therapy room	10 min fluent conversation

*Father was introduced into the therapy setting for the first time. Previous to this mother came alone.

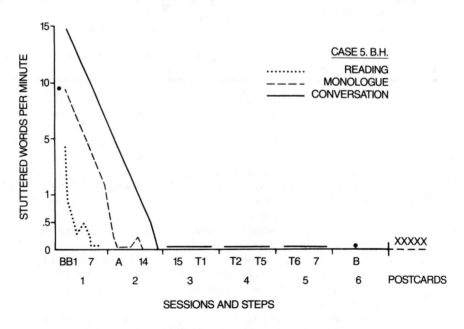

Figure 17-5.   Mean number of stuttered words per minute for Case 5, BH, during a 5-session fluency training program over a 6-month period.

Table 17-8. Summary of five programs for children who stutter.

I	Name	Age	Sex	Program	Reinforcer and Punishers	Transfer	Maintenance
	RA	8	M	DAF	Time off from therapy, social	Spontaneous,	Classroom
	MH	6	M	Programmed densitization	Social and *no*	Spontaneous parent, school speech clinician	Parent, school speech clinician
	CE	8	F	Programed desensitivation	Social	Spontaneous, parent	Parent
	RM	9	M	Gradual increase in length of utterance	Social, counting stuttered words	Unknown, parent	Parent
	BH	9	M	Gradual increase in length of utterance	Points for toys given and taken away	Spontaneous, school speech clinician, parents	Parents

II	Time Sessions	Hours Approximately	Rate of Stuttering (Conversation) pre-	post-	Follow-up (Measured from Beginning of Program)
	51	29.3	16.2	0.4	At 15 months
	88	73.3	14.0	0.3	At 15 months and 23 months
	58	48.3	7.3	0.7	At 9 months and 17 months
	61	30.5	9.0	0	At 9 months and 17 months
	5	15.0	13.0 some? reported by parents	0	At 6 months and 21 months

speech remained fluent with simple maintenance programs. Only further research will demonstrate which of these programs is the most effective.

Operant procedures, that is, systematic therapy programs with small steps and appropriate reinforcement, were demonstrated to be an effective strategy for helping children with stuttering problems. Most of these programs were long (a mean of 39.3 hours). It is hoped that programs in the future will be shorter but equally effective, like that for BH. The value of viewing any program of stuttering therapy as including three phases—establishment, transfer and maintenance—was demonstrated.

There are several implications of this report for the speech clinician working with children who stutter. First, there are many ways to systematically establish fluent conversational speech or to teach children who stutter to speak fluently. Second, most children (four out of five in this report) will spontaneously transfer their new fluent speech to other speaking situations. Third, it is important to continue to recheck children who have completed programs to help them maintain their fluency. The recheck serves the two purposes of evaluating the efficacy of the establishment and transfer programs and of providing for maintenance.

Some speech clinicians may wish to view these programs as only one part of the total treatment process. They may be used in conjunction with other forms of therapy for stuttering. However, interviews with the five children and their parents and teachers revealed that the achievement of fluent speech was enough in itself to eliminate their stuttering problems.

ACKNOWLEDGMENT

The author wishes to acknowledge the work of the following graduate student speech clinicians: Trudee Lewis, Susan Trafton, James Smith, Brooke Belcher, Marion Lea, Bonnie Moon, Kathleen Griffin, Barbara Mervo, Barbara Van Kirk, Suzanne Gowdy, Mary Ann Beggs, JoAnn Cooper, Bill DeMastus, and Gerald Mill.

REFERENCES

Curlee, R. F., and Perkins, W. H. Conversational rate control therapy for stuttering. *J. Speech Hearing Dis., 34,* 245–250 (1969).

Goldiamond, I., Stuttering and fluency as manipulable operant response classes. In L. Krasner and L. Ullmann (Eds.), *Research in Behavior Modification: New Developments and Implications.* New York: Holt, Rinehart and Winston, 106–156 (1965).

Haroldson, S. K., Martin, R. R., and Starr, C. D., Time-out as a punishment for stuttering. *J. Speech Hearing Res., II,* 560–566 (1968).

Leach, E., Stuttering: clinical application of response-contingent procedures. In B. Gray and G. England (Eds.), *Stuttering and the Conditioning Therapies.* Monterey: Monterey Institute for Speech and Hearing, 115–128 (1969).

Martin, R. R., The experimental manipulation of stuttering behaviors. In H. Sloane, Jr., and B. MacAulay (Eds.), *Operant Procedures in Remedial Speech and Language Training.* Boston: Houghton Mifflin Co., 325–347 (1968).

Mowrer, D. E., Evaluating speech therapy through precision recoding. *J. Speech Hearing Dis., 34,* 239–244 (1969).

Perkins, W. H., and Curlee, R. F., Clinical impressions of portable masking unit effects in stuttering. *J. Speech Hearing Dis., 34,* 360–362 (1969).

Rickard, H. C., and Mundy, M. B., Direct manipulation of stuttering behavior: an experimental-clinical approach. In L. Ullman and L. Krasner (Eds.), *Case Studies in Behavior Modification.* New York: Holt, Rinehart and Winston, 268–274 (1965).

Ryan, B. P., The establishment, transfer and maintenance of fluent reading and speaking in a stutterer using operant technology. Paper presented at the Annual Convention, American Speech and Hearing Association, Denver (November 1968).

Shames, G., Verbal reinforcement during therapy interview with stutterers. In B. Gray and G. England (Eds.), *Stuttering and the Conditioning Therapies.* Monterey: Monterey Institute for Speech and Hearing, 99–114 (1969).

Shames, G., Egolf, D. B., and Rhodes, R. C., Experimental programs in stuttering therapy. *J. Speech Hearing Dis., 34,* 30–47 (1969).

Van Riper, C. V., *Speech Correction: Principles and Techniques.* Englewood Cliffs: Prentice-Hall (1954).

Operant Therapy for Children

Bruce P. Ryan

INTRODUCTION

Looking back at clinical research done 12 years ago is bittersweet. Bitter in the sense that one can see how naive one was and how myopic one was because of being too close to the work at that time. Sweet in the sense that the roots of research can be seen and such re-examination provides an opportunity to redirect one's present course.

As I reviewed this clinical research report, I could see themes of findings and directions. Some were overt and need only to be stated again for emphasis. Some were covert and required additional information and inference. Some of these themes were followed up; some were not.

My contribution in this book will be to identify and discuss these themes and their present status. Usually, I prefer to present data and make data-bound statements. Because of the necessary page limitations and the bulk of the data, I will just make statements and refer the reader to the data. My basic source of data is Ryan and Van Kirk (1974) and Ryan and Ryan (1983). These two reports concern a two-year project with one-year follow-up on 40 school-aged children who stuttered, employing various operant establishment, transfer and maintenance programs. At present I have data on several hundred additional children who stuttered from both this country and the United Kingdom (Ryan, Rustin, & Ryan, 1981) but much of that is not published. Other sources of data for the reader to view will be found in the bibliography under my name. I have restricted the bibliography to representative samples of research and, or, discussion of operant therapy or research with children.

Finally, I wish to explain the use of the denotations "I" and "we" in the following pages. The word "I" will denote an observation that is basically mine although the data may have been collected by others under my supervision. The use of "we" commonly will denote the combined data collection or interaction of thoughts between my colleague and wife, Barbara Van Kirk Ryan, and me. She

Postscript   17

helped collect data for the 1971 article and has been involved in much of my research and life ever since. Although fraught with obvious peril I take full responsibility for the correct use of "I" and "we" in the following pages. Because she and I do not always agree on interpretations of data or their implications, occasional "we's" may more accurately represent data collection activities rather than agreement on interpretations. My public recognition of her contribution to my research and thoughts on stuttering is very appropriate and long overdue.

OVERT THEMES

Stuttering as Operant Behavior

The title of the article and almost every page make reference to this observation. Stuttering is operant behavior determined by its consequences (Costello, 1982; Martin, Kuhl, & Haroldson, 1972; Ryan, 1970; 1974; Ryan & Van Kirk, 1974; Ryan & Ryan, 1983; Shine, 1980; Webster, 1980). All of these studies demonstrate that stuttering may be manipulated by arranging appropriate evoking stimuli and providing effective consequences.

One should grow or change lest one become stagnant. However, I suggest that growth can occur in many ways and is not always measured by the adjective "new." The basic operant system (Skinner, 1953) is still very functional and viable, much like the law of gravity, for an interpretation and understanding of stuttering behavior. What is new is the continued and expanded use of the system to refine management programs for children who stutter. Then, at some point in time, a level is reached where "the program works" and attention is to be directed to other activities such as disseminating validated programs, developing programs to train clinicians to operate such programs, and researching operant explanations of the development of stuttering. The basic system is not changed or new, but its applications are.

Measurement

A hallmark of operant conditioning strategies has been careful, continuous measurement, usually of the frequency of occurrence of a behavior such as stuttering. Our metric has been counting stuttered words, total words spoken, and talking time, which are converted to rates per minute (Ryan, 1974). This metric has continued to be extremely helpful in evaluating stuttering behavior before, during, and after therapy. It was and is relatively simple, valid, reliable, and useful.

Fluency Interview. The standard interview of 29 tasks has been revised and now includes only 10 tasks. This resulted from our analysis that indicated there was much overlap and redundancy of information in the earlier procedure. The present form (Ryan & Kirk, 1971) requires approximately 15 minutes to administer and yields 10 minutes of talking time for analysis. The data from the present Fluency Interview do continue to demonstrate that stuttering is variable-contingent on the complexity of the speaking task. For example, children usually do not stutter when reciting a nursery rhyme or poem, but do stutter when they are required to ask questions of the clinician-tester. This continuum of stuttering behavior across tasks has provided some additional measurement of severity. For example a child who stuttered on even the most simple verbal task would be judged more severe than a child who did not. We also used this Fluency Interview as an extra program measure of the generalization of fluent speech (Ryan & Van Kirk, 1974).

Criterion Test.   Casual measures of reading, monologue, and conversation in the 1971 article have evolved into standard 5-minute measures of each, and we are now experimenting with 3-minute samples that will provide more time for therapy. Although the criterion test is similar to and often correlates highly with the Fluency Interview, it continues to be an important in-program test for movement through establishment, transfer, and maintenance.

Counting Stuttering Words.   I continue to count only four classes or types of stuttered words: part-word repetition (syllable or sound repetition), whole word repetition, prolongation, and struggle (a catch-all category comprising the many struggle or tension variants of stuttering). This extremely simple system has worked very well over the years. I have been tempted on several occasions to develop a more sophisticated system, but experience has indicated that one is not necessary. We have taught a very large number of clients to become fluent and clinicians to teach clients to become fluent with this classification system.

Word or Syllable Count.   I did not count words or syllables spoken in the "early days," whereas now we routinely measure either words or syllables spoken per minute. A discussion of the relative merits of both will be found in Ryan (1981). These data have been helpful to verify that the children were speaking at normal rates after therapy. At the time I was working with the cases in the 1971 article I stated "He sounds normal," (an admittedly subjective judgment) as verification. Now, when we use "he sounds normal," we can substantiate that observation with word- or syllable-rate data. Unfortunately, there is a paucity of normative data on normal children's normal speech and disfluency rates so we do not know what our target rate should be.

Severity.   It should be noted that the children in the 1971 study averaged 11.9 stuttered words per minute (SW/M). Our later research demonstrated that a sample population of 40 school-aged children averaged only 7.2 SW/M (Ryan & Van Kirk, 1974). The children in the 1971 article were selected partly on the basis of severity (high rate of stuttering) in order to demonstrate that operant procedures did indeed work well on clients with severe stuttering. Our later research provided evidence that the programs also worked on children who had less severe stuttering. I infer from the 1974 study that the "average" rate of stuttering of children is closer to the 7.2 figure than to the 11.9 figure, but only future research will verify that.

Postscript 17

The metric, SW/M, is a simple, functional measure of severity, but I believe that a more viable measure of severity is a composite score of stuttering rate, speaking rate, and topography of stuttering (Ryan, 1974). Such a measure would be extremely helpful to us in research and planning management programs. Most clinical management programs are presently designed on the institutional constraint basis that requires two-time-a-week therapy, or six weeks of special intensive therapy or semester-bound therapy in university training clinics. I am still working on a measurement of severity that would predict success in therapy and/or hours of therapy required. This measure would be extremely helpful in selecting therapy schedules or time commitment.

Programs

Phases. In the 1971 article it may be noted that therapy was characterized as having three phases: establishment (fluency in the presence of the clinician), transfer (generalization of fluency to other people and environments), and maintenance (continuation of fluency over long-term periods, a lifetime). This conceptualization has continued to be helpful, and these phase demarcations do indeed appear to describe the therapy act. Later research (Ryan & Van Kirk, 1974) demonstrated that important changes in fluency in the natural environment occurred during transfer and maintenance programs.

Establishment Programs. The programs described in the 1971 article were individualized. There were three programs: Programmed Desensitization, Delayed Auditory Feedback (DAF), and Gradual Increase in Length and Complexity of Utterance (GILCU) for five children. Each was slightly different for each of the five children. A close examination of the programs labeled "programmed desensitization" and the programs labeled "gradual increase in length and complexity of utterance" revealed that they could both be described as "gradual increase in length and in complexity of utterance." Although in the article these programs appear to be very different, the underlying core of events was that the client progressed from simple responses and simple stimuli to more complex responses and more complex stimuli with the consequences being held relatively constant. Therefore, the core of these programs is asking the client (SD) to engage in increasingly more complex fluent utterances (R) followed commonly by positive reinforcement for desired responses and "nothing" and, or, some form of punishment (withdrawal of tokens for Case 5, BH) or (Rf) for undesired responses.

At the time of the 1971 article I was experimenting with a variety of establishment programs. The three in the article were a sample of nine other programs that I did not report. These nine programs were eventually reduced to four programs: programmed traditional, punishment, gradual increase in length and complexity of utterance (GILCU) and Delayed Auditory Feedback (DAF). We then tested these four programs against each other (Ryan & Van Kirk, 1974; Ryan & Ryan, 1983). The results of this study revealed that all four were effective, but DAF and GILCU appeared superior in terms of run hours and ease of administration. We also discovered again what we believe to be a "core" of management based on operant conditioning principles. The clinician sets the stage (SD) for the client to respond (R) and then the clinician provides the consequence (Rf). That basic paradigm runs through all forms of establishment programs. The core therapy act may be varied with different evoking or response-contingent stimuli. The response mode may be composed of differing responses (successive approximations) and the clinician may choose to either positively reinforce or punish the responses emitted, or both.

As we observed the variety of programs we ourselves had used over the years and the four programs in the 1974 study, it appeared that there was not as much variation as we had initially perceived. We could indeed write a specific different program for each child, but they all contained certain similar elements. The variations were merely "window dressing" giving the various procedures an appearance of difference.

The question then turned from "How many different operant speech fluency programs can we design?" to "Which programs are best?" and, finally, to "Is there a 'core' of effective therapy imbedded in all successful operant programs?"

The answer to the last question is, "Yes." This core is embodied in our present two establishment programs: GILCU and DAF (Ryan & Van Kirk, 1971; Ryan, in press).

In these two programs we have limited the clinician's initial stimuli to instructions to the client to "speak fluently" in reading, monologue, and conversation. These three oral modes remain in our present programs because they capture the common oral events in most children's lives, and they provide a sequence from "easy" to "hard" for both the client and the clinician. Reading is viewed as the easiest because all the client has to do is read and be fluent. The content is prepared. Of course, children who cannot read skip this mode. The next easiest is monologue, which requires the client to think of something to say and be fluent. The final mode of conversation requires the client to answer questions, ask questions, and engage in the other roles required of normal conversation and be fluent.

The response of the client is varied between the gradual increase in length and complexity of utterance (one word, two words, etc., up to five minutes of fluent conversation) in the GILCU program and the prolonged speech pattern of the DAF program, which is gradually shaped to normal fluency for five minutes of conversation. Several modern programs employ one or the other of these responses: Costello (1982), Mowrer (1975), Shine (1980), and Webster (1980).

The consequences in these two establishment programs are "good" and a token for correct desired responses in either program and, "Stop, speak fluently" for GILCU and "Stop, speak in your slow, prolonged pattern" for DAF contingent on each stuttering behavior. This contingency then is both positive reinforcement for fluency and punishment for stuttering.

Although the core of effective operant speech therapy is in both of our present establishment programs, the clinician must decide which program, DAF or

Postscript 17

GILCU, to use. Because GILCU has proven easier for the child (and the clinician, incidently) and usually effective, we try it first. If it fails, we then turn to the DAF program. Degree of severity is also used in making this decision. Given a child who is older and more severe we would start with the DAF program because it has been shown to be more effective with severe clients than GILCU (Ryan & Van Kirk, 1974). Twelve years of research and observation of several hundred clients employing one or both of these two establishment programs indicate their effectiveness.

The one occasional problem is the inability or lack of desire of clients to engage in monologue or conversation. Out of our 40 subjects in the 1974 study only two demonstrated this behavior. We were able to stimulate these children to talk using pictures, topic ideas, etc. One of the most powerful stimuli for talking is silence by the clinician, and if used carefully, often solves the problem. Incidently, I do not view these special talking-evoking procedures to be new programs, but only a variant on the basic instructional aspects of the two standard programs.

Token Systems. In the 1971 study I used formal token systems with only two clients, RA and BH. Research and casual observations over the past 12 years have suggested that operant speech-fluency programs may be administered without token systems, but that token systems are extremely helpful in obtaining client attention to the task and attendance at therapy sessions. We presently consistently use token systems with children for those reasons.

Criterion Levels. The level of fluent speech has been changed from 0.5 stuttered words a minute to 0 stuttered words a minute. I did not know initially where to set the desired level of fluency. Later research confirmed that 0 SW/M per step for passing was not only possible, but highly desirable. Our present programs include 0 SW/M per step and 0.5 SW/M to pass exit or post-criterion tests. We are seriously considering 0 SW/M for passing criterion tests, also.

Hours of Therapy. In the original work in 1971, I was not concerned with how long therapy took, but only how effective it was. Consequently, establishment programs ranged from 15 to 73.3 hours for completion. Our present establishment programs average 10 hours (Ryan & Van Kirk, 1974). This increase in efficiency has been accomplished through streamlining the programs without reducing their effectiveness. A reduction in hours of therapy in and of itself is not remarkable, but when this fact is applied to inter-program comparison or the servicing of many clients on a large scale, the number of hours of therapy does indeed become very important. For example, if two different programs are demonstrated to be equally effective, but one takes three times as long, it is only logical and good service to clients to select and use the shorter one. If one applies these same data to the service of large numbers of stuttering clients, then it becomes clear that the faster procedure will provide more service to more clients. As we view new procedures coming out of the learning laboratories we continue to apply this metric to determine if they are faster than what we already have. Most have not been.

Somewhat related to this point is the time spacing of therapy sessions. In the 1971 research I used a wide variety of therapy session spacing ranging from two 30-minute sessions a week to three hours once a week. The data suggest that it is not the frequency of therapy sessions but the number of therapy hours that is critical. Two exceptions are that clinical sessions of very brief duration spread out over very long term periods (15 minutes once a month) and overly intensive periods (six hours a day for one week) may not be optimal for effective change. We do not have hard data on this point, but only casual observation.

Normal, Fluent Speech.   I was somewhat ambivalent about whether or not normal, fluent speech could be obtained in the early research. This ambivalence is reflected in the setting of criterion levels discussed above. The results shown in the 1971 article were harbingers of what was to come, i.e., the achievement of normal, fluent speech. Client BH, who moved from our research area, was reported to be a normally speaking child by people in his new environment. He had been one of the most severe of the five clients. Later research (Ryan & Van Kirk, 1974) verified that normal, fluent speech was indeed possible. This observation has been confirmed by other researchers (Shine, 1980, for example). Apparently the achievement of normal, fluent speech in children who stutter is a reasonable goal. Although there continues to be a professional controversy about the feasibility of that goal (Ryan, 1979), the data suggest that it is possible. The paucity of normative data on children's fluency at this time makes it very hard to resolve this issue to everyone's satisfaction.

Transfer Programs

In the 1971 article there was much natural generalization of fluent speech from the clinic setting, both reported and observed. In our 1974 research (Ryan & Van Kirk, 1974) we observed that generalization, measured a number of different ways, varied widely among our 40 subjects. Most showed some level of improved fluency in their natural environment without any formal transfer program. This observation was also made by Shine (1980). Some clients, however, did not show the same high level of fluency in transfer that they did in the therapy setting.

The transfer program we presently use is composed of seven series: different physical environments; increased audience size; home; school; strangers; telephone; all-day, 16-hour; and 32 steps (Ryan & Van Kirk, 1971; Ryan, 1974; Ryan, in press). The transfer program provides for additional, albeit occasionally minimal, improvement in fluency in natural environments. Our early transfer programs (Ryan, 1971) involved parents and teachers, and our present program still does although it can be run without either. Transfer programs are time-consuming to run and difficult to organize but they are apparently necessary for many children to ensure generalization of fluency.

Postscript 17

Maintenance

In the 1971 article I was experimenting with a variety of maintenance programs that involved parents, teachers, local speech clinicians, or combinations thereof who did something to maintain the children's fluency (see RA, for example, on maintenance). Our present standard maintenance program provides only for rechecks, which are gradually faded over a 22-month period (Ryan & Van Kirk, 1971; Ryan, in press). These rechecks provide for continued fluency and permit us to recycle clients who are having difficulty. We did observe that clients who had been on maintenance programs continued better fluency than clients who had not (Ryan & Van Kirk, 1974). Maintenance of fluency in a systematic, formal way is an important aspect of the clinical management of stuttering in children.

Follow-up

Observation of clients after formal therapy is completed is perhaps the most important, if difficult, measure to obtain. It is this measure that verifies the efficacy of our basic establishment, transfer, and maintenance procedures. One could say that *all* therapies should be evaluated and validated by follow-up measures. Any procedure that has not been subjected to accurate and consistent follow-up should be suspect. The follow-up reported in the 1971 article indicated continued fluent speech for the five clients. Our findings of later research (Ryan & Van Kirk, 1974; Ryan, 1980) suggested wider variability, and we did find that some clients had reverted to measurable stuttering behavior. Those clients generally were older children with more severe stuttering. Follow-up measures continue to be an integral part of activities with children who stutter.

Manipulation of Stuttering in the Natural Environment

Client RA, who had originally been on a DAF program, was eventually put into a classroom where his fellow students provided consequences as he publicly practiced fluent reading, monologue, and conversation. His fellow students said, "Remember to use your fluent, prolonged speech," consequent on any stuttering by RA anywhere on the school grounds and during the school day. They also reinforced fluent speaking. In the 1971 article this was defined as a maintenance program because RA had demonstrated a great deal of in-clinic fluency previously but could not maintain it. In retrospect, I view this as a very special demonstration of manipulating stuttering directly in the natural environment. This strategy proved to be extremely successful for RA and a very positive experience for him and his classmates as evidenced by an analysis of a follow-up video-tape recording of him and his classmates. On the video-tape recording the children comment very positively about RA and helping him with his fluency. RA, himself, publicly thanked me and his classmates for helping him with his speech. More than any study I have ever done, this one project demonstrated the humanness of operant conditioning therapy, which is often viewed as cold and dehumanizing.

We have never repeated this particular procedure with another client, but I continue to believe that training in the natural environment might well prove to be both effective (as demonstrated by RA) and efficient because it would obviate the need for a formal transfer program. Possible extrapolations of this procedure could be initially training the parent to manipulate the child's stuttering in the natural environment (the home) with the clinician there as observer and trainer during the early phases. Such efforts are known to be effective in many other phases of early child education and parenting. Another possibility would be use of this procedure initially in the classroom with both classmates and teacher directly involved in the manipulation of fluent speech.

Finally, some combination of in-home and in-school training for school-age children could be very effective. Additional research needs to be done on this procedure.

Self-control or Self-monitoring

Another dimension of treatment that we did not follow up was self-control or self-monitoring. Self-monitoring is defined here to mean attention to one's own behavior, whereas self-control implies that one will both monitor and control or manipulate one's own behavior in some way. These may not be commonly used definitions or distinctions, but I believe they can be useful. Our casual observation was that children often learned to count their own stuttered words (self-monitor), and some children did learn to control their stuttering or more precisely their fluency (self-control). Some children even reported and demonstrated that they could "turn on" fluent speech (self-control). This dimension of stuttering therapy is very popular right now, but careful research has not been done to validate its accurate measurement or its role in stuttering therapy. Our only data came from our 1974 project (Ryan & Van Kirk, 1974). One of the programs tested in that project required that the clients learn to count their own stuttered words. Interestingly enough, we found that all four clients on this procedure had difficulty counting stuttered words at high accuracy (90%) and tended to pass steps by simply becoming fluent.

The concept of self-control or self-monitoring is still not clear. If self-control or self-monitoring is defined as mentalistic attention to or control of the act of speaking (a common definition), then direct observation of it would be extremely difficult, if not impossible. What can be observed are the results of such self-monitoring; that is, slower speech, or more fluent speech, or counting stuttered words accurately, etc.

I do not question the possible importance of such a concept of self-control, but I believe that research exploration of this behavior must necessarily restrict itself to observable events, such as measuring "Raise your hand when you are engaging in monitoring behavior" or the overt results of such monitoring such as fluent speech. If only the overt results of such monitoring can be scientifically

Postscript   17

measured, then inferences concerning the presence or absence of the effect of such a hypothetical, unobservable construct may be nonfunctional.

Of some interest on this point was the behavior of one of our subjects in the 1974 study who was extremely poor at counting his own stuttered words. This client also showed minimal generalization of fluency and a great gap between his in-clinic excellent fluent speaking behavior and his out-of-clinic continued high rate of stuttering. Self-monitoring or self-control is worth additional exploration, but this exploration should be data-bound lest we verbally convince ourselves of something that might be, but can never be, demonstrated scientifically.

COVERT THEMES

Covert themes refer to ideas and procedures that are not readily apparent from reading the original article because they require information that is not generally public knowledge. I list them here because they are of importance, at least to me, and in a larger sense should be of interest to all who have a stake in the eventual solution of the problem of stuttering.

Impact

Impact refers to the influence this article may have had on my colleagues interested in stuttering treatment. Although this may be very hard to measure, I would like to attempt it. First of all, I received over 600 requests for reprints of this article from all over the U.S. and the world. I have never had such a response to an article either before or since.

Second, as I examine the work of Mowrer (1975), Shine (1980), and Costello (1982), among others, I find many direct and indirect references and similarities to the strategies and conceptualizations of therapy, especially the gradual increase in length and complexity of utterance concept, found in the 1971 article. GILCU, incidently, was not of my own creation (Ryan, 1974). It was certainly my hope to share with and inspire my colleagues. Those named above have made my dream come true.

Third, the article had little or no impact on most of my colleagues whom I will not name. These colleagues still go about the treatment of stuttering without any understanding of the import of this early article and collection of data. They continue to express this lack of understanding in a wide variety of ways, which range from simple lack of knowledge of the behavioristic, operant conditioning literature to direct negative statements about operant conditioning therapy.

Children Versus Adults

This theme is also covert. To understand it one must know a great deal about stuttering and its treatment. What was hidden in this article was the obvious positive results of direct speech therapy on the stuttering of children. Long a taboo for most speech-language pathologists, direct therapy for children has become quite popular in the last decade. Professional speech-language pathologists may have been doing direct therapy with children for years but few had written about it with any clarity or data.

The major finding of clinical research on direct therapy with children is that it is extremely effective (Ryan, 1974; 1979; 1981; Ryan & Van Kirk, 1974; Ryan & Ryan, 1983; and Shine, 1980). The achievement of normal, fluent speech in children who stutter, which persists over time, is very common for clinicians using verified operant-based therapy programs. Such therapy is also effective for adults, but is more complicated, takes longer, and produces inconsistent results. It is speculated that somewhere along the age continuum, somewhat related to severity, the older client takes on new behaviors or simply has practiced old behaviors so long that they are very resistant to permanent extinction or elimination. We observed this in the 1974 study. Our best results were for our younger, elementary-school clients, and our worst results were for our older, junior and senior high-school clients.

Operant Methodology as a Research Strategy

Somewhat related to impact discussed previously is the covert theme of the power in the use of operant technology to answer questions about the nature and treatment of stuttering. Is stuttering learned behavior? The data suggest it is. Can stuttering in children be dealt with directly or does that increase the stuttering problem? All of the clients in the article and several hundred clients since then have been treated for their speech problem directly. We have no verified case of one child client becoming worse after treatment. Will fluent speech generated in the clinic transfer to other environments? Yes, both as reported in the 1971 article and observed carefully and measured in the 1974 research. These and a myriad of other questions can be answered by casting the question into operational definitions, observing functional relationships, and, or, manipulating contingencies.

Disseminating Programmed Treatment

One of the results of this early research was the preparation and testing of replicable, validated procedures for managing stuttering in children (Ryan & Van Kirk, 1971). Dissemination efforts thus far have included several hundred clinicians across the United States, Great Britain, Scotland, Ireland, and West Germany (Ryan, Rustin & Ryan, 1981). We have occasionally found some resistance by clinicians to direct therapy for children who stutter as a vestige of earlier theories on the nature of stuttering. Additionally, there have been many clinicians who resisted the necessary structured, restrictive elements of programmed instruction. However, the general results of these dissemination efforts have been positive in that most of the clinicians trained have produced similar results to those of our own experimental studies.

The major problem at this time in dissemination is the lag between the experimental laboratory or field applications of these procedures by clinician-researchers and practicing clinicians and the training of student clinicians in

Postscript   17

university training programs. With few exceptions, university training programs are still producing students with little or no experience in stuttering therapy and even less knowledge or skill in the use of operant technology. This omission is extremely unfortunate and will preclude or at least delay the delivery of effective services to thousands of children who stutter, who may have been helped to become normally fluent had their clinicians been trained in appropriate remediation procedures.

CONCLUSIONS AND SUMMARY

This journey back in time has been refreshing and redirecting for the most part. I appreciate having been asked to participate in this book. Some 12 years later it appears that stuttering may still be usefully viewed as operant behavior, and operant technology (the experimental analysis of behavior) is still alive and well. The basic tenets of operant technology, which include functional definitions of overt behavior, continuous measurement, successive approximation and the analysis and provision of appropriate consequences for behavior to be manipulated, are well illustrated in the literature concerning stuttering.

A number of my colleagues have engaged in, and reported on, the use of effective operant speech therapy with children. Yet, there are still many of my colleagues who have not yet done their homework on operant technology, not read the published literature on the results of such technology, and, worst of all, not yet incorporated such information and training into their university training programs.

Primitive establishment programs of programmed desensitization, gradual increase in length and complexity of utterance (GILCU), and delayed auditory feedback (DAF), among other programs, have been refined to the two establishment programs of DAF and GILCU based on the effective core of operant therapy for stuttering. These present programs have proved extremely effective and efficient (average 10 hours of therapy). The metric of counting four types of stuttered words has been shown to be both adequate and functional.

Data collected over the past years have confirmed the need for transfer, and maintenance programs and the difficult but vital collection of follow-up data all of which were initiated and demonstrated in the original 1971 article. The accurate measure of severity of stuttering with its attendant value of prediction of success in therapy or even spontaneous recovery awaits further research, as does the description of "normal fluency" of children who do not stutter (normative studies). Added to this list of "researchables" is self-monitoring or self-control, which offers bright promise, if it can be reliably described, measured, and manipulated.

Two most interesting and possibly most important studies are of the development of stuttering (its cause) through the use of operant technology, and management of the problem in the child's natural environment (school and home). We are now engaged in this research.

The most important impact of this early research was to demonstrate the value of direct speech fluency therapy for children who stutter. The data collected by us and other clinician-researchers suggest that stuttering may indeed be eliminated through early direct intervention. Children who stutter may become normal, fluent speakers with only a small trace of memory of their stuttering. It behooves all members of the speech-language pathology profession to train clinicians and to provide effective operant speech therapy to all children who stutter.

REFERENCES

Costello, J. (1982). Current behavioral treatments for children. In D. Prins and R. Ingham (Eds.), *Treatment of stuttering in early childhood.* San Diego, CA: College-Hill Press.

Martin, R., Kuhl, P., & Haroldson, S. (1972). An experimental treatment with two preschool stuttering children. *Journal of Speech and Hearing Research, 15,* 743–752.

Mowrer, D. (1975). An instructional program to increase fluent speech of stutterers. *Journal of Fluency Disorders, 1,* 25–35.

Ryan, B. (1970). An illustration of operant conditioning therapy for stuttering. In W. Starkweather (Ed.), *Conditioning in stuttering therapy: Applications and limitations.* Memphis, TN: Speech Foundation of America.

Ryan, B. (1971). Operant procedures applied to stuttering therapy for children. *Journal of Speech and Hearing Disorders, 36,* 264–280.

Ryan, B. (1974). *Programmed therapy for stuttering in children and adults.* Springfield, IL: Charles C. Thomas.

Ryan, B. (1979). Stuttering therapy in a framework of operant conditioning and programmed learning. In H. Gregory (Ed.), *Controversies about stuttering therapy.* Baltimore, MD: Univerity Park Press.

Ryan, B. (1981). Maintenance programs in progress—II. In E. Boberg (Ed.), *Maintenance of fluency.* New York: Elsevier North Holland.

Ryan, B. (In press). Treatment of stuttering in school children. In W. Perkins (Ed.), *Current therapy in communication disorders.* New York: Thieme-Stratton.

Ryan, B., & Ryan, B. V. (1983). Programmed stuttering therapy for children: Comparison of four establishment programs. *Journal of Fluency Disorders, 8:4,* 291–321.

Ryan, B., & Van Kirk, B. (1971). *Monterey fluency program.* Palo Alto, CA: Monterey Learning Systems.

Ryan, B., & Van Kirk, B. (1974). *Programmed stuttering therapy for children.* (Final report, Office of Education Project 0-72-4422) Washington, DC: U.S. Department of Health, Education and Welfare.

Ryan, B., Rustin, L., & Ryan, B. V. (1981, November). Comparison of speech and therapy of English and American stutterers. Paper presented at the American Speech-Language-Hearing Association, Los Angeles.

Shine, R. (1980). Direct management of the beginning stutterer. *Seminars in speech, language, hearing, 1,* 339–350.

Skinner, B. (1953). *Science and human behavior.* New York: Macmillan.

Webster, R. (1980). Evolution of a target-based behavioral therapy for stutterers. *Journal of Fluency Disorders, 5,* 303–330.

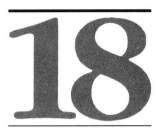

Stutter-Free Speech: A Goal for Therapy

George H. Shames and Cheri L. Florance

Postscript
A Current View of Stutter-Free Speech

George H. Shames

18

Stutter-Free Speech: A Goal for Therapy

George H. Shames and Cheri L. Florance

This book[1] is a description of a particular regime of stuttering therapy that has the goals of developing speech that is free of stuttering and a self-concept that enables the client to view himself as a normal, nonstuttering speaker.

There are philosophical, theoretical, and tactical issues involved in the clinical modification of stuttering behavior. A person's change and growth as a speaker is entwined with his growth and change as a total, social being. Such changes may well impinge on his basic self-identity. Questions such as "Who am I? What have I been? How did I get to be this way? What will I become?" are suggested, if not asked. When entering therapy, a client activates a special system of support to help bring about his growth and change. It is a temporary system; and our goals as therapists include getting that client into and out of these special therapeutic circumstances and back into his nonspecial mainstream of society as quickly, as efficiently, and as effectively as possible.

Of necessity due to the complexities of communication problems, therapy is conceptualized in a multidimensional, interacting framework. Many different things are going on at the same time during therapy. We have the behavioral tactics that focus on the specific communication behaviors to be acquired. We have the therapeutic relationship, which is the context in which these behavioral tactics operate. We have the client and his will to recover, his motivation to learn, his coping styles, and his resistances to change. We have the stutterer's environment in the form of family and friends who remain interactive with him and may serve to facilitate or to impede his therapeutic regime. Finally, we have you, the clinician, as a feeling and reactive participant in the process. The therapy itself is based on the very simple idea of helping the stutterer learn to produce elements of normal speech.

This therapy is strongly based on a great deal of theory and research from the fields of stuttering and behavior psychology. We have tried to selectively translate that theory and research into viable and effective clinical tactics for the problem of stuttering. As a result, we have explored, systematized, and sequenced a number of principles, tactics, and experiences that constitute this particular way of providing therapy for stuttering.

Much of the content of this therapy has come from the stutterers themselves, as they taught us how to help them. Although this book describes a general structure for a program of therapy, its application and tactics are highly individualized as each stutterer moves through his own unique therapeutic experience. Even though many of the tactics and descriptions presented are quite specific and common among a number of the clinical regimes, they provide only our way of looking at the processes of therapy

[1]This previously published material is highlights and excerpts from the book *Stutter-free speech.* It focuses on the principles, rationale, phases, and goals of this particular therapy.

and their underlying principles. There is room and flexibility for the individual reactions of the stutterers within the general process. The tactics are constantly undergoing scrutiny and revision in terms of each stutterer's needs.

The prologue for this therapy was five years of clinical studies involving a number of short-term experiments, revised clinical programming when new ideas about therapy emerged, and long-term follow-up evaluations of stuttering clients (Shames & Florance, 1977).

We have tried to provide an overall therapeutic regime within the contexts of:

1. The application of specific behavioral principles and tactics designed to change specific speech behaviors.
2. Principles and tactics to help the stutterer become responsible for managing his own therapy.
3. Issues in the transfer and "carry-over" process.
4. A clinical therapeutic relationship as it evolves within the context of interviewing and counseling.

In order to discuss such a series of therapeutic processes we have arbitrarily dissected it into its component parts. However, these components are neither static nor independent, neither parallel nor even sequential. At times, the conditioning processes and the relationship processes proceed in tandem; at times, simultaneously. However, our discussion will address each process separately.

Our goals are:

1. To establish speech that is free of stuttering.
2. To establish a speaker's self-perception that is compatible with his speech behavior; that is, as someone who no longer is a stutterer, or as one who no longer stutters (if that is the fact of his speaking behavior).

To reach these goals the stutterer learns to deliberately control the rate of his talking (fast or slow) and to control how he segments his speech acts, so that he continuously phonates and continues his airflow between words as he moves forward through his speech acts. Our focus is on the acquisition of these two behaviors: control of rate, and continuous phonation.

The stutterer is then trained to monitor his new speaking skills in a deliberate and scheduled manner, and to expand his speech monitoring into his entire "talking day." Eventually the stutterer replaces his monitored stutter-free speech with unmonitored stutter-free speech. These processes are systematically scheduled so that he goes through several phases:

Phase 1. Replacing stuttering with volitional control over speech (monitored stutter-free speech).

Phase 2. Training in independent self-monitoring and self-reinforcement.

Phase 3. Transfer and generalization to the nonclinical environment.

Phase 4. Replacing monitored speech with unmonitored speech.

One of the basic principles underlying this therapy is that the client develops a system of behavioral tactics and rules for strategies that enable him to either move progressively and gradually forward toward stutter-free speech, or, if necessary, to back up in a systematic way. A "back-up" system as well as a progressive shaping system is necessary whether we are dealing with the target responses, the occasions and situations, processes of self-reinforcement, or the schedule of reinforcement.

Phase 1, which deals with developing volitional control over speech, has been directly influenced by the early work involving the use of the DAF machine. In the children's program, Phase 1 was additionally influenced by the research on parent-child interactions and the shaping group.

Phase 2, which deals with self-reinforcement and monitoring stutter-free volitional control of speech, evolved from the research on self-regulation, self-reinforcement, and the concepts of internal and external locus of control as well as on the Premack principle of reinforcement.

Phase 3, which deals with environmental transfer and maintenance, is based on the ideas and tactics of therapy on the contract plan coming from the areas of family therapy and marital therapy.

Phase 4, which deals with replacing monitored with unmonitored speech, is based partly on the concept of replacement of stuttered speech and on processes of generalization.

Throughout the therapy is the influence of the information about schedules of reinforcement derived from operant-laboratory research. Similarly, the content and format of the interviews were influenced by the research on the content of what stutterers talk about and the interviewing and counseling strategies and concepts developed by Rogers (1972), Ivey (1975), and Strupp (1962, 1972).

THE CLINICAL RELATIONSHIP

The clinical relationship between the stutterer and clinician is the primary context for behavioral change. At times, other people significant to the stutterer such as parents, teachers, siblings, friends, and other stutterers may be brought into this context, but the basic vehicle for establishing significant and durable changes in the stutterer is the interpersonal, clinical interactions between the two primary participants—the stutterer and the clinician.

The stutterer is more than a laboratory demonstration subject. He is more than a set of push buttons that can abruptly turn on and turn off certain target responses. He is more than an animal running through a maze to reach a reward. As he goes through various phases of behavioral change associated with his problem, he reacts, resists, feels, anticipates, hopes, and dreams. He is suspicious and fearful, and brings his history as a stutterer and as a total person to his therapeutic experience.

In addition to the communication problem of stuttering, the process of therapy and of change can be a problem in and of itself. Changing, even positive change, can be stressful. Recognizing this, clinicians cannot limit their functions to being discriminative stimuli (S^Ds) or to being contingent consequences (CCs) in their attempts to influence the stutterer's behavior. The stutterer needs the human qualities of the clinician as well as her behavioral technological competence. As Fromm-Reichman states about psychotherapy, the patient "needs an experience, not an explanation" (Strupp, 1962, p. 582). The clinical relationship starts to evolve with the first contact between the stutterer and the clinician, developing its style and form, functioning as the stutterer moves through the various behavioral phases of his therapy. It is as though two parallel, interacting processes and experiences go on at the same time, one focusing on the behavioral aspects of changing the stutterer's speech and another focusing on such things as feelings, motivation, trust, support, honesty, affection, and respect between the two participants.

THE PHASES OF THERAPY
Phase 1: Volitional Control

The Basic Program. During Phase 1 the client is trained to produce elements characteristic of normal speech. The elements compete with stuttering behavior and result in stutter-free speech. The training paradigm begins by instructing the subject to produce a very slow rate of speech, stretching each word into the following word to produce continuous phonations throughout the speech act and to eliminate pauses or interruptions that disrupt spontaneous conversational speech. To effectively train a consistent slow rate of speech, we utilize a delayed auditory feedback signal (250 milliseconds). By slowing the linguistic and motoric encoding process down to an abnormal rate, the client gives himself time to concentrate on producing the target behavior: continuous phonation. He must control his rate appropriately and without increasing speed or he will hear the delayed speech signal as a negative reinforcer. The goals of the first phase of the treatment program are:

1. To establish volitional control of continuous phonation, rate, and prosody.
2. To establish a normal response in terms of the suprasegmental aspects of speech.
3. To establish speech that is free of stuttering.

The client is required to complete 30 minutes of conversational stutter-free speech at each of five delay intervals on the DAF machine (250, 200, 150, 100, and 50 msec.). Initially, a period of training is necessary to teach the correct response on DAF. The client is instructed to slow down his speech until he no longer hears the echo through the earphones or until it sounds as if the two voices are speaking at the same rate.

Phase 2: Self-Reinforcement

Introduction. Although each phase of the therapy contributes its own unique features to the overall program, each phase depends on the preceding phase and integrates with the succeeding phase. Phase 2, Self-Reinforcement has a significance that goes beyond the phases of therapy. Eventually, the client finds himself on his own, depending on himself and making crucial judgments about what he should do. He has to reason, problem-solve, and become responsible. These responsibilities are far-reaching.

Some may focus quite specifically on the stuttering problem, but others may deal with general social interactions, education, and occupation. Becoming responsible for one's self in a general way may relate to a general pattern of self-responsibility that each of us over the years may have developed. On the other hand, our tendencies toward self-responsibility may vary with the kinds of situations we find ourselves in and how comfortable we are with ourselves under certain circumstances.

It appears that some people have a strong tendency to manage their affairs with very little outside support, structure, or feedback, while others need a great deal of external control, support, and feedback. One of the features of this therapy for stuttering is that it provides specific and formal training in the processes of self-reinforcement. This is part of a regime of self-regulation that the stutterer faces in the next phase of therapy and may face after therapy is formally terminated.

The structure of this phase of the therapy is based partially on the theory of Kanfer and Karoly (1972). It states that self-regulation has three elements: monitoring, evaluation, and reinforcement.

The goals of Phase 2 are to train the client to independently:

1. Self-instruct behavior responses
2. Self-monitor behavior
3. Self-evaluate behavior
4. Self-consequate behavior

During this training phase, the responsibility for each of the components of the self-regulation process is transferred from clinician to client control. Initially, the clinician presents an overt signal, such as a hand raised to instruct the subject to produce a slow rate with continuous phonation. A hand lowered indicates a faster rate with continuous phonation. This instruction functions as an S^D for the behavior of deliberate monitored speech. The client then produces the instructed speech behavior and it is tape recorded. After listening to the tape-recorded speech behavior, the clinician and client evaluate the production of instructed rate and continuous phonation. After the client successfully produces and evaluates the target behavior, he also assumes responsibility for self-instruction. The self-instruction signal is reduced to a more covert motoric movement (such as a socially acceptable gesture or raised finger) so it becomes totally unnoticeable to a lis-

tener. The very slow rate of speech is faded out systematically, leaving only a socially acceptable rate of talking. The client is now trained to self-instruct, to monitor, and to self-evaluate monitored speech behavior . . . and is now ready to self-consequate his speech behavior. We have arbitrarily selected unmonitored speech as a reinforcer. Premack (1959) states that a high-frequency behavior can function as a reinforcer if it is made contingent on the emission of a low-frequency target behavior. Because unmonitored speech is highly desired by our clients and is a high-frequency behavior for all speakers, we have selected this behavior to serve as a reinforcer for monitored speech. Also, because it is under the control of the stutterer, unmonitored speech is appropriate as a self-reinforcer rather than as an externally provided reinforcer. Therefore, the client is now able to engage in all four self-regulatory behaviors as follows:

1.	Self-Instruction	Motoric signal to emit monitored or unmonitored speech
2.	Self-Monitoring	Client deliberately emits socially acceptable rate and continuous phonation
3.	Self-Evaluation	Client self-evaluates correctness of response
4.	Self-Consequation	Client rewards himself with unmonitored speech

The goals are:

1. To establish independent volitional control of the speech response.
2. To establish a monitored, normal-sounding speech response.
3. To train elements of self reinforcement.

Phase 3: Transfer

Introduction.   Once the client is able to self-instruct, self-monitor, self-evaluate, and self-consequate his newly learned stutter-free speech behaviors, he is ready to address transfer of training. For most clients the first two phases of therapy follow a relatively consistent pattern in terms of time for treatment criterion and manner of response acquisition. However, the transfer of training period tends to vary a great deal from client to client. The purpose of this phase is to facilitate the client's ability to develop strategies for incorporating monitored stutter-free speech into his total life systems. For some individuals this type of transfer requires changes in many other complex aspects of his personality, style, self-concept, and coping mechanisms.

The Emotional Aspects of Transfer. When the stutterer begins to change his speech, other aspects of his life may be subject to change concomitantly. Giving up stuttering may mean giving up his primary coping or defense mechanism for self-protection. Fear of failure may predominate when he considers attempting the social and vocational interactions he has consistently avoided in the past. He has learned to relate to people from a posture of his own weakness, rather than from a posture of his strengths. As a result, he has been reinforced by listeners for playing a role of the weak victim. In this role, he is not threatened nor interrupted in his talking; not only has he lowered his own expectations, but those with whom he interacts have also lowered his expectations. This posture is far different than a posture of strength (normal speech), where expectations are perhaps higher and qualitatively different, where relations develop that involve the unmasked person underneath, the real person that is in each of us. It is a posture of strength where stuttering is not a factor in his success or failure as a human being. A posture of weakness can be deeply imbedded in the stutterer's self-concept, in his overt behaviors, and in his dynamic coping strategies. The rewards of being nurtured by others, of having an excuse for failure, and of feeling helpless and victimized are part of the investment in his problem that the stutterer must make some decisions about. Does he hang on to these rewards of weakness and try to continue to function in this weak mode, or does he give these things up for the rewards that may accrue with stutter-free speech? These decisions are difficult and are usually re-examined throughout therapy, as the stutterer experiences the consequences of stuttered and stutter-free speech. Deciding to change his manner of talking becomes a much bigger choice than merely electing a new motor-speech response. For many clients it means changing every aspect of their lives.

The environmental transfer phase of the treatment program is a particular period where new personality dynamics appear to emerge. As the client accumulates stutter-free speech experiences, he also attempts speaking in situations he may have feared or avoided in the past. These experiences may involve social or vocational interactions unique to the client's history. Thus, as the client continues to increase his transfer activities, components of self-concept and self-perception begin to change in concert with his new experience. The client attempts to remain at a comfortable level at all times while continuing to slowly but steadily shape the response until he is able to successfully monitor his new speech behavior in all communicative interactions.

When we accept the responsibility for dealing with a stutterer's problems, we are accepting a responsibility for more than merely applying some effective conditioning operations or behavioral modification tactics. We are concerned with more than those changes in speech occurring in our office. We are also responsible for helping the stutterer to assimilate these changes and to integrate them into his total intrapsychic and interpersonal condition. What has loosely been referred to as carryover involves the total person, not merely his speech. It involves an environmental generalization of new speaking skills; it also involves the stutterer's reactions to these experiences.

Evoking a single instance of stutter-free speech is a relatively uncomplicated and easy operation for both the clinician and the stutterer. Instating stutter-free speech in a controlled environment may depend more on operant conditioning tactics than any other aspect of therapy. However, environmental transfer may depend mostly on the therapeutic relationship that has evolved. It is in this phase of therapy that client change is most validly facilitated and evaluated.

The Contract. The goal of Phase 3 of the treatment program is to transfer the newly trained speech behaviors environmentally. Because this newly trained behavior is yet somewhat fragile and the possibility of an interruption in the client's ability to concentrate on producing his new complex of behaviors may arise from a number of environmental variables, a highly systematic, preplanned environmental transfer structure has been developed. This transfer plan is in the form of a contract. With the contract, the client predetermines the exact time, place, listener, and his own behavior plan for using his new speech behavior environmentally.

By defining as many variables as he can in formulating the contract, the client is essentially controlling his environment as much as possible. As a result, he is able to focus his concentration on programming his new motor speech responses as self-instructed by his behavior plan. The client's focus or concentration on programming the new behaviors replaces his automatic motor programming of old speech responses. By using the contract the client increases the probability of his instructing and emitting the desired behavior, stutter-free speech (controlled rate, continuous phonation, and forward-moving speech). This contract represents the client's minimal commitment to the transfer of his stutter-free speech to the environment. It is based on the client's comfort level about those activities. The client can go beyond the elements of his contract if he so chooses. However, frequency and duration of monitored speech, speaking situation, and audience are varied until the client's entire talking day is monitored stutter-free speech, and a wide variety of conversational interactions have been successfully completed. Individuals vary in how they implement this phase and in how rapidly they expand their contracts. Typically, the contract is drawn up each morning and the client reviews the day's activities each night, usually by tape-recording his review of the day. This contract activity is reviewed with the clinician during the following therapy session. It is important at this stage in the program for the clinician to satisfy two goals:

1. Permit the client to develop his own problem-solving strategy.
2. Facilitate the client's successful talking experiences.

To satisfy these goals the clinician must move in and out of several roles: counselor, teacher, and speech therapist. Sometimes the tactics of the clinician may conflict with the tactics the client wishes to explore. For example, if the client devises a contract activity that is within the general framework of the program but success seems doubtful, should the clinician as counselor permit the client to attempt the activity and risk failure, or should the clinician as teacher tell the client that his plan could be improved in a particular way? For the most part, we have found that the client will, with extra determination, engage in those activities he has designed and gut-level believes in instead of following the didactic instruction from the clinician. Because we would like to see the client make permanent, durable changes in his speech and self-perception, we believe that the client needs the space and supportive environment for personal decision making and growth. Therefore, although within the session the clinician may nondirectively help the client develop seemingly appropriate problem-solving strategies, the ultimate decisions are left to the client. In this way, the clinician reinforces the client by her belief in the client's ability to solve his own problems, to be responsible for himself, and to be in charge of his environment. It is within this client-centered behavioral context that the transfer process begins.

Expansion of contract transfer activities and the continuation of Phase 3 eventually blend into Phase 4 when the client starts to progressively replace his monitored stutter-free speech with unmonitored stutter-free speech. The process is analogous to the expansion and contraction of an accordion. At first the accordion expands with increasing amounts of monitored stutter-free talking, via the transfer contract. Then at a certain point the accordion is squeezed together as monitored stutter-free speech is replaced by unmonitored stutter-free speech.

Four types of observations signal that the client is ready for the replacement process of Phase 4. These are:

1. He is monitoring easily during his entire talking day.
2. His unmonitored talking that he schedules as a reinforcer is always stutter-free.
3. His unscheduled unmonitored talking is generally stutter-free.
4. His scheduled unmonitored speech and his monitored speech sound similar in terms of rate and continuous phonation to the extent that the clinician cannot differentiate the scheduled unmonitored and monitored speech.

Some clients meet all four criteria for entering Phase 4. However, some clients never reach the point where they monitor their entire talking day. For these clients, the latter three criteria are valid for terminating Phase 3 and starting Phase 4.

Phase 4: Training in Unmonitored Speech

There are several criteria employed for starting a client into Phase 4 of the therapy. The most significant criterion is that the client is able to monitor his stutter-free speech for the entire talking day and in a wide variety of speaking situations. However, in the absence of this criterion, if the client's monitored and unmonitored speech sounds the same and if both are generally free of stuttering, then Phase 4 can be initiated. Monitoring rate and continuous phonation is indeed a very special way of talking. The client has learned to volitionally program certain elements of the motor-speech act at will. Although the client is consistently producing stutter-free normal-sounding speech at this point, he is still paying special attention to the way he speaks. The goal of Phase 4 is to replace these special monitoring behaviors with automatic stutter-free talking.

At the end of the third phase of treatment, the client is using a behavior plan in which he monitors (is deliberate and concentrates on how he talks) 80% of the time and uses unmonitored speech (lets go of his concentration) for about 20% of the time as a reinforcer for monitoring. Thus, he begins a speech act with careful, deliberate concentration on monitoring the rate, continuous phonation, and forward movement of his speech. Then, either toward the end of the speech act or at various times while he is talking, he signals to let the words come out automatically. So during the beginning of a speech response, he pays careful attention to volitionally controlling elements of his motor programming system and relaxes the intensity of concentration on a few words while he is talking, usually at the end of a speech act or semantic-thought unit. The paradigm for the monitored–unmonitored speech pairing is based in part on the findings of David Premack (1959). Premack found that high-frequency behavior, if made contingent on low-frequency behavior, can reinforce low-frequency behavior. By definition, reinforcement increases the probability of the future occurrence of a specific response. Thus, in accordance with the Premack Principle, unmonitored speech was originally used to reinforce monitored speech in this therapy program. However, this high-frequency behavior is also consistently reinforced by the client and by society; this may be the reason that the client consistently emits those behaviors. The basic reason for replacing monitored with unmonitored speech is knowing that unmonitored stutter-free speech will be reinforced by society and by the stutterer himself.

Because of its prior function during Phases 2 and 3 as a self-reinforcer under the scheduled control of the stutterer, and because it is desired by him and has a public representation, unmonitored talking has a good probability for replacing monitored speech. Its scheduled and unscheduled occurrence is already a part of the client's experience. During Phase 1 and Phase 2, we arranged the client's responses so that he produced monitored stutter-free speech. This complex of behaviors under stimulus control (self-instruction) was directly adjacent to the response of a few words of automatic talking (the client's highly desired speech behavior). At that time this unmonitored stutter-free talking was used as a reinforcer for learning to program correct rate, phonation, and forward movement of motor speech behavior.

Because the monitored–unmonitored paradigm is included early in the general therapy plan, there is a base of experience for the goal of Phase 4. In Phase 4 we are ready to alter the learning format so that automatic talking begins to replace monitored speech. The client moves from a schedule of monitored talking 80% of the time and unmonitored talking 20% of the time to a schedule of 50% unmonitored talking, by monitoring every other phrase. He then reduces monitoring further by monitoring just the initial portion of each speech act or phrase and using unmonitored speech for the rest. He may then monitor just the initial portion of every other speech act or phrase. At this point the replacement schedules become highly individualized. We have to keep in mind what the individual is capable of remembering and doing. He may move to a time-block schedule and monitor the first speech act he produces every half-hour, then every hour, and then once in the morning, afternoon, and evening. He might choose to monitor once a day, once a week, or only on payday. At this time, monitored speech may be totally replaced or the client may still elect to monitor speech only during special events, like being on television, asking for a raise, or speaking before a large group. However, it seems that under those conditions, the normal speaker would also pay special attention to his speech; the stutterer's monitoring at special times is similar in forms and intervention to the speech monitoring of nonstutterers.

REFERENCES

Ivey, A. (1975). Microcounseling—innovations in interviewing training. Springfield, IL: Charles C. Thomas.

Premack, D. (1959). Toward empirical behavior laws: 1. Positive reinforcement. *Psychology Review, 66,* 219–233.

Rogers, C. (1972). *Patterns of processes that take place in encounter groups.* Information cassette series. Chicago: Instructional Dynamics, Inc.

Strupp, H. (1962). Patient-doctor relationships: Psychotherapist in the therapeutic process. In H. J. Bachrach (Ed.), *Experimental foundations of clinical psychology* (p. 582). New York: Basic Books.

Strupp, H. (1972). On the technology of psychotherapy. *Archives of general psychiatry, 26,* 270–278.

A Current View of Stutter-Free Speech

George H. Shames

Since the development and refinement of the therapy that has come to be known as "Stutter-Free Speech," it has continued to evolve. As we spend more time with a particular therapeutic perspective, and more time with clients within that perspective, it is to be expected that changes and improvements and individual accommodations should occur.

It might be helpful to review briefly the evolution of this therapy as it was first conceived out of its early and more traditional beginnings in stuttering therapy, and of how behavioral issues and clinical relationship issues of therapy were more directly blended and integrated back in 1973. These derivations do not appear in the originally published material and are included here because they provide a greater depth of understanding of the underlying principles. It would also be productive to trace those experiences up to and through 1980 during which many of the phases of the therapy were refined and resulted in the book *Stutter-free speech.* Finally, I would like to trace things to the present, which has seen still further understandings and therefore changes in the regime of therapy.

Basically, as I look back on all of this I can identify three distinct time-periods of thought and activity.

In 1963 there was a publication by Shames and Sherrick, titled "A discussion of nonfluency and stuttering as operant behavior" in the *Journal of Speech and Hearing Disorders.* This paper was an attempt to translate traditional clinical perspectives, observations, and experiences into the constructs of operant conditioning. It was a mental exercise to see if an operant point of view would expand, clarify, raise questions on, provide answers to, and generate research about the nature and development of stuttering, as well as influence, change, or clarify what we do about the problem in a clinic situation. This time might be thought of as an incubation period during which theory, clinical tactics, and research strategies were being conceptualized. From 1966 to 1973 (the second distinct time-frame), in collaboration with Don Egolf, Robert Rhodes, Joe Carrier and Arlene Kasprisin-Burelli, we researched many of the processes of therapy for stuttering. We applied principles of instrumental conditioning within various perspectives of traditional therapeutic intervention, using the clinical interview and clinical interactions as the vehicle for study.

In one series of studies we looked at the Johnson-Semantogenic theory by systematically increasing and decreasing what stutterers talked about during clinical interviews through strategies of operant conditioning. We also determined that such changes in the content of stutterer's utterances appeared to be related to the frequency of their stuttering in ways that supported Johnson's theoretical ideas. In another series of studies we applied operant conditioning tactics to Van Riper's cancellation therapy. Such procedures seemed to tighten up the procedure and resulted in dramatic decreases in overt stuttering frequency, often to the point that stutterers never had occasion to learn the final stages of the cancellation regime. One interpretation of these results was that we were employing a punishment paradigm that was temporarily suppressing stuttering. These also appear in the *Journal of Speech and Hearing Disorders,* 1969, by Shames, Egolf, and Rhodes.

In a third series of studies we looked at the verbal interactions between parents (primarily mothers) and their stuttering children. This investigation resulted in a therapy that we termed our "mirror-image" therapy, during which the clinician would verbally behave and do just the opposite of what we observed the parents doing during interactions with their children. These studies were heavily based on the thinking of Ginott (1969) about how parent and child relate and interact and on principles of reinforcement. Again, we found that by helping parents and children change the nature of their verbal interactions (eliminating interruptions, reducing competition for talking time, increasing sensitivity to feelings, etc.) there were associated reductions in the overt frequency of stuttering. All of these studies are summarized in the book *Operant conditioning and the management of stuttering* by Shames and Egolf (1976).

Although we were greatly encouraged by the results of these studies, we recognized several areas of concern that needed further attention:

1. The various therapeutic regimes that were studied required a great deal of highly specialized training in observation, interviewing skills and conditioning tactics for the experimental therapists.
2. The therapy regimes were long-term.
3. The reductions in stuttering frequency typically resulted in a residual of low-frequency stuttering.
4. There were inconsistent degrees of relapse after the formal experimental therapy had terminated, perhaps because of too loose a maintenance or carry-over program.

In the third time-period of thought and activity commencing approximately during 1973 and in collaboration with Dr. C. Florance from 1976 to 1980, there were distinct and well-defined shifts. Some were gradual and became operational over a period of time stemming in part from research in areas other than

Postscript   18

stuttering and in part from serendipitous experiences and interactions with colleagues and stuttering clients. Other shifts were quite abrupt and were derived from a need to make things better.

One of the most basic shifts came out of a long-standing consultative relationship with Dr. William Perkins, who had been using a delayed auditory feedback tactic to initially change stutterer's speech. With the adoption of tactics that employed the DAF machine there was a radical change in goals of therapy. Instead of a small residue of stuttering following therapy, the goal became "monitored stutter-free speech." Thus Phase 1 of the stutter-free speech program based on the Curlee-Perkins program came into its earliest form. As I worked with the DAF I came to speculate more about what was going on, especially with regard to developing normal sounding, nonstuttered speech. The DAF per se creates a circumstance conducive to slowing down one's speech by prolonging the syllables. But there is much more to normal-sounding speech; in fact, slowed-down speech, although free of stuttering, is still quite prolonged and abnormal. The stutterer has to learn to do other things with his speech in order to attain normal sounding speech. These include moving forward in the utterance; continuing his airflow for phonation between and within words; using normal stress, accent and melody; and developing a faster rate of utterance. All but the latter are quite independent of the DAF experience, and sometimes are exacerbated by the DAF. These processes and our tactics for dealing with them represent a departure from our initial use of the Curlee-Perkins program. Since the 1980 publication with Florance, I have formalized a pre-DAF conversation stage of Phase 1 that focuses on developing skills of "continuous phonation." A series of phonation exercises are now employed (at 250 ms on the DAF) that provide controlled phonation practice on individual phonemes, nonsense syllables of all combinations of consonants and vowels, single words, continuously phonated two- and three-word units, phrases, sentences, cloze tactics, verbatim repetition of silently read material, and oral summarizations of previously read material. These exercises add about two to four hours of therapy to Phase 1 before the DAF conversational stage of activity is begun. Although slowing down one's speech may be important to developing control over stuttering, it may well be that the real value of slowing speech is that the entire vocal mechanism is temporarily put into slow motion, thereby increasing our awareness of and sensitivity to the integration of respiration, phonation, and articulation. Stutterers have an increased awareness of the continuous vibration of their vocal cords under the slow function conditions.

We have also become aware of some other things that appear to be going on during Phase 1. The stutterer appears to develop a feeling of control over his talking mechanism as he accumulates stutter-free talking time and actually exercises this control by using the DAF machine and controlling his phonation skills. This sense of control seems to be accompanied by an emerging change in what the stutterer expects of himself and what he expects his speech to be like. This expectancy changes from "no control" to "control"; from "stuttering" to "stutter free." These feelings of control and expectancy are enhanced by additional "practice" after each therapy session, starting during Phase 1. Originally, I did not encourage stutterers while in Phase 1 to engage in slow-down, prolonged speech outside of the therapy session. However, our experiences at our residential camps for stutterers have revealed that additional practice, at every stage of Phase 1, even in social situations, is valuable, especially for enhancing the feelings of control and expectancy and perhaps for the motor skill as well. However, such social practice seems more appropriate for socially protected situations, such as a camp, a hospital residential program, or the home, rather than in a general outpatient situation, where outside social use of very slow speech would probably be socially penalized. In its original and early forms this therapy regime jumped from Phase 1 (developing control and changing the speech pattern) to a Transfer Phase (which ultimately became Phase 3). There was no Phase 2 as we now know it. The stutterer took his new skills of monitored stutter-free speech learned on the DAF machine and practiced them outside in social situations. He depended on the social reinforcement of his listeners for the content of what he was talking about. He depended on his own joy of being stutter-free while monitoring his speech and depended on a very few significant people in his environment whom he felt he could count on for verbally reinforcing his new style of talking. But alas, we found that this type of "carryover" program was too loose; that the reinforcements encountered in the clinic from the clinician are not encountered in the real-life nonclinical world of the stutterer; that the stutterer's history of situational anxiety and helplessness made it easy for the fear-ridden stutterer to walk away from this part of his therapy; and that the sporadic emergence of "coincidental fluency" rendered his monitoring as too expensive a price to pay for maintaining stutter-free speech, and therefore monitoring could easily become a "crutch" used only to avoid stuttering.

Recognizing these many problems there appeared to be a strong need to develop strategies that would enable the stutterer to reinforce himself and to use those strategies in his regular life. Thus Phase 2, Training in Self-Regulation, and self-reinforcement, was developed, based on the model of Kanfer and Karoly (1972). Their model involved three components: monitoring, self-evaluation, and self-reinforcement.

I added a fourth component at the beginning of the paradigm, a "signal," which would function as a discriminative stimulus (S^D) for the latter three components. At first this S^D was provided by the clinician. Eventually the client signalled himself in order to take on the responsibility for initiating his monitoring activities. Self-reinforcement was effected through tangible reinforcers (money, privileges, prizes, etc.), but these types of reinforcers proved to be cumbersome and not meaningful. Based on the thinking of Premack, that high-frequency behavior could be used to reinforce low-frequency behavior, very brief insertions of "nondeliberate," "less monitored" speech were used to reinforce longer, more deliberate, monitored utterances by the stutterer. These brief insertions of un-

Postscript 18

monitored speech in the utterances of a stutterer could have had a reinforcing effect because they functioned to relax the stutterer's vigilance over his phonation and rate behaviors. Relaxation has been found to be reinforcing in other behavioral studies (Edmunds, 1974). Phase 2, Self-Responsibility, was thus formalized as a regular and crucial part of the Stutter-Free Speech Program.

The next step was to tighten up the Transfer Phase (Phase 3), to develop a plan and a commitment from the stutterer, and to recognize the stutterer's comfort level and anxieties as important dimensions of this process. The behavioral contract had been in use for some time with the retarded, in family therapy regimes, and in weight-loss and smoking-reduction programs. The idea of a hierarchy of contracts integrates this thinking with the hierarchial approaches associated with systematic desensitization therapies for phobias developed by Wolpe (1958) and used by Brutten (1967) in their work with stutterers. The Hierarchy of Behavioral Transfer contracts became the vehicle of Phase 3, wherein the stutterer integrated his Phase 1 skills into a Phase 2 paradigm of self-reinforcement and ultimately employed his Phase 2 paradigm in his real world through Phase 3 contracting.

At first the contracting was approached gradually and slowly in terms of a hierarchy of difficulty levels. However, since 1980, from my most recent experiences, we have seen that some stutterers can move through this phase quickly, intensively, and with a total immersion in social contracting without regard to a formal hierarchy of difficulty levels. The stutterers develop (with guidance) their own pace, depth, and immersion into this process. There are some who still need the slower approach. At this writing we are trying to identify the optimum schedule of therapy and schedule of behavioral contracting for individual stutterers. Some need to move slowly, some need to move rapidly. Some need a great deal of nurturing and counseling; others do not, and seem to derive a great deal of social reinforcement for the changes in their life and in their speech. Some stutterers assimilate dramatic changes easily, while others resist these changes or are frightened by them. The clinical relationship seems to be very important during Phase 3, Transfer, because the initial changes in speech are now taking form in the person's total life system. The stutterer needs a compassionate, empathic companion in the form of his clinician, as these changes start to take form in the stutterer's interpersonal network and in his own views of himself. Up to this point the three phases of the therapy have provided the stutterer with a structure for a series of behavioral experiences. His responses to this structure and to these experiences—how he assimilates, integrates and changes with them—require a counseling relationship with his clinician. It is difficult and improbable that a stutterer can handle these experiences alone. Clinicians should expect to function as counselors to help these stutterers as they change not only their speech, but also their expectations with people, their goals, how they feel about themselves and value themselves, and also generally help them to integrate these changes in their total life system and intrapersonal views.

Phase 4, as I now see it, was the result of a happy accident. Phase 4 is designed to gradually replace the stutterer's vigilance and monitoring of rate and phonation with nondeliberate, unmonitored speech. The seeds for this replacement process were planted during Phase 2, when brief insertions of unmonitored speech were used to reinforce the stutterer's monitoring activities. Scheduled, unmonitored stutter-free speech was further strengthened during behavioral contracting in Phase 3. During this time I observed that the properties of monitored speech were generalizing to the insertions of unmonitored speech. The unmonitored speech was slower than it had been and contained elements of continuous phonation to the point where the monitored and unmonitored speech during contracts eventually could not be differentiated. This generalization suggested that we might be able to facilitate a generalization process and replace the monitoring with totally nonvigilant, nondeliberate, unmonitored speech. Phase 4 gradually schedules this replacement process, which in a sense reverses the schedule of the Phase 3 Transfer Phase, whereby monitored, deliberate speech is gradually scheduled for progressively less frequency of occurrence. Our experience has shown that this can be accomplished for large numbers of stutterers, and that this phase lays the groundwork for a very real change in self-concept: from that of a stutterer to that of a nonstutterer.

CHANGES IN THE FORMAT OF THERAPY

Several other programmatic changes are worthy of comment. One is that the child program of therapy has been administered on an individual basis quite effectively. The parent counseling and training is still a crucial aspect of the therapy, and lays the foundation for carry-over into the child's home and social environments. We have found that the child's program can be carried out equally well in small groups or individually.

A second experience has been with brief, intensive, residential therapy programming in camp settings. We have been able to integrate children and adults in all phases of the therapy. Also in such protective settings we have been able to provide significantly greater amounts of practice time in real social interactions. This latter type of experience strengthens the control and comfort that the stutterer has with his initial forms of slow, stutter-free monitored speaking and seems to have a generally facilitative effect on later stages of therapy.

SUMMARY OF CHANGES IN TACTICS IN THE STUTTER-FREE SPEECH PROGRAM

1. There is now formalized practice in continuous phonation prior to DAF conversational phase of therapy.
2. There is social use of "slowed-down" speech during all of the DAF phases of therapy, in protected social environments.
3. The clinician and parents engage in the same pattern of speaking as expected of clients when they are talking to one another.

Postscript 18

4. In the Transfer Phase (Phase 3), contracting may not necessarily be accomplished slowly or in a hierarchical pattern. It can be done intensively, pervasively, and without regard to difficulty level of the talking situation.
5. The child program can be carried out effectively on an individual basis.
6. Brief, intensive, residential programs such as in a camp or hospital provide an environment and an atmosphere for social interaction, practice, and motivation that can be powerful and effective for helping a stutterer to get started in working on his problem.

We have been studying the general effectiveness of this program for approximately eight years (1974–82). Recently we did a case-by-case review of the most recent 150 stutterers that have gone through the program in Pittsburgh. Coming out of that review is a list of what we thought were critical variables operating in the degree of success of each individual. It appears as Table 18–1.

What we see here is that success or outcome cannot be reduced to simple group percentages. Outcome is a highly individual issue. The question of outcome is not simply a question about the nature of therapy.

As we review this list, we see at least five classes of variables operating that influence outcome.

1. The client
2. The client's family or support system
3. The client's environment
4. The clinician
5. The therapy

The Client.   The client brings to therapy the unique history of his problem, his current pain and circumstance, his motivation for change, his attitudes, his coping and defending mechanisms, and his expectations and goals. He brings his personality, his fears and anxieties, his history with therapy, his self-perceptions, and sense of his own worth and value as a person as well as his sense of control or helplessness. He brings his readiness for therapy, his readiness to relate to a therapist and his readiness to change.

The Family and Significant Other People.   We live in interactional networks; people in interactions with people. We communicate with people, we emote (love, hate, argue, laugh, smile, caress, fear, approach, avoid, etc.) with people. Some people stand out for us. They are close to and important to us. Our children, parents, spouses, families, and certain friends, may move in and out of emotionally supportive roles with us. When a person enters therapy, he has admitted to himself and accepted the fact that he not only needs to and wants to change, but is on the threshold of doing something about it. At this critical time, he is vulnerable and perhaps requires the support of those people that are close to him. Although therapy is often a private affair between the client and clinician, it can be a lonely experience. As a client takes his new skills out of the clinic and into his real world, he needs nonintrusive understanding from his family and friends. He

Table 18-1.   Variables Influencing Progress

1. Initial dramatic change
2. Changing too fast to assimilate
3. Magic or superstitious behavior
4. Motivation
5. Coasting on initial change
6. Health
7. Money
8. Moving
9. Family and environmental support
10. Continued contact and support of a clinician
11. Resistance to change
    a. fear for change
    b. low self-expectation; acceptance of problem
    c. devaluing of self
12. Denying problem
13. Self-reinforcement tactics
14. Skills of the clinician
15. Automatic generalization
16. Not adhering to elements of the therapy
17. Minimally handicapping problem
18. Prior unsuccessful therapy
19. Personality variables: coping skills
20. Continuous and overwhelming stress: family, job, emotional
21. Maintaining a goal orientation and direction
22. Pay-off of problem; i.e., helplessness
23. Overwhelming effects of panic and anxiety
24. Using therapy as a crutch
25. Using therapy as an avoidance
26. The price of vigilance
27. Other problems: psychosis, mental retardation, brain damage
28. Belief in the program
29. Confidence in the therapist

needs his independence and sense of responsibility, but he needs to nurture these processes in caring interactions with his loved ones.

The Environment.   Although people are a part of the client's environment, we are speaking here of an expanded class of factors, beyond the client's close family and friends. Instead we are including the day-in, day-out circumstances of people, stress, job, excitement levels, social pressures, time pressures, social deprivations and isolation, life style, pace of activities, etc. that a client encounters on a fairly regular basis. Everyone lives with some stress in their lives. Children are forced to conform to the regime of eating, sleeping, and toilet and social graces to be a member of a family. Adolescents live with the stress of seeking their own identities away from the family, escaping the power structure of parents, exploring their emerging sexuality, and maintaining acceptance with their peers.

Postscript   18

Adults live with various stresses of careers, loneliness, and isolation, finding their niche in the world. Even minor changes in daily routine can be stressful. Stress is a normal part of living. However, when stresses mass and impact on us; that is, too many in too short a time frame, people can be overwhelmed by them and not be able to cope with them. At these times, it becomes difficult to integrate any therapeutic change into a life system, because the life system is undergoing radical change, and such integration becomes a task, like trying to thread a constantly moving needle. Also, these other stresses (therapy may also be viewed as a source of stress) may take priority over the issues involved in therapy. In therapy, when we become aware of these stresses, we should either try to help the client to space them out to reduce their massed impact, or give the client a chance to talk about them during therapy as a way of verbally, cognitively, and emotionally unmassing them, even before they may occur (as a post-therapy experience). Overwhelming post-therapy stress can seriously undo the gains achieved during therapy.

The Clinician.   Although all of these factors affect outcome, and no one factor is more important than any other factor, the clinician is a key to getting it all started. The clinician should expect to give almost everything at his command. The clients, the problem, and the therapy are demanding. The clinician should expect to give his intuition, his reasoning, his technical skills, his caring, his beliefs, his values, his goals and his understanding of people. He has to be able to commit himself, to focus on the client, to be available, to empathize. It is a draining commitment—a commitment of love and trust. A commitment that goes beyond the initial changes in speech, carrying through the long and usually difficult process of environmental transfer and integration. It is a commitment to help when resistances surface, when anxieties overwhelm, and if relapse occurs. It is a commitment to go as far as the client may wish, in an honest and therapeutic encounter. It is a commitment to finish what one starts in generating a trusting clinical relationship.

The Therapy.   The therapy itself is also a critical factor in outcome. Usually when a question is raised about the effectiveness of a therapy, it is implicitly a question about the validity of the conceptualization of the process of therapy. We must constantly ask ourselves whether the therapy addresses the pertinent issues of the problems being presented by the client. We must look at the rationale, the logic, the pertinence, and the totality of the therapy. In these instances of problems of stuttering we must consider such things as the stutterer's motor responses, his attitudes and feelings, social interactions, intraphysic problems, the role of the family, and his environmental support. We must consider the tactics of initial change in speech and helping the stutterer to become responsible for maintaining these changes. Finally we must consider strategies for long-term support and evaluation.

Outcome is not merely a measure of pre- and post-therapy status or of changes in the overt frequency of stuttering. Outcome is a longitudinal issue of following clients for a long period of time. Outcome deals with the stability and impact of changes over a period of time as the client integrates these changes into his total interactional network and life system.

Outcome is a blending of each of these five classes of variables (the client, the family, the environment, the clinician, the therapy) into an integrated experience for each stutterer and for each family and for each clinician. The blending and the experience is different for each stutterer. A weakness in any one of these factors can result in a clinical failure. When they each come together in the right way, the result can be a stutterer who is finally free of his problem.

REFERENCES

Brutters, E., & Shoemaker, D. (1967). *The modification of stuttering.* Englewood Cliffs, NJ: Prentice-Hall.

Curlee, R. F., Perkins, W. H. (1969). Conversational rate control therapy for stuttering. *Journal of Speech and Hearing Disabilities, 34,* 245–250.

Edmonds, R. M. (1984). *Relaxation as a reinforcer in desensitization.* Doctoral dissertation, University of Pittsburgh.

Ginott, H. (1969). *Between parent and child.* New York: Avon.

Ivey, A. (1975). *Microcounseling—innovations in interviewing training.* Springfield, IL: Charles C. Thomas.

Kanfer, F., & Karoly, P. (1972). Self control: A behavioristic excursion into the lion's den. *Behavior Therapy, 3,* 398–416.

Perkins, W. H. (1973). Replacement of stuttering with normal speech: II. Clinical procedures, *Journal of Speech and Hearing Disabilities, 38,* 295–303.

Premack, D. (1959). Toward empirical behavior laws: 1. Positive reinforcement. *Psychology Review, 66,* 219–233.

Rogers, C. (1972). *Patterns of processes that take place in encounter groups.* Information Cassette Series. Chicago: Instructional Dynamics, Inc.

Shames, G. H., Egolf, D. B., & Rhodes, R. (1969). Experimental programs in stuttering therapy. *Journal of Speech and Hearing Disabilities, 34,* 30–47.

Shames, G. H., & Egolf, D. B. (1976). *Operant conditioning and the management of stuttering. A book for clinicians.* Englewood Cliffs, NJ: Prentice-Hall.

Shames, G. H., & Florance, C. L. (1977). *Behavioral management of stuttering.* Short course at National Convention of American Speech and Hearing Association, Chicago.

Shames, G. H., & Florance, C. L. (1980). *Stutter-free speech—a goal for therapy.* Columbus OH: Charles E. Merrill.

Shames, G. H., & Sherrick, C. E. (1963). A discussion of stuttering and nonfluency as operant behavior. *Journal of Speech and Hearing Disabilities, 28,* 3–18.

Strupp, H. (1972). On the technology of psychotherapy. *Archives of General Psychiatry, 26,* 270–278.

Strupp, H. (1962). Patient-doctor relationships: Psychotherapist in the therapeutic process. In H. J. Bachrach (Ed.), *Experimental foundations of clinical psychology,* p. 538. New York: Basic Books.

A Point of View about Fluency

Herbert Rubin and Richard Culatta

Postscript
Cognitive Therapy

Herbert Rubin

19

A Point of View About Fluency

Herbert Rubin and Richard Culatta*

University of Pittsburgh

At once the most striking and nagging fact about stutterers is their ability to be fluent. Implicit in this simple statement is a host of clues, positive and negative, about the etiology, maintenance, and therapy for stuttering. Perhaps the most important of these implications are: (1) The stutterer does not have to stutter. (2) There are, therefore, reasons why he does. (3) Organic determination is not one of these reasons. In addition, observing a stutterer's episodic demonstration of normal speech, we can conclude with very little by way of logical legerdemain that complete fluency is a feasible goal of therapy, and that this goal may be attained directly.

Since the desired behavior is already demonstrated by most stutterers in at least some specific situations, it should not be necessary to revert to a series of gradual or successive approximations of that behavior. We need not teach a client to be fluent. That response is already in his repertoire. We do need to help him to bring under conscious control the mechanisms by which he produces fluent speech.

These points are not totally new, nor are they bound to any of the more common philosophies of

*HERBERT RUBIN, Ph.D., is Associate Professor of Speech at the University of Pittsburgh, Pittsburgh, Pennsylvania. RICHARD CULATTA, Ph.D., is Assistant Professor of Speech and Director of the Speech Clinic at the University of Pittsburgh. The essential points of this paper were first presented at the 44th Annual Convention of the American Speech and Hearing Association, at Denver, 1968, under the title "Stutterers' Identification of the Reasons for Their Cures: Turning Points in Therapy."

therapy. On the contrary, it seems to us contradictory to work intensively with a stutterer, teaching him to stutter in a different way and persuading him to modify his symptoms, or in general to use all the tools at our disposal to help him "stutter better" when both he and the clinician know that he is capable of complete fluency. This inconsistent clinical approach to the problem exemplifies much, if not most, of the stuttering therapy conducted throughout the United States. We classify it as symptom-oriented because of its attention to the details of stuttered speech. It is also indirect, because it does not focus primarily on the reasons for stuttering which its relevant theories identify.

A more recent approach to stuttering therapy, originating in the research laboratory and not yet in widespread clinical use, is behaviorally oriented and frequently described as operant conditioning (Goldiamond, 1968; Martin, 1968; Shames, Egolf, and Rhodes, 1969). This is also symptom-oriented, but we classify it as a direct therapy because its relevant theory identifies the overt verbal response as the primary behavior to be dealt with. The stutterer's basic ability to be fluent is not in question, but only what he says, or how he says it at any one moment. This approach is still highly experimental, however, and not yet clinically proven. Because conditioning techniques are not easily extended outside the laboratory into such environments as the home or school, the success of an operant program could be attributed to

---

Note: From *American Speech and Hearing Association, 13,* 1971, pp. 93–116. Reprinted with permission.

the stutterer's consistent confrontation with the fact of his fluency, on the basis of which he does some serious rethinking about the nature of stuttering.

A third approach, which is not symptom-oriented, and not direct, comes to us from the disciplines of psychotherapy. It attempts to focus on the basic problem, the reasons for the individual's other "neurotic" symptoms, as well as his stuttering, but it is necessarily indirect because the clinician usually cannot identify these reasons. He, therefore, relies upon the client to generate the appropriate information, to which the clinician then reacts, hence the term: client-centered therapy (Rogers, 1951). The approach is cumbersome, if nothing else, because stuttering is part of a whole bag of problems, which, if not more than the sum of its parts, is certainly more than just the part with which we are mainly concerned.

A fourth approach is not symptom-oriented, but it is direct in its focus on the primary problem, as defined by theory. Johnson's (1946) semantogenic therapy is a good example of this, and its descendants can be traced through Williams (1957) to Kent (1961). The program we intend to present also falls within this last category and derives in large part from the three authors just mentioned. We will describe seven major principles and attempt to illustrate them where possible with transcribed excerpts from recorded interviews.

THE PROGRAM[1]

The first, and perhaps the most overriding, of the seven principles is that the program is necessarily a cognitive one. Each of the other six points to be made must not only be brought to the awareness of the stutterer. He must acknowledge them, accept them, and ultimately commit himself to them. This is not to say that the clinical experience has to be a fanatical one. But the task of obtaining real commitment, of going beyond the tacit acceptance or reverbalization by the client of the principles espoused by the clinician, is a difficult one in any direct program of therapy. The point is especially pertinent to the program described here, we feel, because much of what we are asking the stutterer to commit himself to he has already considered at a relatively superficial level. An

example of this is the goal of fluency, which most stutterers verbalize readily, but in which they are not likely to place much stock. On the contrary, most of the adolescent and adult stutterers seen for evaluations at the Speech Clinic at the University of Pittsburgh are extravagant in listing their hopes and desires, but quite pessimistic when pressed to set a date for the attainment of complete fluency.

How this commitment is attained, what finally makes sense or appeals to the psychology of any one stutterer, is largely an individual factor. For this reason, much of the content is unpredictable at the outset. The client becomes a constant source of information, of experiences, attitudes, and beliefs, which the clinician must utilize to present the six following principles in a manner acceptable to the stutterer. To the extent that we rely on the client as a source of such information we acknowledge that the program is client-centered. The principles, however, we feel are applicable to all stutterers. On the other hand, the order in which they are considered is not critical, and which of them becomes the focus of any therapeutic session may well be determined by information the client provides.

The second principle is that the stutterer has the basic physiological ability to be fluent. Johnson (1946) states that "it is a big mistake to think that stutterers cannot talk fluently, when they are fluent 80 per cent of the time." Although Johnson was probably referring to a proportion of the total number of words spoken per unit time, his argument can also be applied to the periods, however brief or rare, during which most stutterers report they have been consistently fluent. What has usually been missing from these reports of fluency is the intention or deliberation on the part of the stutterer to speak fluently. He reports it after the fact, is sometimes surprised by it and always grateful for it. He does not, however, take the credit or the responsibility for it. The goal of the program, then, is for the stutterer to acknowledge this ability and to demonstrate it unequivocally in the clinic. Fluency is what he says he wants, and he should not settle for less. The following taped excerpt from the recheck session of a stutterer who was discharged, and has since been fluent, illustrates a client's evaluation of the second principle:

Stutterer: I think that what probably helped more than anything over the long run was coming in here every week and doing it consistently; you know,

[1]A more formal program of therapy based on the following principles is currently being developed at the University of Pittsburgh and will be reported subsequently.

when you do that so much you know you kind of get to believe that maybe you really can do it.
Clinician: You mean the request that you had, you know, to be fluent for an hour; is that what you're getting at?
Stutterer: MmHm.

Another ex-stutterer identified the turning point in his therapy as his appreciation of the significance of control: "Control focuses on two points. One is to be actually fluent, and the other is to be able to have the awareness."

The third principle is that the client must accept the responsibility for his stuttering as well as for his fluency. If he can control his speech mechanism to do the one, he can control it to do the other. The argument simply states that if he does not have control over both fluency and disfluency, he does not have control over either. Together they exhaust the possibilities of speaking, along the dimension of fluency; they represent both sides of the same coin, and are inseparable. This analysis enables us to appreciate that the stutterer is skeptical about his fluent speech and refuses to take credit for it, just as he feels helpless about his disfluent speech and is reluctant to take the responsibility for that. The stutterer's attitude toward his speech is a vital aspect of therapy. Williams (1957) claims that

> many stutterers consider their stuttering to be an "it" that they carry around with them. They feel that it has an entity of its own. As long as he retains this "it" he cannot see his behavior. The belief that stuttering happens to you creates a feeling of helplessness and being trapped.

Johnson (1956) adds to this by stating that a stutterer must recognize his speech behavior as something he himself does. The stutterer should not view his nonfluencies as "things" that somehow happen to him. The vital idea is that if the stutterer "does not do it, there would be no it at all."

In the program we are describing, the stutterer must not only accept the responsibility for his disfluency, he must demonstrate this in the clinic, at least to the extent of initiating and terminating stuttering voluntarily. One ex-stutterer reported:

> The most significant thing was the day you had me start to stutter, and as we both know how much I fought you, and the whole thing there, but that started a lot of wheels turning. . . . because I realized how much, when it was forced upon me, when you said, "All right, now stutter," that when the demand came from outside, it

was a source of embarrassment, and it was making you in control of a weapon that I felt was mine, and I was not going to use it at your will. I was going to use it at my will.

Perhaps not for the same reason, most stutterers balk at the request to stutter deliberately. The patent explanation that they refuse because it is unpleasant and socially disturbing is inadequate, because the same stutterers are readily disfluent in a "normal" speaking situation. We feel that they refuse to stutter deliberately because satisfying the request forces upon them the very responsibility they have been rejecting. If they can be responsible for stuttering at this moment they can be similarly responsible all the time. They must then not only ask themselves the question "Why do I stutter?" but they must justify a history of years of stuttering.

This leads to the fourth principle, which is that stuttering to be maintained must be reinforced. Habit is a completely insufficient explanation because stuttering is invariably more effortful than fluency and must have some pay-off value for the stutterer to choose it above an easier pattern of speaking. Shames and Sherrick (1963) report that contingencies of positive reinforcement may maintain stuttering. Among the gains they suggest are attention, excuse for failure, and, in general, the opportunity to shift responsibility for inadequacies to stuttering rather than to personal shortcomings. Wischner (1950) also discusses the secondary gains or benefits which are derived from stuttering and which serve to reinforce the disfluent behavior. This lends support to the proposed view that stuttering is indulged in by the stutterer to attain or to maintain a desired state. Another popular explanation of this desired state is the expression of hostility in a social situation without fear of retaliation (Abbott, 1947). However, we cannot argue at this time for the commonality among stutterers of the use of their pattern of speaking as a tool of social aggression.

We can, on the other hand, make a related argument in the presentation of our fifth principle, which is the unpleasant and offensive nature of stuttering as perceived by the listener. While we trust this statement comes as no surprise to the reader, few people acknowledge its validity. Goldiamond (1968) probably had it in mind, however, when he noted that "the world can be considered as being in a conspiracy to maintain stuttering out of ingrained decency and respect for others' tribulations." One of his stutterers reported that "polite attention was commanded during stuttering and no one left the group or interrupted him while he was stuttering."

It is our belief that stuttering becomes especially offensive to the listener in light of the evaluation that it is controllable, and therefore unnecessary, behavior. For the clinician to disguise these feelings under a cloak of dispassionate acceptance or, worse still, the insincerity of sympathy, is dishonest and perhaps even unethical. Stuttering should not be acceptable. The fact that it is accepted, and most politely at that, makes Goldiamond's reasoning most convincing. Since we feel it is important to feed back to the stutterer the social impression he makes, our program is not a comfortable one for him, and this point of view may be new to the field. One of our ex-stutterers recalled:

I think what he tried to project to me, and what hit me hardest was that the whole prospect of stuttering was disgusting. I never looked at it in that way before. It was never that revolting to me, but he kind of made me believe that what I was doing was revolting to him, and should have been revolting to me too. And I believe that this was a great help.

Another one agreed:

That was most embarrassing. This made me look like a complete fool, but when I realized this I just recognized that you were telling me the truth. Whenever I make up my mind that I want to talk, this I could do. It's strictly up to me. I made this up in my mind; here I am.

These statements were not made casually or spontaneously by the clients. In addition to providing objective feedback to the stutterer, the clinician can emphasize his own negative evaluation of the stuttering. This kind of confrontation forces the stutterer either to defend the behavior in question or to seriously reexamine it. Either way he is forced to examine his stuttering in an objective manner which he otherwise might not do.

The sixth principle is that while stuttering is undoubtedly related to other problems the stutterer may have, and while he has personally integrated the stuttering into his total evaluation of himself, it is a separable symptom. In other words, the stutterer can remain whatever kind of person he is, even if he no longer stutters. Clinical evidence for this is simply that that there are no personality problems peculiar to stutterers. Except for their disfluency they are no more nor less neurotic than any selected group of "normals" who happen never to have stuttered (Goodstein, 1958; Sheehan, 1958). There are two distinct advantages accruing to the stutterer as he accepts this principle: First, it frees him to examine, if he chooses, other symptoms or behaviors which were previously masked by, or seen as part of or less important than, his stuttering. Furthermore, when the load is lightened by even one significant symptom, the remainder of his problems become more workable and can be handled similarly, that is, one at a time. Second, it dispels the superstition that some other nefarious symptom must spring up, like dragons' teeth, to replace the stuttering and maintain the individual's precarious psychic balance. This superstition appears to be at least as common among speech pathologists as among stutterers, and, while it is given credence by some psychopathologists, does not derive directly from Freud's (Freud, 1966) concept of defense mechanisms.

A former client summed our view when he reported that

I would be able to separate my speech from my general feelings about myself—about my competency in other things . . . and you think this is possible. And that it would be the answer to my [speech] problem. The other things would still have to be worked on.

The seventh and final point focuses upon the stutterer's evaluation of himself and of his ability to be fluent both at the level of the abstract and at the immediate level of the next word to be uttered. The abstract level is concerned with the stutterer's self-image as a stutterer as opposed to himself as a normally fluent person. To work on this self-evaluation we must begin with his recognized ability to be fluent. At a more specific level the client is asked to evaluate, at any moment of speaking, his attitudes toward producing the very next word he will utter. These evaluations are constantly solicited and discussed. The cognitive and directive nature of the therapy is perhaps emphasized most strongly with respect to this point. The fruition of this goal is best exemplified by a former stutterer at a recheck session. When questioned about the turning point in therapy for him he stated,

I was walking along the street one day and I started thinking, you know: just what am I? You know, am I a stutterer or what? And I figured, Well, I'm a stutterer if I think like one. If I don't, I'm not.

RESUMES OF THERAPY

At this writing 15 stutterers have been treated in the program described.[2] A summary of their schedules and results appears in Table 19–1. No specific selective procedures were applied; each stutterer was routinely assigned to one or the other of the authors. Two exceptions, Stutterers H and L, were referred by other clinicians who felt they were suitable for our program. The age range is from adolescent to young adult, and all but one (H) are male. The severity of stuttering at intake varied from mild to severe, although quantification of disfluencies was not performed in every case. Previous therapy also varied from none to many years, and in some cases such therapy was obtained at the university clinic. Rechecks on the consistency of results have been possible in six of the 13 clients who have terminated

therapy, after intervals of 4 to 19 months. The remaining two clients, who have been consistently fluent in the clinic only, have been referred to another program, where they are still receiving treatment.[3] We feel comfortable about declaring nine of the stutterers cured (A, C, D, E, G, L, M, N, O), are optimistic about the outcome of two others (F, K), uncertain about two (B, J), and pessimistic about two (H, I).

Careful inspection of the 15 cases suggests that, within the ranges of the variables represented, age and history of previous therapy are not related to success in the program. With only one female represented we cannot comment on the correlation of success and sex. Severity of stuttering at intake may be a significant factor, however. Of the eleven clients with whom we feel we have been most successful, eight were classified as "mild" stutterers, only one as "moderate," and two as "severe." Of the remaining four, in contrast, three were classified as "severe" and

[2]The following references to their therapy are not intended to provide experimental support for the theory presented. Such experimentation is currently under way. The data pertaining to the 15 subjects is intended merely to supplement the point of view expressed in this paper.

[3]The term *fluent*, as used in this paper, specifically refers to speech that is within normal limits, with no unequivocal blocks or otherwise defined events of stuttering.

Table 19-1.   Histories and results of therapy.

Client	Age at Onset of Therapy	Severity	Total Time (Mos.)	No. Sessions Indiv.	No. Sessions Group	No. Sessions Total	Previous Therapy	First Fluent Sample Sess. No.	Normal Fluency Now	Disposition	Months Between Term. and Reeval.
A	20	mild	12	23	12	35	yes	1	yes	terminated	9
B	23	severe	2	10	6	16	yes	1	yes (in clinic)	terminated & reentered	–
C	29	mild	12	26	0	26	no	1	yes	terminated	8
D	28	mild	8	23	8	31	yes	6	yes	terminated	19
E	34	moderate	9	0	21	21	yes	1	yes	terminated	12
F	35	severe	11	42	2	44	yes	3	?	referred for add. psychotherapy	14
G	34	mild	$\frac{1}{2}$	2	0	2	no	1	yes	terminated	4
H	40	severe	$3\frac{1}{2}$	12	0	12	yes	2	?	withdrew	–
I	18	severe	12	27	7	34	yes	13	no	discontinued	–
J	19	moderate	3	8	0	8	no	1	no	continuing	–
K	19	mild	18	22	0	22	yes	1	yes (in clinic)	referred for psychotherapy	–
L	17	mild	3	9	0	9	no	1	yes	terminated	–
M	15	mild	6	16	0	16	yes	2	yes	terminated	–
N	13	mild	3	4	6	10	no	1	yes	terminated	–
O	13	severe	7	10	8	18	no	16	yes	terminated	–

one as "moderate." If prognosis in this program does correlate negatively with severity of stuttering, a number of possible explanations can be offered. The closer the stuttering may be to normal speech, the readier the stutterer may be psychologically to take the final step. If we consider the stutterer at the moment of intake as already in a state of change, previous progress which brought him to a level of mild stuttering may provide the momentum for further change. Also, the more fluent he is at the time of intake, the more experience he has had with fluency, and the more convinced he may be of his ability to be so. Related to this may be his willingness to separate his stuttering from other symptoms or problems with which it has been associated. Both the observation and the tentative explanations for it merit further study. It is also possible, however, that a negative correlation between severity of stuttering and prognosis is characteristic of all programs of therapy, and not indicative of the one we have presented.

We made no measures of intelligence or of emotional maturity. The teenagers who were successful in the program, however, impressed us as being unusually mature, in being able to seek reasons for their stuttering, to demonstrate control of fluency early in therapy, and to accept the responsibility for their speech. On the other hand, we can also report success with a six-year-old, the only child with whom we attempted this approach, and who does not seem very mature at all. This youngster, who had been exhibiting signs of struggle, prolongation, and pitch change during his blocks, was able to manipulate all of these symptoms, as well as fluency, upon request. His clinician communicated amusement and curiosity as well as mild disapproval of the disfluency, and the boy's father was brought into the sessions soon after intake in order to communicate to them in each other's presence our understanding that the child was in complete control of his speech. We undertook this case with some apprehension and, in spite of its apparent success, are not attempting to generalize to the treatment of the young disfluent child. Environmental manipulation through family counseling works too well and too consistently in such cases to suggest clinical experimentation with alternatives.

CONCLUSION

The seven principles that we have outlined are guidelines of a therapeutic rationale that, we feel, is both valid and pertinent. The order in which the principles have been presented is arbitrary and not vital to the success of the program. The judicious utilization of these principles may enable the client and the clinician to construct a foundation upon which they can directly focus on the problem without unnecessary attention to symptomatology. However, since stutterers and fingerprints have much in common, it would not be efficient for the clinician to attempt to assimilate and apply totally the proposed method to every client, although the basic philosophy would have to be acceptable to all. However he decides to speak is completely under the control of the speaker. While the clinician's commitment is every bit as vital as the client's, it does not provide sufficient impetus to carry the two of them through the program. The client's readiness to accept each principle should determine the pace of the program. We make this statement to avoid, as in all therapy, a completely prescriptive or "cookbook" approach, without regard to the client's receptivity. However, to confront the client, to apply pressure to speed up the pace of therapy, is both reasonable and appropriate. For example, after a client has demonstrated consistent fluency in the clinic it is appropriate to ask him to set a date for termination. While the client may balk at an answer, and too cautiously estimate the date, the important communication is that therapy is a finite process, and that fluency is an immediate goal.

We feel that this view presents a specific set of alternatives by which both the client and the clinician can evaluate behavior and modify it as they wish.

SUMMARY

A rationale for stuttering therapy based on the goal of direct and immediate fluency is presented within the broad framework of current therapeutic theory. The major principles of the program are: (1) it is cognitive; (2) the stutterer has the basic ability to be fluent; (3) he must also accept the responsibility for his stuttering; (4) there are reasons or rewards for his stuttering which are appropriate to investigate; (5) stuttering itself is unpleasant, if not offensive, to the listener; (6) although stuttering is related to other attitudes or problems the stutterer may have, it is a separable symptom; and (7) anticipation of fluency is a necessary precursor to it. Brief resumes of the therapy of 15 stutterers supplement the theoretical presentation.

REFERENCES

Abbott, J., Repressed hostility as a factor in adult stuttering. *J. Speech Dis.* 12, 428–430 (1947).

Freud, Anna, *The Ego and the Mechanisms of Defense.* New York: International Univ. (First published in German, 1936) (1966).

Goldiamond, I., Stuttering and fluency as manipulatable operant response classes. In B. D. Sloane and H. N. Mac-Aulay (Eds.), *Operant Procedures in Remedial Speech and Language Training.* Boston: Houghton Mifflin (1968).

Goodstein, L. D., Functional speech disorders and personality: A survey of the research. *J. Speech Hearing Res., 1,* 359–376 (1958).

Johnson, W., *People in Quandaries.* New York: Harper (1946).

Johnson, W., in E. Hahn (Ed.), *Stuttering.* California: Stanford Univ. (1956).

Kent, L., A retraining program for the adult who stutters. *J. Speech Hearing Dis., 26,* 141–144 (1961).

Martin, R., The experimental manipulation of stuttering behaviors. In B. D. Sloane and H. N. MacAuley (Eds.), *Operant Procedures in Remedial Speech and Language Training.* Boston: Houghton Mifflin (1968).

Rogers, C., *Client-Centered Therapy.* Boston: Houghton Mifflin (1951).

Shames, G., and Sherrick, C., A discussion of non-fluency and stuttering as operant behaviors. *J. Speech Hearing Dis., 28,* 3–18 (1963).

Shames, G. H., Egolf, D. B., and Rhodes, R. C., Experimental programs in stuttering therapy. *J. Speech Hearing Dis., 34,* 40–47 (1969).

Sheehan, J. G., Projective studies of stuttering. *J. Speech Hearing Dis., 23,* 18–25 (1958).

Williams, D., A point of view about stuttering. *J. Speech Hearing Dis., 22,* 390–397 (1957).

Wischner, G. J., Stuttering behavior and learning: A preliminary theoretical formulation. *J. Speech Hearing, Dis., 15,* 324–335 (1950).

Cognitive Therapy

Herbert Rubin

Fourteen years was not so long ago, but as I recall writing "A Point of View about Fluency," the excitement that I shared with Rich Culatta about publicizing our convictions and discoveries about stuttering seems remote. The convictions remain, with very few modifications, and the excitement surprisingly is rekindled with each new clinical experience. Originally, we presented only fragmentary data for 15 clients one or the other of us had worked with, two of whom were still in therapy at the time, and only six of whom had been away from treatment long enough to qualify for reevaluation. Through the years since 1971, and a few dozen stutterers seen directly, with as many observed in therapy with other clinicians, I still subscribe to the seven points we made in the 1971 article, with this modification: I am now ready to rank those principles with respect to importance, hence, emphasis in therapy, and to elaborate some of them and to interrelate others.

The 1971 article owes an obvious allegiance to Dean Williams's "A point of view about stuttering," which appeared in 1957.[1] The contrast between the words "stuttering" and "fluency" in our respective titles represented a deliberate refocusing of both client and clinician toward the normative, positively valenced behavior as a feasible goal of therapy and as a response already in the repertoire of the client. Williams's outstanding contribution in 1957 was the personification of stuttering as an entity, an "it" that each stutterer believes he carries around with him and that bears the sole responsibility for the disfluent behavior, freeing the stutterer from blame and choice alike. Focusing upon that entity, the source and perpetuation of so much pain and embarrassment, seemed to us to blind the stutterer to his real ability and potential, to dwell on the past and to reinforce his resignation to remaining a stutterer. So, acknowledging our debt to Williams, and to Johnson before him, we attempted to reverse the emphasis of therapy and to place the responsibility for both the stuttering and the fluency exactly where it belongs: on the shoulders of the stutterer.

[1]The editors invited Williams to update "A Point of View about Stuttering" for this book, but unfortunately his schedule prevented him from contributing.

The first principle Culatta and I presented in 1971 was the cognitive nature of fluency therapy. We felt it was essential for those clients who identified themselves as stutterers to rethink their identities and their abilities. Seeing oneself as a normal speaker is a necessary component of speaking normally, and recognizing one's ability to control the motor speech apparatus is a necessary precursor to that identity. To that extent, our program is cognitive. Although we have not formally labeled our therapy as such, some of our colleagues have called it cognitive, and it seems that the name has stuck. I still think it is the major characteristic of what we do.

We talked only briefly in 1971 about therapy with disfluent children, and I will address that population later in this update. The qualification regarding young children that I want to make at this time is that they do not usually identify themselves as stutterers, and for them the program must be modified accordingly.

For the adults, who constitute the bulk of the clinical population we see, their identity as stutterers is critical. They do not see themselves as just like the rest of us except that they happen to stutter. They are stutterers. The clinical implications are profound. No matter how fluent they may be in the clinic and no matter how effortless and enjoyable that fluency is, their self-image ensures that sooner or later they will revert to their disfluent behavior, which is the norm for them. All else is either lucky or exceptional. I believe the significant success we have therapeutically with young children can be attributed largely to the fact that they do not yet identify themselves as stutterers and are therefore willing to relinquish the disfluency that adult stutterers require to maintain their self-image. I realize that "require" is a strong word. I have tried suggesting a number of similarly strong words with clients to see which they are willing to accept as descriptive of their feelings and behaviors. I was surprised to hear my clients accepting the concept of an "urge" to stutter. Most of them find that word more palatable than "want" or "need," both of which connote more desire or deliberation than "urge," which describes a force over which they feel they have little or no control. But experiencing that old familiar urge to stutter is virtually a guarantee that they are about to be disfluent. Now what is it about that conviction that can possibly be comfortable or reinforcing? It confounds the behaviorist in each of us. In fact, most clients I know identify an unenviable panic that accompanies each major block. They described a terrifying moment of helplessness, of abandoning themselves to a force over which they have no immediate control. The metaphors abound: downhill skiing on ice, a rudderless ship, a speeding car without brakes.[2] Why would a stutterer generate such aversive feelings when he has the physiological ability to utter the word fluently? He has done so many times before; can say it readily when alone, in unison, or after someone else has uttered it; when talking to a baby or an animal or other nonjudgmental audience. Clearly it's not the word or the sound that's the culprit. I believe the answer has to do with responsibility. Even panic, helplessness, and embarrassment, all genuine feelings,

[2]Wischner, 1952; Sheehan, et al., 1962.

Postscript   19

are preferable to the responsibility of being unaccidentally fluent or deliberately disfluent, which brings us to the second and third principles, respectively, of the 1971 article. These two aspects of responsibility, to be fluent or disfluent at will, still constitute the biggest hurdles in therapy with adults. Most stutterers do not want that responsibility, and therein lies the predicament of therapy. Our clients are convinced that their stuttering is the bane of their lives, the one thing they feel holds them back the most. And they are sincere. But they are equally sincere in their conviction that the means for speaking fluently are not completely available to them. Such is ambivalence. It is also neurotic. I think most stutterers must confront their ambivalence, talk it out and work it out, if therapy is to be successful over the long-term.

PRAGMATICS OF STUTTERING

The fourth principle of our earlier article is that there are reasons worth investigating for why an individual continues to stutter when he doesn't have to. I can't think why Culatta and I did not talk about the pragmatics of stuttering 14 years ago. Perhaps the term was still largely in the province of philosophers at that time. But pragmatics it is, and I would like to underscore the major functions of stuttering at this time. I first want to acknowledge that the scapegoat concept of stuttering is older than I am. Stutterers are able to excuse many failures or shortcomings because of their speech. It is more tolerable to attribute poor performance at school, or the loss of a job or a girl, to stuttering than to intelligence, looks, personality, or effort.

The pragmatics I want to discuss in the current update deal not so much with the stutterer's bruised self-image as with the social dynamics of the situation in which he stutters and with whom. What does the stutterer accomplish by his manner of speaking that fluency cannot? In 1971 we suggested as a fifth principle that stuttering is unpleasant, if not offensive, to most listeners. No one since that time has come forward to indicate otherwise, least of all a stutterer, for whom the prospect of listening to another stutterer is a uniformly aversive experience. Abbott (1947) long ago suggested that stuttering is an indirect way to express hostility, to make a listener uncomfortable, and to do so with impunity. Rarely does a listener interrupt a stutterer, turn away, or otherwise retaliate for the unpleasant and completely avoidable experience. Support for Abbott's analysis comes from most stutterers' acknowledgment that they avoid confrontation, and that when they do express hostility directly they are almost invariably fluent; that is, they do not need to stutter. In this light, stuttering is a very manipulative behavior, one which centers attention on the unusual speaker, keeping others respectfully attentive at the same time they squirm with discomfort, but always tolerant of their offender, too polite to tell him off or to walk away. Interestingly, it is on the telephone, where most stutterers claim to have the greatest difficulty, that they also report that an unseen listener is more likely to escape by hanging up, often anonymously, than is the victim of a face to face encounter with a stutterer to flee.

In addition to the manipulative, potentially hostile functions of stuttering there are other pragmatics of passivity and submissiveness that seem to go together. Stuttering is a nonverbal signal, to speaker and listener alike, that the stutterer is weak, childlike, and in poor control of at least a part of his body. This is very much like waving the white flag of surrender. "I can't hurt you. I'm no threat. I'm handicapped." is the message. At the same time, the stutterer is asking for special consideration. The white banner might well have lettered upon it: "Fragile. Handle with care." Support for this interpretation comes from the consistent observation that stutterers are more likely to be disfluent when asking for something than during any other kind of utterance. Indeed, a pleading, defenseless plaintiff is very likely to receive the support he seeks. No matter that the respondent subconsciously smells a rat, that the social benefactor senses he's being taken advantage of. The discriminative stimuli are loud and clear. "Don't hit someone when he's down. Don't be a bully, even though you suspect at some level that you're the one who's being bullied." For those stutterers who can recognize this child role that they sometimes adopt it is very useful to listen to their voices on tape as the pitch goes up and a tentative, plaintive tone is heard at the very moment they feel so young, innocent, and intimidated by the authority to whom they submit.

Both the hostile-manipulative and the childlike-submissive functions of stuttering are indirect in that it is the *manner* of speech that carries the message. The stutterer does not come out and say what is on his mind. Indeed, as Travis discusses in another part of this volume, the stutterer does not say what is on his subconscious mind either. It is not only confrontation that stutterers avoid; it is the expression, nay, the recognition, of any strong feelings, positive or negative. When I ask the question, "How do you feel about that?" or "What are you feeling right now?" I will most of the time hear what my clients are thinking, almost never how they feel.

Stuttering, then, is the medium of disguise, of deception. What the listener hears and sees is not what he or she gets. Related to and corroborating this interpretation is the negative correlation between stuttering and eye contact. I have become most aware of a stutterer's tendency to break eye contact after he has been fluent for a while. It's a subtle and silent signal that he is anticipating difficulty speaking. With clients who have learned to control their speech in therapy, that difficulty is usually manifested in a reduced rate and a disruption in the prosodic flow (increased pause times and flattened pitch range) rather than overt blocks, but the message is unequivocal. He has been thinking like a normal speaker and suddenly, like the toddler who realizes he has let go, reverts to his conventional self-image and prepares to stumble and fall. He is a stutterer once more. Fascinating are the answers to the question "Why?" at this point: "It was too good to be true, or to maintain." "It couldn't go on forever." (Note the neutral pronoun, "it" rather than "I." "It didn't feel like me." "It wasn't natural." What I hear them saying is that they are uncomfortable with the identity of a fluent speaker communicating openly and freely. They then close up, turn away, and

Postscript   19

hide behind the barrier that is stuttering. If I question their honesty at that moment I find that I've often uncovered a genuine dissimulation. At the moment of stuttering a client frequently blocks mentally as well as physically, suddenly changing topic or unconsciously lying. Like Pinocchio's nose, the signals of eye aversion and shift to disfluency may reveal for all to see what the speaker himself is unaware of. I do not suggest by this that each stuttered word signals a specific falsehood, but rather that the shift from fluent to stuttered speech, the isolated disfluency against a normal background, indicates a change in the mental state of the speaker, most often in the direction of masking his true thoughts and feelings from self and listener alike. And what he very likely needs to mask from consciousness at the moment he is most fluent is the recognition that he has the ability to be a normal speaker, that that fluency is immediately and automatically available to him. Why should that realization be threatening to a stutterer? Would he then have to give up the (unconscious) pretense, to take his place alongside the rest of us, with no convenient screen to hide behind? I think so. Let us remember that stuttering is a very resilient disorder, easy to revert to when the going gets rough, always tolerable, and never fatal. To many stutterers it is a most familiar, if not comfortable, way of life. I suggest that our task as clinicians is rendered doubly difficult by the recalcitrance of our clients: first to overcome their resistance in the rarified therapeutic environment sufficiently to elicit normal speech, and then to facilitate the maintenance of that normal pattern in the outside world and in the face of the social adversity that has become for a particular speaker the discriminative stimulus for stuttering. The latter difficulty, one of transfer and maintenance, is by far the more serious of the two. Most speech pathologists who work intensively with stutterers recognize that obtaining fluency in the clinic is not the major problem. There are many well-publicized techniques for doing so, which can be found elsewhere in this volume, in addition to the direct approach that Culatta and I have advocated. The problem is to strengthen the stutterer's conviction that he can and will remain fluent when confronted with competing signals to raise the white flag, to find the first available telephone booth in which to change back into the mild-mannered Clark Kent, to appear once again to be the ineffectual and unthreatening child for whom stuttering has been a protective cover.

To review what I have referred to as the pragmatics of stuttering, a number of the principles we introduced in 1971 can be seen to be closely related. The pragmatics are the reasons for stuttering. Expressing hostility indirectly, and without fear of retaliation, is one such reason. Not having to acknowledge that hostility, or any other uncomfortably strong feeling, is another; the stutterer can fool himself and at least some of the people, some of the time, about what he thinks and feels and what he is really capable of when he speaks. The third general function of stuttering to which we have referred is the submissive, childlike role the speaker assumes as a stutterer, a role which ensures special handling by a benevolent listener, apparently worth the price of dignity lost.

PSYCHOLOGICAL FACTORS

The sixth principle we raised in the earlier article is that the behavior of stuttering is related, but not inextricably tied to, the attitudes and problems that the stutterer presents. Most of us are intimidated on occasion. We may feel inadequate to a task or inferior to another person. If self-doubts or trepidations were indicators of psychopathology we would have to redefine what we mean by psychologically normal. The point I try to make to a stutterer is that he can be and feel whatever he currently experiences in a social encounter, but without having to stutter. Lots of others experience the same discomforts and remain fluent. Perhaps this point is not so simple as it appears. If stuttering is the name on the mantle that insulates the stutterer from the self-doubts that nag and dog the days of the rest of us, then it may not be realistic to talk of a separable symptom; that is, stuttering. Consequently, one of the goals of fluency therapy is for the stutterer to see speech as something he *does*, not something he *is*. He can be whatever he is and still speak fluently if he chooses. A further implication of this reasoning is that he can also stutter if he chooses. Most stutterers will accept the first statement but balk at the second. Choose to stutter, indeed!

Perhaps the most helpful therapeutic experience for the client who has trouble separating his stuttering from the rest of his self-image is to speak fluently session after session, week after week, in a reliable fashion in the clinic. A substantial base of data is gathered to which clinician and client must both react. What is the significance of the consistently fluent output? Typical answers to this question are "It's easy in here. You understand me (or 'the problem')," "I'm fluent here because I know you won't accept anything else" or "You expect me to be fluent," implying that other people don't expect him to be fluent and/or that they accept stuttering as a viable alternative to fluency. Of course, the client is thus placing the onus for his stuttering or fluency on the listener, a variation of the issue of responsibility raised earlier. But how much simpler this problem is to deal with in therapy than the refusal of the client to be fluent anywhere with consistency. Once control can be demonstrated reliably in a limited context, the remaining task is to extend or generalize the behavior, more a quantitative problem than the qualitative issue of "Do I have the capacity to be fluent in the first place?"

EXPECTANCY

The seventh and final principle raised in the original article is that stuttering (or fluency) results from the expectancy of the speaker to behave in one way or the other. Of course this issue can be examined at three levels, at least. First and most broadly, one's identity as a stutterer suggests a general expectancy to stutter in a speaking situation. Secondly, however, all stutterers are predictably fluent in some situations and disfluent in others, and their expectations probably correlate with their past experiences in similar situations. The third and most specific level of

Postscript 19

expectancy involves a particular word, or even part of a word. In therapy we work on all three levels, the first of which I have already discussed. The situational level is easy if the situation to be worked on is the therapeutic one. I would not go so far as to say that my expectation that my clients be fluent in therapy is a contagious one, but I am serious about it. I am convinced that they are in complete control of their speech organs, just as they are of their arms, hands, and fingers, and I communicate that conviction unequivocally. A block is not the only appropriate occasion for me to interrupt a client to ask "why?" A fluent utterance, or even a fluent word, can also be the occasion for the question. Responsibility for the one is qualitatively no different from responsibility for the other.

Often I will employ a technique I refer to as "overtalk" in which I will ask the client questions as he talks or reads aloud. He is previously instructed to listen, but not to answer, to just continue what he is doing at the same time he pays attention to what I am saying. The task is not as difficult as it sounds, especially if the client has first practiced the technique while reading aloud, which takes so little mental effort. The questions I ask are geared to the level of situational expectancy: "How are you feeling right now? How likely are you to stutter? Is there anything I can do to make you stutter? Is this a stutterer or a fluent speaker I'm listening to?" Of course, I can and do often direct the questions to a more specific level of expectancy: "How certain were you that you would be fluent on that last word? On the next word? Is there any doubt at all? Who is responsible for your performance? Am I doing it to you? Who gets the credit for that word?" etc. The word-by-word level of guaranteeing fluency is what we call monitoring. Like most other techniques I prefer to demonstrate it first for my clients. The argument I make is that we are all disfluent sometimes unless we monitor. I monitor my speech when it is important for me to be fluent. I can then guarantee that each word will be fluent because each word is deliberately uttered. This does not mean my speech is monotonously or mechanically or even painfully slow, although the rate I demonstrate is usually slower than normal. The distinguishing characteristics of monitoring as I demonstrate it are deliberateness and rate. My conviction regarding fluency is such that I am willing to bet money on each word. But I wouldn't talk that way all the time; it requires some mental effort and it does slow me down. However, when it is important enough to me to be fluent, it is a very simple and direct technique. Is it ever important enough for a stutterer to be completely fluent? They say it is. Then is the time to monitor, and probably only then. Shames uses the technique as a precursor to unmonitored fluency, which can be made contingent upon any predetermined duration of monitored speech (1980). But the ultimate goal of Stutter-Free Speech and of Cognitive Therapy is normal unmonitored fluency.

Expectancy is another way of talking about the self-fulfilling prophecy. The three levels of expectancy I have just reviewed differ primarily in their range of focus, from one's self as a stutterer for whom disfluency comes as no surprise, no matter where or when, to a specific word on which the stutterer may be completely convinced that a block is unavoidable. A major goal of therapy, therefore, is to substitute for that negative expectation the more positive attitude of being deliberately fluent, at all three levels. The positive attitude is preemptive. Every client can experience the feeling on at least some verbal task during the first therapeutic interview, perhaps counting, repeating a word over and over, reading aloud, etc. The nature of the task is irrelevant to the goal of experiencing the unequivocal conviction that he will be fluent. That qualitative feeling is what the stutterer must familiarize himself with so that he can employ it in increasingly normal speaking tasks and situations. Beware of words like "try" and "hope" when discussing these tasks with a client. Trying and hoping have nothing to do with the issue. Find a task for which there is no doubt, even if you must resort to a single vowel uttered at intervals of one full second. Eventually, most clients can generate at will the conviction that they will be fluent on the next word they utter. Often I ask them to manipulate that conviction without ever uttering the word, and then to reverse their feeling so that they expect to stutter on the same word, still unuttered. The task of alternating their expectations, without ever testing them through overt speech, is a very useful one, and can proceed through as many cycles as you wish. Stutterers have had so much experience with panic and helplessness that seemed to them to be spontaneous, that to generate these feelings deliberately, to call them forth and then to dispatch them, to substitute for them a feeling of control, of certainty, can be rewarding indeed. Just as the task of alternating indefinitely fluent and disfluent productions of the same word demonstrates control over one's motor abilities, so the task of alternating one's convictions demonstrates control over cognitive states.

MAINTENANCE

Those, then, are the seven principles of "A Point of View about Fluency" revisited at this writing. In addition to elaboration and changes in emphasis, I have included some specific techniques I have found useful when working with clients who stutter. Fluency within the therapeutic context is attainable often in the very first session. It is the first order of business and always an immediate goal. The second order of business is understanding the dynamics that maintain the stuttering behavior. Together these two goals characterize the process of cognitive therapy, but never is the first subordinated to the second. At least in the therapeutic situation there is neither excuse nor justification for stuttering, no matter how great the needs or the payoff may be outside. Too often, however, it is not enough to demonstrate consistent fluency in the clinic and to seem to understand the pragmatics and the psychology of stuttering. Stutterers persist. I am sorry to report no greater long-term success with cognitive therapy than with any other of the procedures for adults that you have read about in this volume. Two doctoral students, Mary Jo Kann and Margaret F. Piehler, have been interviewing clients who have terminated or been discontinued from therapy, and also clients who are still in treatment. The complete results of their follow-up study will be reported

Postscript   19

at a later date, but at this time it appears that about half of those clients who left the clinic as fluent speakers have reverted to stuttering at least some of the time. They have improved since intake to be sure, but qualitatively remain stutterers. Almost all of them claim they can control their speech musculature, but apparently have reverted to abandoning that control when confronted with the old social cues. Two of these clients have since enrolled in a popular, well-advertised program of therapy. Likewise, we often enroll graduates of other programs who have relapsed after their initial successes and have come to us to try something new, something different, "hoping" that they will finally hit upon a permanent success. Shames and I, working in the same clinic, occasionally find ourselves treating clients whom the other has already worked with but who are back in the marketplace, for one reason or another. Perhaps we should be addressing ourselves more to the recalcitrance of stutterers than to the differences in our various approaches to the problem, all of which seem to work in the short-term.

One clue to the solution to the problem of relapse may be that the longer I see a client the more I feel I am engaged in psychotherapy than speech therapy. Stuttering is a simple problem only insofar as it masks other problems. It is analogous to consolidating your loans with a single finance agency. All the client has to worry about is his single installment payment. The rest of his doubts and neuroses can be attributed to the scapegoat, stuttering. Fluency may be achieved at the cost of broken defenses and a host of other concerns that had remained well-hidden. I do not subscribe to Barbara's (1954) or Glauber's (1958) convictions that the cause and, therefore, the preferred treatment for stuttering is psychodynamic. While psychotherapy may be appropriate for those stutterers who do not take the final step toward identifying themselves as fluent speakers; that is, as ex-stutterers, and while I often refer recalcitrant clients for psychotherapy, I believe it is essential that they first come to grips with the issue of their physical potential for fluency. If the stutterer's attitude remains one of victimization and helplessness, if stuttering represents for him an irrational force over which he has no control, I do not recommend psychotherapy. A psychotherapist who is unsophisticted about the subleties of stuttering may unwittingly reinforce the negative attitudes of the client and thereby overlook the simple and direct task of achieving fluency at the same time he or she complicates unnecessarily the task of analyzing the psychodynamics of the problem.

ETIOLOGY

It should be apparent by now that I am convinced that stuttering is an acquired disorder. While I do not deplore research into the hard or soft predisposition to stutter; that is, genetic mechanism or family attitude, I see no relevance of that research for the treatment of the adult stutterer. Unless the client sees himself as fully capable of being a fluent speaker, the best he can achieve is a compromise, a better way of stuttering, or a fatalistic readiness for relapse at any time. I just do not think that is fair to our clients. When what they most need is a realistic conviction of their normal potential, many stutterers get from their well-meaning clinicians only another pessimistic prediction to add to their long-standing self-doubts. Although I have been emphasizing work with adult stutterers, the issue of predisposition can have negative effects upon the treatment of children if they or their families are led to believe that there is a genetic or familial factor that makes them different from other children.

THERAPY FOR CHILDREN

The most important datum for us to recognize about therapy for disfluent youngsters is that when they or their families are seen early enough, recovery is complete in 100% of the cases. That is quite a statement to make. We have yet to lose a preschool client to stuttering when the parents have received counseling, and every speech pathologist I have talked to reports the same success. What are the implications for research into the predispositional factors of stuttering? Obviously, if such factors are ever demonstrated, then we must conclude that they are not completely determining. They can be counter-effected by intervention, often with only a parent of the child, and sometimes in just a single session. It is possible, of course, as Adams (1980), Curlee (1980), Gregory and Hill (1980), and others have suggested that there are not one but two populations of disfluent children, those who are merely developmentally disfluent, as Johnson (1942) claimed and Bloodstein (1961) later reiterated, and another population of children who are prone to stutter, who therefore require early and careful intervention. However, I feel the anguish of stuttering is such that every disfluent youngster who is referred for evaluation requires early and careful intervention, especially when that intervention can be effected as quickly and economically as results have shown.

I indicated early in this paper that I would discuss the application of cognitive theory to therapy with children who stutter. With preschoolers whose disfluency has stabilized, especially if their parents seem so concerned that they are likely, in spite of counseling, to react affectively when their children stutter, it is appropriate to work directly. We neither talk about stuttering with these children nor do we evaluate either their fluency or their disfluency. The preemptive goal of therapy with young children is to prevent their learning to feel helpless and victimized by forces they perceive as beyond their control. To that end we focus primarily on their intention to speak in a certain manner. Satisfying their stated intention, even if it is disfluency, meets with clinical approval, and failing to satisfy their stated intention, even if they speak fluently, is met with disapproval. In other words, the target behavior is to speak as you said you would, no matter whether you intended to be disfluent or fluent. Furthermore, the exact nature of the disfluency or the fluency must satisfy the stated intention. Repetition, being the most discrete and most easily quantified disfluency, is the form we usually suggest to

---
Postscript 19
---

the child, although silent blocks or prolongations can also be utilized. Typically the child is asked to toss a die or to spin a pointer to determine the number of times he must say the word(s) in question. Selecting the number "I" means no repetition, a response that is only quantitatively, not qualitatively, different from any other number. The behavior is first modeled by the clinician, who later alternates roles with the child, who then has the opportunity to assess the clinician's performance. In addition to counting the number of times a word is to be uttered, rate, or even intensity may also be varied, although never through more than two or three degrees, to keep the task manageable. As you will find elsewhere in this book, rate, within certain limits, correlates very closely with fluency, and rate control is a most effective technique to use to attain fluency.

To ensure the child's growing conviction that he can decide how to talk, that he is in control of this behavior and is not subverted in the home environment, the parent is brought in to observe the activity. In this way neither parent nor child feels either helpless or pitying. Both know what the child is capable of and can expect that behavior outside of the clinical setting. In addition, the parent is not likely to allow the child to use disfluency as an indirect means to communicate what he can be encouraged to express directly. If, during spontaneous speech, the child is disfluent, it is appropriate to ask him why. Did he intend to say that word twice? An affirmative answer terminates the issue. A negative answer, however, suggests further probing: "Why, then, did you say it twice? How else could you have said it? Let's practice with that word for a while. Throw the die." etc. If the child is mature enough, probably at least of school age, the clinician can go further and inquire about reasons for disfluency. No matter that the child cannot answer such a question readily. Just as with an adult client, the important message is that the question is an appropriate one, that there are reasons for being disfluent, that it isn't just happening to him. And that message cannot be overemphasized. Initially a client may object to my phrasing, "Why did you choose to say the word that way?" But eventually most of them recognize that control brings with it the responsibility of choice, explicit or implicit.

CONCLUSION

While the behavioral goals of complete fluency are the same for both adults and children, the attitudinal goals are different for the two populations. For children, the briefer and less eventful their fluency therapy is, the better. We neither refer to their speech as stuttering nor to them as stutterers. The sooner this disfluent period in their lives becomes part of their developmental past, the happier we are. Perhaps it is appropriate at this time, however, to say a few words about the concept of complete, or 100% fluency. I have been criticized by my colleagues for establishing a standard for my clients which exceeds the normally observed measure of 97% to 99% fluency. The most stringent goal is one we set for a limited, circumscribed task only, a word, a phrase, a 5-minute sample, etc. In other words, when a speaker is monitoring his or her speech, a 100% success rate is both feasible and appropriate. Indeed, a single disfluency indicates a failure in the task of monitoring. That task, and that goal, are always available to a stuttering client, just as they are to you and to me when fluency is important enough that we exert the effort to ensure it. What my clients do during unmonitored speech is another story, and their exact percentage of disfluency is not as important as their conviction that they can be fluent at will and their freedom from blocks. This is merely another way of saying that they are entitled to be normally disfluent only so long as they are not attempting to be 100% fluent; that is, monitoring.

Monitoring is not a gimmick. It is a very specific form of consciousness-raising, of raising the act of speaking from an automatic level to a very purposeful one. Although I may ask a client what he does when he monitors, I never suggest specific techniques. My own experience at the task is imageless; all I am aware of is the determination that the word I am uttering, and the next word, are fluent. This determination is a very important component of cognitive therapy. It makes the difference between helplessness and control. Although the behavioral manifestations of monitoring are a reduced speaking rate and suprasegmental indications of deliberateness, it is more important how you feel than specifically what you do. Also, while monitoring will preempt stuttering, it is not effective as a technique to employ in response to the urge to stutter. That is too late. Monitoring is an anti-expectancy behavior to be sure. But it functions at all three levels of expectancy: identity, situation, and specific utterance. It is a natural response, one that all of us use at one time or another. Clients may attempt to monitor only after they expect to stutter or have stuttered on a word. At such a time, it becomes a gimmick and guarantees nothing because the speaker has already stuttered, either explicitly or implicitly.

In conclusion then, cognitive therapy for stuttering is a straightforward procedure that begins with the recognition that a stutterer has the physiological ability to be fluent and that he can manifest that ability directly, utilizing the same techniques that fluent speakers do when they want to guarantee fluency. If he resorts to tricks or prostheses to achieve fluency, they will only reinforce his long standing conviction that he cannot control his speech as other people do. The behavioral aspects of the therapy are neither complex nor mysterious. It is the psychological component that gets us every time: the dynamics that maintain the behavior, the resistance to change, the reluctance to assume the responsibility for what one does, and, finally, the fear of confronting the reasons behind the stuttering. I don't think any approach to therapy with adult stutterers can ignore these issues, and only if we deal with them effectively can we be instrumental in accomplishing long-term change.

REFERENCES

Abbott, J. A. (1947). Repressed hostility as a factor in adult stuttering. *Journal of Speech Disorders, 12,* 428–430.

Adams, M. R. (1980). The young stutterer: Diagnosis, treatment and assessment of progress. In W. H. Perkins (Ed.), Strategies in stuttering therapy. New York: Thieme-Stratton.

Postscript   19

Barbara, D. A. (1954). Stuttering: A psychodynamic approach to its understanding and treatment. New York: Julian Press.

Bloodstein, O. (1961). The development of stuttering: III. Theoretical and clinical implications. *Journal of Speech and Hearing Disorders, 26,* 67–82.

Culatta, R. A., & Rubin, H. (1973). A program for the initial stages of fluency therapy. *Journal of Speech and Hearing Research, 16,* 556–567.

Curlee, R. F., (1980). A case selection strategy for young disfluent children. In W. H. Perkins (Ed.), Strategies in stuttering therapy. New York: Thieme-Stratton.

Glauber, I. P. (1958). The psychoanalysis of stuttering. In J. Eisenson (Ed.), Stuttering: A symposium. New York: Harper and Row.

Gregory, H. H., & Hill, D. (1980). Stuttering therapy for children. In W. H. Perkins (Ed.), Strategies in stuttering therapy. New York: Thieme-Stratton.

Johnson, W., et al., A study of the onset and development of stuttering. *Journal of Speech Disorders, 7,* 251–257.

Rubin, H., & Culatta, R. A. (1971). A point of view about fluency. ASHA, 380–384.

Rubin, H. & Culatta, R. A. (1974). Stuttering as an aftereffect of normal developmental disfluency. *Clinical Pediatrics, 13,* 172–176.

Shames, G. H., & Florance, C. L. (1980). Stutter-free speech: A goal for therapy. Columbus, OH: Charles E. Merrill.

Sheehan, J. G., et al. (1962). Guilt, shame, and tension in graphic projections of stuttering. *Journal of Speech and Hearing Disorders, 27,* 129–139.

Williams, D. E. (1957). A point of view about stuttering. *Journal of Speech and Hearing Disorders, 22,* 390–397.

Wischner, G. J. (1952). Anxiety-reduction as reinforcement in maladaptive behavior: Evidence in stutterers' representations of the moment of difficulty. *Journal of Abnormal Social Psychology, 47,* 566–571.

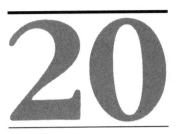

Maintenance of Fluency: A Review

Einer Boberg, Pauline Howie, and Lee Woods

Postscript
Relapse and Outcome

Einer Boberg

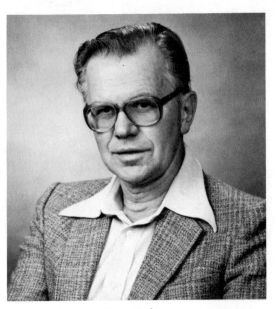

Einer Boberg

Einer Boberg agreed to write a chapter on Relapse and Outcome. For most of us, this would be like keeping an appointment to see our dentist. We anticipate pain and discomfort, and would like to deny any knowledge, experience, or concept of it, except when we consider the work of our colleagues. However, relapse is a fact of life for the stutterer and the clinician and is one of the types of outcomes that each of us has at one time or another come to know.

Boberg comes to his task with a history of scholarly and professional concern for these issues. His earlier publication with Howie and Woods directly addressed these problems. In addition, he has been the organizer of two major conferences dealing with the Maintenance of Fluency and is the editor of a book titled *The maintenance of fluency.*

In his previously published material, Boberg pointed up many of the methodological problems in dealing with relapse, such as definition and measurement and differing therapeutic philosophies and tactics, with a special focus on maintenance strategies to prevent or counteract relapse. There was a recurring pessimism about outcome in part due to the "human condition," in part to presumed genetic factors, and in part to inadequate maintenance strategies. However, most of his pessimism stemmed from the observation that the topics of outcome and relapse were not receiving adequate research attention.

In his update on this topic we see that Boberg attenuates his pessimism with his observation that many of the methodological problems are being researched, and that various programs of therapy are now measuring outcome, identifying factors in relapse, and developing strategies to prevent or counteract relapse. From this standpoint alone, of attention by the profession, Boberg acknowledges that although we haven't eliminated or perhaps even reduced the high numbers of relapses, we are making steady (though slow) progress toward understanding and managing these issues in therapy.

We can talk about relapse in terms of group statistics, but it continues to be a highly individualistic issue, as all clinical outcomes are. Boberg has presented a realistic view of both of these outlooks and has made our painful visit with the reality of our work into both a challenge and an invitation to join in its study.

20

Maintenance of Fluency: A Review

Einer Boberg, *University of Alberta, Edmonton, Alberta, Canada*

Pauline Howie, *University of New South Wales Teaching Hospitals, Sydney, Australia*

Lee Woods, *Klamath Speech and Hearing Centre, Klamath Falls, Oregon*

Three purposes for writing this paper are: to review specific work done on the maintenance of fluency in the post-treatment environment, to abstract and discuss pertinent issues in maintenance, and to present several speculative positions which might account for the relapse phenomenon and stimulate further research.

INTRODUCTION

Clinical treatment programs for stuttering have improved substantially during the past decade. A number of publications (Curlee and Perkins, 1969; Ingham and Andrews, 1973; Perkins, 1973: Ryan, 1974; Mowrer, 1975; Costello, 1975; Boberg, 1976; Shames and Egolf, 1976; Dalton, 1977) have described programs based on behavioral principles which have generally been successful in establishing normal fluency within a clinical setting and transferring that fluency into extra-clinical situations. Unfortunately, establishment and tranfer are only the first two of the required three steps in a complete fluency management program. The third and possibly most important step is to maintain a satisfactory level of fluency in the clients' natural environment after clinical treatment has been terminated.

There is a dearth of published studies providing accurate information on how well fluency is maintained in the post-treatment environment. In a table summarizing results of treatment, Bloodstein (1975) reviewed 58 studies. Only 18 of these studies reported any follow-up results. The few studies that do address this issue indicate that relapse or regression is a common experience for adult stutterers. Cooper (1977) has recently drawn an analogy between stuttering and alcoholism by suggesting that relapse is part of the "human condition . . . regression occurs almost invariably after cessation of treatment for most if not all human behavioral problems."

The problem of maintenance is complicated by certain difficulties inherent in both measurement and development of success criteria. For instance, are covert measurements of speech in the clients' natural environment necessary in addition to the more usual overt measurements obtained in a clinical setting? Covert measurements present technical, logistic, and even ethical problems, in some cases. Must we measure other parameters of speech in addition to frequency of stuttered and nonstuttered syllables? Perhaps we need to develop valid instruments to reliably measure changes in attitudes and social interaction patterns. Can the term "satisfactory fluency" be operationally defined or given more objective meaning? Additionally, we face substantial logistic problems in both arranging for and persuading large numbers of clients to cooperate with evaluation procedures. All of these problems suggest that this last

Note: Reprinted by permission of the publisher from Maintenance of fluency: A review, by Einer Boberg, Pauline Howie, and Lee Woods, *Journal of Fluency Disorders, 4,* pp. 93–116. Copyright 1979 by Elsevier Science Publishing Co., Inc.

step in the management program will indeed be the most difficult.

We have three purposes in writing this paper. The first is to review specific work done in the maintenance of fluency. Second, we will attempt to abstract and discuss pertinent issues in fluency maintenance. Finally, we will present several speculative positions on relapse in the hope that this will provide further discussion, research, and improved clinical strategies.

This paper is not intended to be an exhaustive review of every article on maintenance. We have selected certain papers for their particular contribution and/or because they possess one or more of the following characteristics:

1. Description of clinical strategies used during the post-treatment period.
2. Description of measures used to assess fluency.
3. Description of the author's criteria for evaluating the success of a clinical program.
4. Published results of clients' performance following termination of the clinical program.

We will refer primarily to those sections of published studies which deal with maintenance issues. Other than a brief designation of the type of therapy employed we will not review experimental designs or therapeutic procedures, as these have been reviewed elsewhere (Ingham and Andrews, 1973).

It is necessary to distinguish between the terms "follow-up" and "maintenance." In this paper we will use the term follow-up to refer to the evaluation of a client's long-term, unassisted performance; that is, the evaluation/measurement of his fluency when there has been no clinical intervention. In contrast, maintenance refers to various post-treatment activities aimed at assisting the client in maintaining the fluency gained in the treatment program.

LONG TERM OUTCOME OF BEHAVIORAL TREATMENT PROGRAM FOR STUTTERING

Outcome in the Absence of Maintenance Activities

Several studies have reported follow-up programs which apparently did not involve scheduled maintenance activities. In a paper describing a therapy program, Gregory (1972) included follow-up information. Several teen adult stutterers were assessed nine months after completing what the author described as an "avoidance reduction, anxiety reduction therapy based principally on concepts of learning theory psychology." Two procedures were used in the assessments:

1. Self-report techniques such as the Stutterer's Self-Rating of Reactions and the Iowa Scale of Attitude.
2. Tape recordings of reading and speech samples obtained in the clinic environment. Panels of observers were asked to listen to randomly presented segments from the tapes and then rate stuttering severity on a nine-point equal-appearing interval scale.

Gregory reported that although there was a slight trend toward increased stuttering at the nine-month follow-up, the severity ratings were still significantly below the pre-therapy ratings. No data were presented concerning frequency of stuttering and word output. Clients' self reports revealed a decrease in avoidance, more enjoyment of speaking, decreased stuttering, and a better attitude toward stuttering.

Mowrer (1975) presented follow-up information on 11 of 30 clients who had participated in his stuttering program. Client performance was judged through casual encounters and informal clinic visits rather than in formal assessments. Only two of the 11 clients were considered to be fluent five years after treatment. Mowrer suggests that clinic support should possibly be maintained longer and withdrawn more slowly. He also speculates whether "some basic change in personality must be effected before a lasting change in fluency will result."

Egolf et al. (1972) reported on an experimental program for children using parent-child interaction patterns. Of the nine children treated the authors were able to reevaluate five at periods ranging from two to nine months post-therapy. The data are presented as percentage of words stuttered but no information is given on how the measurements were made. The authors conclude that "in general, therapeutic results were maintained and somewhat improved in both the controlled waiting-room situation and the therapy situation." Shames and Egolf (1976) have also reported encouraging results with small numbers of clients but methodological details are not provided.

Dalton (1977) plans to conduct formal assessments of her clients at one, six, and 12 months after treatment. She obtained an overt speech sample in the clinic setting and administered the revised Erickson S24 scale, the Iowa Avoidance Scale, and the Eysenck Personality Inventory. Speech measures included number of words spoken, and words stuttered per minute, expressed as percentage improvement or regression. Less than 60% improvement was considered inadequate progress. The mean improvement of 31 clients at the end of a four-week treatment using syllable-timed speech was 44%. Forty-eight clients who were treated in a prolonged speech program showed a mean improvement of 73% at the end of treatment. At the time of publication, 25 of the 31 clients in the syllable-timed group had completed the one-month follow-up assessment. The mean improvement was 41%, but only eight clients were above the required 60%. By comparison, 41 of the 48 clients in the prolonged speech group had completed one-month follow-up asessment. Their mean improvement was 68%. Twenty-eight were above the required 60%.

Prins and Miller (1973) reported a study in which they correlated post-therapy regression with personal and social adjustment scores. Sixteen boys and young men were seen in the clinic for follow-up evaluation 10 months after an eight-week intensive period of traditional-type therapy. Since all 16 clients had requested additional therapy, they represented a selected subgroup of the initial 66 clients treated. Adults were asked to complete the Iowa Job Task while children described a cartoon sequence. Speech was assessed in randomly selected speech samples. The mean percentages of words stuttered were 30% in pre-therapy testing, 9% in post-therapy testing, and 21% in the 10-month follow-up evaluation.

In an earlier paper Prins (1970) presented data to suggest that clients perceived maximum regression to occur within six months of therapy termination. He also suggested that an intensive residential program may produce "disfluency overkill." The rapid, dramatic improvements which often occur in intensive programs may result in a fluent speaker who is uncertain as to what he did to accomplish the change. "In this state, even mild difficulty in a post-therapy speaking experience could trigger a regressive sequence from which the stutterer might have little basis for self-extrication." More recently, Prins (1977) has suggested that maintenance should consist of a gradual tapering off so that the individual gradually assumes more and more responsibility for his progress and does not rely on the clinician. Prins'

expectations of stutterers in the post-treatment period are similar to what he would expect from people who set up regimes for controlling other types of behavior. "Some will continue to do it for life; others will fall flat on their faces while the majority will operate somewhere between those extremes."

Outcome of Programs Involving Specified Maintenance Activities

There are several reports in the literature on the long-term outcome of treatment programs which involve specified maintenance activities. However, the design of most of this research does not allow the long-term effects of initial treatment to be distinguished from the effects of the maintenance program. The following section will deal with research which falls into this category.

Ryan and Van Kirk have published several studies which include information about post-treatment performance. Van Kirk (1972) reported that the mean stuttering rate for 18 clients was 0.09 stuttered words/minute at the end of an operant program and 0.08 stuttered words/minute nine months after the therapy was terminated. The maintenance phase involved decreasing clinical contacts in the form of rechecks at intervals of one month, three months, six months, and then yearly. No information was provided concerning the assessment methods used. The author reported that one boy who regressed was successfully recycled through a home program and had maintained fluency for three months at the time of publication.

Ryan (1974), and Ryan and Van Kirk (1974) have described management programs and presented results from post-treatment evaluations. The objective of the maintenance program was fluent speech in a wide variety of settings with many different people over a long period of time. Three activities were pursued during maintenance:

1. Daily self-monitoring of stutters.
2. Intermittent home practice which is gradually faded out.
3. Clinic contact for measurement and reinstruction as necessary.

Post-treatment performance was assessed overtly in the clinic using samples of reading, monologue, and conversation. Client performance outside the clinic was based on self-report. In his book, Ryan presented data for 58 clients who had participated in their programs. He obtained post-treatment data on 24 clients although only nine clients actually completed the formal maintenance program. The mean stuttering rate for the 24 clients, expressed as stuttered words/minute, was 9.9 pre-therapy, 0.3 immediately post-therapy, and 1.7 one year post-therapy. Fourteen of the 24 clients satisfied Ryan's criterion of successful maintenance (1 stuttered word/minute or less). Half of these 14 were children.

Webster (1974) reported follow-up data on 20 clients at a mean of 25 months after treatment. Speech was measured as the percentage of disfluent words during conversational speech. The report does not specify details of the setting in which speech samples were collected. Forty-five percent of clients showed less than 1% disfluent words and 70% showed less than 3% disfluent words. Sixty percent reported satisfaction with their speech. Daly and Darnton (1976) assessed nine clients overtly in the clinic 10 months after a treatment program based on Webster's techniques. They obtained similar self-reports of satisfaction with speech but measures of disfluency (using the Riley Scale) suggested more serious regression than does Webster's data. Webster (1974) argues that if the behaviors necessary for fluency are sufficiently over-learned during intensive treatment, they should be highly resistant to extinction and maintenance should not be necessary. In his client manual Webster (1975) does suggest maintenance activities which aim to maintain the automaticity of the targets acquired during treatment. Daily practice, transfer of targets, self-monitoring, and the self-diagnosis of specific problem areas are emphasized. The effectiveness of these maintenance activities has not been evaluated, however, perhaps because within Webster's theoretical framework maintenance is of secondary importance.

Regular assessments are made of the Prince Henry Program for adult stutterers (Ingham and Andrews, 1973b), in which maintenance has (until recently) involved no more than encouragement to continue practicing prolonged speech and to maintain regular clinic contact. Andrews and Ingham (1972a) reported virtually no stuttering and normal speech rate when clients were evaluated overtly in the clinic three, six, and nine months after treatment, but a covert check 18 months post-treatment produced means of 7.8% syllables stuttered (%SS) and 152 syllables

per minute (SPM). No overt clinic measures were reported at 18 months post-treatment. Guitar (1976) evaluated clients overtly, but in a nonclinic setting, 12 to 18 months post-treatment, and reported an increase in frequency of stuttering from none at the end of treatment to a mean of 2.4% SS. Further analysis of Guitar's data including the subjects in his cross-validation group produced a mean %SS of 4.0 with a mean speech rate of 166.0 SPM. Fifty percent of clients were stuttering at 1% SS or less (with a mean of 180 SPM), 37% were stuttering between 1.1% SS and 10.0% SS (mean of 159 SPM), and the remaining 13% were over 10.1% SS (mean of 102 SPM).

Covert speech samples have been systematically collected in two evaluations of the Prince Henry Program. Ingham (1975) collected overt and covert samples, both in a nonclinic setting for nine clients at three and six months post-treatment. The reported means for %SS and SPM suggest the occurrence of slight relapse within the first six months, which was not apparent in the clinic setting (Andrews and Ingham, 1972a). At three months post-treatment, the covertly recorded speech showed significantly lower SPM and higher %SS than the overtly recorded speech, although at six months the difference was present in speech rate only. A covert—overt difference in speech rate only was also reported by Howie and Tanner (1978) in an evaluation of 43 clients in a nonclinic setting 12 to 18 months post-treatment. These authors report similar distributions of stuttering frequency and speech rate to that of Guitar (1976). Furthermore, 43% of clients reported satisfaction with their speech, and 41% considered that they had essential or good fluency. Seventy-eight percent reported the need to attend to the act of speaking fluently at least 10% of the time, suggesting that, for the majority of clients, fluency had not become automatic. However, clients' attitudes toward their speech, as meaured by the Erikson Scale of Communication Attitudes, were within normal range and showed little evidence of regression to pre-treatment levels.

In the last two years, the Prince Henry Program has expanded its maintenance activities considerably. The present maintenance program involves (1) clinic contact every three weeks for at least nine weeks following treatment, (2) a suggested systematic practice schedule involving formal speech drill and "real-life" assignments in gradually decreasing amounts over the three months following treatment, and (3) weekly self-help groups with structured speech practice and evaluation of self and others. Of course, not all clients carry out the suggested activities.

Perkins and his colleagues have stressed the need for continued deliberate generalization of skills during maintenance as well as the importance of dealing with any negative reactions to fluency from the client's family and friends (Perkins, 1973b). Perkins et al. (1974) have reported the failure of a system of monetary rewards for maintained improvement, but they present no data to support this. At the time of writing, their program offers clients the choice of several maintenance options in an attempt to satisfy the differing needs of clients (Perkins, 1977). These options are:

1. Self-help groups.
2. Bi-weekly two-hour clinic attendance for speech practice and evaluation.
3. Bi-weekly two-hour counseling sessions, exploring attitudes and values associated with speech.
4. Whole day "booster" programs of intensive speech practice.
5. Individual therapy.
6. Retaking the intensive program (permitted only after a period of counseling). These options have been developed on the basis of clinical trial-and-error, and the relative effectiveness of different options has not been evaluated.

Perkins (1973) and Perkins et al. (1974) presented long-term outcome data on two treatment programs, both based on speech-rate control, but one emphasizing DAF-induced prolonged speech (Method 1) and the other emphasizing breath control, phrasing, and prosody (Method 2). It is not clear whether the maintenance options just described were available after these programs. The 27 clients treated by Method 1 reduced their mean stuttering frequency (based on speech samples collected overtly in "real-life" situations) from 16.3% SS pre-treatment to 2.6% SS at the end of treatment. However, stuttering rate had increased to 8.4% SS six months post-treatment, and only 30% of clients had maintained more than 85% reduction in their pre-treatment stuttering frequency. By contrast, the 17 clients treated by Method 2 reduced their mean stuttering frequency from 9% SS pre-treatment to 1% SS at the end of treatment and maintained a mean of

1.7% SS six months post-treatment, with 53% of clients showing at least 85% reduction in pre-treatment levels. The apparent superiority of Method 2 was generally supported by other outcome measures, ranging from subjective judgments by naive listeners of speech rate, fluency, and "expressivity," to self-reports by clients. However, since the two groups were not matched on pre-treatment stuttering severity, the results can only be suggestive.

Research Evaluating Specific Maintenance Activities

The research reviewed above indicates the presence of relapse in the post-treatment environment whether or not maintenance activities are carried out. Since no control groups were used it is not possible to tell whether the success (or failure) of clients is a function of therapeutic activities or merely related to the passing of time.

A few studies have attempted to demonstrate a relationship between specific client/clinician behaviors and measured speech behaviors. For example, Ryan (1974) analyzed the relationship between completion of his transfer/maintenance program and long-term outcome for 17 adults. He reported the data in terms of whether clients skipped the program, did a part of it, or completed the program. A criterion of 1 stuttered word/minute was used to determine success. In a group where there was no transfer and no maintenance program, one out of three clients had maintained. In a group where there was partial transfer and no maintenance, one out of five had maintained. In the partial transfer and partial maintenance group, one out of four had maintained; in the complete transfer but no maintenance group, both clients were maintaining at the three-month follow-up; in the complete transfer and maintenance group, all three clients maintained their fluency on the average of 17 months. Ryan concludes from these limited data that transfer and maintenance programs are necessary to maintain fluency established in the clinical setting.

Daly and Darnton's (1976) data also allow a crude assessment of regular contact and continued therapy as a maintenance activity. They describe a maintenance program carried out with nine adolescents. The program began two months after treatment, when clients had presumably had no clinic contact and their speech was deteriorating. The program involved a 2-hour therapy session each week for six weeks; a total of 12 hours of therapy. This produced an improvement in Riley Severity Scores (from a mean of 14.33 to a mean of 10.14), but clients did not regain their immediate post-treatment level (mean of 6.55), and the improvement was not sustained after the six-week period ended. At 10 months, regression had occurred again (Mean Riley score 15.44).

Boberg and Sawyer (1977) similarly showed arrest and reversal of relapse following "refresher" weekends which began 12 months after treatment. Thirteen clients were assessed 12 months post-treatment and five of these were reassessed six months later. Assessment procedures included video samples of conversation and reading, taped conversations with a confederate outside the clinic, and a telephone call in which a confederate posed as a landlord or personnel manager. Measures of total words stuttered per minute and total words spoken per minute were converted to percentage of words stuttered. In the four testing periods the mean percentage of stuttering was: pre-clinic, 26.5%; immediate post-clinic, 1.95%; 12-month post-clinic, 7.72%; 18-month post-clinic, 4.7% (N = 5). The refresher weekends were held at approximately three-month intervals and consisted of a telescoped version of the intensive clinic program including self-monitoring, prolongation, cancellation practice, and transfer activities. The relapse observed in the 12-month probe was most pronounced in those testing situations involving the use of the confederate. This confirmed the frequent clinical observation that stutterers generally are more fluent within the clinic than outside. The reversal trend observed after the refresher weekends were initiated was quite marked and appeared in all four probe measures. Contributing factors were assumed to be the effect of the refresher weekends and the galvanizing effect of confronting the reality of their relapse as revealed by the 12-month probe.

Holgate and Andrews (1966) attempted to assess the effectiveness of weekly practice and group psychotherapy as maintenance strategies. Twenty stutterers treated in a two-week syllable-time (ST) speech program were given no specific post-treatment maintenance and were compared with 10 stutterers who carried out weekly maintenance activities at the clinic. (Unfortunately, the initial therapy of the maintenance group differed slightly from the no-maintenance group in that it involved 1.5 hours daily nondirective group therapy in addition to ST speech training.) Clinic maintenance activities included ST speech practice (formal drill, play readings, discussion, and debate) and 1.5 hours psychotherapy dealing with anxieties about stuttering. General outside speech assignments were recommended. Frequency of stuttering was overtly assessed prior to intensive therapy and 12 months post-treatment but speech rates were not reported. After 12 months the maintenance group showed considerably better performance than the no-maintenance group. However, these results are difficult to interpret because the two groups were not matched on pre-treatment stuttering severity and were not subjected to identical initial treatment programs.

Using a more careful design, Andrews and Ingham (1972b) compared two matched groups of stutterers treated in identical ST speech programs in order to examine the effect of monthly day-long token system refresher courses versus monthly assessments only. Speech performance (% SS and SPM) was evaluated using the Iowa Job Task. At nine months both groups had maintained their immediate post-treatment level of speech with equal effectiveness: roughly 20% had stutter-free speech at normal rates; an additional 20% had stutter-free speech at slow rates. Although this research is concerned with an essentially outdated treatment method, its results are important in that they suggest that refresher courses may be no more effective in maintaining fluency than simple clinic assessment. Further research is needed to determine whether a regular assessment group can be considered as a control group (no maintenance) or whether regular clinic contact, even without structured practice, is in itself a crucial maintenance activity.

DISCUSSION
Methodological Problems

From the foregoing review it appears reasonable to conclude that relapse or regression following treatment for stuttering is a common experience and that this regression is likely to occur within the first six months. Furthermore, it is likely that the actual amount of regression is higher than the published research suggests. Research reports are likely to be biased in a positive direction if most measures are obtained in the setting in which clients acquired fluency. There is ample clinical and anecdotal evidence to indicate that stutterers experience an observable increase in fluency when they return to the clinical environment. Another source of bias arises if the evaluator is closely involved with the clinical program. When Boberg and Sawyer (1977) positioned a nonclinical confederate in a building away from the clinic the clients demonstrated more disfluency in retesting than when they were retested in the familiar clinical settings.

We have already seen that some measures of stuttering differ depending on whether evaluation is overt or covert (Ingham, 1975; Howie and Tanner, 1978). Assuming that covert as well as overt measures are necessary, under what conditions should these be made, and how often? Ideally, we might wish to record clients speaking in a number of natural situations with no awareness that they were being evaluated. Furthermore, the situations should be standardized for audience size, nature of communication, length of communication, and should be repeatable at intervals of approximately six months. Due to ethical considerations, logistic problems, and limitations on recording technology, we may have to settle for considerably less than the ideal. Ingham (1977a) has suggested that further advances in precision of measurement may have to await further advances in recording technology. However, we might, at the very least, expect that clinical reports include an attempt to measure speech fluency overtly in nonclinical settings with nonclinical audiences. It may also be possible to develop a formula by which "real-life" performance may be predicted on the basis of measures obtained under more artificial conditions (Perkins et al., 1974).

Another problem lies in determining which parameters to measure when assessing speech adequacy. A number of studies report data in percentage of syllables or words stuttered, and number of syllables per minute spoken per unit of time. Other studies present only the number of stuttered words per minute. Still others present severity ratings based on judgments made by an audience. Other researchers use clients' self-ratings on a questionnaire. None of these measures have been demonstrated to measure adequately the client's global capacity to cope with his environment in terms of his speech fluency. It may be necessary to develop an objective means of assessing the stutterer's ability to function within his social and vocational setting. Some recent attempts have been made (Frayne et al., 1977; Ingham and Packman, 1978) to evaluate the "normalcy" of the speech

of treated stutterers in terms of the ability of naive listeners to distinguish it from the speech of normally fluent speakers.

It is also necessary to define what constitutes an acceptable level of fluency. It is most likely that the therapist and client may entertain significantly different criteria for judging success. A client who stuttered severely (more than 30%) may be entirely satisfied with residual stuttering of 3% if he is convinced tht he will not regress. On the other hand, a client may insist that his vocational and social settings require "complete fluency" and that anything less than that is unacceptable. To complicate the matter still further, we must also recognize the client's almost limitless ability to rationalize and accept a greater than necessary level of disfluency as he considers the energy and vigilance required to maintain fluency at the level obtained in the clinic.

A somewhat different issue relates to the difficulty of evaluating the effectiveness of specific maintenance activities. Clients can be encouraged but not forced to carry out prescribed maintenance activities. If the long-term outcome of clients who regularly perform maintenance activities is compared with those who choose not to, differences in outcome may be due to personality factors or learning ability rather than to the maintenance program as such. More generally, any speech behaviors observed sometime after completion of treatment may be attributable to a whole range of influences other than treatment or maintenance activities per se (Ingham, 1977b).

Summary of Maintenance Activities Currently Employed

When considering the relapse problem some clinicians/researchers may be tempted to throw up their hands and ascribe the fluency failures to the inevitable "human condition." We believe that it is most important to view the problem in perspective. Substantial progress has been achieved in the establishment and transfer phases of stuttering management. It now remains for researchers/clinicians to apply their attention to the maintenance phase. As we have seen, research in this area is scant. However, a myriad of "maintenance" techniques are employed, presumably on a trial-and-error basis. These techniques may be classified into four major groups. A brief overview may provide a basis for designing systematic research into their effectiveness. The categories are:

1. Regular clinical contact following treatment. Suggested activities at clinics range from simple assessment and counseling (Ryan and Van Kirk, 1974; Howie et al., 1976; Daly and Darnton, 1976; Perkins, 1977) to the requirement that clients "pass" certain criteria (Ingham, 1977a). In Ingham's program each client initially returns to the clinic on a weekly schedule. During the visit he produces samples of monologue and phone conversations. If his stuttering rate exceeds a rigid criterion, he must return each week until the criterion is passed, at which time he expands the length of time to two weeks, four weeks, and so on. Regular clinical evaluation of tape recordings of speech in a wide variety of situations can provide useful feedback for the client as well as a basis for planning appropriate maintenance activities. There is no definitive research on the relationship between clinic contact and long-term outcome, although Daly and Darnton (1976), and Boberg and Sawyer (1977) have shown that clinic contact can arrest and reverse relapse, even if only temporarily.

2. Emphasis on client self-responsibility. The opinion is often expressed (Mowrer, 1975; Howie et al., 1976; Prins, 1977; Hanna and Own, 1977; Dalton, 1977) that self-therapy must occur after intensive treatment and that the client must be weaned gradually from his dependence on the clinic. Various techniques have been employed to this end. Clients have been trained to self-monitor disfluencies and correct use of fluent speech skills (La Croix, 1973; Ryan and Van Kirk, 1974; Costello, 1975; Boberg, 1976; Ingham, 1977a). Similarly, some clinicians have stressed the importance of developing awareness of "what you do to get fluency" (Prins, 1977; Hanna and Owen, 1977) and an ability to deal effectively with regressive episodes (Prins, 1977). Regular or intermittent speech practice at home is often prescribed (Ryan and Van Kirk, 1974; Howie et al., 1976) usually decreasing gradually as time since treatment increases. The importance of transfer of the practiced skill to real-life situations is often emphasized (Webster, 1975; Howie et al., 1976; Hanna and Owen, 1977). Self-reinforcement for fluency and for completion of maintenance activities is being employed by some clinics (Ryan, 1974; Howie et al., 1976; Hanna and Owen, 1977). A related concept is that of self-help groups (Woods, 1976; Perkins, 1977).

There has been little research on the effectiveness of these kinds of activities. DiGusto et al. (1976) have reported better outcome in clients who regularly self-monitored. At the Prince Henry Hospital there is in progress an evaluation of the effect on maintenance of fluency of detailed daily practice schedule and weekly group self-help meetings. After leaving the intensive treatment program unchanged for one year (30 patients in the revised maintenance program and 30 as controls), one year post-treatment speech evaluations are now being collected.

3. Emphasis on the need for changes in attitudes to speech, self-concepts, etc. The notion that negative attitudes to speaking may prevent adequate generalization of fluency has received some empirical support from Guitar's (1976) and Guitar and Bass' (1978) recent findings of a relationship between pre-treatment attitudes (regardless of stuttering severity) and long-term outcome of treatment. To deal with this problem, systematic desensitization has been built into therapy to deal with fears of speaking (Ingham and Andrews, 1973; Ryan, 1974) and group psychotherapy has been employed during intensive treatment or maintenance (Holgate and Andrews, 1966; Perkins, 1977). Similarly, training in assertiveness and other social skills have been employed (Cohen, 1976; Hanna and Owen, 1977). Cohen (1976) showed that 36 clients with a pretherapy mean of -1 on the Rathus Scale (compared to a norm of $+20$) showed a mean of $+18$ following assertiveness training at the end of a behavioral speech program. Ten clients were contacted six months post-treatment and scored $+34.10$ on the same scale. The author suggested that assertion training was like planting a seed that continued to grow, even after therapy was terminated. Unfortunately, the author did not provide any data on fluency.

Although "attitude" therapy makes intuitive sense, it will be recalled that Ingham et al. (1972) found that regular psychotherapy produced no better long-term performance than simple clinic contact. The effectiveness of maintenance activities related to attitude change has yet to be clearly established.

4. Intensive 'refresher programs' or recycling through the initial program. Recycling has been employed with some success (Van Kirk, 1972; Perkins, 1977; Hanna and Owen, 1977) but failure is also common. Boberg and Sawyer(1977) have shown positive results in a small sample following short, intensive refresher programs, but the experience of two of the authors of the present paper (Woods and Howie) has been that the results of such programs do not justify the time consumed. Relapse following recycling may be due to the fact that clients who seek recycling have additional personality problems (e.g. over-independence on the clinic) or particular difficulties in some of the skills necessary to achieve fluency (e.g. auditory discrimination, general learning ability, coordination, breath control).

SPECULATIONS ON FLUENCY RELAPSE

In this final section we enter the arena of speculation to present some theoretical notions about relapse. In our review we found practically nothing written about why stutterers relapse. Into this vacuum we propose to thrust some speculative concepts in the hope that they may help generate research. The following sections are presented as armchair theorizing and should be viewed as such.

The Role of Micro-Stutters

Wischner (1952) likened stuttering to the instrumental avoidance acts demonstrated in the early experimental animal studies. An animal was trained in a running cage to avoid a shock by running in response to the sound of a buzzer. One of the most important features of a learned avoidance response is that it is unusually difficult to extinguish. Even if the original punishing stimulus is no longer present the animal does not discover this fact because he continues to run whenever the buzzer sounds.

The analogy to stuttering, like most analogies, is not perfect but may still be useful. If the buzzer represents an environmental stimulus to speak and the running response represents struggle behavior, we may be able to better visualize what happens. Furthermore, we need to assume that stutters can and do vary in magnitude from a covert, physiological state of tension so mild that the individual himself is hardly aware of it, to a full-blown, overt, struggle reaction.

When a client leaves an intensive clinic he is likely to speak fluently. Furthermore, he is likely to thoroughly enjoy the fluency feeling and decline an invitation to continue monitoring his speech and disfluencies. We have seen many clients confidently announce at the end of the clinic that they definitely will not stutter again. After the self-confidence and

euphoria generated in the clinic has begun to dissipate, the client will likely begin to experience tensions again in response to environmental cues. We may refer to these as micro-stutterings. At first, these tensions might be so minor that the audience, and possibly even the speaker, may be unaware of them, and therefore they will not be punished. One might hypothesize that the micro-stutters serve the same function as the running response in the experimental animal; they successfully avoid a confrontation with the reality of whether the grid is "still hot." The micro-stutters are reinforced because they help to avoid a further breakdown. The speaker finishes his phrase and is further reinforced. Moreover, the reinforcement is likely provided on an intermittent schedule and thus make the micro-stutterings still more resistant to extinction.

With the passage of time the micro-stutters increase, both in magnitude and frequency, and become overt stutters. By this time they are subject to external social penalty but the speaker is now once again enmeshed in the same vicious circle that played so prominent a part in the initial development of his stuttering (Bloodstein, 1975). A complicating factor in this is that the appropiate ways of dealing with the threat or occurrence of stuttering are unlikely to be reinforced. If the client is fluent when he leaves the clinic he will not have opportunities to practice the appropriate response during the first critical days or weeks. His speech will tend to be spontaneously fluent. By the time the micro-stutters appear he will have had several weeks or even months without practice on the appropriate speech skills.

There are several clinical and research implications in this model. If it can be demonstrated that micro-stutters, initially unnoticed, are reinforced and gradually increase in frequency and severity, the therapy progam should specifically train the client to recognize the micro-stutters, deal appropriately with them, and thus avoid the subsequent build-up. Secondly, it may be unwise to achieve a 100% level of fluency in the clinic. If the client left the clinic with residual stuttering and was taught how to deal appropriately with it he might be more successful when the stuttering reappears in his post-treatment environment.

Is Fluency its Own Reward?

Remaining within the bounds of learning theory but viewing regression at a more global or subjective level, we can ask why regular, conscious control and practice of a speech skill is not sufficiently rewarding to sustain itself. It should be noted that this question assumes first that stutterers do learn a skill in treatment (as opposed to simply changing self-expectations, for example) and secondly that pracice of the skill will help to maintain fluency. Neither of these common assumptions has empirical support.

From this point of view, the post-treatment condition of the stutterer is a clear example of "Catch-22." He is told that in order to continue to speak fluently he must practice religiously, but because he speaks so fluently after treatment he feels no need for practice. As he practices less and less, the experiences and feelings of stuttering increase and cause him either to practice more or to conclude that he or the treatment technique is hopeless. The obvious conclusion usually drawn from this situation is that the treated stutterer should continue to practice in spite of how he feels about his speech. In fact, the clinician may even believe that the improved fluency itself should be sufficient reward to maintain the necessary practice. Furthermore, since improved fluency is often present with no conscious attention from the stutterer (as it has been all his life), it does not constitute a clear reward for practice.

In contrast, practicing is immediately punishing in several ways. First, practicing invariably requires careful monitoring of one's speech and therefore a loss of spontaneity and of the feeling of self-acceptance. In real-life situations, the treated stutterer is often tempted to participate freely in communication when his speech problem requires that he control or compensate. Therefore, hoping to be fluent by accident is chosen over the certainty of being nonspontaneous by design. Accepting responsibility for artificial communication may be internally more punishing than hoping for the normal speech one can produce at times.

A related second reason for the punishing nature of practice is the inherent abnormality of any control technique. The reason for practicing is usually to avoid abnormality, so practice is unpleasant and usually not maintained unless external rewards are used.

The third reason practice is not maintained is that consequences are delayed and intermittent. Missing one day's practice rarely produces results strong and consistent enough to affect long-term speech behavior. Doing something which isn't much fun and isn't clearly necessary is punishing and not likely to con-

tinue. The clinical implications of the punishing aspects of practice are that treated stutterers will practice only if the perceived positive consequences of practice outweigh the perceived negative consequences. Repeated reality testing of relative perceived abnormality of controlled and noncontrolled speech by nonbiased listeners and the stutterer seems essential.

A Physiological Basis for Disfluency

Finally, we may view the problem of relapse not in terms of reward and punishment but rather in terms of the innate capacities of the stutterer. Several writers report empirical evidence of a genetic contribution to stuttering (Andrews and Harris, 1964; Howie et al., 1976; Kidd, 1977; Sheehan and Costley, 1977) although environmental variables are almost certainly involved also. The theoretical speculations offered above can certainly explain why some of the secondary, maladaptive symptoms of stuttering are hard to extinguish, but the assumption of a physiological basis for disfluency adds a new dimension to the problems of maintenance. If treatment is actually providing the skills necessary to compensate for an innate deficiency, it would be predicted that the core behaviors will inevitably reappear unless great care is taken to maintain the acquired skills.

The risk of relapse for any individual may depend partly on the strength of his genetic loading, particulary if the genetic predisposition proves to be a continuum rather than a dichotomy. There is some evidence to suggest that the chance of recovery from stuttering following therapy is lower in individuals with a family history of stuttering (Neaves, 1970; Cooper, 1972). Spontaneous recovery from stuttering (that is, in the absence of therapy) also appears related to family history of stuttering (Sheehan and Martyn, 1966). These authors further showed that spontaneous recovery was more likely in mild stutterers than in severe stutterers, a finding which has since been confirmed by Cooper (1972) for recovery in general, and by Guitar (1976) for recovery following treatment. Whether stuttering severity reflects genetic or environmental factors or a combination of both is unclear at this stage.

The implication of a genetic viewpoint is that, at least for those with a heavy genetic loading for stuttering, the client must accept that maintenance is a life-long process. If such "loaded" individuals can be identified, maintenance programs could be designed specifically to reinforce the strength of the compensatory skill.

SUMMARY

In summary, we have reviewed evidence which suggests that virtually all forms of intensive behavioral treatment of stuttering produce immediate dramatic increases in fluency, but encounter serious relapse problems in the post-treatment environment. The small amount of existing research on the question of the relationship between maintenance activities and relapse suggests that some form of skill practice and/or clinic contact reduces the severity of relapse. Researchers are only beginning to grapple with the methodological problems of choice of speech samples, choice of measures, criteria of success, and control of extraneous variables. The literature provides a rich source of ideas for maintenance strategies, ranging from various forms of clinic contact, emphasis on client responsibility, attitude change strategies, to the retraining programs. However, the rationale for the use of any given strategy is often hazy. In this paper we have offered three different theoretical viewpoints on the relapse problem and considered their implications for planning maintenance strategies. As stated before, these ideas are speculative and represent some of our intuitive and inductive reasoning, which may lead to deducted facts. Maintenance remains the last and possibly most challenging aspect of fluency management. At present, a wide spectrum of maintenance strategies need to be studied, in terms of their effectiveness as therapeutic tools, and also at the level of the power of the theoretical rationale on which their use is based.

The senior author gratefully acknowledges the support of the Divison of Communication Disorders and G. Andrews at the Prince Henry Hospital, New South Wales, Australia, where he was visting scientist in 1977. He would also like to express appreciation to the following for the opportunity to visit and observe during the study tour: R. Ingham, R. Lanyon, D. Mowrer, W. Perkins, and D. Prins.

REFERENCES

Andrews, G., and Harris, M. *The Syndrome of Stuttering.* London: Heinemann Medical Books, 1964.

Andrews, G., and Ingham, R. Stuttering: An evaluation of follow-up procedures for syllable timed speech/token system therapy. *Journal of Communication Disorders,* 1972a, 5, 307–319.

Andrews, G., and Ingham, R. Stuttering: An approach to the evaluation of stuttering therapy. *Journal of Speech and Hearing Research,* 1972b, 15, 296–302.

Bloodstein, O. *A Handbook of Stuttering.* Chicago: National Easter Seal Society, 1975.

Boberg, E. Intensive group therapy program for stutterers. *Human Communication,* 1976, 1, 29–42.

Boberg, E., and Sawyer, L. The maintenance of fluency following intensive therapy. *Human Communication,* 1977, 2, 21–28.

Cooper, E. Recovery from stuttering in a junior and senior high school population. *Journal of Speech and Hearing Research,* 1972, 15, 632–638.

Cooper, E. Controversies about stuttering therapy. *Journal of Fluency Disorders,* 1977, 2, 75–86.

Costello, J. The establishment of fluency with time-out procedures: Three case studies. *Journal of Speech and Hearing Disorders,* 1975, 40, 216–231.

Curlee, R., and Perkins, W. Conversational rate control therapy for stuttering. *Journal of Speech and Hearing Disorders,* 1969, 34, 245–250.

Dalton, P. Research into the effectiveness of intensive group treatment for adult stammerers. *Bulletin of the College of Speech Therapists,* 1977, 303, 8–10.

Daly, D., and Darnton, P. Intensive fluency shaping and attitudinal therapy with stutterers: A follow-up study. Paper presented at the annual convention of the American Speech and Hearing Association, Houston, Texas, 1976.

DiGusto, J., Smith, G., and Ingham, R. Self-monitoring of stuttering: An experimental and therapy evaluation study. Paper presented at the annual convention of the Australian Association of Speech and Hearing, Sydney, Australia, 1976.

Egolf, D. B., Shames, G., Johnson, P., and Kasprisin-Burelli, A. The use of parent-child interaction patterns in therapy for young stutterers. *Journal of Speech and Hearing Disorders,* 1972, 37, 222–232.

Frayne, H., Coates, S., and Marriner, N. Evaluation of post-treatment fluency by naive subjects. *Australian Journal of Human Communication Disorders,* 1977, 5, 48–54.

Gregory, H. An assessment of the results of stuttering therapy. *Journal of Communication Disorders,* 1972, 5, 320–334.

Guitar, B. Pre-treatment factors associated with the outcome of stuttering therapy. *Journal of Speech and Hearing Disorders,* 1976, 19, 590–600.

Guitar, B., and Bass, C. Stuttering therapy: The relation between attitude and change and long-term outcome. *Journal of Speech and Hearing Disorders,* 1978, 43, 392–400.

Hanna, R., and Owen, N. Facilitating transfer and maintenance of fluency in stuttering therapy. *Journal of Speech and Hearing Disorders,* 1977, 42, 65–76.

Holgate, D., and Andrews, G. The use of syllable-timed speech and group psychotherapy in the treatment of adult stutterers. *Journal of Australian College of Speech Therapists,* 1966, 16, 36–40.

Howie, P. Andrews G., and Woods, L. *Therapist Manual for the Stuttering Treatment Program.* Sydney, N.S.W.: The Prince Henry Hospital, 1976.

Howie, P., and Tanner, S. An intensive behavior modificaiton treatment program for adult stutterers: Description and evaluation of outcome. Paper presented at the Annual Conference of the Australian Behavior Modification, Sydney, Australia, May, 1978.

Ingham, R. A comparison of covert and overt assessment procedures in stuttering therapy outcome evaluation. *Journal of Speech and Hearing Research,* 1975, 18, 345–354.

Ingham, R. Personal communication, 1977a.

Ingham, R. Towards an accountability model for the management of stuttering. Paper presented at the Victorian Dept. of Education Speech Therapists' In-Service Training Meeting, Melbourne, Australia, May, 1977b.

Ingham, R., and Andrews, G. An analysis of a token economy in stuttering therapy. *Journal of Applied Behavioral Analysis,* 1973a, 6, 219–229.

Ingham, R., and Andrews, G. Details of a token economy stuttering therapy program for adults. *Australian Journal of Human Communication Disorders,* 1973b, 1, 13–20.

Ingham, R., and Andrews, G. Behavior therapy and stuttering: A review. *Journal of Speech and Hearing Disorders,* 1973c, 38, 405–411.

Ingham, R., Andrews, G., and Winkler, R. Stuttering: A comparative evaluation of the short term effectiveness of four treatment techniques. *Journal of Communication Disorders,* 1972, 5, 91–117.

Ingham, R. J., and Packman, A. C. Perceptual assessment of normalcy of speech following stuttering therapy. *Journal of Speech and Hearing Research,* 1978, 21, 63–73.

Kidd, K. K. A genetic perspective on stuttering. *Journal of Fluency Disorders,* 1977, 2, 259–269.

LaCroix, Z. Management of disfluent speech through self-recording procedures. *Journal of Speech and Hearing Disorders,* 1973, 38, 272–274.

Mowrer, D. *Technical Research Report S-1: Reduction of Stuttering Behavior.* Tempe, Arizona: Arizona State University Bookstore, 1975.

Neaves, R. To establish a basis for prognosis in stammering. *British Journal of Disorders of Communication,* 1970, 5, 46–58.

Perkins, W. Behavioral management of stuttering. Final report, Social and Rehab Service Research Grant, 1973a.

Perkins, W. Replacement of stuttering with normal speech: II. Clinical procedures. *Journal of Speech and Hearing Disorders,* 1973b, 38, 295–303.

Perkins, W. Personal communicaiton, 1977.

Perkins, W., Rudas, J., Johnson, L., Michael, W., and Curlee, R. Replacement of stuttering with normal speech: III. Clinical effectiveness. *Journal of Speech and Hearing Disorders,* 1974, 39, 416–428.

Prins, D. Improvement and regression in stutterers following short-term intensive therapy. *Journal of Speech and Hearing Disorders,* 1970, 35, 123–135.

Prins, D. Personal communication, 1977.

Prins, D., and Miller, M. Personality, improvement and regression in stuttering therapy. *Journal of Speech and Hearing Research,* 1973, 16, 685–690.

Ryan, B. *Programmed Therapy for Stuttering in Children and Adults.* Springfield, Illinois: Charles C. Thomas, 1974.

Ryan, B., and Van Kirk, B. The establishment, transfer, and maintenance of fluent speech in 50 stutterers using delayed auditory feedback and operant procedures. *Journal of Speech and Hearing Disorders,* 1974, 39, 3–10.

Shames, G., and Egolf, D. *Operant Conditioning and the Management of Stuttering.* Englewood Cliffs, New Jersey: Prentice-Hall, 1976.

Sheehan, J., and Costley, M. A re-examination of the role of heredity in stuttering. *Journal of Speech and Hearing Disorders,* 1977, 52, 47–59.

Sheehan, J., and Martyn, M. Spontaneous recovery from stuttering. *Journal of Speech and Hearing Research,* 1966, 9, 121–135.

Van Kirk, B. Operant therapy programs for stuttering conducted in a rehabilitation center. *Rehabilitation Literature,* 1972, 33, 107–108.

Webster, R. A behavioral analysis of stuttering: Treatment and theory. In Calhoun, K. et al. (eds.). *Innovative Treatment Methods in Psychopathology.* New York: John Wiley and Sons, 1974.

Webster, R. *The Precision Fluency Shaping Program.* Client Manual, 1975, Vol. II.

Webster, R. Personal communication, 1977.

Wischner, G. Anxiety-reduction as reinforcement in maladaptive behavior: Evidence in stutterers' representations of the moment of difficulty. *Journal of Abnormal Social Psychology,* 1952, 47, 566–571.

Woods, L. Manual for the Speakeasy Clubs: Fluency maintenance groups for the stuttering treatment program. Sydney, Australia: Prince Henry Hospital, 1976.

Relapse and Outcome

Einer Boberg

In the previous paper we reviewed articles that focused on the difficulty of maintaining fluency in the post-treatment period. We concluded that although most behavioral treatments produce dramatic increases in fluency in a short time, many stutterers experience some degree of relapse in the post-treatment environment. We also noted that the amount of research on maintenance issues and the inherent methodological problems were negligible. 1979 was also the year of the Banff International Conference on the Maintenance of Fluency (Boberg, 1981). This event brought people together to share their concerns and discuss research and clinical strategies.

In this paper I will try to summarize and integrate some developments since the 1979 paper and conference. I will consider whether there is evidence that researchers and clinicians are generally more aware of the maintenance issues, whether the methodological issues have been addressed or new approaches developed. Are there new experimental investigations in this area? Is there new information about etiology that has implications for maintenance? What clinical strategies have emerged from the literature? What are the general prospects for the long-term maintenance of fluency? Does the benighted stutterer have any more reason for optimism than he did some years ago? These questions will be examined in the following pages.

INCREASED INTEREST IN MAINTENANCE?

Let us start by looking back at previous reports of clinical programs. Bloodstein (1981) has conveniently summarized the results of 117 studies reported between 1928 and 1979. Only 46 of these studies, less than 40%, provided any information about post-treatment performance. Furthermore, those that did often use vague terms such as "improvement maintained," which contribute very little to our understanding of the long-term effects of therapy. Bloodstein noted that most of the studies made little attempt to evaluate the stutterer's progress outside the clinic

Postscript 20

or determine whether the results were lasting. He sadly concludes that the assessment of therapy results is a "process fraught with opportunities for error and self-delusion."

Bloodstein listed 11 tests that a therapy method must meet before it can be considered successful. The fifth item in this daunting list is that "the stability of the results must be demonstrated by long-term investigations" (pp. 336–337). He suggests 18 months as the minimum time period that must elapse before treatment results can be considered stable. He also emphasized what others have noted (Ingham, 1975; Boberg & Sawyer, 1977), that speech performance must be measured in nonclinical settings with nonclinic staff. Most clinicians are aware that clients will typically speak more fluently in the clinic when talking to their clinicians. Although this is one of the best-known facts about stuttering, it is also the most frequently ignored when clinicians report the results of treatment.

What evidence is there that the situation has improved in the last five years? In a major book published in 1979 Gregory explored controversial issues in stuttering therapy. He asked several prominent writers to comment on the long-term results of therapy and the problem of relapse. It is beyond the scope of this paper to review the many useful contributions included in this book other than to applaud the recognition that such a publication gives to the importance of maintaining fluency.

Another influential volume appeared the following year: *Strategies in stuttering therapy* (Perkins, 1980). Many of the contributors to this book dealt generally and even specifically with maintenance. Adams (1980) admitted that in the past the major responsibility for maintenance had been placed on the client, but that more and more, clinicians were now recognizing that they must play an active part in maintenance. Costello (1980) also stated that the client and clinician share joint responsibility for assuring that fluency is maintained. She points out that if relapse occurs, "both parties suffer: the client for losing fluency after a long period of devotion and hard work, and the clinician for believing certain techniques to be effective when reinforcement was still needed" (p. 321). Shine (1980) referred to a maintenance program that is continued for at least a year after therapy with gradual decreasing frequency of clinic visits. Gregory and Hill (1980) reported that they analyze factors that interfere with maintenance of normal fluency and take the appropriate steps to improve the program. Boberg (1980) described how he and his colleagues prepare clients for a maintenance program of home assignments and clinic visits. Florance and Shames (1980) described some variables that operate in maintenance, how they train clients in self-responsibility, and the tactics used in their maintenance programs.

In addition to the two books already mentioned, numerous articles appeared as journals, chapters in books, and topics at conferences. In a paper presented to the Annual Multidisciplinary Approach to Stuttering at Baylor College of Medicine in May 1979, Webster (1980) described the evolution of his treatment program and provided data on 200 randomly selected cases at a mean follow-up time of 10 months. Other examples are a recent paper by Kamhi (1982) and a short course presented by St. Louis at the annual American Speech and Hearing Association conference (1982). When all of these items are considered together it does indeed seem reasonable to conclude that maintenance is beginning to receive the attention it deserves. We now need to examine whether this flurry of activity has generated anything of value.

METHODOLOGICAL ISSUES

In the 1979 paper we addressed the problem of measuring long-term outcome and suggested that such measures might differ depending upon where and when and under what conditions they were made, and whether they were done overtly or covertly. One general assumption has been that post-treatment clients display more disfluencies when measured covertly than when measured overtly. A few experimental studies have addressed this issue.

The results from some studies appeared to suggest that when covert and overt studies are compared the differences are so small that overt procedures should be sufficient for routine clinical assessments. Andrews and Craig (1982) tested 56 subjects at an average time of 18 months after intensive treatment at the Prince Henry Hospital in Sydney. They used three assessment measures:

1. Clinic overt assessment. A clinic staff member made an unannounced telephone call to the subject. The call was recorded and analyzed for percentage of syllables stuttered and speech rate in syllables per minute. The subject knew that he was being recorded.
2. Client covert assessment. Another client, enrolled in the transfer phase of a current program, made an unannounced call to the subject and said that he was making the call as part of his transfer assignments. The subject was not aware that he was being recorded.
3. Nonclinic covert assessment. A stranger telephoned a randomly chosen subgroup of the clients and conducted a public opinion survey. The clients were not aware that they were being recorded or assessed. The authors report that the group data for the covert measures were not significantly different from the overt measures, and that covert measures may not be necessary for a realistic assessment of group progress. However, in single case studies, individual differences probably require overt and covert assessment across standardized speaking situations in order to describe the behavior fully.

Howie et al. (1982) conducted covert and overt assessments immediately before and after an intensive treatment program. The pre-treatment covert sample was obtained during routine hospital admission procedures, where an interviewer posed as a psychologist to obtain samples of monologue and conversation. In the post-treatment covert sample clients were invited to participate as a control group of normals in research on the thought processes of schizophrenics.

Postscript 20

The overt samples were obtained during pre- and post-treatment evaluations in a different part of the hospital with interviewers not associated with the clinic program. The results revealed no significant pre-treatment differences between the covert and overt assessments. However, immediately after treatment the covertly assessed stuttering frequency was significantly higher than the overtly assessed frequency. All but three of the 15 clients stuttered more during covert than overt assessment. The differences were small but consistent.

These results present interesting comparisons with other research. In an earlier study Ingham (1975) showed that three months after treatment, covertly assessed stuttering was higher and speech rate lower than when overtly assessed. However, at six months Ingham's clients did not show a clinical or statistically significant difference between overt and covert measures. This trend agreed with another study by Howie et al. (1981), in which they tested clients 15 months post-treatment and found no group differences between overt and covert measures of stuttering frequency. Howie et al. (1982) offered the hypothesis that as time since effective treatment increases, the discrepancy between covert and overt measures decreases. They suggest that this change is related to the decreasing power of clinic-associated cues to influence the speech of treated stutterers. To the clinician they offer the suggestion that before treatment, and 18 months or more after treatment, covert evaluations may be unnecessary. However, during the first few months after treatment, reliance on overt assessments may exaggerate the gains of therapy. In conclusion the authors state that whether or not covert assessments should be done depends on the stage of treatment when assessment occurs and the aims and designs of the research. It can never be automatically assumed that a level of stuttering frequency observed in one situation will be the same in another situation. The researcher and clinician should assess how valid it is to generalize in a given situation. I must also add the reminder that the term "overt assessment" in these studies refers to objective measures of client performance obtained in a nonclinic situation with interviewers who were not associated with the treatment program. It definitely does not include casual evaluations done in the clinic by the clinicians who administered the treatment program

A second methodological issue raised in the 1979 paper revolved around which parameters to measure in post-treatment speech. It is difficult to obtain agreement on what to count as a disfluency in speech samples. Different clinics use different rules governing which disfluencies will be counted as stuttered and which will be considered as normal disfluencies. For instance, some clinics may count all disfluencies as stuttered, including interjections, phrase revisions, pauses, etc., while other clinics may regard disfluencies within those categories as within normal range. While published articles now routinely report high reliability scores between independent clinicians when rating speech samples, there is no assurance that such high reliability exists between clinics. It is not surprising to find high reliability between clinicians if they were trained and/or work in the same institution. However, that does not indicate that high agreement would be found with a clinician from another institution. If differences in counting strategies do exist we would expect them to be manifest in the scores reported on follow-up studies. A review of the literature reveals a dearth of definitions that specify in sufficient detail how a particular clinic analyses and categorizes disfluencies in a speech sample. We obviously need much better agreement in this area before we can make meaningful comparisons of clinical results from different clinics. This issue is considered in another publication (Boberg & Kully, 1983), where we have described our rule system for counting and a training program for clinicians.

In addition to the disagreements just outlined, there is also marked disagreement over what other measurements should be made in order to properly assess treatment outcome. Some writers insist that only objective measurements should be considered, while others attempt to measure many other parameters. For instance, Shames and Florance (1980) include 17 measures on an experimental basis in order to determine the "permanence of changes in speech, self-concept, perceptions of others, self-reinforcing tendencies, motivation, and coping styles." Adams and Runyon (1981) also take the position that there is much more to a stutterer's speech problem than can be determined by measuring frequency and topography of stuttering and accessory behaviors. In a recent article these authors review the research that demonstrate that the "fluent" speech of stutterers can be differentiated from the fluent speech of normal speakers. Judges apparently can do this through the use of cues such as longer syllable durations, low vocal intensity, inappropriately placed pauses, vocal tremor and tension, and imprecise articulation. They suggest a joint effort between clinicians and speech scientists to more accurately describe the post-treatment speech of stutterers. Such an endeavor might suggest further clinical strategies to eliminate those residual abnormalities in the speech and help the clinician decide when the client can be dismissed. Adams and Runyon believe that the stutterer who is most ready for dismissal and who is most likely to maintain his improvement is the one whose speech is objectively and perceptibly indistinguishable from normals. It should be free of stuttering, produced at an acceptable rate, sound natural, and be free of perceptible signs of tenuous fluency. Those patients who are largely or completely free of stuttering but who continue to exhibit objective and perceptible signs of tenuous fluency are more likely to relapse. Ingham (1982), however, cautions that there are no data to indicate that stutterers whose fluency remains objectively and perceptibly different from normals tend to relapse more than those clients who are indistinguishable from normals. Ingham argues convincingly that all such clinical recommendations must be built on a solid base of research data.

There is also a critical coterie who doubt that we can ever adequately measure the outcome of therapy. Sheehan (1980), displaying more than the usual amount of skepticism, suggests several principles that we should keep in mind when evaluating outcome reports:

1. The more trivial the criteria for improvement, the higher the resulting percentage of success.

Postscript 20

2. The experimenter evaluating his own results will tend to report more success, however defined, than will be confirmed by later independent evaluation.
3. The more poorly controlled a study is, the higher the probability of a success claim resulting from it.

Sheehan insists that in a complex disorder such as stuttering, outcome measurement must include many more dimensions than objective frequency counts of stuttering.

Yet another issue revolves around what constitutes a reasonable target for therapy, in terms of disfluency. Some clinicians maintain that 100% fluency is a legitimate and achievable target in therapy (Howie et al., 1981; Goldberg, 1981) while others accept some level of disfluency as the final target (Boberg, 1980; Webster, 1980). The resolution of a part of this question obviously relates to the preceding issue: what should be counted as a disfluency. Another aspect of this question is whether it is clinically sound to ask people, who have stuttered for many years, to achieve a target of 100% fluency. In commenting on this question Sheehan (1980) maintains that to argue that because the stutterer can be fluent part of the time, he should be able to be fluent all of the time is like saying that if a shortstop in a baseball game plays several consecutive games without error there is no reason he should not play all games without error. To talk about "stutter-free speech" is like talking about error-free baseball. Just because a client has a skill in his repertoire does not mean that he will always be able to use it. Sheehan insists that the motivational and individual elements in the treatment of a complex disorder such as stuttering makes it inevitable that stutterers will sometimes fail. Martin (1981) also states that "it is probably unrealistic or even undesirable to expect a successfully treated stuttering client to speak without emitting any disfluencies" (p. 18). Kamhi (1982) also fervently hoped that clinicians who use fluency-oriented therapy programs would "cease pretending that the majority of stutterers will be able to maintain fluent or stutter-free speech on a long-term basis." He suggests that if we reduce our expectations we will be able to confront the relapse problem more honestly and effectively.

It seems fair to conclude that we are not yet on the threshold of a broadly based agreement on what items to include in our definition of stuttering, what parameters to measure in outcome, and what goals should be established for therapy.

EXPERIMENTAL INVESTIGATIONS IN MAINTENANCE

Although many articles have outlined numerous methods that may be useful in maintaining treatment effects, very few have experimentally demonstrated that a post-treatment performance trend could be altered by adding or modifying a maintenance procedure. Boberg and Sawyer (1977) showed that "booster" sessions that followed treatment were effective in arresting and reversing a deterioration in post-treatment performance. Ingham has now added two experimental studies on maintenance. In one study (1980) he tried to determine whether a particular maintenance schedule was effective in maintaining treatment gains. Two schedules of return visits to the clinic were devised. In the performance contingent schedule (PC), clients returned to the clinic with decreasing frequency, starting with weekly visits, and then expanding the interval between visits to 32 weeks. If the client failed the criterion test on any given visit he was returned to the beginning of the cycle. Thus the client's performance during the clinic visit determined when he would be required to come for the next visit. In the nonperformance schedule (NPC) clients continued on an assigned schedule regardless of speech performance. Criterion performance was achieved if the clients spoke with 0% syllables stuttered at a rate between 170 and 210 syllables per minute. All measures were made by a clinician using an electronic button-press counter from either on-line assessment or recordings of telephone calls. Assessments of speech performance were made in three ways: (a) within-clinic assessments; (b) outside-clinic assessments, where clients collected samples of their speech while talking to family members and making telephone calls; (c) covertly recorded telephone calls to the clients by a hospital staff member who was ostensibly inquiring about conditions during the client's stay in the hospital. The group data indicated that the performance-contingent schedules were associated with a higher level of performance during assessment than the nonperformance schedules. The suggestion is made that the clinician can improve post-treatment fluency in some subjects by manipulating the maintenance schedule.

In a second study using single-subject design, Ingham (1982) combined training in self-evaluation of speech performance with a self-managed, performance-contingent maintenance schedule. In Stage 1, the adult subject was required to count the number of stutterings and estimate speech rate during daily speech tasks. If his scores agreed with the clinician's scores and his performance was within the target range on four consecutive days he moved to the second stage. Now the client could choose to decrease the schedule of daily speech tasks if he determined that he reached the target on two consecutive days. If he scored himself as failing to achieve the target behavior on any speech task he would then return to an earlier schedule. He might also fail the second stage if random checks by the clinician, on a sample of recordings, revealed that he had not reached his target. Covert and overt assessments indicted that whenever the self-evaluation training was introduced to the maintenance schedule it was associated with substantially reduced stuttering, and that this reduction was maintained over a period of at least six months. The clinical significance of this study is that it demonstrated that training in self-evaluation and self-management can be associated with improved speech performance in the post-treatment period. I hope that we will see more such well-controlled demonstrations of clinically important strategies.

In an experimental study on a related topic Martin and Haroldson (1982) investigated the effect of contingent self-stimulation for stuttering. In this study

---

Postscript 20

---

and a similar earlier study by Boberg (1969), stutterers were given time-out contingent on each stuttering. Another group of stutterers administered time-out to themselves, contingent on each stuttering. Stutterers in both time-out conditions showed marked reductions in stuttering compared with base rates. Stutterers who administered their own time-outs, however, showed significantly less extinction of reduced stuttering following the time-out period, and significantly greater generalization to telephone speaking, than did the stutterers who were timed-out by the experimenter. The significance of these and the Ingham studies is a strong indication that if self-management skills were properly and systematically taught to clients, the benefit might be substantial in transferring and maintaining treatment gains.

NEW SPECULATIONS

In the 1979 article we offered three speculations on why stutterers relapse after successful treatment. One possibility is that there exists a physiological basis for stuttering. An implication of this position is that maintenance might be a life-long process. Stutterers who maintain treatment gains do so because they continue to exercise those skills that successfully compensate for the underlying physiological or neurophysiological condition. Recent evidence has persuaded me that this is the most plausible of the three speculations presented in the earlier paper.

A plethora of papers have appeared in recent years reporting evidence of discoordination in the laryngeal and oral areas. Adams (1981) and Zimmerman (1980) have integrated much of this material, and Zimmerman et al. (1981) have developed a sophisticated model to account for the findings. Although this material is useful in understanding more precisely the manifestations of stuttering, it remains to be seen whether it will contribute substantially to our eventual unscrambling of the etiological puzzle. Even if the difficulty is most easily observed at the laryngeal level, it is highly unlikely that the problem originates there but rather involves higher neurophysiological centers. In an integrative and summarizing lecture, Perkins (1981) reviewed the evidence for and against organic disfunction in stuttering and concluded that the disfunction almost certainly involves some neural component that controls the larynx, but that the control does not reside in the larynx. He indicated that there is evidence of mistiming of neural control of the speech mechanism, particularly as it affects the airstream. Recent EEG studies by Moore and Haynes (1980), Boberg et al. (1983), and Moore (1984) provide persuasive evidence that the discoordination observed at laryngeal levels originates in disfunction at the level of the right and left hemispheres. The current data suggests that the right hemisphere is overly active in stutterers and that disfluent verbal behavior may result from differences in hemispheric processing. These differences may be related to an inability of the right hemisphere to handle the segmentation aspects of language. If these early indications are confirmed by subsequent research it will certainly affect how we approach the problem of stuttering. As Perkins (1981) pointed out, if stutterers are constitutionally limited in the facility with which they can achieve fluency, they will then need to rely more heavily than normal speakers on compensatory skills such as rate control, rhythm, and breath flow in order to speak fluently. Expectations of eventually attaining fluency will need to be attenuated somewhat. Such a development may relieve the pressure for complete fluency that is currently put on some stutterers.

PROSPECTS FOR THE FUTURE

Two recent studies are particularly relevant when trying to gain some perspective on where we are, what progress we have made, and what prospects the future holds. Howie et al. (1981) studied the short-term (3 to 9 weeks) and long-term (12 to 18 months) outcome of 36 adult stutterers after an intensive treatment program. For the short-term study telephone calls were made and recorded in the clinic and analyzed for percentage of stuttering and speech rate in syllables per minute. For the long-term study overt speech samples were collected by a stranger in an unfamiliar setting. Covert speech samples of a telephone call were also obtained.

The short-term results showed that for the group as a whole there was no significant deterioration of treatment gains although 4 of the 36 clients stuttered at more than 3% in the overt clinic evaluation. In the long-term study the authors reported that clients are still "significantly more fluent and their attitudes to speaking are significantly more positive than before treatment, but that signs of relapse are present in 30–60% of clients, depending on the stringency of the criterion applied for normal fluency" (p. 107). They went on to report that almost all the clients reported improved speech, though only half of the clients were satisfied with their improvement. Most clients indicated that fluency was not automatic and often required deliberate attention: 24% of the clients reported that they had to attend to the act of speaking 100% of the time. About 97% of clients reported improved speech on questionnaire, and 86% reported increased confidence 15 months after the intensive treatment.

Howie et al. believe that their data permit them to estimate the long-term odds for a client seeking therapy. They suggest that a client has a 70% chance of gaining substantially improved speech and increased speaking confidence 12 months after treatment. If the client is aiming for "normal" fluency the odds are lower. The client has a 40% chance of stuttering 1% or less, of being satisfied with his speech, and of reporting good fluency. The authors said that the majority of their clients find such odds acceptable. Since these treatment effects have been demonstrated on a large group of clients in a well-established program and since they are similar to results from other intensive programs, there does appear to be a basis from which we can offer clients a reasonable prediction of outcome. It is refreshing to read a study in which the authors are prepared to make a prediction about outcome and base their predictions on data rather than wishful thinking. Even some deterioration of fluency following intensive treatment does not negate

Postscript   20

the equally clear evidence of the substantial and lasting changes produced with the majority of clients.

Another paper by Andrews et al. (1980) exudes optimism and confidence in the efficacy of treatment, in sharp contrast to the many papers in the gloom-and-doom school. These authors challenged the widely held notions that stuttering is poorly understood and difficult to treat. They employed a new mathematical technique, meta-analysis, to demonstrate that stuttering treatment is effective and reasonably stable over time.

In meta-analysis the effect of treatment, or effect size, is calculated as the difference between the mean pre-treatment and post-treatment scores on a measure, divided by the standard deviation of the pre-treatment scores. This effect-size statistic allows different treatments to be compared and different outcome measures to be related. The authors used this procedure to determine: (a) how effective is the treatment; (b) which methods are most effective; and (c) what are the implications for the clinician.

Forty-two studies were assembled in which it was possible to calculate an effect size; these were then classified according to the principal treatment used. In answer to how effective was the treatment, the authors reported that the mean of the 116 effect sizes was 1.3, indicating that the average treated stutterer was more normal-speaking than 90% of his/her untreated fellows. Stuttering treatment is clearly effective.

In answer to which treatment procedure produced the best results, the meta-analysis revealed that prolonged speech and gentle onset were the strongest treatments, both in the short- and long-term. These two clinical procedures have produced similar results when used by different clinicians in different clinics in different countries, so the results cannot easily be attributed to spurious findings or methodological flaws, according to the authors.

The clinical implications of this meta-analysis are that treatment will require approximately 100 hours to produce substantial improvement and should include some form of prolonged speech and gentle onset with gradual shaping of the normal speech to normal rates. An effective program must also include a systematic transfer of new speech into the normal environment, possibly some counseling to improve attitudes, some cooperation from family and friends, and, finally, a planned maintenance program to consolidate all these activities. In comparing the treatment of stuttering to treatment programs in other health science areas the authors maintain that there is little room for pessimism.

> The standard of research in studies reporting data is good, and reliable and adequate follow-up periods are common . . . Relapse over time is slow, certainly slower than with some other treatments for chronic conditions. Some stuttering treatments are clearly beneficial and their effects are comparable with treatments for other chronic problems in the health sciences. (p. 305)

While such optimism is a pleasant relief from the more usual lamentations in review articles, we may wish to postpone our victory celebrations for yet awhile. No matter how sophisticated a meta-analysis might be, it is still subject to the law that states that the quality of output is governed by the quality of input to a system. Many of the 42 studies used in this analysis have not escaped the methodological problems described earlier in this paper. This fact must be taken into account when evaluating the results of the meta-analysis. Nevertheless, the authors are to be applauded for presenting an exciting new perspective and injecting a note of refreshing optimism.

In conclusion, this re-examination of the maintenance issues has been a relatively happy one. Although many difficulties abound and much research has yet to be done there does appear to be evidence of substantial progress during the last few years. Clinicians and researchers alike are paying more attention to the long-term outcome of treatment, some of the methodological issues have been addressed with varying degrees of success, exciting prospects have been revealed through experimental and innovative studies, and new clinical strategies have been suggested that now must be extensively tested. If this present trend continues, I believe that it is reasonable to anticipate even more progress in the next few years on this most challenging aspect of the treatment of stuttering.

REFERENCES

Adams, M., & Runyan C. (1981). Stuttering and fluency: Exclusive events or points on a continuum? *Journal of Fluency Disorders, 6,* 197–218.

Adams, M. (1980). The young stutterer: Diagnosis, treatment and assessment of progress. In W. Perkins (Ed.), *Strategies in stuttering therapy.* New York: Thieme-Stratton, Inc.

Adams, M. (1981). The speech production abilities of stutterers: Recent, ongoing and future research. *Journal of Fluency Disorders, 6,* 311–326.

Andrews, G., & Craig, A. (1982). Stuttering: Overt and covert measurement of the speech of treated subjects. *Journal of Speech Hearing and Disorders, 47,* 96–99.

Andrews, G., Guitar, B., & Howie, P. (1980). Meta-analysis of the effects of stuttering treatment. *Journal of Speech Hearing and Disorders, 45,* 287–307.

Bloodstein, O. (1981). *A handbook on stuttering.* Chicago, IL: National Easter Seal Society.

Boberg, E. (1969). The effects of self-administered and experimenter-administered "time-out" on stuttering. *Dissertation Abstracts, 30 B,* p. 884.

Boberg, E. (1980). Intensive adult therapy program. In W. Perkins (Ed.). *Strategies in stuttering therapy.* New York: Thieme-Stratton, Inc.

Boberg, E. (Ed.). (1981). *Maintenance of fluency.* New York: Elsevier.

Boberg, E. & Kully, D. (In press). *Alberta comprehensive stuttering program.*

Boberg, E., & Sawyer, L. (1977). The maintenance of fluency following intensive therapy. *Human Communication, 2,* 21–28.

Boberg, E., Yeudall, L., Schopflocher, D., & Bo-Lassen, P. (1983). The effect of an intensive behavioral program on the distribution of EEG alpha power in stuttering during the processing of verbal and visuospatial information. *Journal of Fluency Disorders, 8:3,* 245–263.

Costello, J. (1980). Operant conditioning and the treatment of stuttering. In W. Perkins (Ed.), *Strategies in stuttering therapy.* New York: Thieme-Stratton, Inc.

Postscript   20

Florance, C., & Shames, G. (1980). Stuttering treatment: Issues in transfer and maintenance. In W. Perkins (Ed.), *Strategies in stuttering therapy.* New York: Thieme-Stratton, Inc.

Goldberg, S. (1981). *Behavioral cognitive stuttering therapy.* Tigard, OR: C.C. Publications.

Gregory, H., & Hill, D. (1980). Stuttering therapy for children. In W. Perkins (Ed.), *Strategies in stuttering therapy.* New York: Thieme-Stratton, Inc.

Gregory, H. (Ed.). (1979). *Controversies about stuttering therapy.* Baltimore, MD: University Park Press.

Howie, P., Tanner, S., & Andrews, G. (1981). Short and long-term outcome in an intensive treatment program for adult stutterers. *Journal of Speech and Hearing Disorders, 46,* 104–109.

Howie, P., Woods, C., & Andrews, G. (1982). Relationship between covert and overt speech measures immediately before and immediately after stuttering treatment. *Journal of Speech and Hearing Disabilities, 47,* 419–422.

Ingham, R. (1975). A comparison of covert and overt assessment procedures in stuttering therapy outcome evaluation. *Journal of Speech and Hearing Research, 18,* 346–354.

Ingham, R. (1980). Modification of maintenance and generalization during stuttering treatment. *Journal of Speech and Hearing Research, 23,* 732–745.

Ingham, R. (1982). The effects of self-evaluation training on maintenance and generalization during stuttering treatment. *Journal of Speech and Hearing Disabilities, 47,* 271–280.

Ingham, R. (1982). Letter to the editor. *Journal of Fluency Disorders, 7,* 303–307.

Kamhi, A. (1982). The problem of relapse in stuttering. *Journal of Fluency Disorders, 7,* 459–468.

Martin, R., & Haroldson, S. (1982). Contingent self-stimulation and stuttering. *Journal of Speech and Hearing Disabilities, 47,* 407–413.

Martin, R. (1981). Introduction and perspective: Review of published research. In E. Boberg (Ed.), *Maintenance of fluency.* New York: Elsevier.

Moore, W. (1984). CNS characteristics of stutterers. In W. Perkins and R. Curlee (Eds.). *The nature and treatment of stuttering: New directions.* San Diego, CA: College Hill Press.

Moore, W. & Haynes, W. (1980). Alpha hemispheric asymmetry and stuttering: Some support for a segmentation dysfunction hypothesis. *Journal of Speech and Hearing Research, 23,* 229–247.

Perkins, W. (Ed.). (1980). *Strategies in stuttering therapy.* New York: Thieme-Stratton, Inc.

Perkins, W. (1981). Implications of scientific research for treatment of stuttering—a lecture. *Journal of Fluency Disorders, 6,* 155–162.

Shames, G., & Florance, C. (1980). *Stutter-free speech: A goal for therapy.* Columbus, OH: Charles E. Merrill.

Sheehan, J. (1980). Problems in the evaluation of progress and outcome. In W. Perkins (Ed.), *Strategies in stuttering therapy.* New York: Thieme-Stratton, Inc.

Shine, R. (1980). Direct management of the beginning stutterer. In W. Perkins (Ed.), *Strategies in stuttering therapy.* New York: Thieme-Stratton, Inc.

St. Louis, K. (1982). Transfer and maintenance of fluency in stuttering clients. Short course presented at the *Annual Convention of the American Speech and Hearing Association,* Toronto.

Webster, R. Evolution of a target-based behavioral therapy for stuttering. *Journal of Fluency Disorders, 5,* 303–320.

Zimmerman, G. (1980). Stuttering: A disorder of movement. *Journal of Speech and Hearing Research, 23,* 122–136.

Zimmerman, G., Smith, A., & Hanley, J. (1981). Stuttering: In need of a unifying conceptual framework. *Journal of Speech and Hearing Research, 24,* 25–31,

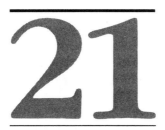

Concluding Remarks

George H. Shames and Herbert Rubin

Concluding Remarks

George H. Shames and Herbert Rubin

INTRODUCTION

As editors, we have probably enjoyed working on this book more than any of you have reading it. The personal contact with each of the contributors and the stimulation that the process provided evolved into an intellectual adventure for us. Our enjoyment would have been even greater had we been able to conclude this work with a simple and final interpretation of the diverse contributions included herein. We fully intended to do so at the outset of this adventure. However, we soon became aware that this was not an appropriate thing for us to do, given the richness of the diversity, the information presented, and the different rates and patterns of change reflected among the contributors over such varying periods of time.

It would be nice if we could take responsibility for the wisdom contained in this volume. We read many things we wished we had said. We also read things we do not agree with, but feel we have neither the right nor the responsibility to alter or to interpret. One reason for this is our dual roles of contributors and editors who bring to these tasks our own biases. Differences among the contributors are real, and their significance should not be distilled or edited, insofar as they reflect serious conceptual issues. They should not be glossed over, hidden, or de-emphasized. However, throughout the book in our introductory chapters to each section, we have attempted to highlight important issues and to ease the reader's task in relating content in the various chapters and points of view. The content of each chapter is distinctly and distinctively the product of the contributor, with the sole qualification of those authors who have updated someone else's material. It should also be noted that some contributors represent disciplines outside speech pathology and thus reflect different theoretical and clinical perspectives in their work with stutterers.

Patterns of Change

It is interesting in the format of a book such as this to track the patterns of change of the different contributors over the respective intervals of time represented here. At the simplest level we can identify three categories: essentially no change in the thinking of the contributor, expansion or refinement of a point of view that is still basically intact, and significant change or rejection of the previously held point of view. This system of analysis also holds for those contributors who are updating someone else's original material, because the current contributors were selected on the basis of their earlier compatibility with the original author's perspective.

As we track patterns of change we will try to identify the specific issues that we examine for change and that have been addressed by the contributors. Each of the three original chapters in this book (Matthews, Wingate, and Boberg) presents a historical perspective that lends itself to the same system of examination for change as those chapters that include reprints and updates. We will explore the significant issues addressed by the contributors according to the general format of the book.

Matthews necessarily addressed theoretical, research, and management issues dating back to the beginnings of our profession in the 1920s. As a prologue, his chapter leads us up to the current controversies and state of the art from Matthews's perspective as student and later as professional psychologist and speech pathologist. His point of view is probably less biased than most because stuttering has not been his major interest and because he brings to the task a critical mind and a background in scientific method. Having first been drawn to physiological explanations of stuttering, and later to psychodynamic explanations, Matthews has become a healthy skeptic, apparently despairing of finding *the* answer to the problem of stuttering. Perhaps by implication he is suggesting multiple answers to the problem but with a sharp call for a strong data base. As an issue, searching for a single answer to questions about causation, therapeutic goals, and strategies seems to characterize the historical period about which Matthews is writing. From our current perspective, the problem of stuttering appears to be more complex, suggesting multiple solutions and perhaps multiple populations. Matthews, possibly representing others whose professional experience spans half a century, has clearly rejected a number of previously held points of view, based upon equivocal or insufficient supporting data. As a scientist, he remains open to new data, but from the perspective of the null hypothesis. The null hypothesis is a statement of expectation of no difference, and therefore no conclusive, answers.

In contrast to Matthews, who never had an axe to grind with respect to the theory or therapy for stuttering, most of the contributors in the second section of this volume would be more likely to reject the null hypothesis in favor of experimental hypotheses, reflecting their bias, their enthusiasm, and their hopefulness of finding answers to the problem of stuttering. Although these characteristics can be motivating and infectious they carry with them the risk of a commitment that welcomes confirming data but may ignore contradictory data. In the absence of confirming data one can cling to a theoretical perspective by criticizing the work of others or by interpreting the failure of another's research as support for one's own position. One solution to the trap of theoretical rigidity is to ask of ourselves what we expect of others: to generate research information that will provide data relevant to our own theories. Such data can result in a confirmation and strengthening of a theoretical position or, if negative, should result in a reformulation of the theory.

As we look at the contributors to Part Two on Theories of Causation and Dynamics we find that they distribute themselves across all three categories of patterns of change over time. Where we find essentially no change, or little change, in the thinking of a theorist over a period of years we should be able to identify the reasons for the stability of that theory. Either there are experimental and clinical data (positive or negative) that support the theory, or the theory has generated significant researchable hypotheses stimulating research activity in others, or there simply have been no data brought forth to support or to infirm the theory, or, finally, the commitment of the theorist or his followers has been so strong that any major change might be interpreted as sacrilege. Often the originator of a theory is more amenable to change than his disciples who, in addition to their theoretical commitment, may have developed a personal loyalty to the theorist.

It appears that the Approach-Avoidance Conflict Theory as developed by Sheehan, the Two-Factor Theory as interpreted by Brutten, and Wingate's discussion of the physiology and genetics of stuttering have remained essentially the same over long periods of time. Brutten's earliest explication of his theory appeared in 1967, but Sheehan's goes back to 1953, and Wingate reviews material as far back as 1916 regarding conditioned reflexes and the physiology of stuttering in the 1920s, although specific reference to the genetics of stuttering is not found until 1935. With respect to both Brutten and Sheehan we are presented with intriguing theories that have captured the fancies of many students of stuttering but which have not generated researchable hypotheses to produce data that directly address the theory.

In comparison with the three chapters just mentioned, the contributions of Perkins and of Shames in Part Two reflect considerable refinement over time in their perspectives with regard to stuttering. While they have not changed their original points of view, they have expanded their frameworks and have addressed more specific dynamics of the problem of stuttering. For example, Perkins still holds to his discoordination hypothesis, involving the coordination among articulation, respiration, phonation, and breathstream management as reflecting an underlying neurological timing process. He has expanded this to include the effects of these discoordinations, with resulting emphasis on the stutterer's uncertainty about voice onset. As certainties (confidence) about voice onset increase, stuttering appears to decrease. Perkins views therapy as a compensatory activity that is designed to achieve more certainty about voice onsets. In a similar vein, Shames retains his original point of view. He still feels that many aspects of the problem of stuttering can be understood through the perspective of operant behavior. He has gone further within that perspective to emphasize those events that precede instances of stuttering and their consequences. Specifically, he is concerned about the stutterer's internal events of thinking, feeling, and evaluating with respect to himself and the external environment. These internal events could function as discriminative stimuli for stuttering, and therefore should be addressed both theoretically and in therapy.

Striking contrasts appear in the chapters of Travis, Johnson (updated by Bloodstein), and Flanagan between their reprints and their current points of view. In the case of Travis, we see a fascinating pattern of change, where in 1957, as a lay psychoanalyst, he initially emphasized the psychodynamics of stuttering. At that time, he viewed stuttering as the repression of unacceptable feelings, and he viewed therapy as basically psychoanalytic. At the present time, however, Travis appears to have reverted to his original thinking that lack of cerebral dominance with a probable genetic base is the etiological explanation for stuttering, as originally published in the 1920s and 1930s. However, with regard to therapy, he embraces the thinking of Perkins that the management of stuttering is designed to compensate for the genetically based problem. The behavioral techniques of DAF, rate control, and counseling function to deal with the effects of stuttering rather than its etiology. He seems to have come full circle with respect to stuttering theory, but has embraced current compensatory management practice.

Johnson's theory of the cause of stuttering has probably enjoyed greater popularity among clinicians than any other theory of etiology. It gave clinicians working with young stutterers the clinical focus on environmental manipulation. It also provided an impetus via semantic therapy for dealing with the faulty belief systems of adult stutterers, in particular the feelings of helplessness and victimization. Later, others embraced this focus on belief systems to include counseling in the management of stuttering in adults. As a student and disciple of Johnson, Bloodstein describes his own change of thinking relative to the semantogenic theory of stuttering. As such, this chapter qualifies as one that represents significant change from the date of the original publication to the present update. The reasons that Bloodstein offers for his change in perspective are several: he feels that the theory cannot ultimately be proved or disproved, instances of the original appearance of stuttering and reactions to it cannot be directly observed or experimentally manipulated, and Johnson's original research was vulnerable to distortions of memory and report bias. In addition, there are data indicating that calling attention to stuttering can have a therapeutic effect upon young children (Wingate, 1959) and that in some instances the initial appearance of stuttering involves significant muscular tension, and not merely effortless repetition (Bloodstein, 1960, 1961). However, Bloodstein points out that Johnson's original ideas generated a great deal of thinking and research. Johnson's basic message of the normalcy of stutterers was the backdrop of much of the research on personality, physiology, and birth and developmental histories of this population. Evidence of Johnson's influence appears in Bloodstein's own theory of anticipatory struggle (1958), in Williams's significant semantically oriented article "A Point of View about Stuttering" (1957), and in Rubin and Culatta's publication, "A Point of View about Fluency" (1971).

The Flanagan, Goldiamond, and Azrin research was the pioneering experimental effort in applying principles of operant conditioning to the problem of stuttering. It provided the impetus for major research programs by Curlee and Perkins (1969), by Perkins (1973), by Webster (1980), by Siegel (1970), by

Shames, Egolf, and Rhodes (1969), and by Shames and Egolf (1971). Perhaps the most striking contribution of the original publication of Flanagan et al. was the observation that the overt frequency of stuttering can be reduced in the laboratory by the application of punishment, and without addressing the stutterer's anxiety or any other covert aspect of stuttering. Flanagan appears to have changed his thinking radically in the recognition that punishment is not a viable clinical tactic and has very limited application to therapy and prevention.

In Part Three, two of the chapters reflect unchanged views between the original publications and the current updates. Gregory reviewed the rationale, tactics, and values of parent counseling and concluded that they appear to have been, and will continue to be, effective strategies for dealing with the environment of stutterers. He focuses on how events in the home appear to relate to specific instances of increase or decrease in the occurrence of disfluencies in children's speech. In contrast to Gregory's emphasis on disfluency, Seeman's update of Rogers's original views continues to focus on the underlying feelings of the stutterer with little or no reference to the stutterer's manner of speaking. The nature of counseling continues to be broader than and independent of the complaint presented by the client. This approach to therapy involves experiencing a relationship in which the client undergoes a process of growth in self-responsibility with potential application for resolving future problems beyond the original complaint.

The majority of contributors to the section on therapy present in their updates extensions and refinements of the original points of view. Some of these refinements appear to reflect the influences that many of these individuals are having upon one another through their respective research and publications. For example, Luper predicts that there will be a greater recognition and acceptance by clinicians who practice the tactics developed by Van Riper of the value of fluency in changing the attitudes of stutterers. Similarly, Wolpe acknowledges the value of fluency in desensitizing the stutterer's anxiety about talking. In this instance, he specifically refers to fluency attained through devices such as a metronome or regulated breathing to provide rhythmic stimulation. Shames and Rubin have had the advantage of working in the same setting wherein the cognitive and behavioral perspectives are shared. We observe each other's therapy and consult regularly, which results in the mutual adoption of certain aspects and components of each other's point of view. For example, Rubin now utilizes unmonitored fluent speech as a consequence of successfully monitored fluency, and Shames had placed greater emphasis on the later phases of his Stutter-Free Speech program, which deal with the same counseling issues that characterize cognitive therapy.

The refinements presented in the chapters by Ryan and Webster remain strictly within a behavioral framework and reflect continued improvement of their formal programs designed to be used with little individual variation. Each of these contributors is attempting to make his program more effective by simplifying procedures and reducing the number of tasks, thereby making them more manageable for the stutterer.

Boberg, in his consideration of outcome and relapse in therapy, reflects a general evolution and sophistication in the tactics of measurement of variables related to outcome, including attitude, as well as behavior. He has placed special emphasis upon the representativeness of data, based upon regular and continuing sampling. Armed with this information, Boberg feels we are now in a position to study different strategies in order to facilitate maintenance and to prevent relapse.

UNRESOLVED ISSUES

As we have discussed earlier in this book it would be nice to have conclusive answers to the problems presented herein. The fact that we do not have conclusive answers but instead are faced with a number of unresolved issues should be viewed as a challenge rather than as defeat. Two interrelated issues are therapeutic success and the independence of theory, research, and therapy for stuttering. Still the biggest challenge to our profession is the poor record of success in therapy with adult stutterers. In fact, the ultimate validating criterion of the diverse theories and research programs presented here will be a therapeutic success rate that approximates 100%. The very reason for the existence of the profession of speech pathology is the clinical service we provide. Even basic speech science as studied in our various institutions is an outgrowth of speech pathology, without which it could as easily be housed in psychological, physiological, acoustic, or engineering laboratories. The ultimate focus of theory, research, and training must keep in the forefront our major professional function: successfully treating people with communication disorders. Not only are we not getting outstanding results in therapy with adult stutterers, but much of the theory and research in this field has only limited application to problems of therapy. An example of this issue is the recent resurgence of interest and research in the alleged genetic basis of stuttering. There appears to be no feasible clinical application aside from the questionable role of genetic counseling. This is not to say that such research is unimportant but rather that it does not address our primary professional concern.

When we examine, on an individual basis, those factors that appear to influence the success of any therapy, we find that outcome is a function of a number of researchable variables of unquestionable relevance. Such issues as the client's age, motivation, coping and defense mechanisms, history of therapy, family support, and stress in the environment must be taken into account as well as the more obvious variables related to the therapeutic program. Judicious case selection and how you define criteria for success can result in enthusiastic reports of outcome independently of what happens to the stutterer.

To summarize what we have just discussed, there is a need to sharpen our focus on therapy by resolving a number of relevant issues. Our record of therapeutic success with adult stutterers is poor; much of our theory and research is not directed toward improving that record; there is little uniformity among clinicians with regard to reporting criteria for case selection or outcome.

Diversity of opinion is a fact in the area of stuttering, as evidenced by the contributors to this volume. This diversity can mean that we have more than one answer to the problem of stuttering, or that we have no answer as yet to that problem. In the event of the first interpretation, the diversity may lie primarily in the varied populations of stutterers, each amenable to a different treatment approach. In the event of the second interpretation we may have an explanation for the strong challenge that the problem of stuttering poses for so many speech pathologists. We seem to need to find answers for long standing troublesome questions, and are joined in this need by stutterers themselves and the people who know them, who are quick to respond to any report in the popular media about anything new or different in treatment. The fact that the combination of enthusiasm and novelty works for at least a short while for almost everyone compounds the diversity in our field and diverts some of us from more thorough-going data gathering and analysis. It also diverts many stutterers from the long term commitment that is probably essential for therapeutic success.

Most therapies have a history of some success and of some failure. Most therapies resemble one another in certain ways in spite of differences in the theoretical perspective. A historical example of this comes from the 1940s when voluntary stuttering was the therapy of popular choice, but was explained by different theorists through the principles of negative practice, anti-avoidance, cancellation, anxiety reduction, shifting from thalamic to cortical control, or fluent stuttering. The chapter in this volume by Sheehan, which explicates the Suppression Hypothesis, is a more current justification for the tactic of voluntary stuttering. Each of these rationales was presented for the very same therapeutic tactic.

When we look at current therapeutic procedures we may also be able to identify some processes that are generic to successful outcome. Either by accident or by design, at some point in the therapy, either with awareness or without it, for longer or for shorter periods, stutterers slow their speech. When the rate of talking becomes the main focus of therapy it is usually described as "rate control," although the process can be observed in other therapies where it has been not so identified. Another generic component of most current therapies is monitoring some feature of speaking. Monitoring refers to awareness, but in therapy for stuttering also includes the deliberate emission of a particular predesignated speech behavior. Some of the features so addressed are rate, breath-stream management, phonation, prosody, and deliberate stuttering. A third generic process in therapy is the elimination of avoidance behaviors at both the situational and speech levels.

In addition to these behavioral aspects of speech, many current therapies further address the cognitive issues of self-responsibility, helplessness versus control, and degree of conviction. However, these attitudinal factors do not seem to be as universal as the behavioral ones that may suggest that the first three components are more critical to successful therapy, while the latter three components may be essential for some stutterers but not all.

Similar to the attitudinal variables in therapy for stuttering are a number of deeper psychological issues not unique to stutterers, and not necessarily critical for all stutterers, which are addressed in some current therapies. These include components of the therapeutic relationship such as trust, caring and support, attention to feelings, and the psychodynamics of the problem, including the individual etiology, current maintaining factors, and how the stutterer copes with and adapts to his problem.

One example is understanding what impact changing the way he talks can have upon the stutterer's basic psychological makeup. Change works in two directions, however, and some clinicians feel that since the stutterer's psychological makeup influences the extent and rate of change of behavior, we must address the stutterer's personality as part of the therapeutic process. As another example, it may be necessary to distinguish between psychosocial withdrawal for reasons other than speech and self-imposed isolation because someone stutters. What is our role, and how far do we go in attempting to increase a client's socialization whose history and style of interacting suggests a very different disposition?

Each of these three classes of variables, with their varying degrees of utilization and effect on outcome, need to be explored in therapeutic research. We should go beyond judging the effectiveness of therapy solely on the basis of how the initial change in speech was accomplished, to include the stability of that change over time as well as attitudinal change during the process of therapy.

As we continue to review unresolved issues in therapy for stuttering, we can identify at least five variables that relate to process rather than the content. One of the most practical issues in any therapeutic regime is the determination of an optimal schedule for seeing a client. It would seem that such an obvious issue would have been resolved experimentally a long time ago. However, it would be necessary to hold all other therapeutic variables constant. Some of these variables are: sequencing and tactics of the program; use of the same clinician; use of the same criteria for progression; use of the same assessment procedures, including when and how such assessments are made; and the client's psychological as well as physical availability. Can we hold all of these variables constant, manipulating only the schedule of attendance? In spite of the difficulties in designing such clinical experimentation, it should be done.

A second process variable in therapy is determining the function and the effects of early dramatic change, the sudden reduction in stuttering, and the accompanying euphoria. This effect is occasionally associated with unexplained fluency outside of therapy, sometimes labeled as "false fluency." Some explanations for this phenomenon are: the stutterer has a need for the process to seem easier and simpler than, in fact, it will be; he is adapting to and becoming more comfortable with the process of therapy; a "honeymoon effect" results from the relationship with a new clinician, from belief in the therapy and from the feelings that he is finally doing something about his problem, and successfully; and the feeling of confidence that comes from being in control of one's behavior. Everything we have been talking about here is very positive. Why then do we see this as an unresolved issue? For one thing the stutterer may consider his fluency to be permanent; for another, the windfall of unearned fluency can deter him from working on his problem. Such episodes of fluency reinforce the stutterer's conviction that in some mystical way stuttering happens to him, and he is not directly responsible for it. The sudden increase in fluency, in light of a long history of stuttering, can also raise serious questions in the mind of the stutterer about his prior investment of time and energy, and how he has permitted his stuttering to have such an impact on him. The initial euphoria can lead to eventual doubts about the value and adequacy of the new therapy. Some of the tactics introduced to resolve the problem of early dramatic change are immediate monitoring, voluntary stuttering, and counseling, but it should be dealt with in some fashion. Having described this early fluency as temporary, we must necessarily next deal with the regression that inevitably follows, and which may characterize therapy in general as an uneven process. The stutterer's fluency is only one issue of many. Different therapies organize different experiences for the stutterer, to which each stutterer reacts in different ways. At times the stutterer moves forward easily; at times he resists; at times he moves backward. Each of these different experiences may generate different reactions, not all of which are conducive to the forward flow of therapy. For example, release of anxiety and reluctance to take responsibility may cause regression, while social reinforcement and the feeling of being in control may move the client forward. The issue of early dramatic change and the unevenness of therapy may be reduced to the question of advising the client in advance. Such forewarning can have both negative and positive effects. On the negative side, not all clients experience a sudden increase in fluency; such forewarning can be discouraging; expecting regression can lead the client to fulfilling the prophecy of the clinician. On the positive side, forewarning can provide an understanding and an emotional acceptance of what might otherwise be a devastating experience; the tactics involved in preparing the client for handling adversity can be useful to him outside of the clinical context; and finally, for some clinicians the issue becomes an ethical one of sharing with the client what they are likely to experience during the therapeutic process.

The third class of process variables deals with carry-over or transfer. These two terms refer to the use of behaviors and attitudes relevant to those behaviors, outside the clinical context in which they were originally established. Unresolved issues here involve the relative responsibilities of the client and the clinician in the process of carry-over; the formal or systematic structure of carry-over versus the casual or unsystematic structure; when to begin the process; the role of the family and other members of the immediate environment participating in that carry-over structure; whether or not to attempt to attenuate stress in that environment; the use of information from other kinds of therapies, such as weight control, smoking reduction, and substance abuse, relative to self-management versus external controls; the schedule and nature of contact between the client and clinician during the process of carry-over; and finally, determining the criteria for the termination of formal therapy, including the attainment of previously agreed-upon goals. That aspect of therapy that we call carry-over remains the biggest hurdle and the single most important unresolved issue in the clinical management of stuttering. When comparing the clinical effectiveness of different therapeutic strategies the process of carry-over merits as much scrutiny as the establishment of fluency or any other aspect of therapy.

The fourth process variable is relapse, the reappearance of the original or substitute behaviors and attitudes after therapy has been successfully terminated. The unresolved issues relative to deciding whether or not a relapse has occurred are the frequency of the behaviors in question and the time intervals between the appearance of these behaviors. Having determined that relapse has occurred, we are still faced with the unresolved issue of what to do about it, whether to recommence formal therapy, and, if so, at what stage in the process.

The last process variable we wish to discuss is the measurement of speech behaviors. We see this issue as second in importance only to that of carry-over and transfer. Measurement is important to research, to clinical diagnosis, and to the assessment of therapeutic effectiveness both within and across programs. Unresolved issues here include what to measure, how valid and reliable those measures are, how representative they are, and whether to include covert measures in addition to the overt. A specific example of the problem of what to measure is stuttering versus fluency. The former behavior is easier to define and to measure but leaves us with a target behavior that is undefined except as the absence of stuttering. That the problem of assessing fluency is not simply a semantic one is evidenced by questions such as the naturalness or normal-soundingness of the client's speech as judged by impartial observers. Some of the components of speech such as rate and pause time are more easily measured than others and relate to the global judgment of fluency as do more confounding instances of normal disfluency such as interjections and whole-word and phrase repetitions. In other words, can we determine from the nonstuttered speech of an individual whether that person is a stutterer or a normal speaker? This determination must also enter into the assessment of the effectiveness of therapy programs and generally in the description of the stutterer's speech.

Thus far we have discussed unresolved issues that focus on variables that deal with the content of therapies on the one hand and with the processes of therapy on the other. At this point let us examine some of the population variables that theorists in the area of stuttering have been struggling with for half a century. Two questions that these variables can help us to answer are: whether stutterers differ from normal speakers in the first place, and whether stutterers differ from one another in ways so significant that we may have to arrange for different goals and management strategies for each group. The first question is most important at the time of early diagnosis, when we attempt to distinguish between developmentally disfluent children and incipient stutterers. The second question becomes important after the decision has been made that we are dealing with a stutterer, when we either attempt to select a therapeutic program that is most appropriate to a particular stutterer or, after unsuccessful treatment, to find an alternative program. Ideally, we should be able to select strategies to preclude therapeutic failure, rather than use that failure as the basis for matching a client to a particular program.

One population variable that may help us answer the first question relative to whether stutterers differ from normal speakers is the reported spontaneous recovery of fluency without professional intervention. Some studies have indicated as many as 80% of normal-speaking individuals questioned report having stuttered at some time or other in their lives, but have never had therapy. (Andrews & Harris, 1964) Are these people different in some ways from those who stuttered but did not recover, and from those who were developmentally disfluent and never identified as having stuttered? We know far too little about the phenomenon of spontaneous recovery. Too much of the relevant information has come from anecdotal report. We would like to be able to use spontaneous recovery prognostically, and we would like to observe it directly and to determine correlates such as family history and home environment. Similar to spontaneous recovery is the episodic nature of both developmental disfluency and later stuttering, where periods of fluent speech lasting for weeks or months appear unpredictably against a background of disfluency. Both of these phenomena are characterized by long intervals of fluency during which the stutterer experiences feelings of well-being and a sense that his speech problems are over. The major difference between the two seems to be the apparently unpredictable reappearance of stuttering in the case of episodic disfluency.

Similar in its unpredictability is the nature of stuttered speech in general, insofar as specific discriminative and reinforcing stimuli have not been identified, at least outside of the laboratory. The experience for the stutterer is one of confusion and apparent randomness of the occurrence of stuttering, which leads him to feel helpless and victimized. We must keep in mind that the majority of the time stutterers speak without stuttering, and it is against the backdrop of fluency that we should attempt to study those variables that correlate with specific moments of stuttering. Some of these variables that have been identified prospectively in the literature are: the various levels of conflict proposed by Sheehan; excitement levels and state of affect as suggested by Travis; expectation on the part of the stutterer, based on his history with specific sounds and words; anxiety reactions triggered by abrupt change as well as by certain discriminative stimuli, as contained in the theories of both Wolpe and Brutten; and the progressive build-up of fear and of the expectation to stutter that accompanies periods of fluency. The study of these variables in relation to the moment of stuttering may well render what appears to be random a more understandable and systematic phenomenon.

The third population variable we want to consider, age, relates interestingly to the issues of spontaneous recovery and the episodic nature of early stuttering, both of which seem to characterize the young stutterer rather than the adult. Bloodstein has often said that stuttering is a disorder of childhood. The apparent basis for this observation is that stuttering is much more common in children than in adults. A more subtle and interesting implication of that statement, however, is that stuttering is a childlike or regressive behavior. We have observed earlier that the therapeutic success record is enviably better with children and best with preschoolers. The same cannot be said of adult stutterers. Do those children who recover spontaneously or who respond successfully to treatment differ from those who grow up continuing to stutter? Another way of framing this question is to inquire whether the longer history of stuttering is a sufficient explanation of the differences we observe, or whether some children who stutter are in fact qualitatively different from those who respond well to treatment or who recover spontaneously.

Perhaps the most puzzling population variable is the significantly greater number of male than of female stutterers. This unexplained fact has stimulated hypotheses ranging from genetic and neurophysiological explorations through psycho-developmental and socio-cultural ones. Interestingly, to date none of these investigations has proven conclusive.

Apparently related to the uneven sex ratio among stutterers is the observation that stuttering seems to run in families. Geneticists have been exploring this issue with results as yet as unsatisfying as the investigations into the sex ratio.

In spite of the lack of conclusive data there appears to be strong feeling among speech pathologists, as represented in this volume, that at least for some stutterers there is a genetic basis for the disorder. Familial incidence does not necessarily prove a genetic argument and, in fact, can be as useful in supporting alternative arguments, but until geneticists determine chromosomal differences between stutterers and nonstutterers, incidence is the only form of relevant data directly available. For this eminently pragmatic reason familial incidence has been cited in support of such diverse research perspectives as cultural, semantic, and anthropological, as well as genetic.

This volume represents an anthology of diverse thought and practice in the area of stuttering in which the contributors were asked to re-examine significant contributions to the literature they made years ago. What is clear is that we have become more demanding of both ourselves and of each other insofar as we expect our research and our therapy to yield a firm data base. We are no longer in a circumstance where one philosophy carries the burden and the responsibility for the profession, serving as a model for the rest of us. We should acknowledge the pioneering role of Van Riper in developing an elaborate and descriptive program of therapy for working with adult stutterers. It was that very systematic organization that made his program attractive to the rest of the profession. Today we have a number of similarly well thought-out and highly structured programs available to us, some of them described herein. Not only is detailed descriptiveness appealing, but it also enables us to replicate programs and evaluate them, and to train student clinicians to deliver responsible service to larger numbers of stutterers. The very specificity and descriptiveness of these programs, which is a part of the heritage from Van Riper and of the behavioral movement, creates an openness of the therapeutic process that facilitates comparisons of outcome.

There is one qualification of programmatic therapy that we should consider here. While perhaps not so intended by the originator of a therapeutic program, a sequence of management strategies may be viewed by some practitioners as unalterable, when, in fact, they were designed to be skeletal outlines that permit more spontaneous interactions or branching from the original sequence, based on the stutterer's reaction to therapy. Such spontaneity and freedom to diverge from protocol underscores the human element in clinical interaction. We are working with people who stutter.

Individual differences suggest one kind of variability. That we may be dealing with more than one kind of stutterer, however, is strongly suggested by the differences in theory of causation, by the fact of spontaneous recovery, by differences in the effectiveness of therapeutic strategies, and by the rate of relapse associated with different therapies. Our challenge is to study and to understand these differences, not with a view to arriving at a single explanation or therapeutic strategy, but to further identify these differences in order to better match each client to that therapy that will most effectively deal with his needs. In order to accomplish this goal our study must be organized into a system that integrates information among the activities of highly controlled laboratory research, clinical and field studies, and therapeutic practice.

REFERENCES

Andrews, G., & Harris, M. (1964). The syndrome of stuttering. London: Heinemann.

Bloodstein, O. (1958). Stuttering as an anticipatory struggle reaction. In J. Eisenson (Ed.), *Stuttering: A symposium.* New York: Harper.

Bloodstein, O. (1960). The development of stuttering: I.   Changes in nine basic features. *Journal of Speech and Hearing Disabilities, 25,* 219–237.

Bloodstein, O. (1961). The development of stuttering: III.   Theoretical and clinical implications. *Journal of Speech and Hearing Disabilities, 26,* 67–82.

Curlee, R., & Perkins, W. H. (1969). Conversation rate control therapy for stuttering. *Journal of Speech and Hearing Disabilities, 34,* 245–250.

Perkins, W. H. (1973). Replacement of stuttering with normal speech: I. Rationale. *Journal of Speech and Hearing Disabilities, 38,* 283–294.

Rubin, H., & Culatta, R. (1971). A point of view about fluency. *American Speech and Hearing Association, 13,* 380–384.

Shames, G., & Egolf, D. (1971). *Experimental therapy for school age children and their parents.* USOE Final Report, Project No. 482130, Grant No. OEG-0-8-080080-3525. Washington, DC: Department of Health, Education, and Welfare.

Shames, G., Egolf, D., & Rhodes, R. (1969). Experimental programs in stuttering therapy. *Journal of Speech and Hearing Disabilities, 34,* 30–47.

Siegel, G. (1970). Punishment, stuttering and disfluency. *Journal of Speech and Hearing Research, 13,* 677–714.

Webster, R. (1980). Evolution of a target based behavioral therapy for stuttering. *Journal of Fluency Disorders, 5,* 303–320.

Williams, D. (1957). A point of view about stuttering. *Journal of Speech and Hearing Research, 22,* 390–397.

Wingate, M. (1959). Calling attention to stuttering. *Journal of Speech and Hearing Research, 26,* 326–335.

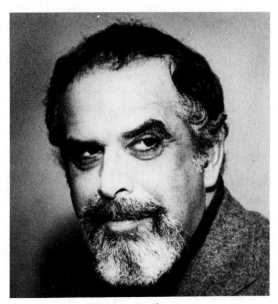

George H. Shames

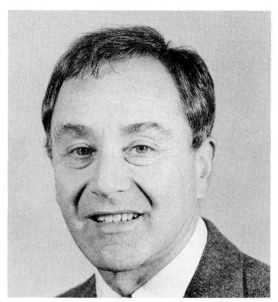

Herbert Rubin

George H. Shames, Ph.D., is Professor of Psychology and Communication Disorders at the University of Pittsburgh. He is the Coordinator of the Division of Communication Disorders. Dr. Shames is a Fellow of the American Speech-Language-Hearing Association and holds the Certificate of Clinical Competence in Speech. In addition, he is a licensed psychologist in the Commonwealth of Pennsylvania. He is also licensed in Speech Pathology in North Carolina and Florida. He is the author of numerous articles in the periodical literature and of two books: *Operant conditioning and the management of stuttering* and *Stutter-free speech—a goal for therapy.* He is also the Senior Co-Editor, with Elizabeth Wiig, of a new introductory text on speech pathology: *Human communication disorders—an introduction.*

Dr. Shames has been a guest lecturer, visiting faculty member, and workshop leader at universities, colleges, hospitals, international meetings, and public school programs in the United States, Great Britain, Canada, Australia, Israel, and Mexico. He also directs intensive, residential summer camps for stutterers throughout the country.

Herbert Rubin, Ph.D., is Professor of Communication Disorders at the University of Pittsburgh, where he also serves as Associate Dean of the Graduate School of Arts and Sciences. A Fellow of the American Speech-Language-Hearing Association, he holds a Certificate of Clinical Competence in Speech and has been an Education and Training Board Site Visitor since 1975. Dr. Rubin has been a consultant for Educational Testing Service, Pittsburgh Public Schools, Western Pennsylvania School for the Deaf, Pittsburgh Veterans Administration Hospitals, Pittsburgh Hearing and Speech Society, and a member of the Legislative Council of ASHA.

Dr. Rubin has taught numerous graduate and undergraduate courses, including theories of Language Development, Verbal Behavior, Cybernetics, Voice and Diction, and the Psychology of Speech. He has also conducted graduate seminars in Aphasia, Stuttering, Voice Disorders, Family Counseling, and Self-Communication.

Dr. Rubin has contributed a number of journal articles on stuttering, speech, and audibility to the professional literature. He is also the author of chapters in *Symposium on the perception of language, Communication disorders related to cleft lip* (with George H. Shames), and *Principles of pediatrics: Health care of the young.*

Name Index

Abbott, J. A., 191, 263, 469, 476
Abramovitz, A., 345
Adams, M. R., 26, 27, 39, 62, 73, 76, 77, 79, 80, 87, 160, 162, 165, 172, 174, 175, 483, 502, 505, 508
Agnello, J. G., 165, 174
Ainsworth, S., 283
Alfonso, P. J., 62
Allen, E., 227
Allen, G. D., 62
Anderson, B. F., 178
Anderson, L. O., 49, 54
Andrews, Gavin, 17, 61, 62, 86, 167, 174, 175, 177, 347, 353, 354, 489, 490, 492, 494, 496, 498, 499, 503, 510, 526
Appel, J. B., 225
Atkinson, G. J., 223
Azrin, Nathan H., 175, 203, 212, 213, 217, 219, 220, 224, 225, 228, 230, 355, 356, 357, 520

Baer, D. M., 221, 224, 227
Bandura, A., 285
Barbara, D. A., 482
Barber, V. B., 353
Baruch, D., 100
Bass, C., 392, 496
Bell, Jody, 73, 87
Berlin, L., 15
Berndt, L. A., 228
Berry, M. F., 58
Biggs, B. E., 203, 221, 222
Bijou, S. W., 221
Bilger, R. C., 223
Birns, B., 158
Blanchard, E., 31, 42
Blanton, M. G., 188
Blanton, S., 188
Bloodstein, Oliver N., 6, 10, 11, 27, 32, 35, 36, 61, 81, 124, 130, 134, 162, 168, 186, 190, 191, 204, 223, 241, 276, 380, 381, 407, 483, 489, 497, 501, 502, 520, 527
Bluemel, C. S., 35, 125, 131, 136, 188
Boberg, Einer, 10, 17, 40, 173, 175, 270,

488, 489, 494, 495, 496, 501, 502, 505, 506, 508, 518, 521, 522
Boren, M. C. P., 223
Boudreau, L. A., 358
Bower, G., 95
Brady, J. P., 353, 354, 355, 357
Brenner, N., 76, 80
Bridger, W. H., 158
Broad, D., 74
Brookshire, R., 25
Brown, S., 34, 87
Brown, S. F., 192, 193
Brutten, Gene J., 36, 40, 41, 42, 142, 143, 155, 156, 157, 158, 159, 160, 161, 162, 163, 164, 166, 168, 169, 172, 173, 176, 186, 252, 253, 336, 350, 352, 353, 458, 519, 527
Bryant, A. F., 58
Bryngelson, Bryng, 8, 9, 14, 58, 92, 187, 195, 196, 248, 381
Burgi, Ernest J., 15
Burns, D., 353

Cady, B., 223
Carrier, Joe, 454
Case, H. M., 193, 196
Cherry, C., 352
Clark, T. B., 58
Cohen, 496
Colburn, N., 34
Colombat de l'Isere, M., 353
Cooper, E. B., 176, 223, 224, 277, 279, 281, 386, 489, 498
Cooper, M. H., 62
Cortese, P., 202
Costello, J. M., 163, 228, 432, 435, 440, 489, 496, 502
Costley, M., 498
Cousins, Norman, 262
Cowan, D. W., 193
Cox, N. J., 63
Craig, A., 503
Cross, D. E., 62, 165
Culatta, Richard, 467, 474, 475, 476, 478, 520

Culbertson, S. A., 217, 223, 229
Cullinan, W. L., 165
Curlee, R. F., 76, 78, 175, 417, 418, 422, 456, 483, 489, 520
Curry, F. K. W., 61
Cutler, J., 174

Dalton, P., 489, 490, 496
Daly, D. A., 223, 224, 492, 493, 496
Daniloff, R., 74
Darley, F., 34, 35
Darnton, P., 492, 493, 496
Davis, Dorothy M., 125, 128, 129, 238, 239
Decker, T. N., 62
Denhardt, 133
DiGusto, J., 496
Dollard, J., 99, 100, 103, 186, 187, 188, 190, 194, 197
Doob, L., 103
Draper, M., 76
Dunlap, Knight, 33, 188, 191, 193, 196, 202

Edmonds, R. M., 458
Egland, George O., 125
Egolf, Don B., 26, 170, 228, 273, 276, 278, 285, 417, 454, 455, 467, 489, 490, 521
Eisenson, J., 190
Emerick, L. L., 281
England, G., 350
Epstein, L., 42
Everson, Richard, 15
Eveslage, R. E., 25
Eysenck, Hans J., 52, 349, 353

Felty, 221, 223
Fenichel, O., 187, 191, 192, 197
Ferster, C. B., 217, 218, 219, 220, 221, 223, 224, 226, 227, 229
Fishman, H. C., 193
Fitzsimons, R. M., 275, 281
Flanagan, Bruce C., 27, 42, 203, 212, 213, 217, 222, 224, 251, 520, 521
Fletcher, J. M., 49, 53, 54, 57, 188, 191,

Fletcher, J.M., *continued*
    197
Florance, Cheri L., 43, 174, 281, 387, 392,
    447, 448, 455, 456, 502, 505
Floyd, S., 168
Font, M. M., 54
Frank, J., 94
Frantz, S. E., 175
Fraser, Malcolm, 381
Frayne, H., 495
Freeman, F. J., 62, 76
Freud, Anna, 470
Freud, Sigmund, 13, 50, 51, 56, 189, 194
Freund, H., 133
Frick, J. V., 190, 219
Froeschels, Emil, 35, 125, 130, 131, 133,
    188, 189
Fromm-Reichman, 449
Fuller, J. L., 60

Garside, R. F., 62
Gendlin, E. T., 317, 318, 319
Gilbert, H. H., 165
Ginott, H. G., 283, 455
Gladstein, K. L., 63
Glasner, H. G., 275, 276
Glasner, P., 35
Glauber, I. P., 187, 188, 482
Glauber, P., 34
Goldberg, S., 506
Goldiamond, Israel, 203, 212, 213, 217,
    222, 223, 224, 229, 237, 245, 246, 263,
    346, 348, 352, 398, 417, 418, 422, 467,
    469, 470, 520
Goldman-Eisler, F., 33
Goodglass, H., 61
Goodstein, L. D., 470
Gould, E., 202, 203
Gray, B. B., 350
Gray, M., 58, 59, 60, 61
Gregory, Hugo H., 26, 61, 272, 273, 277,
    278, 279, 280, 281, 283, 284, 285, 287,
    391, 407, 483, 490, 502, 521
Gronhovd, K. D., 170, 175
Grusec, J. E., 225
Gruss, J., 283
Guitar, B., 42, 383, 392, 492, 496, 498

Hadley, R., 202, 203
Hake, D., 225
Haley, J., 94
Hall, J. W., 62
Halle, M., 49
Halvorson, J., 25
Hand, C. R., 165
Hanna R., 496
Haroldson, S. K., 160, 221, 228, 417, 432,
    507
Harris, B., 52
Harris, F., 227
Harris, M., 62, 347, 354, 498, 526
Hasbrouck, J., 221
Hayden, P., 76, 79, 160
Haynes, S. N., 160
Haynes, W. O., 62, 508
Heath, 319
Hebenstreit, M. B., 54
Hegde, M. N., 168, 172
Hege, Keith, 402
Hersen, M., 31
Hilgard, E. R., 95

Hill, D., 26, 277, 279, 283, 284, 287, 483,
    502
Hill, H. E., 57, 165, 188, 195
Hillman, R. E., 165
Hirschman, P., 160
Hixon, T., 74, 76
Holgate, D., 494, 496
Holland, J. G., 219, 229
Holz, W. C., 224, 225, 228, 230
Hood, S. B., 278, 281
Horowitz, E., 190
Howie, Pauline M., 173, 489, 492, 495,
    496, 497, 498, 503, 504, 506, 509
Hudgins, C., 74
Hull, C. J., 16, 33, 57
Hull, Clark L., 54, 132
Hurst, M. R., 163
Hutchinson, R., 226

Ingham, R. J., 80, 175, 177, 489, 490, 492,
    494, 495, 496, 499, 502, 504, 505, 507
Inness, M., 193
Isserlin, 133
Ivey, A., 449

Jacobson, Edmund, 345
Jaeger, W., 134
James, J. E., 228
Janssen, P., 162, 163, 175
Jastrow, Joseph, 54
Jeffrey, C. J., 358
Jerger, J., 62
Johnson, Linda, 26, 27, 73, 87, 284
Johnson, Wendell O., 6, 8, 11, 13, 14, 23,
    25, 27, 34, 35, 36, 37, 38, 39, 40, 48,
    54, 55, 56, 57, 58, 61, 87, 92, 119, 124,
    125, 130, 131, 132, 133, 134, 135, 136,
    137, 138, 158, 162, 168, 187, 188, 189,
    190, 193, 194, 195, 196, 219, 241, 248,
    249, 264, 273, 274, 380, 381, 455, 468,
    469, 474, 483, 520
Johnston, J. M., 217
Johnston, M., 227
Jost, H., 158

Kamhi, A., 502, 506
Kanfer, F. H., 160, 246, 450, 457
Kann, Mary Jo, 481
Karoly, P., 450, 457
Kasprisin, Arlene, 278, 454
Kasprisin-Burrelli, Arlene, 26, 278, 454
Katkin, 252
Kay, D. W. K., 62
Kent, L., 468
Kent, Ray, 87
Kidd, J. R., 158
Kidd, Kenneth K., 61, 63, 158, 498
Kimble, G. A., 163, 170, 177
Kimbarow, M. L., 223, 224
Kimmel, H. D., 252
Knott, J. R., 55, 56, 57, 61, 119, 187, 190,
    193
Korzybski, A., 6, 9, 10, 11, 131
Kraaimaat, F., 162, 163
Kraepelin, 133
Krasner, L., 246
Krych, D., 172
Kuhl, P., 80, 228, 432
Kully, D., 505
Kurtzke, J. F., 15

LaCroiz, Z., 496
Ladefoged, P., 76
Lang, P. J., 336, 345
Lanyon, R., 336, 458, 499
Lazarus, A. A., 336, 345
Lazovik, A. D., 336, 345
Leach, E., 172, 417
Lemert, 277
Lenneberg, E., 74
Leutenegger, R. R., 54, 55
Levy, David, 197
Lewin, K., 187, 189
Liebert, R. M., 166
Lindsley, O. R., 219
Lingwall, J. B., 223
Long, K. M., 165
Lubker, Bobby Boyd, 398
Luper, Harold L., 62, 165, 270, 274, 280,
    362, 380, 388, 391, 521
Lussenhop, A. J., 61

MacNeilage, P. F., 61
Mair, J. M. M., 353
Makuen, G. H., 58
Malamud, W., 55
Mallard, A. R., 165, 175
Malmo, R. B., 164
Martin, R. R., 80, 160, 221, 222, 223, 224,
    228, 263, 417, 432, 467, 506, 507
Martyn, M. M., 203, 498
Masters, J. C., 169
Matthews, Jack, 4, 5, 15, 17, 518
Meader, Clarence, 6
Mecs, H. L., 227
Meissner, J. H., 193
Meyer, L. A., 175
Meyer, V., 353
Meyer, W. H., 165
Michael, J., 224
Migler, B., 346, 348
Milisen, R., 192
Miller, G., 74
Miller, M., 491
Miller, Neal E., 99, 100, 103, 132, 186,
    187, 188, 189, 190, 194, 197, 252
Moeller, D., 54, 56
Moncur, J., 116
Moore, P., 76
Moore, W. H., Jr., 62, 508
Mordecai, D., 278
Morgan, J. J. B., 52
Morgenstein, 277
Mowrer, D. E., 418, 435, 440, 489, 490,
    496, 499
Mowrer, O. H., 192
Mulder, R. L., 274, 280, 391
Mundy, M. B., 36, 417, 420, 422
Murphy, A., 275, 281
Murray, 252
Muyskens, John, 6, 7, 8, 10, 13
Myers, N., 165
Mysak, E., 34

Neale, J. M., 166
Neaves, R., 498
Nelson, L., 284
Nelson, S., 58
Netsell, R., 76
Nunn, R. G., 175, 355, 356, 357
Nye, R. D., 230

Oehlert, G.,
Orton, Samuel T., 9, 55, 117, 118
Owen, N., 496

Packman, A. C., 175, 495
Paul, Gordon L., 345, 348, 349
Pavlov, 143
Pennypacker, H. S., 217
Perkins, William H., 7, 8, 26, 27, 72, 73,
    74, 76, 78, 82, 87, 121, 168, 170, 174,
    175, 179, 391, 417, 418, 422, 456, 489,
    493, 495, 496, 499, 502, 508, 519, 520
Perls, 319
Perozzi, Joseph A., 64
Peters, T. J., 383, 392
Phillips, J. S., 160
Piehler, Margaret F., 481
Pillsbury, Walter, 6
Pisoni, S., 246
Porter, H. K., 190
Premack, David, 450, 453, 457
Pressman, J., 74
Prins, D., 491, 496, 499

Quist, R. W., 223

Rayner, R., 52
Records, M. A., 158
Reed, C. J., 223
Reich, A., 62
Reis, R., 62, 76, 77, 160
Reynolds, D. J., 345
Rhodes, Robert C., 417, 454, 455, 467,
    521
Rice, L. N., 317, 318, 319
Rickard, H. C., 36, 417, 420, 422
Riley, G., 283
Riley, J., 283
Rimm, D. C., 169
Risley, T. R., 227
Robbins, J., 223
Robbins, S. D., 49
Rogers, Carl R., 14, 264, 281, 294, 295,
    316, 317, 319, 320, 449, 468, 521
Rosenfield, D. B., 61
Rubin, Herbert, 23, 261, 467, 474, 517,
    520, 521
Rudas, Joanna, 73
Runyan, C. M., 165, 175, 505
Rupp, R. R., 62
Russell, G. Oscar, 10, 11
Rustin, L., 277, 431, 441
Ryan, Bruce P., 16, 43, 172, 264, 376, 391,
    416, 417, 431, 432, 433, 434, 435, 436,
    437, 438, 439, 440, 441, 489, 491, 492,
    493, 496, 521
Ryan, Barbara Van Kirk, 431, 432, 434,
    441

Salter, 336
Salzinger, K., 246
Sapon, S. M., 219
Sargent, W., 51
Savoye, A., 165
Sawyer, L., 494, 495, 496, 502, 506
Sayers, B., 352
Sayles, D. G., 62
Schaef, Robert, 17

Schoonover, Reggie, 402
Schwartz, D., 177
Schwartz, M., 80, 355, 357
Sears, R., 103
Seashore, Carl E., 117
Seeman, Julius, 294, 316, 521
Seider, R. A., 63
Seligman, M. E. P., 52
Seltzer, H., 228
Shames, George H., 23, 27, 31, 33, 36, 40,
    41, 43, 133, 158, 170, 174, 228, 229,
    237, 248, 251, 252, 261, 268, 273, 276,
    278, 281, 285, 376, 387, 391, 392, 417,
    447, 448, 454, 455, 467, 469, 480, 482,
    489, 490, 502, 505, 517, 519, 521
Shapiro, A. J., 62
Shaw, C., 36
Shaw, C. K., 172
Sheehan, Joseph G., 27, 32, 40, 41, 132,
    186, 187, 201, 202, 203, 204, 207, 208,
    209, 221, 222, 264, 275, 276, 278, 281,
    391, 470, 498, 505, 506, 519, 523, 527
Sheehan, Vivian M., 186, 201, 204
Sherrick, Carl E., Jr., 33, 36, 133, 158, 237,
    248, 251, 252, 278, 454, 469
Shine, R., 432, 435, 437, 440, 441, 502
Shoemaker, D. J., 36, 42, 142, 155, 156,
    158, 159, 161, 162, 163, 164, 166, 169,
    172, 252, 253, 350, 352, 353
Shrum, W. F., 36, 172
Shulman, E., 193
Sidman, M., 217, 222
Siegel, G. M., 42, 158, 223, 224, 251, 263,
    520
Skinner, B. F., 16, 133, 217, 218, 220, 221,
    223, 224, 225, 227, 229, 230, 237, 238,
    239, 245, 252, 253, 432
Soderberg, G., 76
Solomon, M., 188
Solomon, R. L., 225
Sontag, L. W., 158
Sortini, A. J., 49, 50
Spence, Kenneth, 16, 54
Spriestersbach, D. C., 34
Springer, M. T., 165
St. Louis, K., 221
Starkweather, C., 172
Starkweather, C. F., 174
Starkweather, C. W., 160, 165, 392
Starr, C. D., 228, 417
Stassi, E. J., 165
Steer, M. D., 56, 125
Stetson, R., 74
Stewart, 277
Stocks, J., 87
Stromsta, C., 62
Strupp, H., 449
Sullivan, Harry Stack, 13, 100
Sussman, H. M., 61

Tannenbaum, R. S., 160
Tanner, S., 357, 492, 495
Taylor, I., 61
Ten Cate, M. J., 49
Thompson, W. R., 60
Thorndike, E. L., 226
Tompkins, E., 133
Toscher, M. M., 62
Travis, Lee Edward, 8, 9, 27, 32, 49, 54,

55, 56, 73, 92, 93, 100, 117, 131, 132,
    187, 191, 192, 193, 194, 195, 196, 248,
    263, 264, 477, 520, 527
Tureen, J., 134
Tuttle, W. W., 193

Ulrich, R. E., 226
Ushijima, T., 62, 76

Van Houten, R., 224, 230
Van Kirk, Barbara, 43, 416, 431, 432, 433,
    434, 435, 436, 437, 438, 439, 441, 491,
    496
Van Riper, Charles, 8, 13, 14, 34, 35, 43,
    57, 73, 77, 92, 119, 125, 136, 155, 158,
    159, 160, 165, 174, 175, 187, 188, 189,
    190, 191, 192, 193, 194, 195, 196, 219,
    223, 229, 248, 249, 270, 273, 274, 281,
    285, 362, 363, 367, 373, 380, 381, 382,
    383, 384, 385, 386, 387, 388, 389, 390,
    391, 392, 393, 397, 407, 420, 455, 521,
    528
Vermilyea, F., 35
Viek, P., 192
Voas, Robert B., 193, 202

Wahler, R., 276
Waters, G. C., 225
Watson, B. C., 62
Watson, John B., 50, 51, 52, 54
Webb, W. B., 224
Webster, L. M., 172, 177
Webster, Ronald L., 174, 177, 229, 383,
    386, 391, 396, 397, 399, 402, 405, 407,
    408, 432, 435, 492, 496, 502, 506, 520,
    521
Wells, C., 190
Wendell, M., 174
Wepman, J. M., 58
West, Robert, 8, 58, 131, 135
Wexler, D. A., 317, 318
Whitteridge, D., 76
Williams, Dean E., 243, 278, 399, 427,
    468, 469, 474, 520
Wingate, Marcel E., 27, 48, 49, 57, 61, 62,
    63, 64, 76, 81, 165, 168, 174, 407, 518,
    519, 520
Winitz, H., 238
Winkler, R., 175
Wischner, G. J., 16, 32, 35, 132, 186, 188,
    196, 251, 264, 469, 497
Wolf, M., 227
Wolff, H. G., 346
Wolpe, Joseph, 52, 142, 264, 336, 337,
    343, 345, 350, 353, 384, 385, 458, 521,
    527
Woods, Lee, 173, 488, 489, 496, 497
Wyatt, C., 273, 275
Wyneken, C., 133, 187, 188
Wynne, L. C., 225

Yairi, E., 34
Yates, 336

Zenner, A. A., 170, 172, 175
Zimmerman, G. N., 61, 62, 160, 165, 174,
    508
Zwitman, D. H., 279

Subject Index

Adaptive behavior, stuttering as, 32, 33
Adult stutterers, 41, 267, 475, 522, 528
  vs. children, and operant therapy,
    440–41
Aggression.(*see* Hostility)
Airstream management, 84–86, 121, 508
  (*see also* Breathing control;
    Respiration)
American Speech and Hearing Association,
  92, 503
Analytical psychiatry, 13–14
Anatomy and stuttering, 7
Anatomy of an illness, 262
Anger, and fear in stutterers, 103, 115–16
Antecedent events, and behavior, 254
Anticipatory struggle theory, 27, 35, 124,
  133
Anxiety, and stuttering, 41, 42, 104, 134,
    213, 216, 264, 330, 351, 399–400,
    527
  and behavior acquisition, 213, 216, 237
    (*see also* Fear)
  deconditioning neurotic, 343–49
  heirarchy of, 337, 339
  reduction of, 31, 32, 194, 249
Approach-avoidance conflict theory and
    therapy, 27, 28, 186, 187–210
  analysis of therapy techniques, 205–207
  clinical contributions of, 207–208
  conflict hypothesis, 188–192
  fear reduction, 192–95
  problem definition, 187–88
  recent developments in, 208–209
  treatment, 195–98
Articulation, discoordination of, with
    respiration and phonation, 73–81,
    82–89
Assertive responses, 344–45, 347
Attitudinal changes, and behavior, 263–65,
    391–93, 496
  and cognitive therapy, 468, 479, 484
Audiology, 50, 54 n.5, 55
Authority, and punishment, 203
Autonomic nervous system, 42, 253
Aversive stimulus (*see* Punishment)

Avoidance, 119, 373–74, 382, 386

Banff International Conference on
    Stuttering, Second (1984), 208
Banff International Conference on the
    Maintenance of Fluency, 501
Behavior theory of stuttering, 28, 31,
    143–46, 157–68
Behavior therapy for stuttering
  deconditioning emotional factors,
    343–49
  modifying behavior. 363–93
  two-factor, 146–53, 155–57, 168–78
Behaviorism, 50, 52, 249
Biofeedback, 42, 142, 253, 390
Breathing control, 353, 355–57, 403 (*see
    also* Airstream management;
    Respiration)

Calming the stutterer, 367–71
Cancellation therapy, 249, 455 (*see also*
    Modification of stuttering behavior)
  using to alter speech response, 378–79
Case studies of stutterers
  and client-centered therapy, 320–34
  of emotion fear and repression, 106–15
  family counseling, environmental
    manipulation and, 286–89
  of operant therapy for children, 418–27
Causes of stuttering, 6 (*see also* Etiology of
    stuttering; Theories of stuttering)
  treating, vs. treating symptoms, 13,
    14–15
Cerebral dominance, and stuttering, 9, 56,
    117–19, 121, 389, 508 (*see also*
    Laterality; Handedness)
Child management questionnaires and
    checklists, 279
Children as stutterers, 9, 29, 37–38, 250,
    283–84, 309, 475 (*see also* Parents of
    stutterers)
  cognitive therapy for, 483–84
  and developmental disfluency, 33–37
  differences between onset and
    development of, 125–29

environmental manipulation and family
    counseling for, 273–89
  interaction with parent, 26, 35, 93, 99,
    104, 250, 272, 276, 279, 281, 455
  nonfluency as operant behavior, 238–45
  operant therapy for, 417–30, 431–43
  prevention of, 25–27
Choral readings (*see* Speech arts)
Classical conditioning, 42, 142, 253
  and behavioral theory, 143–45
  and behavioral therapy, 146–49
Client-centered therapy, 14, 294, 295–315,
    316–34
  basic hypothesis, 296–97, 312–15
  case analysis, 320–34
  theoretical variants of, 317–19
Client/therapist relationship, 14, 309–11,
    449, 493
Clients, 460 (*see also* Attitudinal changes)
  capacity for self-direction, 296–97,
    312–15
  expectations of therapy, 261–63
  experience of therapist, 303–304
  individual needs, and therapy strategy,
    176, 407–408
  internal frame of reference, 301, 306
  self-responsibility, 469, 476, 496
Clinical contact after therapy, 496
Clinical imperative, 407
Cognitive-affective reprocessing, 318
Cognitive therapy, 28, 318, 400, 467–86
  for children, 483–84
  etiology of stuttering, 482–83
  maintenance of, 481–82
  program principles, 468–70
  resumes of history and results of,
    471–72
Communicative responsibility, 80, 469,
    476, 496
Computer evaluation of voice onsets,
    402–403, 409, 411
Conditioning in stuttering therapy, 376
Conditioning theory, 36 (*see also* Behavior

theory; Classical conditioning; Instrumental conditioning; Operant conditioning)

Confidence (*see* Self-confidence)

Conflict, 187 (*see also* Approach-avoidance conflict theory; Fear)
  hypothesis and stuttering, 188–92, 196, 201
  levels of, 191–92

Content of speech, 26, 249, 455

Contract, behavioral transfer, 451–52, 458

Control stuttering techniques, 206, 208

Conversation
  modifying stuttering behavior with, 365
  pauses and interruptions in, 240

Corrective feedback, and speech, 275

Counseling and psychotherapy, 294, 316

Counselor (*see* Therapist)

Counterconditioning, 148–49

Covert and overt measurements, 503–505

Crying in children, and emotional repression, 100–101

Cues, as initiators of stuttering, 95–96, 100

Cures, 7, 12–13, 15–16, 43

DAF (*see* Delayed auditory feedback)

Deconditioning, 146–48

Deconfirmation, 368

Defence mechanisms, 31

Delayed auditory feedback, 80–81, 121, 222, 398, 419 (table), 434–36, 449, 456

Desensitization, 272, 362, 367–71, 384–85, 434 (*see also* Systematic Desensitization therapy)

Developmental disfluency, 33–37, 39

Diagnosis of stuttering, 128–129

Diagnosogenic Theory, 6, 25, 124, 125–29
  evaluation of, 138
  influence on later theories, 132–33
  influence on research, 133–36
  influence on therapy, 136–38
  origin of, 130–32

Differential reinforcement, 41

Disfluency, 26, 250, 251 (*see also* Developmental disfluency)
  categories of, 38
  charting, 284
  reinforcing competing responses, 28
  in voicing, whispering, and lipped speech, 78 (table)

Distraction effect, 80, 221

Dramatic readings (*see* Speech arts)

Drugs to control stuttering, 206

"Easy" stuttering, 229, 377–78, 387

Ego protection, and the stutterer, 192

Effective-planning-time hypothesis, 86–87

Emotional factors and stuttering, 11, 93–116, 117–21, 252–53, 367, 382
  deconditioning, 343–49
  and need for individual diagnosis and therapy, 352–53
  and transfer of fluency, 450–52

Emotional reactions, 330 (*see also* Negative emotions)
  genetic factor of, 158–59, 164
  learned, 52, 144–45
  release of, 197
  to words, 191

Endocrinology and stuttering, 6–7, 8

Environmental factors and stuttering, 461–62
  evaluation of, 277–79
  interaction with genetic factors, 157–59
  manipulation of, in therapy, 272, 273–89

Erickson S24 Scale, 491

Etiology of stuttering, 24–25
  and cognitive therapy, 482–83

Expectancy of stutterer's behavior, 479–81

Experiencing, and personality change, 317–19, 322, 330, 331

Extinction of behaviors, 42

Eye contact, as therapy, 368–69

Eyedness, 127 (table)

Eysenck Personality Inventory, 491

Family of stutterer, 267, 460
  counseling, 272, 273–91

Fear, 52, 527 (*see also* Anxiety)
  and emotional repression, 97, 98, 100, 103, 105 (fig.)
  reduction, and stuttering, 192–98, 202
  of specific words, syllables, or situations, 188, 191
  of silence, 190, 202–203
  in therapy, 261
  of "unspeakable feelings", 106–15

Feeding children, and emotional repression, 101

Fluency, 437 (*see also* Disfluency; Nonfluency)
  as its own reward, 497–98
  charting, 284–85
  explanations of, 34, 37, 84
  failures of, 161–64 (*see also* Relapse)
  false, 208, 524–25
  as the goal, 467, 468, 484, 506
  perceptions of, 128–29, 134, 495
  reinforcing, 28, 172, 469
  standards of, 134

Fluency-shaping, 383, 386–88, 391, 392 (*see also* Precision Fluency Shaping Program)

Fluent stuttering, 375–76

Focusing in therapy, 319

Follow-up, 438, 490

Freezing sounds, 370

Frequency counts of stuttering, and therapy, 205

Frustration, learning to tolerate, 369

Functionalists, 14

General semantics, 9–10, 56, 131 (*see also* Diagnosogenic Theory; Semantogenic theory)

Genetics and stuttering, 23, 49–69, 127, 527
  emotions and, 158–59, 164
  interaction with environmental factors, 157–59
  interest in, vs. psychology, 58–61
  pedigree of Huntington's chorea, 59, 60 (fig.)
  pedigree of a stuttering family, 58, 59 (fig.)
  and relapse, 498–99

Glutamic acid treatment, 15

Gradual Increase in Length and Complexity of Utterance Program

(GILCU), 416, 425 (table), 427 (table), 434–36, 440

"Habit" characterization of stuttering, 32, 33

Handbook of speech pathology, 92

Handbook on stuttering, 124

"Handedness" and stuttering, 8, 9, 118, 127 (table), 128 (*see also* Cerebral dominance; Laterality)

Hawthorne effect, 13, 16

Heredity (*see* Genetics)

Hollins Communications Research Institute, 413

Hostility of stutterers, 107, 192–93, 197, 226, 263, 324, 325, 469, 476

Human perspectives in speech and language disorders, 72

Huntington's chorea, genetics of, 59, 60 (fig.)

Incipient stuttering, 35, 274

Information
  for parents of stutterers, 281, 282–83
  organizing, 318
  as stimuli, 172–73

Instrumental conditioning (*see also* Operant conditioning)
  behavioral theory and, 145–46
  behavioral therapy and, 149–53

Interactionism of genetic and environmental factors, 157–59

Interpersonal context of stuttering, 94, 98, 104, 116, 275

Iowa Avoidance Scale, 491

Iowa Job Task, 491, 494

Iowa Scale of Attitude, 490

Iowa therapy, 11, 13, 14, 15, 195, 196, 197, 380–81

Isoniazid treatment, 15

Journal of Speech and Hearing Disorders, 72, 248, 454

Labels, 10, 331

Laryngeal function, 62, 74, 76
  role in stuttering, 82–86, 508

Laterality, 9, 55, 56

Learned behavior, stuttering as, 40–44, 62, 95–98, 132

Learning
  conditions of, 99–104
  counterconditioning and, 148
  theory, 16, 40, 41

Lipped speech, 83
  physiological adjustments for, 74, 75 (fig.)
  syllable disfluencies and, 78 (table)

Listener, 37, 168
  negative experience of stuttering, 469–70, 476
  parents as. 274
  as reinforcer, 218, 230, 238
  and speaker interaction, 93, 94, 96, 120, 191

MIDVAS therapy, 387, 390 (*see also* Modification of stuttering behavior)

The maintenance of fluency, 488 (*see also* Relapse; Outcome of therapy)

Maintenance of fluency, 489–500

Maintenance of fluency, *continued*
and cognitive therapy, 481–82
evaluating specific maintenance
activities, 493–94
experimental investigations in, 506–508
future trends in, 509–511
increased interest in, 501–503
long-term outcome, 90–94
methodological problems, 494–95
summary of current techniques, 495–97
of therapeutic gains in children, 286,
438
Maintenance of stuttering, 24–25, 196
Maladaptive behavior, stuttering as, 32, 33
Management (*see* Clinical management)
Manding, 239
Mass therapy, 177, 352
Measurement of speech behaviors,
433–34, 439–40, 503–505
Medical model of stuttering, 31
Meta-analysis of therapy, 510
Metronome therapy, 13, 353–55
Mirror image therapy, 455
Model of speech, clarifying, 376–77
Modeling procedures in therapy, 285–86
Modification of stuttering, 142
Modification of stuttering behavior,
363–79, 380–94
basic steps of therapy, 389–90
calming and toughening the client,
367–71, 383–85
cancellation of old speech responses,
378–79, 386–88
eliminating avoidance and
postponement, 373–74, 385–86
exploring the problem, 363–66,
382–83
future trends in, 388–93
Molecular analysis of stuttering, 159–61,
171
Moments of stuttering, 159–60
Monitoring speech, 449–50, 480, 485
Multidisciplinary Approach to Stuttering,
annual meeting of, 502

The nature of stuttering, 380
Negative emotions, and stuttering, 10,
164–66, 172 (*see also* Hostility)
classical conditioning and, 144–45
Negative reinforcement, 42, 253, 374–75
(*see also* Punishment, negative)
Neuromotor breakdown and stuttering,
160–61, 162
Neurophysiology, and stuttering, 8, 62, 92,
508
Neuropsychiatry, 13, 15
Neurosis, 14, 31–32, 133
and conflict, 189
decondition habits of, 343–49
rejected as reason for stuttering, 470–71
Neutral stimuli, 143–44
Noise, as punishment, 213–16, 220, 221
Nondirective therapy (*see* Client-centered
therapy)
Nonfluency as operant behavior, 238–39
contingencies between, and stuttering,
241–43
states of deprivation and punishment,
239–41
Nonreinforcement therapy, 151–52, 193,
201, 203

Normal disfluency, 25, 33, 37–38, 131,
162 (*see also* Developmental
disfluency)

One-population theory of stuttering, 27,
36, 39
"Open Letter to the Mother of a Stuttering
Child," 25, 137
Operant behavior analysis, applied to
speech, 217–19, 237–38
Operant behavior, stuttering as, 212,
213–34, 237–55, 432 (*see also*
Punishment)
and changing speech responses, 241–43
contingencies between stuttering and
nonfluency, 241
implications of, 230–31
initial study indicating, 213–16, 219–20
related research, 222–24
replication studies, 221–22
representative paradigms for, 242
(table), 243
research implications, 245–46
respondent conditioning, 245
self-reinforcement, 244–45
specific stimuli and, 243–44
Operant conditioning, 16, 36, 42, 61, 212,
353, 455 (*see also* Instrumental
conditioning)
*Operant conditioning and the
management of stuttering,* 455
Operant therapy for stuttering children,
416, 417–30, 431–43
case studies, 418–27
disseminating treatment, 441–42
establishment programs, 417, 421
(table), 423 (table), 424 (table),
434–37
follow-up, 438
impact on other programs, 440
maintenance phase, 417, 419, 438,
439–40
measurement of disfluency, 432–33
self-monitoring, 439–40
summary of five programs, 429 (table)
transfer phase, 417, 428 (table), 437,
438
vs. adults, 440–41
Oral reading, 365, 398, 400
Outcome of therapy, 16, 268–69, 286,
462–63, 501–11 (*see also*
Maintenance; Relapse)
in absence of maintenance activities,
490–91
evaluating reports, 505–506
methodological issues in, 503–506
with maintenance activities, 491–93
Over-talking technique, 480
Overt and covert measurements, 503–505
Overt behavior, 249

Parent Attitudes Toward Stuttering
Checklist, 279
Parents of stutterers
counseling of, 9, 25, 40, 136–37,
273–89
information for, 280, 282–83
interaction with child, 26, 35, 93,
99–104, 250, 276, 279, 281, 455
modeling for, 285–86
perceptions of stuttering, 128–29, 134

therapist's understanding the concern of,
280–81
Passivity of stutterers, 476–77
Peckham Experiment, 313–15
Perceptions of Stuttering Inventory (PSI),
405
Person-centered approach, 319–20 (*see
also* Client-centered therapy)
Phonation, 48
discoordination of, with articulation and
respiration, 73–81, 82–89
Physiology of stuttering, 6–7, 8, 9, 49–69
(*see also* Genetics; Neurophysiology)
interest in, vs. psychological, 49, 50
(fig.), 51–57
irregularities in stutterers, 53–54
and relapse, 498–99, 508
Positive reinforcement, 26, 42, 212, 244,
374–75, 469
Practice in therapy, 177–78, 498
Precision Fluency Shaping Program,
397–406
overview, 404 (table)
pre-, posttreatment, and follow up, 405
(table)
and technology, 408–411
Prefrontal lobotomy treatment, 15–16
Primary stuttering, 35
Prince Henry Program, 492–93, 503
Professional researchers and therapists, as
stutterers, 24
Pseudostuttering, 368–69, 389
Psychoanalysis, 28, 92
applied to stutterers, 98–116
Psychology, and stuttering, 10–15 (*see
also* Psychoanalysis)
interest in, vs. physiological, 49, 50
(fig.), 51–57
Psychotherapy for stutterers, 195–98,
201–202 (*see also* Client-centered
therapy)
Punishment of disfluency, 26, 28, 42, 96,
190, 202, 203, 249, 253, 374–75, 455
(*see also* Time out as punishment)
B. F. Skinner on, 229–30
as behavioral therapy, 152–53, 172, 212
negative, 226–29, 238
positive, 224–26
practice as, 498
with aversive stimuli (study), 213–16,
219–20, 221, 222, 223–24

Reciprocal Inhibition Theory, (Wolfe), 142
Redundancy in linguistic processing, 37
Refresher programs, 494, 496–97
Reinforcement therapy, 150–51
Relapse, 31, 43, 174, 269, 482, 488, 493,
494, 501–11, 525–26
and fluency as a reward, 497–98
new speculations on, 508–509
physiological basis for, 498–99
role of micro-stutters, 497
Relaxation, 206, 458
and Systematic Desensitization, 337–342
Repression of emotions, 100, 103–106,
344
case studies of "unspeakable" feelings,
106–15
Research on stuttering, 28, 29–30, 441
evaluating maintenance activities,
493–94

and operant behavior, 245–46
influence of Diagnosogenic theory on, 133–36
openness and accountability in, 212
physiological vs. psychological, 50 (fig.)
Residential therapeutic programs, 460, 491
Resistance to therapy, 13
Respiration, discoordination of, with articulation and phonation, 73–81, 82–89 (*see also* Airstream management; Breathing control)
Response-contingent control study, 213–16, 219–220 (*see also* Operant behavior, stuttering as)
aversive periods, 213, 215 (figs.)
escape periods, 213, 214 (fig.), 221
related studies, 222–24
Response-suppression hypothesis, 204–205
Responses
alteration of, through cancellation, 378–79
conflict in, 97–98, 100
fatigue, 152
inhibiting through competing, 344–45
shaping, 412
Rhythm therapy, 87, 347, 353–55
Riley Severity Scores, 494
Role theory, 203

Science and sanity, 9, 131
Secondary gain from stuttering, 31, 32
Self-confidence, and stuttering, 7–8, 9, 88, 195, 262
Self-disclosure as therapy, 369
Self-editing and correction in speech, 240–41
Self-image as a stutterer, 28–29, 40, 197–98, 203, 447, 470, 475, 479 (*see also* Expectancy of stutterer's behavior)
and client-centered therapy, 320–23, 331–33
Self-reinforcement, and stutter-free speech, 244–45, 449–50, 457
Self-study of stuttering problem, 363, 382, 383
Semantogenic theory of stuttering, 11, 23, 27, 28, 124, 249, 455 (*see also* Diagnososgenic Theory; General semantics)
Sex ratio of stutterers, 158–59, 527
Sex training, and emotion repression, 102–103
Shadowing, 352
Shaping of behaviors, 41–42
Silence, fear of, 190, 202–203
in conversation, 240, 243
Slide technique, 196, 202, 377
Social heredity, 58, 60
Speaker/listener interaction, 93, 94, 120, 191
Speech, 94–95
normal response schema, 346 (fig.), 351 (fig.)
stuttering response schema, 347 (figs.), 351–352 (figs.)
Speech arts, 7, 9, 81
Speech correction: Principles and methods, 136, 380, 385

Speech Foundation of America, 363, 380, 381
Speech pathology, 6, 50, 54, 55, 92
Spontaneous recovery, 7, 43, 526–27
State University of Iowa, 23, 92
Status-gap hypothesis, 203
Stimulus-response concept, 54 n. 7, 143–44, 238
Strategies in stuttering therapy, 502
Strengthening of behaviors, 42
Stress, 36, 253
Studies in stuttering, 55
Studies in the psychology of stuttering, 57
Stutter-free speech, 454
Stutter-free speech therapy, 250, 391, 447–63
changes in, 459–63
client/therapist relationship, 449
evolution of, 454–59
goals of, 447, 448
phases, 448, 449–53
Stutterer's Self-Rating of Reactions, 490
Stutterers (*see* Adult stutterers; Children as stutterers; Clients; Professional researchers and therapists as stutterers; Self-confidence; Self-image)
Stuttering
behavior vs. symptoms, models of, 30–33
compound stimulus and, 347 (fig.)
definitions of, 48, 166–68
emotional factors and, 93–16, 117–21
measurement of, 433–34 (*see also* Measurement)
nonspecific tenseness and, 347 (fig.), 348
onset and development of, 125–29
as operant behavior, 212, 213–34, 237–55
overview of studies on, 5–17
physiology and genetics of, 49–69
pragmatics of, 476–78
response of nonspecific tenseness, 347 (fig.)
Stuttering: An integration of contemporary therapies, 383
Stuttering and personality dynamics, 275
Stuttering bath as therapy, 370–72
Stuttering: Differential evaluation and therapy, 278
Stuttering in children and adults, 132 n. 1
Symptom substitution, 31
Symptoms of stuttering
treating, vs. treating causes, 13, 14–15
Systematic Desensitization Therapy, 142, 336, 350–59
based on relaxation, 337–42, 345, 346

Target behaviors, 401–405, 414 (*see also* Precision Fluency Shaping Program)
Technology, and stuttering therapy, 407–14 (*see also* Precision Fluency Shaping Program)
conditions necessary for, 412–13
general properties of, 408–412
limitations of, 413–414
and scientific principles, 412
Theories of stuttering, 23–44 (*see also*

Causes of stuttering; Etiology of stuttering; *and individual theories, e.g.* Diagnosogenic Theory)
influence of Johnson's Diagnosogenic theory on later, 132–33
Therapists, 414, 462
attitudes of, 295–98
bias of, 305–306
client's experience of, 303–304
developing empathy, support, and honesty, 281–82, 322
expectations of therapy, 265–70
as model for parents, 284–86
in parent role, 104
providing information to parents, 281, 282–83
relationship with client, 309–11, 449, 493
role and funtion of, 298–309, 322–23
structure provided by, 318–19
techniques of, 300–302, 326 n.9
understanding parental concern for stutterer, 280–81
Therapy for stutterers, 381 (*see also* Clinical management of stuttering; Modification of stuttering behavior, *names of individual therapies*)
Therapy for stuttering
behavioral, 146–53
criteria for success, 268, 403, 489
effect of Diagnosogenic Theory on, 136–38
evaluating, 15–17, 438, 502 (*see also* Outcome of Therapy)
goals, 17, 447, 448, 467, 484–85
impact of, on the individual, 352–53
individual's capacity for self-direction in, 296–97, 312–15
outcome (*see* Outcome of therapy)
patterns of change in, 518–22
schedules of, 268, 524
unresolved issues in, 522–28
variables affecting, 460–63, 524–27
Time out as punishment, 227, 228–29, 508
Timing, disrupted motor, and speech, 73, 86–87
To the Stutterer, 363
Toilet and cleanliness training, and emotional repression, 101–102
Transfer of fluency, 399, 400, 403–404, 428 (table), 437, 438, 450–52, 525
Transitional stuttering, 35, 274
The treatment of stuttering, 380, 381
Two-Factor theory and therapy, 28, 36, 142, 143–83, 252
classical conditioning, 142, 143–45, 146–49
definitional issues and stuttering, 166–68
fluency and failed fluency, 161–64
instrumental conditioning, 145–46, 149–53
interactionism genetic and environmental factors, 157–59
molecular viewpoint of, 159–61
stuttering and negative emotion, 64–66
therapy, 146–53, 168–78
Two-population theory of stuttering, 27, 38–40

Unconditional stimuli and responses, 143
University of Iowa, 131
University of Pittsburgh, 11, 249
Unmonitored speech, training in, 452–53, 458–59

Variables
  effecting therapy, 460–63, 524–27
  phonation as independent, 74–76
Veteran's Administration, 15
Vocal apparatus and stuttering, 350–52

Vocational Rehabilitation Administration, 343
Voice onset
  gentle, 400, 402
  time, 83, 84, 87
Voice reaction time, 83, 84
Voice termination time, 83
Voicing, 62, 72
  physiological adjustments for, 75 (fig.)
  syllable disfluencies and, 78 (table)
Voluntary stuttering, 206, 381

Whispering, 7
  physiological adjustments for, 74, 75 (fig.)
  and reduction in stuttering, 79, 83
  syllable disfluencies and, 78 (table)
Willoughby Neuroticism Schedule, 337, 348
Word substitution, 32–33
Words stuttered per minute, 419 (table), 422 (table), 424 (table), 426 (table), 428 (table), 433